CW01512582

OXFORD HANDBOOK OF

Trauma and Orthopaedics

Published and forthcoming Oxford Handbooks

OXFORD HANDBOOK OF

Trauma and Orthopaedics

SECOND EDITION

EDITED BY

Kunal Kulkarni
Consultant Trauma and Orthopaedic Surgeon, University
Hospitals of Leicester NHS Trust, UK

Randeep Aujla
Consultant Trauma and Orthopaedic Surgeon, University
Hospitals of Leicester NHS Trust, UK

Jeremy Granville Chapman
Consultant Trauma and Orthopaedic Surgeon, Frimley Health
NHS Foundation Trust, UK

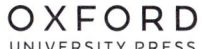

OXFORD
UNIVERSITY PRESS

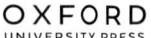

OXFORD
UNIVERSITY PRESS

Great Clarendon Street, Oxford, OX2 6DP,
United Kingdom

Oxford University Press is a department of the University of Oxford.
It furthers the University's objective of excellence in research, scholarship,
and education by publishing worldwide. Oxford is a registered trade mark of
Oxford University Press in the UK and in certain other countries

Published in the United States of America by Oxford University Press
198 Madison Avenue, New York, NY 10016, United States of America

British Library Cataloguing in Publication Data
Data available

Library of Congress Control Number: 2024943823

ISBN 978–0–19–873865–7

DOI: 10.1093/med/9780198738657.001.0001

Printed and bound in China by
C&C Offset Printing Co., Ltd.

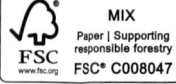

MIX
Paper | Supporting
responsible forestry
FSC® C008047

The manufacturer's authorised representative in the
EU for product safety is Oxford University Press
España S.A. of El Parque Empresarial San Fernando
de Henares,Avenida de Castilla, 2 – 28830 Madrid
(www.oup.es/en or product.safety@oup.com). OUP
España S.A. also acts as importer into Spain of
products made by the manufacturer.

Contents

Detailed Contents

Part 3 **Adults**

11 Adult orthopaedics: rheumatology *311*

12 Adult orthopaedics: pathology *339*

Part 4 **Paediatrics**

Foreword

The more that you read, the more things you will know. The more that you learn, the more places you'll go.

Dr. Seuss

When a new edition of a much-loved textbook arrives on your desk, it is akin to an unexpected visit from a long-lost friend. You are delighted to see them; you scan them quickly to look for differences and are often reassured that they are still the person you have always known. Then, as the conversation develops, as the pages are turned, it is clear that life and the passing of time have added nuance to your relationship, outlooks have broadened, interests have been honed, ideas have changed, and philosophies moved on. Conversation flows, the pages turn, and your happiness in the renewal of the friendship grows.

While this book is inherently written for the 'new' trainee, older trainees will welcome this new edition too as an old friend. They will recognize its worth, note its improvements, and be reminded that there are always points to remember or relearn. In so doing, they too will pass the message on to their friends and colleagues: here is a book that shows you what you need to know.

As a paediatric orthopaedic surgeon, I am inherently in favour of growth and development, of change over time, and of adapting to new ideas and new ways of conveying facts and philosophies. The ability to distil these changes into bite-size pieces of knowledge, easily digestible 'chunks of knowledge', and simple ideas on how to make things better is a great skill and this book does it well. The updated and customized drawings make it easy to read, easy to dip in and out of sections of interest. The sections on anatomy and surgical approaches are particularly helpful.

This new edition is more diverse in its authorship, giving a breadth of national and international viewpoints, in keeping with our globally connected community of trauma and orthopaedics. The editors have worked hard to simplify the content by concentrating on points of clinical relevance and highlighting where the evidence base lies. New content has been included, in keeping with the ever-increasing understanding that the practice of trauma and orthopaedic surgery cannot take part in isolation—our patients deserve us to be working as part of a multidisciplinary team that provides 'best care'.

Despite these changes, the tried and tested basics of '*Look, Feel, Move*' and '*History, Examination, and Appropriate Investigations*' to come to a diagnosis and a management strategy remain. This book continues to provide an impressive introduction to the fascinating world of trauma and ortho-paedics and should be an essential component of your reading list.

Deborah Eastwood

Consultant Paediatric Orthopaedic Surgeon
Great Ormond St Hospital for Children and the Royal National
Orthopaedic Hospital,
Associate Professor, University College London
Past President of the British Orthopaedic Association and European
Paediatric Orthopaedic Society

Preface

Welcome to the second edition of the (subtly retitled) *Oxford Handbook of Trauma and Orthopaedics*!

The Oxford Handbook series has been an immensely popular staple for generations of healthcare professionals worldwide. With over a decade since the first edition of this book was published, we are proud that our specialty has evolved significantly, to pave the way for this update. An increasingly rigorous evidence base has provided renewed content through which we can deliver better care to our patients. This second edition has an entirely refreshed manuscript, alongside new chapters and illustrations, with the goal of providing an overview of the fundamentals of adult and paediatric trauma and orthopaedic practice for readers of differing clinical experiences. With musculoskeletal disorders contributing to a significant proportion of global disability, we hope that a growing number of healthcare professionals will find this much-needed second edition of benefit in helping to understand the foundations of trauma and orthopaedic care.

With a growing armamentarium of randomized controlled trials published in leading international journals, our (biased!) view is that orthopaedics has served as a leader among the surgical specialties in trying to help guide more ways of mapping better certainty in our clinical care decisions. Despite the inevitable uncertainty of applying 'rules' to broad populations, orthopaedic surgery continues to strive for the practice of individualized medicine. Over the years, there have been ongoing strides in standardizing and developing pathways, guidance, protocols, and registries, with the goal of leading the drive to 'Get It Right First Time'. While none of these approaches are without their limitations (and, consequently, critics), their core principles are to be applauded: to enhance and standardize the delivery of the best possible patient care for all.

Since the first edition was published in 2010, the world—and subsequently clinical practice—has experienced ongoing challenges. A mix of growing populations that live longer (i.e. rising demand for lifesaving and quality of life-enhancing orthopaedic healthcare), with the evolution of scientific knowledge and more effective, but also more expensive, technologies (i.e. the need to deliver more subspecialist care in a resource-constrained world that requires more generalists), alongside the unique adaptations necessitated by the COVID-19 pandemic, has led to an increasingly complex world for healthcare professionals to navigate. With changes to medical education and training, including rising numbers of allied healthcare professionals across the globe, the way in which we deliver care has evolved and will continue to do so. For those navigating this increasingly blurry healthcare landscape and needing to make swifter, safer, and better clinical decisions in increasingly challenging working conditions, there remains a need for reliable resources to guide; we therefore hope that this second edition can serve as one of the many useful overarching maps that can assist healthcare professionals in their delivery of the patient care journey.

Most importantly, we would like to express our gratitude to all our expert collaborators who have made this book possible. It is thanks to their hard work that this second edition exists. We are indebted to you all. For our readers—we truly welcome all of your feedback and opinions (please submit this via the book's page on the OUP website ℛ http://www.oup.com), and we will endeavour to incorporate suggested changes into future editions.

Kunal Kulkarni, Randeep Aujla, Jeremy Granville Chapman

Contributors

Usman Ahmed
Consultant Orthopaedic Surgeon
Worcestershire Acute Hospitals
NHS Trust, Worcester, UK

Sultan Alkaalbani
Spine Fellow
Queen's Medical Centre,
Nottingham University Hospitals
NHS Trust, Nottingham, UK

Robert Ashford
Professor and Consultant
Orthopaedic Sarcoma Surgeon
University Hospitals of Leicester
NHS Trust, Leicester, UK

Randeep Aujla
Consultant Trauma and
Orthopaedic Surgeon
University Hospitals of Leicester
NHS Trust, Leicester, UK

James Berwin
Hip Fellow
Southmead Hospital, North Bristol
NHS Trust, Bristol, UK

Kate Brown
Consultant Hand and Peripheral
Nerve Injury Surgeon
Pulvertaft Hand Centre, University
Hospitals of Derby and Burton
NHS Foundation Trust, Derby, UK

David Bruce
Consultant Knee Surgeon
Cardiff and Vale University
Health Board, University Hospital
Llandough, Llandough, Wales

Priyanka Chandratre
Assistant Professor in
Rheumatology
The Ottawa Hospital, Ottawa,
Ontario, Canada

Philip Darcy
Consultant in Emergency Medicine
St George's University Hospitals
NHS Foundation Trust, London, UK

Nicholas Eastley
Consultant Orthopaedic Sarcoma
Surgeon
University Hospitals of Leicester
NHS Trust, Leicester, UK

Victoria Naomi Gibbs
Trauma and Orthopaedic Academic
Clinical Lecturer
Oxford University Hospitals NHS
Foundation Trust and University of
Oxford, Oxford, UK

Jeremy Granville Chapman
Consultant Trauma and
Orthopaedic Surgeon,
Frimley Health NHS Foundation
Trust, Slough, UK

Nicholas Johnson
Consultant Orthopaedic Hand
Surgeon
Pulvertaft Hand Centre, University
Hospitals of Derby and Burton
NHS Foundation Trust, Derby, UK

Michail Kokkinakis
Honorary Senior Clinical Lecturer,
Kings College London and
Consultant Paediatric Orthopaedic
Surgeon
Evelina London Children's Hospital,
Guys & St. Thomas' NHS Trust,
London, UK

Kunal Kulkarni
Consultant Trauma and
Orthopaedic Hand and Wrist
Surgeon
University Hospitals of Leicester
NHS Trust, Leicester, UK

Kim Lammin

Consultant Trauma and
Orthopaedic Surgeon
University Hospitals of Leicester
NHS Trust, Leicester, UK

Chris Lavy

Professor of Orthopaedics and
Tropical Surgery
Oxford University Hospitals NHS
Foundation Trust, Oxford, UK

Shahbaz Malik

Consultant Orthopaedic Surgeon
Worcestershire Acute Hospitals
NHS Trust, Worcester, UK

Nyengo Chiswakhata Mkandawire

Professor of Orthopaedic Surgery
and Head of Surgery Department
College of Medicine, University of
Malawi, Blantyre, Malawi

Aoife Caulfield

Senior Neuro-Physiotherapist
Queen Elizabeth Hospital,
University Hospitals Birmingham
NHS Foundation Trust,
Birmingham, UK

Chang Park

Locum Paediatric Orthopaedic
Consultant
Oxford University Hospitals NHS
Foundation Trust, Oxford, UK

Simon Parker

Hand Surgery Fellow
Fremantle Hospital, Perth, Australia

Shakil Patel

Consultant Spine Surgeon
Queen's Medical Centre,
Nottingham University Hospitals
NHS Trust, Nottingham, UK

Parag Raval

Post CCT Shoulder and
Elbow Fellow
Royal National Orthopaedic
Hospital NHS Trust, London, UK

Daniel Reed

Consultant Paediatric Orthopaedic
Surgeon,
Evelina London Children's Hospital,
Guys & St. Thomas' NHS Trust,
London, UK

Frances Rickard

Consultant Geriatrician
Southmead Hospital, North Bristol
NHS Trust, Bristol, UK

Katie Samuel

Consultant Anaesthetist
North Bristol NHS Trust,
Bristol, UK

Khaled Sarraf

Consultant Paediatric and
Adolescent Orthopaedic Surgeon
Imperial College Healthcare NHS
Trust, London, UK

Siddarth Shah

Consultant Spine Surgeon
iSpine Clinic, Breach Candy Hospital
& Saifee Hospital, Mumbai, India.

Nomaan Sheikh

Consultant Trauma and
Orthopaedic Surgeon
Kettering General Hospital NHS
Foundation Trust, Kettering, UK

David Shipway

Consultant Physician &
Perioperative Geriatrician
North Bristol NHS Trust,
Bristol, UK

Faiz Shivzi

Orthopaedic Surgeon and
Associate,
McKinsey and Company,
London, UK

Bobby Siddiqui

Consultant Trauma and
Orthopaedic Surgeon
Sheffield Teaching Hospitals NHS
Foundation Trust, Sheffield, UK

Muaaz Tahir

Specialty Registrar in Trauma and
Orthopaedics
Birmingham Orthopaedic Training
Programme, Knowledge Hub, The
Royal Orthopaedic Hospital NHS
Foundation Trust, Birmingham, UK

Ahmad Tarawneh

Spine Fellow
Queen's Medical Centre,
Nottingham University Hospitals
NHS Trust, Nottingham, UK

Lauren Thomson

Consultant Orthopaedic Foot and
Ankle Surgeon
The Rotherham NHS Foundation
Trust, Rotheram, UK

Helen Tunnicliffe

Consultant and Advanced Practice
Physiotherapist
University Hospitals of Leicester
NHS Trust, Leicester, UK

Sam Weston-Simons

Consultant Paediatric Orthopaedic
Surgeon
The Cure Children's Hospital of
Zimbabwe, Bulawayo, Zimbabwe

Andrew Wheelton

Consultant Hip and Knee
Arthroplasty and Trauma Surgeon
Northern Care Alliance NHS Trust,
Manchester, UK

Alex Woods

Locum Consultant Shoulder and
Elbow Surgeon
Oxford University Hospitals NHS
Foundation Trust, Oxford, UK

Symbols and abbreviations

➲	cross-reference		ACT	atypical cartilaginous tumour
℘	website address		ACTH	adrenocorticotrophic hormone
>	greater than		ADH	antidiuretic hormone
<	less than		ADL	activity of daily living
≥	equal to or greater than		AED	antiepileptic drug
≤	equal to or less than		AF	atrial fibrillation
°	degree		AFB	acid-fast bacilli
°C	degree Celsius		AFO	ankle–foot orthosis
→	leading to		AFP	α-fetoprotein
↓	decreased		AI	acetabular index
↑	increased		AIIS	anterior inferior iliac spine
~	approximately		AIN	anterior interosseous nerve
™	trademark		AJCC	American Joint Committee on Cancer
®	registered		AKI	acute kidney injury
♂	male		AKP	anterior knee pain
♀	female		ALIF	anterior lumbar interbody fusion
2D	two-dimensional		ALL	acute lymphocytic leukaemia
3D	three-dimensional		ALP	alkaline phosphatase
AAOS	American Academy of Orthopaedic Surgeons		ALVAL	aseptic lymphocyte-dominant vasculitis-associated lesion
AARS	atlanto-axial rotatory subluxation		AMBRI	Atraumatic, Multidirectional instability, Bilateral involvement, Rehabilitation vital, and Inferior capsular shift
ABC	associated both columns		AMTS	Abbreviated Mental Test Score
ABG	arterial blood gas		ANA	antinuclear autoantibodies
ABPI	ankle–brachial pressure index		anti-ds	anti-double-stranded
AC	acromioclavicular		AO	Arbeitsgemeinschaft für Osteosynthesefragen
ACDF	anterior cervical discectomy and fusion		AP	anteroposterior
ACE	angiotensin-converting enzyme		APL	abductor pollicis longus
ACEI	angiotensin-converting enzyme inhibitor		APTT	activated partial thromboplastin time
ACF	antecubital fossa		ARB	angiotensin receptor blocker
AChEI	acetylcholinesterase inhibitor		ARDS	acute respiratory distress syndrome
ACI	autologous chondrocyte implantation		ARMD	adverse reaction to metal debris
ACJ	acromioclavicular joint		ARR	absolute risk reduction
ACL	anterior cruciate ligament; anticardiolipin		AS	ankylosing spondylitis
ACP	advance care planning		ASA	American Society of Anesthesiologists
ACR	albumin:creatinine ratio; American College of Rheumatology			
ACS NSQIP	American College of Surgeons National Surgical Quality Improvement Program			

ASIA	American Spinal Injury Association		CABC	catastrophic haemorrhage, airway, breathing, and circulation
ASIS	anterior superior iliac spine		CAM	controlled active movement
AT	anaerobic threshold		CBG	capillary blood glucose
ATFL	anterior talofibular ligament		CBS	cystathionine β-synthase
ATLS	advanced trauma life support		CBVA	chin–brow vertical angle
aTOS	arterial thoracic outlet syndrome		CC	coracoclavicular
AV	arteriovenous		CCF	congestive cardiac failure
AVN	avascular necrosis		CCH	collagenase Clostridium histolyticum
AVPU	Alert, Voice, Pain, Unresponsive		CCP	cyclic citrullinated peptide
β-HCG	beta-human chorionic gonadotrophin		CCST	certificate of completion of specialist training
BAPRAS	British Association of Plastic Reconstructive and Aesthetic Surgeons		CER	control event rate
			CES	cauda equina syndrome
BASDAI	Bath Ankylosing Spondylitis Disease Activity Index		CFL	calcaneofibular ligament
			CFS	Clinical Frailty Scale
BASK	British Association for Surgery of the Knee		CFU	colony-forming unit
			CI	confidence interval
BASS	British Association of Spine Surgeons		CIA	carpal instability adaptive
			CIC	carpal instability combined
BD	twice daily		CID	carpal instability dissociative
BESS	British Elbow and Shoulder Society		CIND	carpal instability non-dissociative
BGS	British Geriatrics Society		CIWA	Clinical Institute Withdrawal Assessment for Alcohol
BHS	British Hip Society			
BLRS	British Limb Reconstruction Society		CK	creatine kinase
			CKD	chronic kidney disease
BMA	British Medical Association		CLD	chronic liver disease
BMD	bone mineral density		CMCJ	carpometacarpal joint
BMI	body mass index		CMT	congenital muscular torticollis; Charcot–Marie–Tooth (disease)
BMP	bone morphogenetic protein			
BNF	British National Formulary			
BOA	British Orthopaedic Association		CMV	cytomegalovirus
			CNC	calcaneonavicular coalition
BOAST	BOA Standards for Trauma and Orthopaedics		CNS	central nervous system
			CONSORT	CONSORT, Consolidated Standards of Reporting Trials
BOFAS	British Orthopaedic Foot and Ankle Society			
			COOL	COSECSA Oxford Orthopaedic Link
BP	blood pressure			
bpm	beat per minute		COPD	chronic obstructive pulmonary disease
BPSD	behavioural and psychological symptoms of dementia			
			COSECSA	College of Surgeons of East Central and Southern Africa
BSCOS	British Society for Children's Orthopaedic Surgery			
			COVID-19	coronavirus disease 2019
BSR	British Spine Registry		COX	cyclo-oxygenase
BSSH	British Society for Surgery of the Hand		CP	cerebral palsy
			CPAP	continuous positive airway pressure
BTS	British Thoracic Society			
Ca2+	calcium			

	cardiopulmonary exercise testing
CPIP	Cerebral Palsy Integrated Pathway
CPK	creatine phosphokinase
CPPD	calcium pyrophosphate deposition disease
CPR	cardiopulmonary resuscitation
CR	cruciate retaining
CrCl	creatinine clearance
CRP	C-reactive protein
CRPS	complex regional pain syndrome
CS	chondrosarcoma
CSF	cerebrospinal fluid
CT	computed tomography
CTA	computed tomography angiography
CTD	connective tissue disease
CTEV	congenital talipes equinovarus
CVA	cerebrovascular accident
CVT	congenital vertical talus
CXR	chest X-ray
DAIR	debridement, antibiotics, implant retention
DAPT	dual antiplatelet therapy
DAS	Disease Activity Score
DASH	Disabilities of the Arm, Shoulder, and Hand (score)
DCO	damage control orthopaedics
DDH	developmental dysplasia of the hip
DECT	dual-energy computed tomography
DEXA	dual-energy X-ray absorptiometry
DF	desmoid fibromatosis
DH	drug history
DHS	dynamic hip screw
DIC	disseminated intravascular coagulation
DIPJ	distal interphalangeal joint
DISH	diffuse idiopathic skeletal hyperostosis
DISI	dorsal intercalated segment instability
DKA	diabetic ketoacidosis
DM	dermatomyositis
DMAA	distal metatarsal articular angle
DMARD	disease-modifying antirheumatic drug

DNA CPR	Do Not Attempt Cardio-Pulmonary Resuscitation
DOAC	direct oral anticoagulant
DRAFFT	Distal Radius Acute Fracture Fixation Trial
DRUJ	distal radioulnar joint
DVT	deep vein thrombosis
EBM	evidence-based medicine
ECG	electrocardiogram
ECRB	extensor carpi radialis brevis
ECRL	extensor carpi radialis longus
ECU	extensor carpi ulnaris
ED	emergency department; extensor digitorum
EDC	extensor digitorum communis
EDL	extensor digitorum longus
EDM	extensor digiti minimi
EEG	electroencephalography
EER	exposure event rate
eFAST	extended FAST
eGFR	estimated glomerular filtration rate
EHL	extensor hallucis longus
EI	extensor indicis
EIP	extensor indicis proprius
EMG	electromyography
EPB	extensor pollicis brevis
EPL	extensor pollicis longus
EPO	erythropoietin
EQ-5D	EuroQoL Five Dimensions
ER	external rotation
ERA	enthesitis-related arthritis
ERAS	enhanced recovery after surgery
ERT	emergency resuscitative thoracotomy
ESR	erythrocyte sedimentation rate
ESRF	end-stage renal failure
ETC	early total care
EUA	examination under anaesthesia
EULAR	European League Against Rheumatism
FABER	flexion, abduction, and external rotation
FADIR	flexion, adduction, internal rotation
FAP	familial adenomatous polyposis
FAST	focused assessment with sonography for trauma
FBC	full blood count

FCR	flexor carpi radialis	HEPA	high-efficiency particu
FCU	flexor carpi ulnaris	HIV	human immunodeficiency .
FD	fibrous dysplasia	HLA	human leucocyte antigen
FDB	flexor digitorum brevis	HME	hereditary multiple exostoses
FDG	fluorodeoxyglucose	HMSN	hereditary motor and sensory neuropathy
FDL	flexor digitorum longus		
FDP	flexor digitorum profundus	HPA	hypothalamic–pituitary–adrenal (axis)
FDS	flexor digitorum superficialis		
FES	functional electrical stimulation	HPC	history of presenting complaint
FFD	fixed flexion deformity		
FH	family history	HR	heart rate; hazard ratio
FHL	flexor hallucis longus	HRCT	high-resolution computed tomography
FLS	fracture liaison services		
FNCLCC	Fédération Nationale des Centres de Lutte Contre le Cancer	HRQoL	health-related quality of life
		HSMN	hereditary sensory motor neuropathy
FPB	flexor pollicis brevis	HU	Hounsfield unit
FPL	flexor pollicis longus	HUJ	humeroulnar joint
FSH	follicle-stimulating hormone	HVA	hallux valgus angle
FVC	forced vital capacity	ICBD	International Criteria for Behçet's Disease
G	gauge		
GABA	γ-aminobutyric acid	ICD	implantable cardioverter–defibrillator
GCS	Glasgow Coma Scale		
GCT	giant cell tumour	ICP	intracranial pressure
GFR	glomerular filtration rate	ICU	intensive care unit
GH	growth hormone	IFRC	International Federation of Red Cross and Red Crescent Societies
GHJ	glenohumeral joint		
GI	gastrointestinal		
GIRFT	Getting It Right First Time	IgE	immunoglobulin E
GMFCS	Gross Motor Function Classification System	IgG	immunoglobulin G
		IgM	immunoglobulin M
GP	general practitioner	IGRA	interferon-gamma release assay
GRADE	Grading of Recommendations, Assessment, Development, and Evaluation		
		IHD	ischaemic heart disease
		IIM	idiopathic inflammatory myositis
GRAFO	ground reaction ankle–foot orthosis		
		IL	interleukin
GRF	ground reaction force	ILAR	International League of Associations for Rheumatology
GT	greater trochanter		
h	hour	ILD	interstitial lung disease
HACEK	*Haemophilus, Actinobacillus, Cardiobacterium, Eikenella, Kingella*	ILS	immediate life support
		IM	intramuscularly
		IMTA	intermetatarsal angle
HAGL	humeral avulsion of the inferior glenohumeral ligament	INGO	international non-governmental organization
		INR	international normalized ratio
HAS	human albumin solution	IPA	interphalangeal angle
HASO	hip abduction spinal orthosis	IPJ	interphalangeal joint
Hb	haemoglobin	IQ	intelligence quotient
HbA1c	glycated haemoglobin	IR	internal rotation
HDU	high dependency unit		

IRMER	Ionising Radiation (Medical Exposure) Regulations
ISS	Injury Severity Score
ITB	iliotibial band
ITU	intensive therapy unit
IU	international unit
IV	intravenous
IVC	inferior vena cava
IVDU	intravenous drug use
IVIG	intravenous immunoglobulin
JBDS	Joint British Diabetes Societies
JIA	juvenile idiopathic arthritis
JVP	jugular venous pressure
K+	potassium
KAFO	knee–ankle–foot orthosis
KCl	potassium chloride
LA	local anaesthetic
LABCN	lateral antebrachial cutaneous nerve
LCL	lateral collateral ligament
LDH	lactate dehydrogenase
LFT	liver function test
LH	luteinizing hormone
LMA	laryngeal mask airway
LMIC	low- and middle-income country
LMN	lower motor neuron
LPA	lasting power of attorney
LR	likelihood ratio
LUCL	lateral ulnar collateral ligament
LV	left ventricular
LVF	left ventricular failure
MARS	metal artefact reduction sequence
MBD	metastatic bone disease
MCID	minimum clinically important difference
MCL	medial collateral ligament
MCPJ	metacarpophalangeal joint
MC&S	microscopy, culture, and sensitivity
MD1	myotonic dystrophy type 1
MD2	myotonic dystrophy type 2
MDR-TB	multidrug-resistant tuberculosis
MDT	multidisciplinary team
MET	minimal energy technique; metabolic equivalent
Mg2+	magnesium
MG	myasthenia gravis
MIPO	minimally invasive plate osteosynthesis
MM	multiple myeloma
mmHg	millimetre of mercury
MODS	multiorgan dysfunction
MOU	memorandum of understanding
MPFL	medial patellofemoral ligament
MRA	magnetic resonance angiography
MRC	Medical Research Council
MRI	magnetic resonance imaging
MRSA	meticillin-resistant Staphylococcus aureus
MSCC	metastatic spinal cord compression
MSU	monosodium urate
MTC	major trauma centre
MTHFR	5,10-methylenetetrahydrofolate reductase
MTPJ	metatarsophalangeal joint
MUA	manipulation under anaesthesia
MUST	Malnutrition Universal Screening Tool
N	Newton
NAHR	Non-Arthroplasty Hip Register
NAI	non-accidental injury
NBM	nil by mouth
NCA	nurse-controlled analgesia
NCS	nerve conduction studies
NDORMS	Nuffield Department of Orthopaedics, Rheumatology and Musculoskeletal Sciences
NF	neurofibromatosis
NG	nasogastric
NGT	nasogastric tube
NHANES	National Health and Nutrition Examination Survey
NHFD	National Hip Fracture Database
NHS	National Health Service
NICE	National Institute for Health and Care Excellence
NICU	neonatal intensive care unit
NIPE	Newborn and Infant Physical Examination
NIV	non-invasive ventilation
NJR	National Joint Registry
NLR	National Ligament Registry

NMBA	neuromuscular blocking agent	PET	positron emission tomography
NMDA	N-methyl-D-aspartate	PFFD	proximal femoral focal deficiency
NNH	number needed to harm		
NNT	number needed to treat	PHEM	pre-hospital emergency medicine
NPV	negative predictive value		
NSAID	non-steroidal anti-inflammatory drug	PHS	Parkinsonism–hyperpyrexia syndrome
NSCISC	National Spinal Cord Injury Statistical Center	PIN	posterior interosseous nerve
		PIPJ	proximal interphalangeal joint
nTOS	neurogenic thoracic outlet syndrome	PJI	periprosthetic joint infection
		PL	palmaris longus
NT-proBNP	N-terminal pro-B-type natriuretic peptide	PLC	posterolateral corner
		PLL	posterior longitudinal ligament
OA	osteoarthritis	PLS	posterior leaf spring
OATS	osteochondral autologous transfer system	PMH	past medical history
		PMMA	polymethylmethacrylate
OBPP	obstetric brachial plexus palsy	PMN	polymorphonuclear leucocyte
OC	osteochondroma	PMP-22	peripheral myelin protein 22
OCD	osteochondritis dissecans	PO4	phosphate
OD	once daily	POP	plaster of Paris
ODEP	Orthopaedic Data Evaluation Panel	PPD	purified protein derivative
		PPE	personal protective equipment
ODP	operating department practitioner	PPI	proton pump inhibitor
		PPM	permanent pacemaker
OLIF	oblique lateral interbody fusion	P-POSSUM	Portsmouth-Physiologic and Operative Severity Score for the Study of Mortality and Morbidity
OM	overlap myositis		
OR	odds ratio		
ORIF	open reduction and internal fixation		
		PPV	positive predictive value; pes planovalgus
OS	osteosarcoma; Osgood–Schlatter (disease)		
		PQ	pronator quadratus
OSA	obstructive sleep apnoea	PR	per rectum
OSIS	Oxford Shoulder Instability Score	PRC	proximal row carpectomy
		PRISMA	Preferred Reporting Items for Systematic reviews and Meta-Analyses
OTA	Orthopaedic Trauma Association		
PA	posteroanterior		
PACS	picture archiving and communication system	PRN	pro re nata (as required)
		ProFHER	Proximal Fracture of the Humerus: Evaluation by Randomisation (trial)
PAINAD	Pain Assessment in Advanced Dementia		
		PROM	patient-reported outcome measure
PAO	peri-acetabular osteotomy		
PC	presenting complaint	PRP	platelet-rich plasma
PCA	patient-controlled analgesia	PRUJ	proximal radioulnar joint
PCL	posterior cruciate ligament	PSA	prostate-specific antigen
PCR	protein:creatinine ratio; polymerase chain reaction	PSIS	posterior superior iliac spine
		PSO	pedicle subtraction osteotomy
PD	Parkinson's disease	PT	prothrombin time
PE	pulmonary embolism	PTH	parathyroid hormone
PEG	percutaneous endoscopic gastrostomy	PTU	propylthiouracil
		PVD	peripheral vascular disease

PVL	Panton–Valentine leucocidin
PVNS	pigmented villonodular synovitis
QDS	four times daily
QoL	quality of life
RA	rheumatoid arthritis
RBC	red blood cell
RCJ	radiocapitellar joint
RCT	randomized controlled trial
RF	radiofrequency
RhF	rheumatoid factor
RICE	rest, ice, compression and elevation
RNP	ribonucleoprotein
ROM	range of movements
ROTEM	rotational thromboelastometry
RR	relative risk
RRR	relative risk reduction
RTA	road traffic accident
RVAD	rib vertebral angle difference
SA	septic arthritis
SAC	space available for the cord
SACH	solid ankle cushioned heel
SAI	subacromial impingement
SAPHO	synovitis, acne, pustulosis, hyperostosis, and osteitis
SBP	systolic blood pressure
SCFE	slipped capital femoral epiphysis
SCI	spinal cord injury
SCIWORA	spinal cord injury without radiographic abnormality
SCJ	sternoclavicular joint
SCM	sternocleidomastoid
SDR	selective dorsal rhizotomy
SEMLS	single-event multilevel surgery
SF-36	Short Form 36
SH	social history
SHBG	sex hormone-binding globulin
SHS	sliding hip screw
SIADH	syndrome of inappropriate antidiuretic hormone secretion
SIJ	sacroiliac joint
SINS	Spinal Instability Neoplastic Score
SIRS	systemic inflammatory response syndrome
SIS	subacromial impingement syndrome

SLAP	superior labrum from anterior to posterior (tear)
SLE	systemic lupus erythematosus
SLIC	Subaxial Cervical Spine Injury Classification
SLJ	Sinding–Larsen–Johansson (disease)
SLR	straight leg raise
SLT	speech and language therapy
SMN	survival motor neuron
SNAC	scaphoid non-union advanced collapse
SOL	space-occupying lesion
SONK	spontaneous osteonecrosis of the knee
SORT	Surgical Outcome Risk Tool
SPECT	single-photon emission computed tomography
SPO	Smith–Peterson osteotomy
SR	systems review
SRN	superficial radial nerve
SSc	systemic sclerosis
SSEP	somatosensory evoked potential
SSRI	selective serotonin reuptake inhibitor
STIR	short-tau inversion recovery
STROBE	Strengthening the Reporting of Observational Studies in Epidemiology
STS	soft tissue sarcoma
SUA	serum uric acid
SUFE	slipped upper femoral epiphysis
SVR	systemic vascular resistance
T	tesla
T3	triiodothyronine
T4	thyroxine
TARN	Trauma Audit and Research Network
TB	tuberculosis
TBSA	total burn surface area
TCC	talocalcaneal coalition
TCL	transverse carpal ligament
TDR-TB	totally drug-resistant tuberculosis
TDS	three times daily
TEG	thromboelastography
TENS	transcutaneous electrical nerve stimulation

TFCC	triangular fibrocartilage complex
TFL	tensor fasciae latae
TFT	thyroid function test
TGCT	tenosynovial giant cell tumour
THA	total hip arthroplasty
THR	total hip replacement
TIA	transient ischaemic attack
TKR	total knee replacement
TLICS	thoracolumbar injury classification and severity score
TNF	tumour necrosis factor
TORUS	Trauma and Orthopaedic Unifying Structure
TOS	thoracic outlet syndrome
tRNA	transfer RNA
TSH	thyroid-stimulating hormone
TTG	tissue transglutaminase
TT-TG	tibial tubercle to trochlea groove (distance)
TU	trauma unit
TUBS	Traumatic aetiology, Unidirectional instability, Bankart lesion present, and Surgical management
U&Es	urea and electrolytes
UCL	ulnar collateral ligament
UCS	unified classification system
UKKOR	UK Knee Osteotomy Registry
UL	ulnolunate
ULT	urate-lowering treatment

UMN	upper motor neuron
US	ultrasound
USS	ultrasound scan
UT	ulnotriquetral
UTI	urinary tract infection
UV	ultraviolet
VCL	volar carpal ligament
VDRO	varus derotation osteotomy
VISI	volar intercalated segment instability
VLP	volar locking plate
VMO	vastus medialis oblique
VRIII	variable-rate intravenous insulin infusion
VTE	venous thromboembolism
vTOS	venous thoracic outlet syndrome
WAD	whiplash-associated disorder
WCC	white cell count
WHO	World Health Organization
WOC-UK	World Orthopaedic Concern UK
WOMAC	Western Ontario and McMaster Universities Osteoarthritis Index
WTD	wall–tragus distance
XDR-TB	extensively drug-resistant tuberculosis
XLIF	extreme lateral interbody fusion

Part 1

Principles of trauma and orthopaedics

History and examination

General principles of history and examination

A thorough history and examination are key to the diagnosis of musculo-skeletal disorders. A comprehensive clinical approach will help to establish a list of differential diagnosis if a specific diagnosis is not immediately evident, and help to focus on further investigations.

History

This is often the most useful aspect of clinical assessment. A succinct, de-tailed history will often suggest a provisional diagnosis. A focused clinical examination may then be used to confirm any specific pathology. Start with open-ended questions to allow the patient to describe their problem in their own words ('what happens when you try to run?'), later focusing on specific differentials with more closed questioning as appropriate ('do you trust your knee?' or 'does your knee give way while you walk?'). Remember to ask the patient about their expectations from the consultation and sub-sequent management.

The summary below provides a generic overview but does need to be tailored for each group of specific pathologies/systems:

- *Introduction:* introduce yourself; confirm patient identity and age.
- *Presenting complaint (PC):* broadly, the anatomical region(s) and primary symptom(s) (e.g. 'left knee pain and stiffness'). Elicit via an open introductory question (e.g. 'what problem can I help you with today?'). Refine through subsequent history.
- *History of presenting complaint (HPC):* details about the presenting problem(s), including:
  - Aetiology (traumatic or non-traumatic), including mechanism of injury
  - Duration (acute or chronic; congenital or acquired), frequency (number of episodes), time course/pattern (e.g. worse on walking), relieving and exacerbating factors (e.g. particular movements or positions)
  - Previous episodes and treatment (including dates, details of healthcare professionals involved, and efficacy)
  - Other associated symptoms (e.g. rash, swelling), 'yellow/red flag' features (associated with severity and malignancy), including unremitting night pain/unexpected weight loss/fever/systemic upset
  - For pain histories, the mnemonic 'SOCRATES' is helpful (Site, Onset, Character, Radiation, Associations, Time course, Exacerbating/relieving factors, Severity)
  - Do not forget referred (e.g. hip to knee), radicular (e.g. spinal nerve root impingement), and neurological (e.g. compression neuropathy, local ischaemia, peripheral neuropathy) causes.
- *Past medical history (PMH):* other medical comorbidities, previous trauma, previous surgery, prior hospital admissions, anaesthetic history (including adverse reactions), previous venous thromboembolism (VTE). The goal is to consider anaesthetic fitness/risk. In paediatric cases, ascertain any problems during pregnancy/birth, siblings, and developmental milestones.

- *Drug history (DH):* medications taken (dose, frequency/timing, route, duration), drug/other allergies (including metals or dressings). If appropriate, enquire about recreational or non-prescription drugs.
- *Social history (SH):* age, occupation, hand dominance, other household members, nature of home (e.g. house vs bungalow; can they manage stairs?), additional care or support (e.g. warden-controlled flat, carers twice daily, residential home), current/ex-smoking (in pack years), alcohol intake (units/week, duration if high intake), sexual history (if appropriate, e.g. young patient with joint pain/swelling).
- *Functional history/activities of daily living (ADLs):* premorbid ability to perform day-to-day activities (e.g. shopping, cooking, washing, dressing, lifting shopping bags), fine motor control (e.g. writing, buttons). Ask about specific difficulties with performing certain activities. Have any adaptations been made to their home/car/work because of functional limitation? Walking aids (e.g. sticks—in which hand, frame, rollator). Exercise tolerance (maximum distance, flat vs uphill, what stops them—differentiate between breathing difficulty and joint pain). Specific sporting activities/hobbies and performance level (e.g. semi-professional).
- *Family history (FH):* similar problems in other relatives? Other systemic/ significant medical problems (e.g. connective tissue disorders, skeletal dysplasia, neurofibromatosis (NF)).
- *Systems review (SR):* top-to-toe (i.e. neurological, cardiovascular, etc.) overview of any other symptoms that might be relevant (e.g. headache, dizziness, chest pain, shortness of breath), any other 'yellow/red flags' (see earlier).

Examination

'Look, feel, move, special tests'—Apley's (modified) basic principles can be applied to most orthopaedic examinations.

The examination begins the moment you lay eyes on the patient— posture, gait, and ease of movement can all be observed as the patient walks in from the waiting room. Always examine in a room with adequate light and privacy. The patient may need to undress, so provide a gown, sheet, and chaperone, as appropriate. Examine the relevant part of the body gently, systematically, and thoroughly. Start with the good limb first, and then compare with the symptomatic one. Always examine the joints above and below the site of pathology.

- *Look.* Often the most useful step. Note any scars, trophic/skin changes (erythema, ulcers, pressure areas, bruising), swelling, sinus tracts, asymmetry in size/alignment (measure true/apparent limb lengths and girth for wasting), deformity, gait, balance, posture, muscle wasting, fasciculations, systemic features, uneven shoe wear, aids. Systematically define any lumps (size, site, shape, surface, colour, contour).
- *Feel.* Temperature, tenderness, joint effusion (minimal, moderate, significant), abnormal movement, abnormal anatomy (e.g. gapping of ruptured tendons), true/apparent limb length discrepancy, crepitus. Systematically define any lumps (tenderness, temperature, tethering, transilluminance, texture, fluctuance, pulsatility). Note regional lymphadenopathy.

- *Move.* Active (range the patient can achieve by muscular contraction—if less than the passive range, there is a 'lag') and passive range of movements (ROM). Note abnormal/excessive movement. Power (Medical Research Council (MRC) scale; see ➲ Neurological history and examination, pp. 26–30). Stability of joints. Beighton score if hyperlaxity evident (e.g. patellar/shoulder dislocation; Fig. 1.1).
- *Special tests.* A myriad exists to elicit specific signs or assess for specific pathology. Remember and use only a select key few (e.g. Lachman test for anterior cruciate ligament (ACL) laxity, Hawkins–Kennedy test for shoulder impingement). In general, the goals of these are to: (1) test a particular aspect of a musculo-tendinous unit—may require a specific movement/position (e.g. supraspinatus); (2) perform a provocation test to detect impaired function when force is applied in a particular direction (e.g. shoulder apprehension); (3) apply local anaesthetic to remove pain disinhibition (e.g. Neer's test); and (4) to identify instability secondary to soft tissue laxity (e.g. Lachman).
- *Neurovascular examination.* Always indicated. Neurology = tone, power, coordination, reflexes, sensation (specific nerves/dermatomes as appropriate, e.g. anterior interosseous nerve (AIN) branch of the median nerve with supracondylar fractures). Perfusion = pulses/other perfusion markers (capillary refill, temperature). Significant pain on passive movement following trauma should raise suspicion of compartment syndrome.

Tips

- Compare with the other side, whenever possible.
- Assess function (e.g. ability to dress/undress, grip objects comfortably, hold a pen, do up buttons, reach hair, compensatory movements).
- Do not forget site-specific tests (e.g. joint movement or stability).
- Remember systemic examination (i.e. systemic manifestations of relevant conditions such as café-au-lait spots in NF).

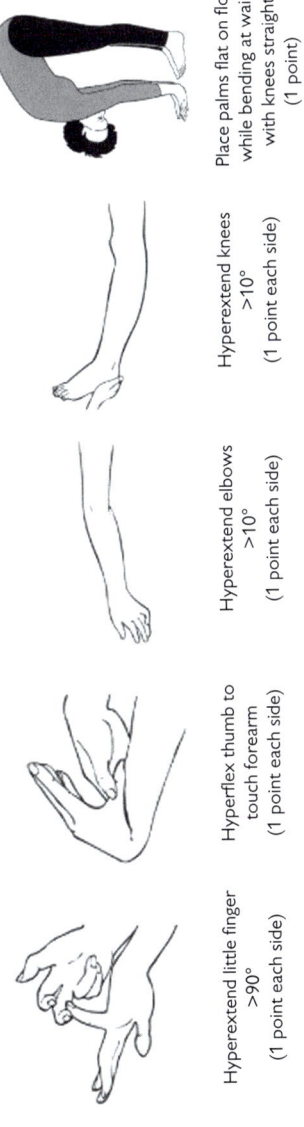

Fig. 1.1 Beighton score. Hyperlaxity is defined as 5/9 (adults) or 6/9 (children).

Hyperextend little finger >90° (1 point each side)

Hyperflex thumb to touch forearm (1 point each side)

Hyperextend elbows >10° (1 point each side)

Hyperextend knees >10° (1 point each side)

Place palms flat on floor while bending at waist, with knees straight (1 point)

Presentation of musculoskeletal disorders

Musculoskeletal disorders are common, with a diverse route of presentation, including to the general practitioner (GP), emergency department (ED), and other specialties. They may present as problems with an isolated limb/joint (e.g. septic arthritis), multiple (e.g. polytrauma), or associated with systemic disease (e.g. rheumatoid arthritis (RA), seronegative arthropathies, gout, metabolic bone disease). They can affect all age groups, ethnicities, genders, and socio-economic groups.

Typical presenting features

- Pain.
- Swelling (acute/chronic, variable/constant, associated pain).
- Stiffness.
- Deformity (loss of normal alignment).
- Loss of function (e.g. weakness, instability, locking).
- Neurological disturbance (central vs peripheral nervous system, sensory vs motor deficit, paraesthesiae, loss of function).
- Developmental issues/delay (associated with 'congenital' problems).
- Trauma (including delayed/missed presentations and sequelae).
- Iatrogenic problems or complications.

Acquired disorders

Presentations may be broadly categorized as either 'acquired' (not present at birth, but developing thereafter) or 'congenital' (present from birth). A 'surgical sieve' helps to consider differential causes (an aide-memoire is the mnemonic 'INVITED MD'):

- Infection (e.g. osteomyelitis, septic arthritis)
- Neoplasia (benign vs malignant tumours)
- Vascular (e.g. osteonecrosis, compartment syndrome, ischaemia)
- Inflammatory/autoimmune (e.g. RA) and iatrogenic (e.g. nerve injury)
- Trauma (bony vs soft tissue, isolated vs polytrauma)
- Endocrine (e.g. ulcers and Charcot joint due to diabetes mellitus)
- Degenerative (e.g. osteoarthritis)
- Metabolic (e.g. osteomalacia, Paget's disease)
- Drugs (e.g. steroids and osteonecrosis).

Trauma

Trauma may affect bone, muscle, soft tissues, nerves, and vessels. Mechanism of injury and initial management are key (see ➋ Initial assessment of the trauma patient: ATLS, pp. 64–66):

- Isolated injury or multiple injuries (polytrauma)
- Soft tissues (closed vs open, clean vs contaminated, haematoma)
- Neurovascular status (injury to peripheral nerves or vasculature)
- Blunt (e.g. blast, road traffic accident (RTA), sports)
- Penetrating (e.g. shotgun, stabbing)
- Burns (nature of causative agent—acid vs alkali chemical, electrical)
- Sequelae of previous trauma (e.g. non-union, malunion, arthritis)
- Systemic complications (e.g. fat embolus, pulmonary embolism (PE) or deep vein thrombosis (DVT)) or sequelae (e.g. psychological).

Shoulder examination

Ensure adequate exposure (men removing tops, women undressing to bra). Examine from the front, the sides, and behind (including axillae). The examiner stands in front; the patient turns. Compare both sides.

Look

- *Skin:* scars (note small arthroscopic portals), sinuses, erythema.
- *Soft tissues:* sulcus sign, wasting of deltoids/rotator cuff fossae/hands/pectorals, 'Popeye' sign with ruptured long head of biceps.
- *Bones:* let the arms hang down in resting position—is there an anteromedial mass (anterior glenohumeral dislocation) or internal rotation (posterior dislocation)? Note sternoclavicular joint (SCJ) and acromioclavicular joint (ACJ) deformity/prominence (dislocation/osteoarthritis (OA)), and any scapular prominence (medial/lateral winging, protraction).

Feel

- *Skin:* general warmth/tenderness.
- *Soft tissue:* rotator cuff fossae (defects/wasting), tendon to long head of biceps, subacromial bursa.
- *Bone:* SCJ, clavicle, ACJ, acromion, greater and lesser tuberosities, glenohumeral joint (GHJ)—anterior and posterior aspects, spine of scapula, and coracoid process.

Move

Examine strength and ROM (Fig. 1.2). Normal: abduction 0–180°, flexion 0–170° (in sagittal plane), extension 0–40°, external rotation 0–60° (arm by side, elbow flexed 90°), internal rotation 0–55° (at 90° shoulder abduction). Observe abduction in front and behind through full range—note difficulty with initiating or painful arc. Assess relative movements of scapulothoracic joint and GHJ.

Special tests

A multitude of tests exist, but only a few are commonly used.

Rotator cuff tests

- *Supraspinatus:* shoulder flexed 30° and abducted 30° (plane of scapula/GHJ), thumb pointing down. Resisted abduction to assess strength—also palpate muscle belly (may also be weak with impingement/pain).
- *Subscapularis (Gerber's lift-off test):* dorsum of hand against lower back, push back against resistance. Alternative is belly press test (both palms on belly, push elbows forward against resistance).
- *Infraspinatus and teres minor:* arm by side of body, elbow at 90°, external rotation against resistance. Hornblower's sign (compensatory shoulder abduction and elbow flexion when reaching mouth due to weak external rotation of teres minor).

Other muscles

- *Biceps:* elbow flexion against resistance. Speed's test (pain on resisted flexion of elbow, with arm supinated).
- *Serratus anterior:* push against wall (? medially winged scapula).
- *Trapezius:* push against wall (? laterally winged scapula).

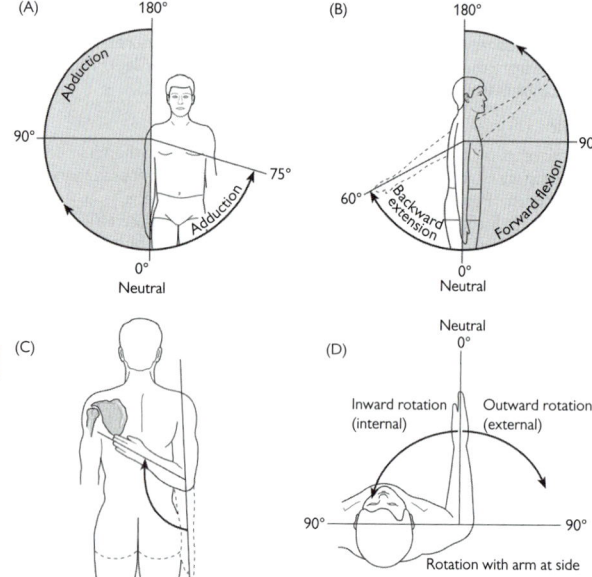

Fig. 1.2 Range of movement. (A) Abduction. (B) Flexion. (C) Internal rotation. (D) External rotation.

Reproduced from Bulstrode et al., Oxford Textbook of Orthopaedics and Trauma, with permission from Oxford University Press.

- *Deltoid (three heads):* abduct shoulder to 90°, and test resisted flexion (anterior), abduction (lateral), and extension (posterior).

Instability tests
- *Load and shift:* stabilize scapula, translate humeral head forward/ backward.
- *Anterior apprehension:* patient seated/supine, abduct, externally rotate, and extend shoulder; then push on head of humerus (from behind) with opposite hand, paying close attention to patient's face to spot pain/ anxiety and prevent in-clinic dislocation. Subluxation and protective muscle contraction with discomfort indicate anterior instability. Abolished by anterior pressure over humeral head when arm in same position.
- *Posterior apprehension:* patient supine, horizontal adduction of internally rotated arm with axial load along humerus.

Impingement syndrome tests
- *Neer's sign:* painful mid-arc abduction (60–120°) while stabilizing scapula, worse with thumb pointing down (empty can), better with

thumb up (full can). Abolition of pain after injection of local anaesthetic (e.g. 10mL of 1% lidocaine) into subacromial space suggests a positive Neer's test.
- *Hawkins–Kennedy test:* 90° shoulder flexion, elbow flexed to 90°, support elbow and internally rotate arm—pain is a positive result.
- *Jobe's test:* supraspinatus muscle test produces pain.

Acromioclavicular joint
- *Scarf test:* take arm across opposite shoulder, with a bent elbow. Pain over ACJ is positive result.

Elbow examination

Look

From the front, with both arms fully extended and supinated, then with elbows fully flexed. From medial and lateral sides. Also inspect from behind. Note:

- Resting posture and any deformity or asymmetry
- Carrying angle (normal 10–15° valgus; compare both sides)
- Skin for scars, sinuses, and erythema
- Soft tissues for swellings (e.g. rheumatoid nodules)/muscle bulk.

Feel

- *General:* warmth, swelling/masses (e.g. enlarged olecranon bursa, rheumatoid nodules, gouty tophi, effusion).
- *Lateral:* lateral supracondylar ridge to lateral epicondyle. Common extensor origin and lateral collateral ligament. Radial head and capitellum (pronate and supinate forearm).
- *Anterior:* biceps tendon, brachial artery, median nerve.
- *Medial:* medial epicondyle, common flexor origin, ulnar nerve (assess subluxation with flexion/extension, Tinel's test).
- *Posterior:* olecranon and triceps tendon.

NB bony prominences of the medial and lateral epicondyles and the olecranon tip should form a line with the arm straight, and an isosceles triangle with the elbow flexed to 90° (between the lateral epicondyle, olecranon, and radial head is a region where more subtle effusions/synovial thickening are palpable). Altered by posterior dislocation or fractures (Fig. 1.3).

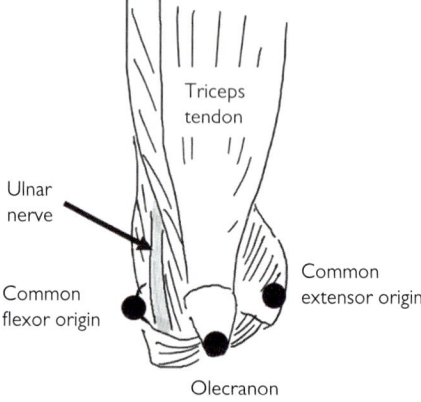

Fig. 1.3 Posterior anatomy, with the elbow flexed to 90°. The olecranon, extensor, and flexor origins (black dots) form a triangle.

Move—active

- *Flexion:* fully extend both elbows and then touch shoulders with fingertips. Normal range: 0–150°.
- *Pronation and supination:* elbows flexed 90° and arms at side to assess pronation and supination. Normal range: 180° of rotation.
- *Golfer's elbow (medial epicondylitis):* pain on resisted wrist flexion in supination.
- *Tennis elbow (lateral epicondylitis):* pain on resisted wrist extension in pronation, or resisted extension of middle finger (extensor carpi radialis brevis (ECRB)).

Special tests

- *Impingement:* pain at extremes of flexion/extension range.
- *Medial collateral ligament (MCL) laxity:* valgus stress with the elbow flexed to 30° and the humerus externally rotated.
- *Lateral collateral ligament (LCL) laxity:* varus stress with the elbow flexed to 30° and the humerus internally rotated (i.e. abduct and internally rotate the shoulder).
- *Posterolateral rotatory instability:* posterior drawer test, or support body weight on elbow with forearm supinated (e.g. lift body weight out of an armchair). Pivot–shift test (anaesthetized patient), similar to the knee, with patient supine and arm above the head, and apply valgus and supinating force while flexing.
- *'Hook' test:* inability to hook finger over distal biceps tendon in the antecubital fossa (ACF) from lateral side (? distal biceps tendon rupture).

Wrist and hand examination

Look

- *General:* posture, finger cascade, wasting, deformity, erythema.
- *Skin and nails:* colour, scars, wounds, clubbing, ridges, pitting.
- *Soft tissue:* swelling, muscle atrophy, contractures, lumps, nodules.
- *Bones/joints:* deformity, OA (distal interphalangeal joint (DIPJ)—Heberden's nodes; proximal interphalangeal joint (PIPJ)—Bouchard's nodes), RA (ulnar deviation, rheumatoid nodules, boutonnière (flexed PIPJ, hyperextended DIPJ)/swan neck (flexed DIPJ, hyperextended PIPJ)/Z deformity of thumb), mallet finger (inability to extend DIPJ), rotational deformity (in extension, look at the nail beds end on; in flexion, look for scissoring of fingers).

Feel

- *Swelling/deformity:* of or near tendons or joints.
- Identify any tender areas (Fig. 1.4): scaphoid tenderness is elicited in anatomical snuffbox or scaphoid tubercle, or on axial loading of thumb (cf. thumb base OA); ulnar fovea tenderness may represent a triangular fibrocartilage complex (TFCC) tear or ulnar abutment.
- *Crepitus:* on joint movement (e.g. with OA).
- *Dupuytren's disease:* palpate palmar fascia for nodules or cords.

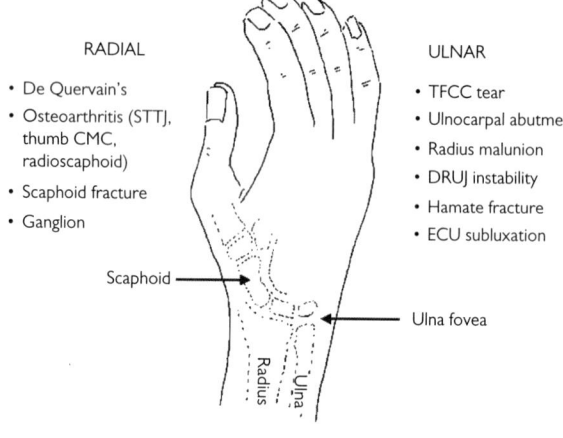

RADIAL

- De Quervain's
- Osteoarthritis (STTJ, thumb CMC, radioscaphoid)
- Scaphoid fracture
- Ganglion

ULNAR

- TFCC tear
- Ulnocarpal abutment
- Radius malunion
- DRUJ instability
- Hamate fracture
- ECU subluxation

Scaphoid

Ulna fovea

Radius   Ulna

- Osteoarthritis
- Rheumatoid arthritis
- Kienbock's
- Ganglion
- Carpal instability

Fig. 1.4 Common wrist pathologies and location of pain.

- *Vascular examination:* capillary refill time, radial pulse at the wrist. Allen's test (occlude both radial and ulnar arteries by direct pressure while making tight fist, open fist, and release pressure over one artery, repeat with the other artery. Assesses each contribution to palmar arch); can also be adapted to test digital arteries of a finger.
- *Sensation:* especially in context of penetrating trauma (2-point discrimination is most sensitive). Test both sides of digit.

Move

Careful examination is required, as subtle abnormalities can produce significant functional impairment.

- *Digits:* assess flexion, extension, abduction, and adduction of all fingers, and circumduction and opposition of thumb. Extension of index and small fingers, while keeping middle and ring fingers flexed, tests extensor indicis proprius (EIP) and extensor digiti minimi (EDM). Cascade with wrist extended/flexed—tendon injury.
- *Wrist*: assess flexion (0–80°), extension (0–70°), radial (0–20°) and ulnar (0–30°) deviation, pronation (0–90°), and supination (0–90°). Note supination and pronation also limited by elbow pathology.
- *Flexors:* isolate separate action of flexor digitorum superficialis (FDS) and flexor digitorum profundus (FDP) on fingers: splint middle phalanx to assess flexor action of FDP at DIPJ; hold other fingers in full extension to assess flexion of FDS at PIPJ of each isolated finger.
- *Power:* assess in main nerve territories. As a screen:
  - *Radial:* wrist and metacarpophalangeal joint (MCPJ) extension
  - *Ulnar*: first dorsal interosseus and small finger abduction (cross fingers)
  - *Median*: with palm upward, abduct (antepose) the thumb
  - *AIN:* OK sign (supracondylar fracture).
- *Functional assessment:* ask patient to write their name, hold a key, drink from a glass, do up a button, and pick up a small object.

Special tests

- *Tinel's test:* 30s tap over median (carpal tunnel) or ulnar (cubital tunnel) nerve.
- *Phalen's test:* fully flex wrist for 30s (reverse prayer)—suggests carpal tunnel syndrome if pain and paraesthesiae develop in med n. fingers.
- *Kirk-Watson's test (scaphoid shift test):* hold forearm with one hand, while other thumb presses on scaphoid tubercle and resists its movement on radial and ulnar deviation of the wrist. Painful click with scaphoid instability.
- *Froment's test:* hold paper between thumb and radial border of index, with interphalangeal joint (IPJ) straight—if weakness in ulnar-innervated adductor pollicis, then patient will grip by flexing the thumb IPJ (uses flexor pollicis longus (FPL)).
- *Finkelstein's test:* flex thumb into palm and clasp with fingers; ulnar deviation of the wrist produces pain in De Quervain's disease.

Hip examination

Undress to underwear. Watch the patient walking (is there a limp?). First examine standing.

Look

- *Around:* walking aids, shoe wear pattern, ease of movement, and posture.
- *Skin:* pelvis, hips, and legs—ischaemic/trophic change, scars, sinuses.
- *Swelling/masses* (e.g. lipoma, trauma, tumour, infection, hernia).
- *Muscle atrophy* (especially buttocks) or hypertrophy.
- *Deformity*: leg length inequality, pes cavus, scoliosis; position and degree of rotation of the leg.

Feel

- *Tenderness:* bony landmarks (greater trochanter (GT), trochanteric bursitis), anterior superior iliac spine (ASIS), ischial tuberosity.
- *Leg lengths:* while standing, palpate ASIS to assess pelvic obliquity. If one side is higher, then place blocks under the patient's foot on the lower side to assess if this is corrected (leg length discrepancy) or is fixed (lumbosacral disease).
- *Trendelenburg's test:* identify and hold the ASIS on both sides, with patient standing. Ask patient to lift one leg off the ground by flexing the knee, while supporting themselves on your forearms. If the contralateral abductors fail to hold the pelvis level (e.g. due to pain or weakness), the pelvis (and ASIS) will tilt downwards on the ipsilateral side ('lifted leg lags'). The patient will compensate by moving their body weight over the standing leg and/or seek support by putting more force through the contralateral arm, similar to use of a walking stick (manifests as more force felt through your forearm) (Fig. 1.5).

Move

- Ask patient to walk, and assess their gait (see ➲ Gait analysis, pp. 32–33).
- Then examine the patient lying down on the couch.

Look

- *Leg lengths: apparent* length discrepancy accepts the contribution of pelvic tilt (thus, one leg appears longer, but the skeletal length of the lower limbs may actually be equal). It can be measured as the distance from the umbilicus to the medial malleoli. *True* leg length discrepancy means the bone(s) on each side are of different lengths. It is measured clinically by holding the pelvis level and the legs symmetrical, and measuring from the ASIS to the medial malleolus. If fixed deformity on one side, place both legs in the same position first.
- *Galeazzi's test:* flex both knees to 90°, with both heels together. This determines whether any leg length discrepancy is below or above the knee (i.e. is the tibia or femur short?).
- *Bryant's triangle:* (perpendicular line dropped from ASIS; note length of horizontal line going proximally from GT tip to this line, and compare both sides); shortening indicates supratrochanteric femoral shortening.

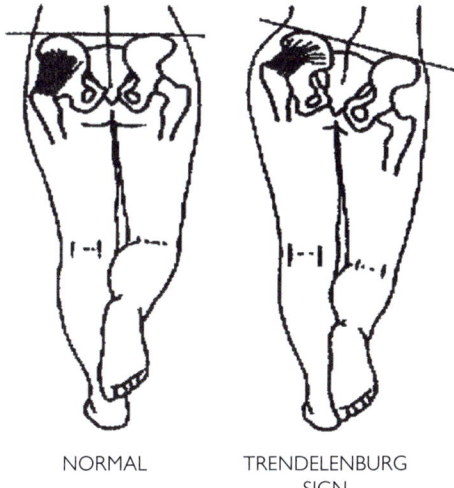

NORMAL

TRENDELENBURG
SIGN

Fig. 1.5 Trendelenburg sign: left abductor pathology, so the right side sags (right 'lifted leg lags').

Feel

- As above. Joint is deep in the groin; palpation is of limited value.

Move

- *Log roll:* gently roll each straight leg (screen for intra-articular pain).
- *Thomas' test:* flex contralateral hip, such that lumbar lordosis is eliminated (place a hand flat under the lordosis to assess this). The hip under examination should be able to extend fully (leg flat on bed); otherwise, a fixed flexion deformity (FFD) is present.
- *Flexion:* normal 0–120°. Flex knee to relax hamstrings.
- *Extension (0–10°):* assess with patient prone or by using Thomas' test.
- *Rotation:* normal 0–40° internal/0–60° external. Perform with the hip in extension, and also flexed at 90° (detects early hip pathology).
- *Abduction:* normal 0–40°. *Adduction:* normal 0–25°. Assess with hip and knee extended, and a hand on the contralateral ASIS to keep the pelvis neutral.
- *Straight leg raise (SLR):* assesses iliopsoas strength. May cause discomfort in certain conditions (e.g. fracture, intra-articular pathology).
- *Anterior impingement test (flexion, adduction, internal rotation (FADIR)):* patient supine, flex hip to 90°, adduct and internally rotate. Femoroacetabular impingement will cause discomfort.
- *FABER test:* flex, abduct, and externally rotate the leg (the 'figure-of-4' position). Sacroiliac joint (SIJ) and posterior hip pathology causes discomfort.

- *Ely test:* patient lies prone and the knee is flexed passively. If the hip on the same side spontaneously rises off the couch, the rectus femoris is contracted.
- *Ober's test:* patient on side, bottom hip/knee flexed. Flex upper leg while stabilizing GT, then extend and abduct upper hip. Then adduct; if difficult/painful, suggests tight iliotibial band (ITB)/tensor fasciae latae (TFL).
- *Clicking:* iliopsoas tendon (groin, internal) vs ITB (over GT, external).

Knee examination

Undress to shorts. Assess limb alignment while standing. Watch patient walk (see ➲ Gait analysis, pp. 32–33). Look for varus or valgus thrust (knee pushes into varus/valgus during stance due to OA or ligament laxity). Initially, inspect while standing, from the front, sides, and back.

Look

- *General:* walking aids. Beighton score if instability/laxity concerns.
- *Alignment of leg:* varus/valgus deformity (measure intermalleolar distance if valgus) and rotation (position of patella and foot).
- *Skin:* wounds, scars, erythema, sinuses.
- *Swelling:* supra-/infra-/prepatellar (? bursitis). Popliteal fossa/calf swelling (DVT, cellulitis; ? ruptured Baker's cyst).
- Knee joint: effusion (? OA; ? fracture; ? ligament injury), synovial thickening or meniscal cyst.
- *Muscle bulk:* quadriceps and calf muscles.

Feel

With the patient supine, assess:
- *Temperature* (using dorsum of hand)
- *Tenderness with knee extended:* suprapatellar pouch, patella, patellar tendon, tibial tuberosity, condyles of femur and tibia, including attachments of collateral ligaments (? tendinopathy, tear, fracture)
- *Tenderness with knee flexed to 90°:* medial and lateral joint lines (? meniscal pathology, ? OA)
- *Popliteal fossa:* palpate for Baker's cyst, aneurysm, lymph nodes
- *Effusion or haemarthrosis:* three methods to assess this:
  - *Sweep test*—for a small effusion, squeeze to occlude the suprapatellar pouch and then move any fluid by stroking it from the medial to lateral side of the knee. Look for a subtle bulge on the medial side where the sweep began
  - *Patellar tap*—for a medium effusion, occlude the suprapatellar pouch; push down on the patella, and try to feel it tap against the femur
  - *Ballottement test*—for a large amount of fluid, pressure from one side of the knee is transmitted to a hand placed on the other side.

Move

- *Patella:* tracking assessed with patient sitting on the side of a high couch, with legs dangling (do before getting patient to lie supine).
- *Patella glide test:* knee flexed to 30°, move medially/laterally. Apprehension on lateral movement suggests recurrent dislocation (movement laterally one quadrant is normal; two suggests laxity).
- *Clarke's test:* apply gentle pressure to superior pole of patella and ask patient to contract quadriceps. Pain indicates pathology.
- *Active ROM:* normal 0–140° (few degrees of symmetrical hyperextension may be normal).
- *SLR:* tests integrity of extensor mechanism.
- *Quadriceps lag:* lack of full knee extension on quadriceps contraction.
- *Crepitus:* passively flex and extend the knee, with hand gently placed over patella to feel for crepitus. Commonly an incidental finding.

- *Collateral ligaments:* varus and valgus stress testing in extension and 30° of flexion—painful minimal joint opening (grade 1), moderate opening with firm end point (grade 2), gross opening with soft end point (grade 3).
- *Cruciate ligament tests* (Table 1.1):
    - *Anterior and posterior drawer:* flex knee to 90°. Look from the side to see if any posterior sag (posterior cruciate ligament (PCL) injury), then pull proximal tibia forward while stabilizing the foot—assess amount of anterior displacement and quality of 'end point' (for ACL injury). If posterior sag, ask patient to contract quadriceps on affected side—*quadriceps active test* is positive if lower leg pulls forward.
    - *Lachman test:* variant of anterior drawer performed at 20° flexion. Stabilize femur with one hand and draw tibia forward. Placing your knee behind the patient can help if you have small hands.
    - *Pivot–shift:* valgus force and internal rotation of the tibia (can lock patient's foot in examiner's axilla/flank) sublux joint, then moving from extension to flexion reduces the joint, with a visible/palpable jump. Best performed under anaesthesia (needs relaxed hamstrings, can cause pain). Glide (grade 1), clunk (grade 2), explosive (grade 3).
- *Menisci:* joint line tenderness most sensitive. Tests involve loading the meniscus. *McMurray's test:* patient supine, knee flexed, one hand on joint lines, other hand under heel, stress joint with internal/external rotation while moving leg from flexion into extension. Positive if painful click. *Thessaly test:* stand on one leg, flex knee to 20°, and rotate trunk medially and laterally.

Table 1.1 Knee tests and pathological examination findings

Structure injured	Tests and findings
ACL	Lachman test
	Pivot–shift test
	Haemarthrosis
PCL	Posterior sag and drawer test
	Haemarthrosis
MCL	Valgus instability
	Tenderness medially
LCL	Varus instability
	Tenderness laterally
Meniscus	Joint line tenderness
	McMurray's test
	Thessaly test
Patella	Patella glide test
	Clarke's test

ACL, anterior cruciate ligament; LCL, lateral collateral ligament; MCL, medial collateral ligament; PCL, posterior cruciate ligament.

Ankle and foot examination

Expose the whole lower leg and foot (shorts/underwear). Inspect front/back/sides/sole of foot, initially with the patient standing and then sitting on an examination couch, with legs dangling over the side.

Look

- *Footwear:* signs of asymmetrical wear, orthotics (e.g. ankle–foot orthosis (AFO)), heel raises.
- Lower limb overall alignment.
- *Gait:* note the presence of all three rockers (see ➲ Gait, pp. 31–32).
- *Heel alignment:* normal 5° valgus. Ask patient to stand on tiptoes while looking from behind—assesses competence of gastrosoleus complex. Normal: hindfoot should swing from valgus to varus.
- *Skin:* scars, swelling, vascular disease, ulcers, gangrene, callosities.
- *Nails:* colour, deformity, infection (paronychia), pitting (psoriasis).
- *Soft tissue:* masses/swelling/muscle atrophy or hypertrophy.
- *Foot size:* unilaterally foot/calf hypotrophy (? congenital talipes equinovarus (CTEV)), bilaterally large foot (? marfanoid).
- Foot shape and position—common variants include:
  - *Neutral* ('rectus') foot
  - *Pes cavus* (high arch): high medial arch, hindfoot varus, adducted forefoot
  - *Pes planus* (flat foot): low medial arch, hindfoot valgus, abducted forefoot ('too many toes sign').
- Toe deformities:
  - *Mallet:* flexion deformity at DIPJ only
  - *Hammer:* flexion at PIPJ, extension at DIPJ
  - *Clawing:* hyperextended metatarsophalangeal joint (MTPJ), flexed IPJs
  - *Hallux valgus* (bunion): valgus deformity at greater toe MTPJ.

Feel

- *Palpate:* systematically to define areas of tenderness. Start proximally and medially, then move around the ankle and then distally to the mid- and forefoot (e.g. tibia/fibula, syndesmosis, lateral malleolus, anterior talofibular ligament (ATFL), anterior ankle joint, medial malleolus, etc.).
- *Pedal pulses* (dorsalis pedis, posterior tibial). Capillary refill.
- *Sensation:* dorsal (superficial peroneal nerve, except first webspace—deep peroneal nerve). Lateral (sural nerve). Plantar medial (saphenous nerve), central (medial/lateral plantar nerve).

Move

- Assess movements sequentially, proximally to distally (Fig. 1.6).
- One hand supports the calf; the other grips the heel and places it into neutral varus/valgus. Then assess ankle dorsiflexion (normal 0–25°) and plantar flexion (normal 0–45°).
  - If the ankle is in neutral and flat to the floor, it is described as *plantigrade*; however, if it remains dorsiflexed, it is in *calcaneus*, and if it remains plantar flexed, it is in *equinus*.
- Continue to grip the heel, but with the other hand, now feel the neck of the talus (anterior to the ankle). With the foot in slight plantar flexion, invert/evert the hindfoot to assess subtalar joint motion (<5°).

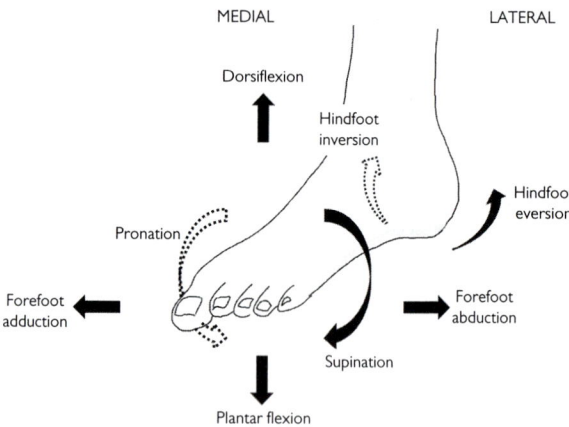

Fig. 1.6 Foot movements. Supination/pronation are a complex triplanar motion of the foot about an oblique axis.

- Continue to grip the heel, but with the other hand, move the mid-/ forefoot to assess midfoot (mid-tarsal) motion.
- Flexion/extension of toes—MTPJ and IPJs (especially first ray—*hallux rigidis*).

Special tests

- *Too-many-toes sign:* patient stands with both feet together in neutral position. Look from behind to see if there are more than two toes visible laterally, which usually indicates pes planus.
- *Silfverskiöld test:* maximally dorsiflex ankle, with knee extended and then flexed. More dorsiflexion on knee flexion indicates gastrocnemius tightness.
- *Double and single heel raise:* patient stands next to wall (for support) and is asked to stand on tiptoes, first with both feet, then with one foot and the other lifted off the ground. Observe from behind. Weakness or rupture of tibialis posterior is a common cause of the heel remaining in valgus and difficulty in performing the manoeuvre.
- *Coleman block test:* with a cavovarus deformity, the patient places the lateral foot on a block (e.g. thick book), with the first ray unsupported and off the block—varus will correct if deformity is flexible and driven by the forefoot. No correction means a fixed hindfoot.
- *Mulder's sign:* for Morton's neuroma. Painful click on compression of toes across MTPJs.
- *Anterior drawer test:* for ATFL. Hold the tibia and heel; with foot in slight plantar flexion, pull the heel anteriorly and assess for laxity.
- *Thompson's/Simmonds test:* assesses tendoachilles integrity. Calf squeeze should produce foot plantar flexion if intact.

Spine examination

Ask the patient to undress down to underwear and put on a hospital gown, untied at the back. Observe walking, standing from sitting, and ease of movement. 'Move' may be easier to perform with the patient sitting at the end of a couch rather than supine.

Look

- *Skin:* scars (remember chest and abdomen from anterior approaches to the spine), sinuses/erythema, midline hair tuft/dimpling (e.g. spina bifida), café-au-lait spots or nodules (e.g. NF).
- *Soft tissues:* masses, paravertebral and limb musculature.
- *Bone:* assess sagittal and coronal balance. A 'plumb line' from the occiput should drop to the natal cleft. Shoulders and pelvis should be level (correct any limb length discrepancy with blocks). Look from the side at lumbar lordosis/thoracic kyphosis.
- *Adams forward bend test:* observe from behind as the patient bends forward. If one-half of the ribcage elevates, this demonstrates structural scoliosis (axial plane deformity).

Feel

- *Tenderness:* may be midline or paravertebral. Non-specific.
- *Abnormalities:* define any masses/asymmetry/steps.
- *Examine the* abdomen: neurogenic bladder.

Move

- *Gait:* often useful to do during 'look'. Ask patient to walk normally, then on tiptoes (S1/2 power), then on heels (L4/5 power).
- Assess movement of cervical and thoracolumbar spine separately (Fig. 1.7). When assessing the neck, ensure shoulders are immobilized. When assessing movements of the trunk, ensure that the pelvis is immobilized. All movements should be symmetrical.

Normal cervical spine movements
- *Flexion* such that chin touches chest, extension to 30°.
- *Lateral rotation* should be to 70–90° on either side.
- *Lateral flexion* ('put ear on shoulder') should be to at least 40°.

Normal thoracolumbar movements
- *Flexion/extension:* occurs mainly in the lumbar spine. Screening assessment made by asking patient to touch toes.
- *Schober's test:* mark two points, 15cm apart, on lumbar spine when erect—should ↑ by 5cm on forward flexion.
- *Rotation:* mainly in thoracic spine—normal 60°.
- *Lateral flexion:* measure reaching down lateral aspect of each thigh.
- *Chest expansion* (limited in ankylosing spondylitis (AS)): normal expansion ≥5cm on full inspiration.

Neurological examination
Mnemonic: *Two People Can't Resist Sex.*
- *Tone:* hypotonia, normal, hypertonia. Note number of clonus beats.
- *Power:* motor strength in all myotomes. Grade 0–5 on MRC scale.

- *Coordination:* point from finger to nose (note past pointing), heel–shin, heel–toe walking (in straight line).
- *Reflexes:* biceps (C5), supinator (C6, brachioradialis), triceps (C7), in upper limbs. Abdominal reflex (T7–10, stroke from lateral to umbilicus and observe contraction—helps to determine level of spinal injury). Knee (L3/4), ankle (S1), and extensor plantar response in feet. *NB variation in reported nerve root responsible between sources.*
- *Sensation:* all dermatomes, light touch and pinprick.
- *Additional:* perianal pinprick sensation and anal tone (present vs absent) if appropriate (e.g. cauda equina compression). Bulbocavernosus reflex (S2–4, anal sphincter contraction with squeezing penis/clitoris, marks end of spinal shock following spinal cord injury).

Special tests

In the CERVICAL spine:
- *Spurling's test:* cervical nerve root compression—exacerbation of pain on axial compression of the head, with the neck extended and rotated to the side of the radicular pain.
- *Lhermitte's test:* placing the chin on the chest causes pain in the spine, radiating into the occiput. Assesses C-spine canal stenosis.
- *Hoffman's sign:* flicking DIPJ of the index finger causes reflex thumb IPJ flexion, with myelopathy (upper motor neuron (UMN) lesion).
- *Romberg's test:* patient stands with feet together and closes eyes. Positive if loses balance (dorsal column proprioception impaired).

In the LUMBAR spine:
- *SLR test:* limitation because of sciatic (leg) pain suggests radiculopathy. Crossed SLR = pain-free leg causes pain down the opposite leg. This is more specific for disc herniation.
- *Lasegue sign:* perform SLR test, then lower the leg slightly from uncomfortable position. Dorsiflex ankle. Positive if pain reproduced.
- *Femoral stretch:* patient prone, hip extension with knee flexed produces pain.
- *Waddell's signs:* suggestive of non-organic low back pain (e.g. non-anatomical tenderness, overreaction, non-dermatomal sensory disturbance). Interpret with caution.

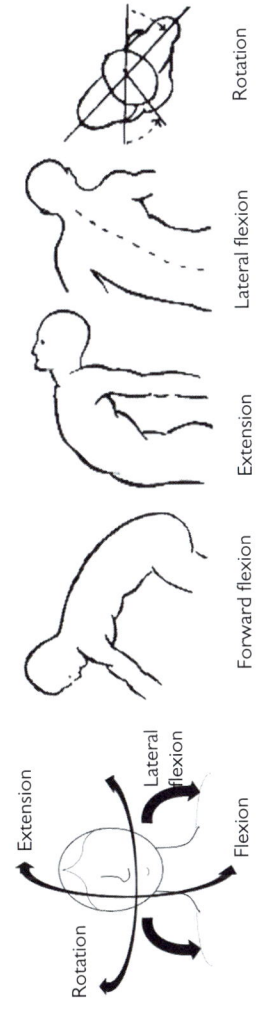

Fig. 1.7 Describing spine movements.

Neurological history and examination

History

A relevant neurological history is important in completing a full assessment of numerous musculoskeletal conditions. The history should be directed by presenting symptoms, location of symptoms, and their severity. It is essential to have a sound knowledge of underlying disorders that cause, or are associated with, musculoskeletal problems. The neurological assessment should help establish the *site of the lesion* and *likely pathology*. This will guide management and outcome/prognosis.

Common presentations

- *Pain:* for mnemonic SOCRATES (see ➡ General principles of history and examination, p. 4). Note extent and direction of radiation. What is more severe (e.g. back vs buttock vs leg)? With claudication, is leg pain worse (suggests vascular) or better (suggests spinal) when walking uphill? Trigger (e.g. neck movements).
- *Numbness (sensory loss) and paraesthesiae:* distribution and change in sensation.
- *UMN signs:* ↑ tone, brisk tendon reflexes, Babinski sign (hallux extends with stimulation of sole of foot), Hoffman's sign (flicking finger DIPJ induces thumb flexion). *Myelopathy (cord injury):* unsteady gait, difficulty with fine motor control (handwriting worse, struggles doing up buttons).
- *Lower motor neuron (LMN) signs:* ↓ tone, areflexia or hyporeflexia, fasciculation, fibrillation, paresis or paralysis.

Neurological symptoms

- *Higher functions:* cognition/memory deterioration (consider underlying central cause).
- *Sensory symptoms:* altered sensation (e.g. numbness, paraesthesiae, hyperalgesia). Distinguish between acute and chronic symptoms. They may be due to disorders of the central or peripheral nervous system, or of both. Symptoms may develop as a neurological manifestation of systemic disease. If pain associated with trophic changes and sensory disturbance following injury/surgery, consider complex regional pain syndrome (CRPS)—*Budapest Criteria* for diagnosis.
- *Motor symptoms:* establish if there is myotomal/nerve root vs peripheral nerve distribution (Table 1.3; also see ➡ Chapter 20). Acute or chronic, fluctuating, static or progressive, exacerbating or remitting? Results of prior treatment and therapeutic response are important.

Examination

Level of consciousness

'AVPU' can be used as a quick screen (Alert, Voice, Pain, Unresponsive) in the acute setting. The Glasgow Coma Scale (GCS) is a more detailed, objective assessment that should be repeated over time to note serial changes in mental status. 'Pain' can be triggered by fingertip or supraorbital pressure or by trapezius squeeze. Mnemonic for the three components: Mental State Examination (MSE)—for Motor (6), Speech (5), Eyes (4) (Table 1.2).

Table 1.2 Adult Glasgow Coma Scale (GCS; scoring min. 3, max. 15)

Revised scale	Score
Eye opening (E)	
Spontaneous	4
To sound	3
To pressure	2
None	1
Non-testable	NT
Verbal response (V)	
Oriented	5
Confused	4
Words	3
Sounds	2
None	1
Non-testable	NT
Best motor response (M)	
Obeys commands	6
Localizing	5
Normal flexion	4
Abnormal flexion	3
Extension	2
None	1
Non-testable	NT

Higher functions and speech

Mental status assessment

This is relevant when determining capacity for consent. Several tools include:

- *Screen:* alert and orientated in time, place, and person?
- *AMTS* (Abbreviated Mental Test Score /10: <6/10 is suggestive of dementia): age, time to nearest hour, repeat and recall an address, year, location, recognize two people, date of birth, date of World War II end, name of monarch, count backwards from 20 to 1.
- *AMT4:* abbreviated version of test—age, date of birth, place, year.

Speech

- *Dysphasias:* distinguish by command, repeat statement, naming object.
  - *Conductive:* repeat statements and names poorly, follows commands
  - *Expressive:* often hesitant and non-grammatical, but comprehension usually preserved (Broca's lesion)

- *Receptive:* fluent, nonsensical, with poor comprehension (Wernicke's lesion)
- *Nominal:* cannot specifically name objects.
- *Dysarthria:* difficulty of articulation only (alcohol, cerebellar, bulbar or pseudobulbar palsy, extrapyramidal).

Cerebellar signs

Mnemonic '*DANISH*':
- **D**ysdiadochokinesia (alternating dorsal/palmar claps of one hand into palm of other hand, with big truncal movements, i.e. from shoulder).
- **A**taxia (Romberg's).
- **N**ystagmus (follow examiner's finger in 'H' pattern).
- **I**ntention tremor (dysmetria when attempt to touch nose to finger).
- **S**lurred speech (dysarthria, staccato speech).
- **H**ypotonia/Heel–toe walk impaired (tandem gait)/Heel–shin coordination impaired/poor.

Cranial nerves (must be examined)
- I (olfactory): assess smell.
- II (optic): mnemonic 'AFRO': Acuity, Fields, pupillary Reflexes (react to light and accommodation), Ophthalmoscope (fundoscopy).
- III (oculomotor), IV (trochlea), VI (abducens): assess movements of eyes and eyelids (aide-memoire 'LR6 (lateral rectus, VI), SO4 (superior oblique, IV)').
- V (trigeminal): assess muscles of mastication and facial sensation (ophthalmic, maxillary, mandibular divisions); afferent arc for corneal reflex.
- VII (facial): assess facial muscles; efferent arc for corneal reflex (note: forehead creases spared with UMN lesions, lost with LMN lesions).
- VIII (auditory): assess hearing (differentiate between conduction and sensorineural hearing loss with Rinne's and Weber's tests) and vestibular function.
- IX (glossopharyngeal): assess swallowing/gag reflex, uvula deviation.
- X (vagus): assess for palatal deviation.
- XI (accessory): assess shoulder shrug.
- XII (hypoglossal): assess tongue movement and wasting (mnemonic 'TT': Tongue deviates Towards side of lesion; uvula away from lesion).

Limbs

Motor system

Examine both upper and lower limbs. Compare both sides. Note tone, power, coordination, and reflexes.
- *Inspection:* look for muscle wasting, attitude of the limb, trophic changes, fibrillation, fasciculation, asterixis, and choreiform movement.
- *Tone:* grasp under elbow and at wrist, and rotate the two joints to assess resistance. Parkinson's disease has lead pipe rigidity (shake hands and pronate/supinate while flex/extending). Clonus with UMN lesions.
- *MRC grading power* (NB this must be through full range of motion):

0	No voluntary contraction
1	Flicker of contraction
2	Movement with gravity eliminated
3	Movement against gravity
4	Movement against partial resistance
5	Full strength

Myotomes

A myotome is a group of muscles innervated by a specific spinal root (Table 1.3). In addition:

- C3–5: supply the diaphragm ('C3/4/5 keep the diaphragm alive')
- T2–12: supply the chest wall and abdominal muscles
- S3–5: important in bladder/bowel control and sexual function.

Table 1.3 Myotomes and reflexes

Root	Movement	Reflex
C5	Shoulder abduction	Biceps
C6	Wrist extension	Brachioradialis (supinator)
C7	Elbow extension	Triceps
C8	Finger flexion	
T1	Finger abduction	
L2	Hip flexion	
L3	Knee extension	
L4	Foot dorsiflexion (tib ant)	Knee (patellar)
L5	Hallux extension (EHL)	
S1	Foot plantar flexion	Ankle (Achilles)

EHL, extensor hallucis longus; tib ant, tibialis anterior.

Deep tendon reflexes

These are elicited by a short, sharp strike to the tendon of the muscle (Table 1.3). Reflexes may be: absent, elicitable with reinforcement (Jendrassik manoeuvre, e.g. jaw clench), present, or brisk.

Superficial reflexes (muscle contraction on stroking skin)

- Abdominal (T7–12).
- Cremasteric (L1, 2) and anal (S4, 5).

Sensory system

(Fig. 1.8)

- Test for light touch (cotton wool), pinprick (pin or 'millinery' wheel) sensation, and vibration sense (128Hz tuning fork).

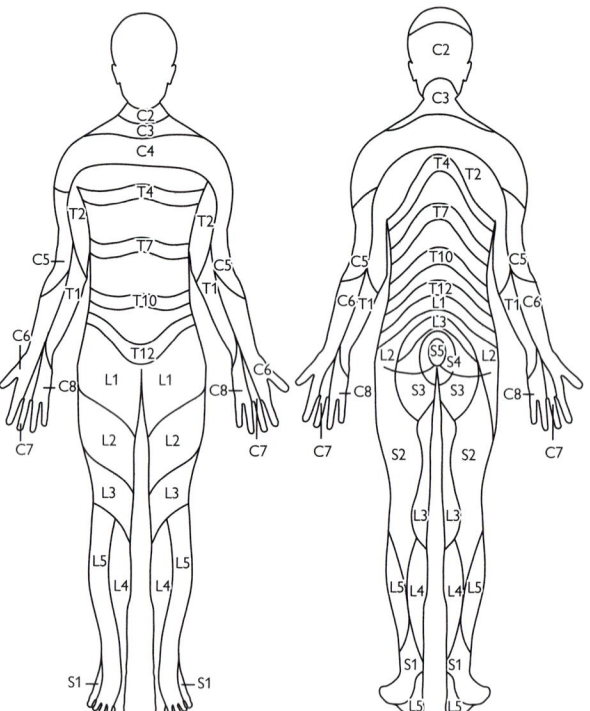

Fig. 1.8 Dermatome chart.

Reproduced from Bulstrode et al., *Oxford Textbook of Orthopaedics and Trauma*, with permission from Oxford University Press.

- Assess proprioception.
- Always assess sensory distribution: dermatomal, peripheral nerve, or glove and stocking.

NB signs of meningeal irritation include painful SLR, Babinski sign (dorsiflexion of hallux after plantar foot stimulation), Kernig's sign (inability to extend knee with hip flexion), and bowstring sign (pressure on popliteal fossa with flexed knee causes radicular pain).

Gait

- Neurological abnormalities can manifest as altered gait (see ➔ Gait, pp. 31–32) (e.g. hemiparetic, ataxic, shuffling, high-stepping, Trendelenburg—note this can also be due to L5 lesion).

Gait

In normal gait, there is complex coordination of movements and muscular contraction involving the lower limb, pelvis, and spine, as well as secondary movements of the upper limbs.

Gait cycle

This is divided into the *stance* (the foot is on the floor, ~60%) and *swing* phases (the foot is in the air, ~40%) (Fig. 1.9):

* *Stance phase:* begins with 'initial contact' as the foot contacts the ground. Initial contact is usually with the heel but may be with the forefoot in pathological gait (e.g. an equinus foot in cerebral palsy). During the 'loading response', the foot takes weight and flattens to the ground. Muscle contractions during walking tend to be eccentric, controlling movement of the limbs: eccentric tibialis anterior contraction follows the loading response, followed by eccentric calf contraction to decelerate the body ('braking') and bring the centre of mass in front of the knee, causing passive knee extension. Fixed flexion of the knee may prevent passive extension during the stance phase, and the quadriceps will need to remain active throughout stance (which is inefficient). NB the stance phase can also be described in relation to the *three 'foot rockers'*: heel (initial contact, impaired in foot drop), ankle (mid stance, impaired in ankle arthritis), and forefoot (terminal stance/ toe off, impaired in hallux rigidus) (Fig. 1.9).

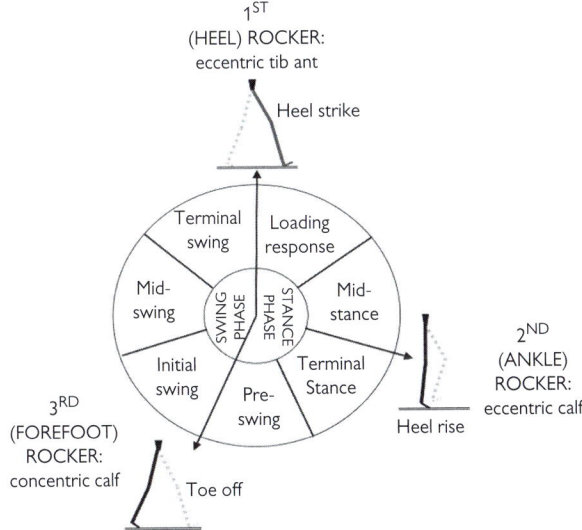

Fig. 1.9 The three rockers of gait.

- *Double limb support:* (~10% of cycle) occurs at the end/beginning of stance, as the opposite foot strikes the ground. During running gait, both feet are in the air at this point instead ('double float').
- *Swing phase:* occurs after the calf muscles contract to plantar flex the ankle and generate 'heel rise' and 'toe-off' into the swing phase. Concentric calf contraction locks the Chopart joints, permits heel rise, and provides a small forward propulsion. Concentric contractions of the hip flexors swing the limb forward, and of the tibialis anterior allow foot dorsiflexion, so the foot clears the ground.

Gait analysis

Walking is too complex a cycle to analyse fully by simple observation. At its simplest level, a video recording of the individual walking is taken from the front and side. Three-dimensional analysis involves having markers placed on the limbs and body, which are tracked by special sensors to record limb/joint movements (kinematics), and force sensors on the ground can measure forces generating movement (kinetics). Surface electrodes can record muscle contractions. This allows quantitative comparison of gait patterns. Calorimetry or measurement of oxygen consumption can be used to assess the energy cost of walking.

Gage described five prerequisites for normal gait:
- Stability in stance
- Foot clearance in swing
- Adequate step length
- Ability to preposition the foot prior to initial contact and loading
- Energy efficiency over the whole cycle.

These factors are considered in order to inform appropriate intervention in patients with pathological gait. Muscles which are contracted or overactive can be relaxed and stretched, with botulinum toxin and physiotherapy, or surgically lengthened. Muscle tendons can be transferred to correct flexible deformities and to provide additional power to supplement weak muscles. Bony deformity can be addressed by corrective osteotomy. Holistic information provided by gait analysis facilitates complete prescription for primary and secondary abnormalities at multiple levels. This avoids the 'birthday syndrome' described by Mercer Rang when an isolated procedure at a joint uncovers a problem at another joint, leading to multiple separate interventions during a child's development. Usually annually.

Gait abnormalities

- *Antalgic:* reduced time in stance phase in affected leg.
- *Short leg:* centre of gravity drops and shifts to short side.
- *Trendelenburg:* pelvis drops on unaffected side during stance, with trunk lurching towards affected side (see ➲ Hip examination, pp. 16–18).
- *Gluteus maximus:* hip extensor weakness, trunk lurches backwards.
- *Quadriceps weakness:* 'back kneeing' to prevent knee collapsing.
- *Hemiparetic gait:* shoulder or leg flexed, internally rotated, forearm pronated, knee flexed, and equinus foot (e.g. post-cerebrovascular accident (CVA)).
- *Ataxic gait:* legs spread, wide base, staggering gait (e.g. cerebellar).

- *Shuffling gait:* very short steps. Occurs in cerebral or long tract disease (e.g. Parkinson's disease).
- *High-stepping gait:* high steps, ↑ knee flexion in swing (e.g. foot drop).
- *Calcaneus 'peg' gait:* weak calf, heel contact throughout stance.
- *Crouch gait:* due to calf weakness, ankles in dorsiflexion in stance.

Chapter 2

Investigations

Haematological and biochemical tests

The choice of investigations should be guided by clinical assessment. Routine preoperative investigations are usually not required in healthy patients; however, some investigations are necessary before major surgery, particularly in those with relevant known or suspected medical comorbidities. For elective surgery, local guidance should be followed, based upon National Institute for Health and Care Excellence (NICE) guidelines.

Interpretation of results

Inter-laboratory measurements vary, and local reference levels must be known when interpreting results.

Haematological tests

Full blood count

Useful if:

- Emergency/major surgery in patients >50 years of age
- Surgery is likely to lead to significant blood loss
- History of significant recent bleeding or cardiorespiratory disease
- Infection suspected.

Clotting profile

- Prothrombin time (PT): measures extrinsic pathway components. ↑ when on warfarin, and in liver disease and disseminated intravascular coagulation (DIC).
- Activated partial thromboplastin time (APTT): measures intrinsic pathway components. ↑ in haemophilia and DIC, and in patients on heparin.
- International normalized ratio (INR): derived from PT (ratio of patient's PT to control PT); this is useful in patients on anticoagulants, particularly vitamin K antagonists (e.g. warfarin).

Erythrocyte sedimentation rate (ESR)

Non-specific marker of inflammation. Useful when normal, less so when abnormal. Not universally available; plasma viscosity is an alternative used in some units.

Sickle cell test

Although most affected patients are of Afro-Caribbean or African origin, those of Middle Eastern, Asian, and some Mediterranean heritage may also be affected and should be screened if appropriate.

HbA1c

Should be checked in patients with diabetes undergoing elective surgery, unless already checked in the last 3 months. Raised HbA1c correlates with a higher post-operative periprosthetic infection rate. Many units have an upper limit cut-off to permit safe major elective surgery without the risk of additional complications (e.g. 8%).

Biochemistry

Urea and electrolytes

Check if:
- Over 65 years of age
- Known cardiopulmonary, renal, or hepatic disease
- Taking diuretics, steroids, or cardiac medications.

C-reactive protein (CRP)

Acute phase protein and general marker of inflammation/infection. Trend often more useful than a one-off value.

Bone profile

Liver and renal function tests may be necessary in certain patients. In patients with metabolic disorders affecting bone (e.g. malignancy), it is important to measure levels of calcium (Ca^{2+}), phosphate (PO_4), and alkaline phosphatase (ALP). Serum vitamin D levels may also be helpful in certain patients.

Further reading

Duggan SM, Tillotson L, McCann PA. Routine laboratory tests in adult trauma: are they necessary? *The Bulletin of the Royal College of Surgeons of England*. 2011;**93**(7):266–72.

National Institute for Health and Care Excellence (2016). *Routine preoperative tests for elective surgery.* NICE guideline [NG45]. Available from: ℬ www.nice.org.uk/guidance/

Joint aspirate and microbiology

Local intra-articular injections (usually local anaesthetic ± steroid) may be both diagnostic and therapeutic. Diagnostic injections can help to identify sources of pain and predict future outcomes of surgery (joint replacement or fusion). Commonly used in the foot and ankle to localize pain and in the hip joint to confirm the primary pain generator location. Injections can be used therapeutically also. Examples include spinal injections around nerve roots and for cases where inflammation is the focal pathological issue.

Aspiration of a joint, or fluid collection, may be diagnostic or therapeutic; often the aim is to confirm or exclude infection. The procedure must be strictly aseptic; never aspirate a joint through an area of cellulitis. Radiographic guidance ± contrast may be needed for a joint that is small or deep (e.g. hip, SIJ). Ultrasound (US) guidance is helpful for deep soft tissue collections and joint aspirations in children. Computed tomography (CT) may be required for deep, inaccessible areas (e.g. paraspinal abscesses).

Consider likely organisms and discuss with a microbiologist, particularly in complex cases (e.g. granulomatous disease). Following joint aspiration, request urgent Gram staining, microscopy, and crystal analysis, with subsequent culture and sensitivities with the microbiology laboratory (telephone them, and mark samples as urgent).

Indications for synovial fluid aspiration

Diagnostic
- Suspected intra-articular infection (i.e. septic arthritis), and need to differentiate from a crystal (gout/pseudogout) or inflammatory arthropathy.

Therapeutic aspiration
- Osteoarthritis or inflammatory arthropathy (may be followed by a local anaesthetic ± steroid injection).
- Acute haemarthrosis (for symptomatic benefit in tense haemarthrosis or to aid in clinical assessment in unclear cases, but not routinely).
- The aspirate appearance and microscopic laboratory findings can aid in diagnosis (Table 2.1).

Table 2.1 Synovial fluid interpretation

Condition	Opacity	Leucocyte count (per mm³)
Normal	Clear	<200
Osteoarthritis	Clear	1000 (<50% PMNs)
Rheumatoid	Cloudy/turbid	1–50,000 PMNs
Crystal arthropathy*	Cloudy/turbid	5–50,000 PMNs
Septic arthritis	Cloudy/pus	10–100,000 PMNs
Fracture	Blood + fat	
Bleeding disorders	Blood only	

PMNs, polymorphonuclear leucocytes.

*Urate crystals in gout (hyperuricaemia causing recurrent attacks of synovitis) show *negative* birefringence on polarized light microscopy. Calcium pyrophosphate deposition is a condition of the elderly; it is usually asymptomatic but sometimes causes synovitis mimicking gout, with *positively* birefringent crystals seen on polarized light microscopy.

Further reading

Coakley G, Mathews C, Field M, *et al.*; Society for Rheumatology Standards, Guidelines and Audit Working Group. BSR & BHPR, BOA, RCGP and BSAC guidelines for management of the hot swollen joint in adults. *Rheumatology*. 2006;**45**(8):1039–41.

Biopsy principles and histology

The purpose of biopsy is to obtain tissue for histological diagnosis. Remember the adage: 'biopsy all infections, culture all tumours'. (See ➲ Chapter 12, Primary malignant bone tumours—principles, pp. 360–361.)

Indications for biopsy

- Suspected primary bone or soft tissue lesion.
- Solitary lesion with a history of carcinoma.
- Unclear diagnosis on imaging.
- Identify microorganism in bone infections.

Principles of biopsy

- Biopsy should be preceded by a thorough clinical and radiological evaluation in the presence of a specialist multidisciplinary team (MDT).
- Affected tissues should be imaged appropriately to enable planning of the approach and the most representative area(s) to sample.
- If there are multiple lesions or metastatic disease, then staging should be undertaken with whole body imaging surveys prior to biopsy.
- The biopsy tract must be planned carefully (performed through as few anatomical compartments as possible) to avoid seeding any tumour into adjacent uninvolved tissues.
- Key neurovascular structures should be protected. Ensure meticulous haemostasis (use a tourniquet without exsanguination, if required).
- Avoid drains, but, if used, should be brought out skin adjacent to the biopsy tract/incision.
- Multiple tissue samples should be collected from the periphery of the tumour for histology and microbiology (as centrally, the region may just contain necrotic tissue). Ideally this should be performed in the centre (and by the surgeon) that will ultimately manage the definitive resection.
- Specimens must be analysed in a laboratory with expertise in bone and soft tissue tumours.
- All biopsy tracks/incisions/drain sites should be excised en bloc with the tumour during definitive surgery.

Biopsy techniques

Tissue specimens can be obtained by percutaneous (fine-needle/core-needle) or open (incisional/excisional) biopsy techniques (Table 2.2). The technique utilized is based on the size, location, and potential diagnosis of the lesion, as well as on the expertise of those performing the biopsy. Needle biopsies are commonly performed under US or CT guidance, which allows accurate sampling of the target tissue.

Table 2.2 Comparison of different biopsy techniques

Technique	Tissue yielded	Pros	Cons
Fine needle	Cells for cytology	Least invasive, low complication risk	Inadequate sampling
Tru-cut needle	Core soft tissue biopsy	Tissue fragments with preserved architecture	Risk of seeding, longer tissue fixation and processing time
Jamshidi needle	Core bone biopsy		
Incisional/ excisional	Large tissue sample(s)	Highest diagnostic accuracy	Risks of complications, local dissemination

Imaging: plain radiographs

Wilhelm Roentgen (hence the term 'roentgenogram') stumbled upon radiographs in 1895. Since then, their use has become commonplace, as they are cheap and readily available, with relatively low radiation exposure.

How are radiographs produced?

(Fig. 2.1)
- X-rays are produced by sharp deceleration of high-speed electrons, which are emitted when a high voltage is placed between a heated tungsten cathode (~2200°C) within a vacuum.
- Via the process of 'thermionic emission', free, negatively charged electrons are generated; these are emitted towards a positively charged tungsten anode. Some hit the outer electrons (with energy lost as heat; hence the anode often spins to cool down); some hit the inner electrons (generating X-rays), and some hit the nucleus (emitting most of the X-rays generated via 'braking radiation' or 'bremsstrahlung').
- The X-ray beam is then concentrated and passed through the patient's body, with differing attenuation (absorption) by different tissues. For example, calcium-containing materials like bone appear radiodense (bright) as they have high attenuation (absorb more X-rays), whereas gas and water absorb virtually no X-rays and hence appear radiolucent (dark). Some X-rays are lost as scatter, with the job of the operator being to minimize and protect themselves and others, including by wearing lead gowns and maintaining a safe distance from the machine.
- In modern practice (digital radiography), there is no 'film'—instead digital receptors convert the differing X-ray attenuation to an electrical signal, which is then processed by a computer and displayed and stored via a picture archiving and communication system (PACS).

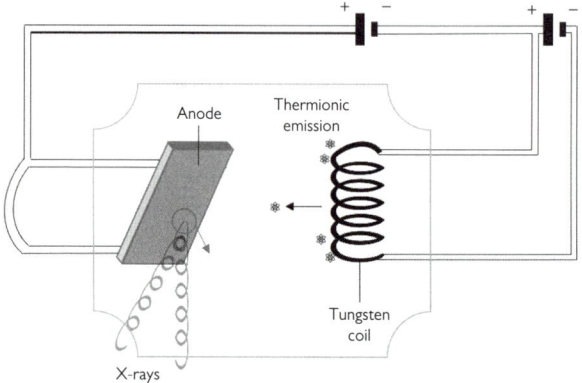

Fig. 2.1 How X-rays are produced.

- When passing through tissue, X-ray beams produce free radicals that can damage cellular DNA. There is a risk that altered cellular DNA can result in neoplastic change, with the risk proportional to the cumulative concentration of X-rays absorbed by the body over a lifetime. X-rays are also teratogenic.
- *Terminology note:* 'radiograph' is the correct term to describe the images we use in clinical practice ('X-rays' are a form of high-energy electromagnetic radiation with a shorter wavelength than light that are generated to help produce the radiographs!).

Radiation protection

As radiographs are not risk-free, guidelines on their safe use are based on the principles of the Ionising Radiation (Medical Exposure) Regulations (IRMER), with responsibilities placed upon organizations and individuals involved in requesting, performing, and supervising procedures involving radiation exposure. The principles are:

- Necessity—will the radiograph influence the patient's treatment?
- Minimizing the irradiated area—what is the smallest irradiated area that will provide the necessary information? Aim to localize the body area to be imaged and minimize irradiation of unnecessary areas.
- Minimizing repeat irradiation—limit repeat radiographs to minimize the cumulative X-ray dose. Make sure that the request form clearly conveys to the radiographer what you are looking for, so that an adequate radiograph is obtained with the least exposure.

Requesting radiographs

1. Always request radiographs in two orthogonal views. A radiograph is a two-dimensional (2D) representation of a three-dimensional (3D) structure. The depth of the structure is assessed by taking a second radiograph at right angles to the first. The most common request for most joints is an anteroposterior (AP) and a lateral projection.
2. When assessing a suspected fracture, include the joint above and below the fracture for a complete appreciation of the injury. This practice avoids missing further pathology such as a second fracture or a joint dislocation associated with a displaced fracture (e.g. a distal radioulnar joint dislocation with a radial shaft fracture—a Galeazzi fracture).
3. State whether the body part to be imaged contains implants (metalware), as this influences the X-ray penetration setting used by the radiographer to achieve the best-quality film.
4. When requesting emergency chest radiographs of a seriously unwell patient, consider a 'mobile' or 'portable' request where the radiographer takes a mobile machine to the patient who remains in a safer environment.

Dual-energy X-ray absorptiometry (DEXA)

This utilizes two X-ray beams of varying energies via a modified scanner. It is used to measure bone mineral density (BMD) via imaging of predetermined anatomical areas (e.g. lumbar spine vertebra, proximal femur). This is used to determine the T- (sex- and ethnicity-matched) and Z- (age-, sex-, and ethnicity-matched) scores. The World Health Organization (WHO) defines the BMD T-score ranges of: ≥ -1.0 SD, normal; -1.5 to 2.0 SD,

osteopenia; and ≤−2.5 SD, osteoporosis. The T-score is generally applicable to secondary fragility fracture prevention in older (aged >60 years or
post-menopausal) patients, whereas the Z-score is more useful in identifying
secondary osteoporosis/metabolic bone pathologies, for example, in children and younger adults (premenopausal women or men aged <50 years).

Imaging: computed tomography

Introduced to clinical practice in the 1970s, a CT scan is a set of images produced by combining multiple radiographs.

How are CT scans obtained?

- The patient passes (usually supine) through a large ring (gantry), which contains a rotating X-ray source that projects a fan-shaped X-ray beam towards a gas or crystal collimated X-ray detector (Fig. 2.2). This allows a much higher-resolution image to be produced than with standard radiographs, with a greater range of greyscale densities (i.e. differing shades of grey for different tissues). This yields higher-definition 3D images, enabling better differentiation between different tissues based upon their differing tissue attenuation.
- Attenuation is measured in Hounsfield units (HU), with water having a reference value of zero. Attenuation of other tissues includes that of fat (−100HU), air (−1000HU), cerebrospinal fluid (CSF) (15HU), blood (30HU), muscle (10–40HU), and cortical bone (1000HU); note that air is darkest (black), and cortical bone is lightest (white). Contrast (iodine ± air) is injected intra-articularly, intravascularly, intrathecally, or intradiscally to aid in soft tissue differentiation.
- A computer combines each individual 2D component (pixel) into a 3D component (voxel), with the depth of each voxel termed the 'slice thickness'. An axial section of the scanned body part is taken with a slice thickness of between 1mm and 10mm. The thicker 10mm-sliced CT images produce a lower-quality image but involves less radiation exposure. The thinner sectioned CT images are used to detect subtle pathology, for example undisplaced vertebral fractures, whereas thicker slices are used to screen for larger lesions, for example, to rule out an intracranial haematoma.

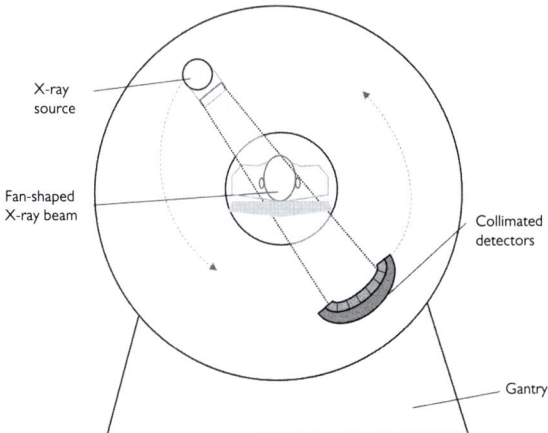

X-ray source

Fan-shaped X-ray beam

Collimated detectors

Gantry

Fig. 2.2 CT scanner.

CT reconstructions

Horizontal, or axial, images are converted into coronal or sagittal sequences by using a computer. This facilitates 3D visual interpretation of the body part under investigation via multiple 2D image sequences. Sophisticated computer manipulation can also construct a 3D reconstructed image that can be rotated 360° to further facilitate interpretation and planning of, for example, operative fixation of displaced fracture fragments in complex trauma; however, the image resolution is reduced.

Applications

- *Intra-articular fractures:* CT can help make treatment decisions. Higher-resolution CT images, compared to plain radiographs, can help diagnose more subtle fractures and ascertain the extent of a fracture and the degree of displacement, alongside identifying other parameters not always readily visualized on plain radiographs (e.g. comminution or intra-articular extension). This information is then used to decide how best to manage fractures and whether surgical intervention can improve outcomes. CT is therefore also helpful in preoperative planning, with fractures involving the calcaneum, acetabulum, proximal tibia (plateau), or distal tibia (pilon) commonly undergoing CT evaluation. Use of CT is ↑ due to improved access, reduced cost and radiation exposure, and better understanding of the principles of fracture fixation.
- *Infection:* CT is used to assess the extent of bone involvement in osteomyelitis.
- *Tumour surgery:* used to assess bony involvement and destruction. Also, while investigating a bony lesion suspected of being a malignancy, CT chest/abdomen/pelvis is performed to detect any metastases that may be undetectable on plain radiographs.
- *Major reconstruction:* CT is used to assess bone stock, which may affect surgical options in major reconstruction/arthroplasty.
- *Spine:* plain radiographs tend to under-represent the extent of bony injury, compared with CT, so high-energy spine fractures are usually investigated by CT. Certain sites are also more difficult to clearly visualize on radiographs and CT is therefore employed (e.g. the cervicothoracic junction and high thoracic spine—commonly overlapped by the shoulders on lateral view radiographs).

Imaging: magnetic resonance imaging

How does MRI work?

(Fig. 2.3)

- Magnetic resonance imaging (MRI) utilizes a large, stationary superconducting magnet and radiofrequency (RF) coils to produce a high-resolution and high-contrast image by manipulation of hydrogen protons. Hydrogen nuclei are spinning protons that rotate in a specific direction. In an MRI scanner, the direction of spin aligns with the direction of the magnetic field.
- When a brief RF pulse is directed at a tissue, proton alignment and the direction of rotation changes (i.e. they lose alignment or 'parallelism' to the magnetic field and then begin to spin or 'precess' in a synchronized manner).
- As the RF pulse is stopped, they 'relax' as they return to their previous state and realign with the magnetic field. The relaxation phase is associated with the release of any absorbed energy, which can be detected by a detector coil.
- As water has a high concentration of protons and different tissues have different water saturations, a highly detailed soft tissue and bony image is constructed by computer interpretation of the differential radiosignals detected with each RF pulse.
- Two basic image weightings are produced—T1 and T2—based upon some important timings: the 'T1' image is based upon the time taken to realign with the magnetic field, whereas the 'T2' image is based upon the time taken for protons to stop their synchronized spinning.

MRI safety

- No ionizing radiation—hence no known risk of malignancy.
- Contraindications to scanning:
  - Cardiac pacemakers (although modern devices are compatible)
  - Internal hearing devices
  - Intracranial aneurysm clips
  - Retained metal fragments—ask the patient and obtain plain radiographs to confirm (e.g. fragments in the eyes/orbit in sheet metal workers/grinders)
  - Joint replacements, fracture fixation, and spinal implants are generally safe. Some departments require a minimum period from implantation.

Different MRI sequences and adjuncts

By adjusting the frequency and timing of RF pulses, different tissues are highlighted on MRI via differential 'weighting'.

T1-weighted: useful for anatomy
- Dark—fluid (e.g. CSF), bone, air.
- Bright—fat.

T2-weighted: useful for pathology
- Dark—cartilage, bone, air.
- Bright—fluid ('water (H_2O) is white on T2').

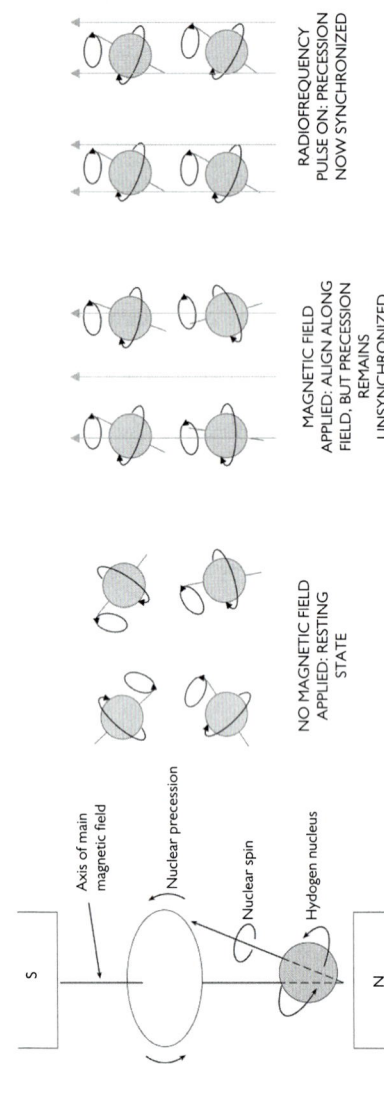

Fig. 2.3 MRI principles.

Other
- Short-tau inversion recovery (STIR)—like T2, but fat appears dark (fat suppression sequence).
- Metal artefact reduction sequence (MARS)—useful to reduce distortion caused by metallic implants.
- Magnetic resonance angiography (MRA)—uses gadolinium or the flow of blood to highlight vessels.
- Gadolinium (contrast)-enhanced—intravenous (IV) contrast agent for MRI (↑ signal on T1-weighted images) aids in differentiation of solid vs fluid-filled soft tissue lesions.
- Proton density—cartilage appears grey (high signal).

The resolution of MRI has improved significantly in recent years with the advent of 3T (3 Tesla) scanners. Bone structure, cartilage, tendons, and ligaments can be more clearly visualized, hence expanding the application of MRI in detection of musculoskeletal pathology.

Applications

- *Spine:* prolapsed disc, spinal stenosis, cord/cauda equina pathology.
- *Knee:* ligament injuries, meniscal tears, cartilage lesions.
- *Hip:* labral pathology, avascular necrosis, undisplaced fractures.
- *Shoulder:* rotator cuff anatomy, labrum and biceps pathology.
- *Hand and wrist:* scaphoid fractures, ligament injuries, osteonecrosis.
- *Other:* tumours and infection (any site).

Imaging: bone scintigraphy

Also known as 'radionuclide imaging', 'nuclear medicine imaging', or a 'bone scan', radioisotope-based imaging was developed in the 1960s. Technetium-99m (99mTc) is the most common tracer used, although others are available such as gallium-67 and indium-111.

How is a bone scan produced?

Radiolabelled tracer elements (radioisotopes) emit gamma radiation, which can be detected by a gamma ray detector. The element chosen is injected and usually preferentially taken up by specific organs. For example, calcium hydroxyapatite ($Ca_5(PO_4)_3OH$) is the calcified mineral content of bone; hence 99mTc-tagged phosphate compounds will be taken up by metabolically active bone. If there is ↑ bone turnover at a particular site, more 99mTc accumulates locally.

A gamma camera detects subsequent radioactive decay in three phases:
- *Flow:* immediately post-injection; shows arterial flow (areas of high perfusion).
- *Blood pool:* 5min post-injection; shows inflammation (pooling of blood in soft tissues/bone secondary to sluggish capillary flow)
- *Static:* 3h post-injection; shows bone activity.

Safety

99mTc has a half-life of 6h and emits low doses of gamma radiation. Hence, the effective radiation dose is less than that of CT pulmonary angiography.

Applications

- Diagnosis of stress fractures.
- Diseases of high bone turnover (e.g. Paget's disease).
- Detection of most types of primary bone tumours or bone metastasis (but may fail to detect some lesions, e.g. multiple myeloma).
- Arthroplasty implant loosening/infection.

Imaging: positron emission tomography

Positron emission tomography (PET) is a type of nuclear imaging that utilizes fluorodeoxyglucose (FDG)—a radiolabelled compound containing glucose that is metabolized in the same manner. ↑ metabolism of any kind involves ↑ glucose metabolism; there is therefore ↑ FDG uptake in regions of high metabolic activity. PET is currently thought to be the most sensitive imaging modality for identifying and surveillance of tumour metastases, as well as for benign tumours with little metabolic activity. A cyclotron produces a PET isotope (e.g. nitrogen-13, oxygen-15, carbon-11) that is tagged to glucose. This is injected into the patient, with subsequent radioactive decay detected by a camera. Resultant activity data are usually superimposed upon a CT or MRI scan to aid in visualization of the relevant anatomy.

Imaging: ultrasound

Developed as a medical diagnostic tool in 1940, US scanning utilizes high-frequency sound waves (>20kHz) that are beyond the human audible range. It is a real-time dynamic procedure (hence useful for evaluating moving structures such as soft tissues across joints, e.g. tendons/ligament) that is safe (with no ionizing radiation involved). However, US is operator-dependent and to obtain and interpret images accurately requires a skilled practitioner.

How does ultrasound work?

(Fig. 2.4)
- High-frequency sound waves are produced by a transducer. These travel until they reach a border between two tissues of differing sound conductivity. At this point, the sound wave will either pass through the tissue or get reflected back to the transducer.
- Fluids allow sound waves to easily pass through, so very little is reflected back to the transducer. However, calcified structures, such as bone, reflect most sound waves back to the transducer.
- The returning sound waves are processed and converted into an electrical signal by a computer, producing a 'real-time' moving image on the monitor.
- Fluid flow can be detected by the 'Doppler effect' (change in frequency of sound waves due to motion), for example, when investigating deep vein thrombosis or ischaemia.

Application of ultrasound

- Investigation of a lump—is it solid, cystic, or vascular?
- Assessment of tendon integrity (e.g. Achilles tendon rupture).
- Delineation of a deep abscess.
- Detection of lower limb venous thromboembolism.
- Evaluation of the cartilaginous neonatal skeletal system.

eFAST

(Extended) focused assessment with sonography for trauma (FAST) scanning is point-of-care ultrasonography, usually performed by a trained ED clinician, primarily designed to identify intraperitoneal free fluid (sensitivity/specificity >90%, but generally requires >500mL for a positive scan). The 'extended' FAST scan also visualizes the anterior thorax. It is usually performed as an adjunct to the 'C' component of the primary survey to guide management in patients unable to have a CT scan (e.g. too unstable).

Further reading

Malik SS, Hall A, Stevenson JD, Cribb GL. Radiological investigations in orthopaedic oncology. *Orthopaedics and Trauma*. 2017;**31**(3):161–72.

Miller M, Thompson S. Basic science. In: *Miller's Review of Orthopaedics*, 8th edition. Elsevier Health Sciences, 2019; pp. 119–26.

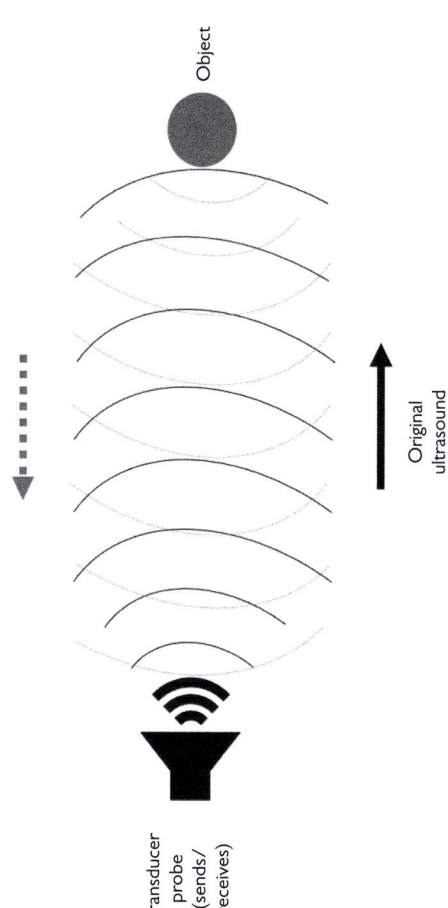

Fig. 2.4 Ultrasound.

Paediatric radiology

The immature skeleton differs from that of the skeletally mature adult in that the growing skeleton undergoes ossification of a cartilage precursor, followed by lengthening via growth plates (endochondral ossification) and widening via the periosteum (appositional, intramembranous growth).

Are radiographs useful?

The neonatal skeleton is often investigated by US, rather than by radiographs, because cartilage is radiolucent. For example, when investigating a suspected dysplastic hip, US is preferred up to the age of 6 months, because the femoral head does not ossify (and then become identifiable on radiographs) until the age of 4–6 months. Neonates with suspected brain abnormalities, such as hydrocephalus, can undergo US of the brain via the anterior fontanelle, which remains open until the age of 2 years. This may be preferable to irradiating the brain with CT scanning or to anaesthetizing the baby for an MRI scan.

Joints are often incompletely seen on radiographs, as they have not fully ossified in younger children. This is especially relevant with elbow fractures, as a severely displaced lateral condylar fracture may be missed on radiographs as the lateral condyle does not fully ossify until around the age of 13 years. Arthrography (under anaesthesia), US, or MRI may therefore be more useful. Paediatric patients are also more vulnerable to radiation-induced malignant neoplasms than adults due to higher radiosensitivity of their tissues, body size, and relatively longer lifespans during which radiation effects may develop.

Beware ligamentous laxity and different 'normal ranges'

Children tend to have greater ligamentous laxity, compared with adults. This is relevant when assessing the paediatric cervical spine where vertebrae appear to be misaligned, or 'pseudosubluxed'. Subluxation is physiological in children due to ligamentous laxity, but also due to the more horizontal facet joint alignment, compared with adult facet joints. This is especially common at C2–3 and C3–4 levels.

Consider patient compliance for imaging

A younger child (under the age of 5/6 years in general) will not tolerate a lengthy investigation such as an MRI scan without either sedation or a general anaesthetic to help them keep still and therefore enable high-quality images to be obtained. This requires consideration when planning investigations. US scanning or plain radiographs are therefore usually easier to perform without the need for sedation/anaesthesia.

Further reading

Hall EJ. Intensity-modulated radiation therapy, protons, and the risk of second cancers. *International Journal of Radiation Oncology, Biology, Physics*. 2006;**65**(1):1–7.

Neurophysiological tests

Neurophysiological tests can supplement clinical examination to aid in diagnosis of abnormalities in nerve conduction. They are most commonly used in investigation of peripheral nerve compression (e.g. carpal/cubital tunnel syndromes) or nerve injury. Tests include:
- Nerve conduction studies (NCS)
- Electromyography (EMG)
- Electroencephalography (EEG)
- Evoked potentials.

Nerve conduction studies

These allow evaluation of peripheral nerves and their sensory and motor response anywhere along their course. NCS involve stimulation of peripheral nerves via depolarizing electrical pulses delivered by a 'stimulating' electrode, with the resultant response recorded from either the same nerve distally (nerve action potential) or the muscle fibres supplied by the nerve (compound muscle action potential) via a 'recording' electrode (Fig. 2.5). These can be recorded with surface or needle electrodes. Measurements can be taken from sensory, motor, or mixed nerves. Conduction depends on many factors (age, skin temperature, nerve size). NCS measure several parameters:
- *Latency:* time from start of stimulation to start of response (ms)
- *Amplitude:* size of the response (µV)
- *Conduction velocity:* speed of the impulse (i.e. distance between stimulating and recording electrodes/time (m/s)).

Other parameters include:
- *F response:* late motor response (i.e. tests axons proximal to the stimulation site); helps to identify root injuries (e.g. brachial plexus)
- *H reflex:* electrophysiological equivalent of a deep tendon reflex; helps to identify polyneuropathies or radiculopathies.

Electromyography

EMG studies the electrical characteristics of muscle and is often performed alongside NCS. The recording electrode is usually a hollow needle with an insulated wire inside (coaxial needle) that is inserted into the muscle under investigation. The electrical activity of the muscle can be recorded at rest (normally silent—upon denervation, may show spontaneous activity, e.g. fibrillation), during voluntary contraction, and during stimulation.

Indications for NCS and EMG

- Localized weakness or altered sensation (e.g. radial nerve palsy following a humeral fracture).
- Unclear history (i.e. 'non-classic' case) or potential multiple sources of peripheral nerve compression (e.g. carpal/cubital tunnel).
- Generalized weakness or altered sensation (peripheral neuropathy vs spinal lesion).
- Weakness alone (motor neuron disease, neuromuscular disease, motor neuropathy, or myopathy).

Timing of NCS and EMG

Optimal timing for electrodiagnostic studies varies according to clinical circumstances. Testing at 7–10 days after a nerve injury may be useful for localization of a lesion and differentiating neuropraxia (mild injury with focal demyelination) from axonotmesis (axon and myelin sheath disruption). However, delayed studies at 3–4 weeks post-injury can provide much more prognostic information.

Nerve conduction study results

Neurophysiological findings with different pathologies are shown in Table 2.3.

Electroencephalography

- Used in diagnosis of cerebral disease by detection of abnormal electrical brain activity.

Evoked potentials

- Stimulus may be light (visual evoked potentials), sound (brainstem auditory evoked potentials), or electrical stimulation (somatosensory evoked potentials).

Table 2.3 Neurophysiological findings with different pathologies

Condition	Latency	Conduction velocity	Evoked response
Normal	Normal	>40m/s	Biphasic
Axonal neuropathy	↑	Normal	Prolonged or ↓ amplitude
Demyelinating neuropathy	Normal	↓	Normal
Anterior horn disease	Normal	Normal	Normal or prolonged
Myopathy	Normal	Normal	↓ amplitude
Neurapraxia—stimulus proximal to lesion	Absent	Absent	Absent
Neurapraxia—stimulus distal to lesion	Normal	Normal	Normal
Axonotmesis—stimulus proximal to lesion	Absent	Absent	Absent
Axonotmesis—stimulus distal to lesion	Absent	Absent	Normal
Neurotmesis—stimulus proximal to lesion	Absent	Absent	Absent
Neurotmesis—stimulus distal to lesion	Absent	Absent	Absent

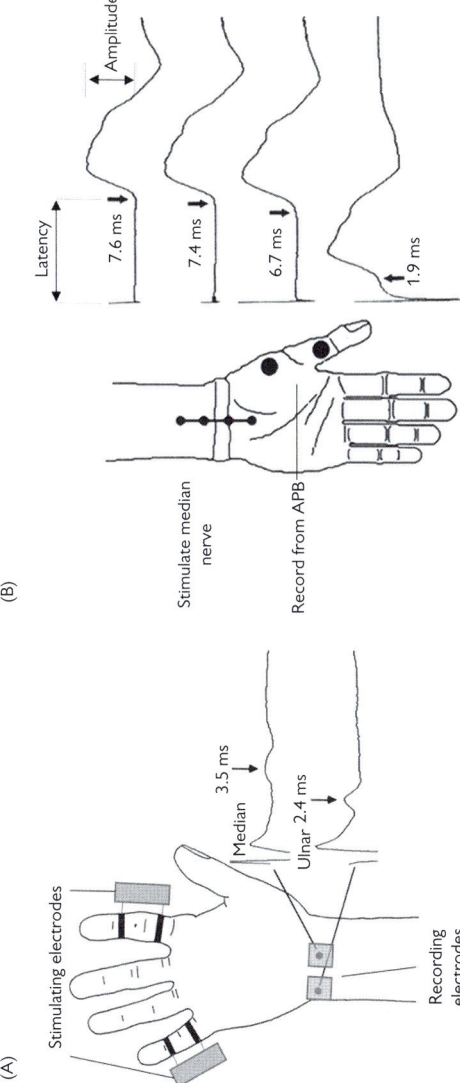

Fig. 2.5 Neurophysiological testing. (A) Sensory study. (B) Motor study.

• Somatosensory evoked potentials (SSEPs) or motor evoked potentials may be used to monitor spinal cord function during spinal surgery or to investigate proximal lesions.

Further reading

Chong HH, See A, Kulkarni K; ELECTS Collaborators. National trends in the initial diagnosis and management of carpal tunnel syndrome: results from the ELECTS (ELEctrophysiology in Carpal Tunnel Syndrome) study. *Annals of The Royal College of Surgeons of England.* 2024;**106**(1):64–9.

Feinberg J. EMG: myths and facts. *HSS Journal.* 2006;**2**(1):19–21.

Robinson LR. Traumatic injury to peripheral nerves. *Supplements to Clinical Neurophysiology.* 2004;**57**:173–86.

Chapter 3

Initial assessment and management

Pre-hospital care and major trauma networks

Pre-hospital care

Pre-hospital emergency medicine (PHEM) is a subspecialty of emergency medicine and anaesthetics. It provides clinicians with clinical and non-clinical skills required for rapid and expert assessment of critically injured or ill patients in an out-of-hospital setting. The goal of care is prompt and safe pre-hospital stabilization prior to transfer to a definitive care setting.

Major trauma networks

A UK-wide system established in 2012 to centralize the care of multiply injured patients to high-volume centres that are best equipped at dealing with patients with the highest injury burden. The networks enable ambulances to bypass local hospitals and take patients to the nearest regional major trauma centre (MTC). Evidence suggests that these networks have improved the flow and care of the most severely injured patients, resulting in reduced morbidity and mortality, particularly in the working-age population most affected by major trauma.

The trauma network broadly comprises two types of hospitals:
- *MTC:* a designated hospital within a region delivering 24/7 consultant-led care with facilities and expertise to provide care for the most critically injured patients. Care is delivered via an MDT approach, with on-site specialties including emergency medicine, anaesthetics and intensive care medicine, cardiothoracic surgery, orthopaedic surgery, plastic surgery, general surgery, neurosurgery, paediatric surgery, and interventional radiology. Care is coordinated by major trauma leads, alongside trauma coordinators, and is delivered on dedicated major trauma wards for those with the most serious injuries (e.g. polytrauma).
- *Trauma unit (TU):* a hospital with the ability to manage patients with a lower Injury Severity Score (ISS). These units have clear systems and protocols via which patients requiring more specialized care can be transferred to the regional MTC.

Transport of the injured patient

Definitive trauma care may warrant patient transfer to a centre with additional resources than those available at the presenting unit, for example, due to the severity of the injuries or the need for specialist management.

Pre-hospital to receiving hospital priorities

- Airway maintenance.
- Control of external haemorrhage and shock.
- Appropriate temporary immobilization.
- Rapid, safe transfer to closest appropriate facility.

Informing receiving hospital to enable preparation

- Time and nature of accident and mechanism of injury.
- Number/age/sex of people involved.
- Condition of victims and injuries sustained.
- Expected time of arrival.

Transfer to definitive care from receiving hospital

Most patients receive all care in the receiving hospital; some need transfer for definitive treatment. Aim to treat life-threatening injuries prior to transfer—catastrophic haemorrhage, airway, breathing, and circulation (CABC)—without delaying through unnecessary investigations. Timing of transfer depends on:

- Distance of transfer
- Available skill levels for transfer
- Circumstances and facilities of local institution
- Intervention required prior to safe transfer.

Arrangement of transfer (referring doctor)

- Initiate transfer: communicate identity, history, and initial assessment.
- Stabilize prior to transfer.
- Select mode of transportation and level of care for transfer.
- Inform transferring personnel of patient's condition and needs.
- Ensure medical notes/investigations go with patient.

Receiving doctor

- Ensure receiving facilities are appropriate.
- Clarify interventions made and current care needs.
- Ensure receiving unit is willing to accept. Prepare team for arrival.

Transportation

This can be potentially hazardous. It is important to ensure:

- Patient is optimally stabilized
- Adequately trained personnel and provision for unexpected crisis.

Adequate monitoring and ongoing management

These include:

- Vital signs, pulse oximetry, end-tidal capnography
- Continued cardiorespiratory support
- Continued blood volume replacement, if required
- Use of appropriate medications.

Meanwhile, communication must be maintained with the receiving hospital, along with ongoing adequate and contemporaneous documentation. On arrival, a complete handover is vital, including details of any problems during transfer.

Communication in the emergency department

Precise communication enables rapid transfer of information between teams to coordinate efforts and optimize care. The ED can be a stressful environment; good communication skills in high-pressure scenarios can relieve situational anxiety and reduce the potential for error. Standardized systems (e.g. 'SBAR' - Situation, Background, Assessment, Recommendation; ATLS - Advanced Trauma Life Support) help to keep information succinct and minimize errors, and help with prioritization based upon imminent threats.

Pre-trauma planning

- Set up and train a trauma team (ideally all ATLS certified).
- Devise and practise a major incident plan.

The ambulance service will generally warn the ED of the impending arrival of major trauma. A receiving team should be assembled, briefed, and prepped according to the expected scenario. The team leader should allocate roles to each member of the team.

Typical roles include:

- *Team leader:* coordinates the whole team
- *Airway and monitoring:* often by an anaesthetist and operating department practitioner (ODP)
- *Primary doctor:* conducts the primary survey
- *Procedure doctor:* prepares for, and performs, procedures
- *ED nurse:* removes clothes and prepares drugs
- *Porter/runner:* collects blood products, transfers patient for imaging
- *Scribe:* documents findings and procedures performed
- *Radiographer:* for portable radiography as directed by the team leader
- *Specialty doctors:* e.g. cardiothoracic, orthopaedic, general.

Resuscitation room

Upon arrival, the team requires succinct, but clear, handover from the paramedic crew: time and mechanism of injury, basic observations and injuries, interventions performed, and allergy status ('AMPLE': Allergies, Medications, Past medical history, Last ate/drank, Events).

Communication may be improved by:

- Contemporaneous notes made by the scribe
- Environment (e.g. team leader ensuring silence at handover)
- Use of digital images of the scene or injuries
- Relatives often accompanying the patient and who may have useful information about the patient's medical history. It is important that someone talks to the relatives and updates them on progress.

Decision-making

Once stabilized, subsequent management options include:

- Transfer to theatre for damage control surgery
- Transfer to CT for further imaging
- Admission ± transfer to theatre/interventional radiology
- Transfer of patient to an MTC
- Observation ± discharge with or without follow-up.

Initial assessment of the trauma patient: ATLS

Prompt assessment, triage, and treatment of trauma patients can save lives. Treatment initiated during the initial stages following injury is the most important in determining outcomes and is termed the 'golden hour'. Note this is a concept rather than an exact time frame. ATLS provides a systematic, standardized algorithm that prioritizes life-threatening injuries, based around the 'ABCs' of the primary survey, followed by a secondary, and then a tertiary survey. The primary survey diagnoses and treats life-threatening injuries. Any compromise in A–E is treated sequentially before moving on to the next step. Note that alternative approaches are increasingly recognized (e.g. the European Trauma Course).

Primary survey

The principles of the ATLS primary survey are summarized below.

Team brief and handover

In a hospital setting, put out appropriate 'calls' (e.g. 'trauma', 'blue' call) to summon appropriate resources. Identify the team lead and members (and skill sets) in advance of patient arrival. Prepare equipment and resuscitation bay. Take a succinct handover from the paramedic team at outset. A scribe should document events and timings.

Airway with cervical spine control

- Stabilize the neck manually (inline immobilization) or with hard collar, sandbags, and tape (triple immobilization).
- Inspect and clear the airway with suction or forceps (remove visible obstructions). Open the airway with jaw thrust if compromised.
- Maintain with oro-/nasotracheal or definitive airway if required.
- Give 100% oxygen through a non-rebreather mask with a reservoir.

Breathing and ventilation

- Look, listen, feel for respiratory effort; auscultate and percuss.
- Inspect chest for wounds, bruising, and asymmetrical chest expansion.
- Palpate for position of trachea, surgical emphysema, and rib tenderness.
- Treat life-threatening issues (e.g. decompress tension pneumothorax, 3-sided dressing over open pneumothorax, chest drain for haemothorax).
- Oxygen saturations, (portable) chest X-ray (CXR).

Circulation and haemorrhage control

- Control external haemorrhage: direct pressure, tourniquet, pelvic binder.
- IV access: two wide-bore cannulae or intraosseous access. Blood tests (including cross-match), venous blood gas. Major hemorrhage protocol.
- Assess central/peripheral pulses, blood pressure (BP), capillary refill.
- Assess sources of bleeding—'blood on the floor and four more'—chest (done in 'B'), abdomen (palpate), pelvis (urogenital bruising, gentle palpation), long bones (palpate, check pulses).
- Initiate warmed fluid resuscitation or haemorrhage control.

Go back and reassess from 'A' after each intervention. Solo providers should not move on from A→B→C, unless life-threatening issues have been dealt with. In clinical practice (i.e. with a skilled trauma team), the stages are often performed in parallel.

Disability (neurological evaluation)
- Conscious level screen—*AVPU*: Alert, responding to Verbal stimuli, Painful stimuli, Unresponsive.
- Assess GCS, pupil size, and reaction to light.
- Can the patient move all arms and legs? Screen neurology before sedation/intubation.

Exposure (and environmental control)
- Remove all clothing.
- Check for hypothermia. Use blankets/Bair Hugger™, warmed fluids.

Adjuncts to primary survey
- Continuous electrocardiogram (ECG), pulse oximetry (oxygen saturations), ventilation rate monitoring, arterial blood gas (ABG) measurement (including lactate), urinary catheters (urine output), gastric catheters (decompress, assess for blood), X-rays (C-spine—more historical, CXR, pelvic X-ray)—now largely superseded by trauma series CT (head, neck, chest, abdomen, pelvis), extended FAST scan.
- *History*: take a succinct AMPLE history.

Secondary survey

The secondary survey can start once the primary survey is complete and any necessary treatment has commenced. It is a top-to-toe examination of the patient to identify all other injuries. This is generally the time when other orthopaedic injuries are identified and managed. In practice, this phase often starts after trauma series CT.

It is useful to have a scribe to document while you examine, as this is a detailed survey.

Head, face, and neck
- Scalp lacerations; visual acuity and movements; hearing and otoscopy.
- Facial fractures.
- Neck movements and tenderness (depending on state of spine).

Chest
- Repeat inspection, palpation, and auscultation of entire chest.
- Palpate sternum.
- Heart sounds.

Abdomen and pelvis
- Inspect, palpate, and auscultate abdomen.
- Assess genitalia for bruising/bleeding.
- Ensure passing urine normally.
- Rectal examination if indicated (e.g. spinal injury).

Musculoskeletal system
- Palpate and move all limbs.
- Be thorough—do not miss small extremity fractures.
- Neurological examination: use the American Spinal Injury Association (ASIA) form to document neurology (see ➲ Chapter 20).

- Log roll and palpate all vertebrae, and perform a per rectum (PR) examination (may not be required if no abnormal neurology/pain and normal spine on CT).
- C-spine 'clearance' if appropriate.

Adjuncts to secondary survey
- Image/investigate anything abnormal (e.g. X-rays).
- Refer to relevant specialties for review/advice.
- Initiate acute treatments (e.g. analgesia, antibiotics, wound dressing, splints).

Initial assessment of the trauma patients: clerking

AMPLE history

Although ATLS assessment will commonly be conducted without any formal 'clerking' of the patient, if the patient is able to give a history, a quick clerking is recommended following the 'AMPLE' approach.

Allergies
- Especially to antibiotics.

Medications
- β-blockers in the elderly may give a false impression to an otherwise shocked patient.
- Anticoagulants may need reversing.
- Recreational drugs/alcohol.
- Prescribe regular medications if indicated.

Past medical history (including pregnancy)
- May be able to find out from family or via medication list.
- Request β-human chorionic gonadotrophin (HCG) blood samples if patient unconscious/confused.

Last ate/drank
- Important to know prior to intubation/surgical procedures, etc.
- Not uncommon for patients to have gastric stasis and require nasogastric tube decompression (or vomit).

Events
- Mechanism of injury: gives multiple clues as to injuries one should expect (e.g. vehicles involved, speed, seatbelt, helmets, vehicle damage, etc.).
- Important to find out if hazardous materials present (e.g. chemicals).

Once the patient is stable and treatment initiated, standard (full) medical clerking may be performed; there is no harm in repetition, as missing details can be picked up. After at least 24h post-admission, a tertiary survey should be performed, which is a complete re-examination of the patient and a review of imaging reports and any other investigations. It is not uncommon to find new pathologies as patients gradually recover from their life-threatening injuries. Do not forget the patient's longer-term rehabilitation and neuro-psychological needs. Early planning is key.

Initial assessment of children

Assessment of children who experience trauma follows the same overall ATLS process as for adults. However, there are some anatomical, physiological, and practical differences that must be considered.

General
- Smaller body mass: more force per unit area from impact.
- Less soft tissues, closer proximity of organs: multiple injuries.
- Fewer ossified bones: fractures less likely than in adults.
- Psychological impact: can lead to regression in milestones.

Airway
- Large occiput (especially in the young) flexes C-spine and closes airway. Place spine board or 1-inch padding under the torso to prevent this. Keep head/airway in a 'neutral' position—the plane of the face should be parallel to the board. Can still use jaw thrust.
- Tongue/tonsils relatively larger than in adults—obstructs larynx.
- Shorter trachea; therefore, risk of intubating right main bronchus.
- Oropharyngeal airway inserted directly, not by using 180° technique. Preoxygenate before mechanical airway insertion.

Breathing
- Different respiratory rates, depending on age.
- Use paediatric bag–mask for ventilation, not adult (different shape).
- Needle decompression: over third rib, mid-clavicular line.
- Chest drain: tunnel under skin and over top of rib above incision. Site as in adults (fifth intercostal space, anterior to mid-axillary line).

Circulation
- Tachycardia, narrow pulse pressure (<20mmHg), slow capillary refill, and cool peripheries may be only signs of shock.
- Hypotension is a late sign.
- Use Broselow® Pediatric Emergency Tape (or similar) to aid with equipment sizes and resuscitation volumes for different ages/weights.
- May require interosseus access.

Disability
- Use paediatric GCS.
- Check glucose concentration.

Exposure
- Keep warm—highest body surface area:body mass ratio at birth, so rapid development of hypothermia.

Adjunct imaging
- Head CT used if GCS score <14 in ED or <15 at 2h post-injury, or any signs of skull fracture.
- X-rays: CXR, spine ± MRI if concern.
- Abdominal ultrasound scan (USS) rather than contrast CT.

Resuscitation of the injured patient

Haemorrhage is the commonest cause of shock in trauma patients. In *hypovolaemic shock*, ongoing circulating volume loss can rapidly result in multiple organ failure due to impaired tissue perfusion—recognize and treat early. Significant volume losses may be well compensated until late in a fit, young patient (particularly children), so it is important to remain vigilant and 'rule out' bleeding. Waiting until the late signs (tachycardia and hypotension) to develop until initial resuscitation will lead to adverse outcomes. The traditional ATLS table detailing classes of shock and associated signs has been demonstrated to not reflect reality. Do not forget the other categories of shock: distributive (septic, anaphylaxis, neurogenic), cardiogenic, and obstructive (massive PE, tamponade, tension pneumothorax).

Clinical features suggestive of hypovolaemic shock

- *Mechanism:* high-energy injury, open wounds, penetrating injury.
- *Signs:* cool peripheries, tachycardia, hypotension, confusion.
- *Shock index* (heart rate (HR)/systolic BP (SBP)) of >0.6.
- *Lactate* >2mm/L or high base deficit.
- *Response* to fluid/blood resuscitation.

Management

- *'Turn off the tap':* direct pressure on wounds with haemostatic dressings, tourniquet (last resort), splint fractures, pelvic binders, angiography, damage control orthopaedics (DCO).
- *Reduce loss:* permissive hypotension—aim for SBP 90mmHg (110mmHg if brain injury is the most serious injury).
- *Restore loss:* warmed red blood cell (RBC):plasma ratio of 1:1 to achieve target BP. Avoid crystalloid.
- *Blood:* O-negative (major haemorrhage protocol) or type-specific/cross-matched if time.
- *Investigations:* consider use of thromboelastography (TEG) and rotational thromboelastometry (ROTEM) to guide transfusion.
- *Tranexamic acid:* 1g over 10min and 1g over 8h (CRASH-2 trial) within 3h of injury if SBP <90mmHg or pulse >110bpm.

Further reading

Graham CA, Parke TR. Critical care in the emergency department: shock and circulatory support. *Emergency Medicine Journal.* 2005;**22**(1):17–21.

National Institute for Health and Care Excellence (2016). *Major trauma: assessment and initial management.* NICE guideline [NG39]. Available from: ℘ https://www.nice.org.uk/guidance

Olldashi F, Kerçi M, Zhurda T, *et al.* Effects of tranexamic acid on death, vascular occlusive events, and blood transfusion in trauma patients with significant haemorrhage (CRASH-2): a randomised, placebo-controlled trial. *The Lancet.* 2010;**376**(9734):23–32.

Paull B. Transfusion of plasma, platelets, and red blood cells in a 1:1:1 vs a 1:1:2 ratio and mortality in patients with severe trauma: the PROPPR randomized clinical trial Holcomb JB, Tilley BC, Baraniuk S, et al. JAMA. 2015;313:471–82. *Journal of Emergency Medicine.* 2015;**49**(1):122.

Polytrauma

Damage control orthopaedics

Polytrauma refers to multiple injuries across different sites secondary to (blunt) trauma. It is a leading cause of mortality in young patients. Multiply injured patients present a management dilemma. Full recovery can only occur once definitive management of injuries is complete. However, the surgery involved in this definitive management is a secondary trauma ('second hit') in itself, leading to further haemorrhage, hypothermia, acidosis, coagulopathy, VTE, fat emboli, and systemic inflammatory response syndrome (SIRS), resulting in sequelae such as acute respiratory distress syndrome (ARDS), multiorgan dysfunction syndrome (MODS), and death. A 'window of opportunity' (days 5–10 post-injury) is quoted for unstable patients, with early total care (ETC) <5 days or >15 days resulting in MODS.

DCO can limit this physiological 'second hit' and subsequent complications. It involves temporary stabilization of orthopaedic injuries to control haemorrhage and allow optimization of the patient's physiology and soft tissues. Temporary stabilization is performed by using the least invasive/physiologically disruptive method. It comprises:

- *Haemorrhage control:* direct pressure, dressings, tourniquet, surgery
- *Soft tissue management:* debridement, splints, foot pumps
- *Temporary fracture stabilization:* casts, traction, external fixators
- *Physiological stabilization:* transfusion, avoiding coagulopathy, warming, intensive care.

Early Total Care (ETC)

ETC is the definitive treatment of all skeletal injuries at the first surgery. Even if a patient is deemed fit enough for ETC, it is essential the patient's physiology and biochemical markers (e.g. lactate) are monitored throughout surgery. It is not uncommon for surgery to start with the aim of ETC (e.g. intramedullary nailing of bilateral femurs) and then to convert to DCO (e.g. after nailing one side) and then temporarizing (e.g. ex-fix) of the other side due to patient deterioration.

Use of DCO or ETC depends on the patient's condition. Patients who are haemodynamically unstable require resuscitation and DCO. The dynamic lactate trend can aid in decision-making, while cut-offs vary, with either <2 or <4 permitting ETC. The base excess is another helpful parameter in management.

Further reading

Roberts CS, Pape HC, Jones AL, Malkani AL, Rodriguez JL, Giannoudis PV. Damage control orthopaedics: evolving concepts in the treatment of patients who have sustained orthopaedic trauma. *Journal of Bone and Joint Surgery.* 2005;**87**(2):434–49.

Vallier HA, Moore TA, Como JJ, et al. Complications are reduced with a protocol to standardize timing of fixation based on response to resuscitation. *Journal of Orthopaedic Surgery and Research.* 2015;**10**(1):1–9.

Principles of non-operative management

The goal of fracture management is to restore correct length, alignment, and rotation of a bone, while allowing early mobilization.

Enabling early mobilization takes greater precedence in certain fractures (e.g. neck of femur in older patients), with complications of injury and subsequent immobility being too great; hence, in these injuries, management is invariably operative.

For intra-articular fractures, the joint surface must also be anatomically restored. If these goals can be achieved best with non-operative management, then surgery should be avoided.

In some instances (e.g. paediatric distal radius buckle fractures, undisplaced distal radius fractures), there is evidence to suggest it may be possible to avoid plaster immobilization altogether in favour of removable splints or supportive bandages.

For some injuries (e.g. mid-shaft clavicle fractures, dorsally angulated distal radius fractures or olecranon fractures in older, low-demand patients, many proximal humerus fractures), non-operative management remains a valid option to consider with appropriate patients.

Remember that non-operative management does not mean no treatment, hence this is better described as 'active surveillance' rather than 'conservative' management. The following points should be considered when following active, non-operative management:

- Reduce fracture: restore length, alignment, and rotation
- Hold fracture: use splint/cast/traction to maintain reduction
- Rest, ice, compression, and elevation ('RICE')
- Consider the need for venous thromboprophylaxis (risk-assess)
- Rehabilitate: early mobilization with physiotherapy
- Medication: analgesics and anti-inflammatory drugs are the mainstays. Also, disease-modifying drugs in inflammatory arthropathy, bisphosphonates ± calcium/vitamin D for secondary fracture prevention in the elderly
- Pain management: referral to specialist pain management services may help to manage symptoms for which there is no simple curative surgical solution (e.g. back pain)
- Radiotherapy: consider for palliation of painful bony metastases—promotes tumour cell necrosis, collagen proliferation, and osteoblastic activity with formation of new woven bone

Soft tissue injuries

Closed fractures

Following the adage 'a fracture is a soft tissue injury with a broken bone beneath', it is important to remember that almost all fractures will have an associated soft tissue injury. This soft tissue response to blunt injury involves microvascular/inflammatory processes with local hypoxia/acidosis and tissue death. Significant crush injury may institute a syndrome of muscle ischaemia, rhabdomyolysis, and severe metabolic derangement requiring aggressive fluid resuscitation ± renal support (elevated creatinine kinase concentration and dark urine may be clues).

Tscherne classification of closed fractures and soft tissue injury

- *C0*: low-energy mechanism; little or no soft tissue injury.
- *CI*: low to moderate energy; superficial abrasion, mild to moderately severe fracture configuration.
- *CII*: high energy; deep, contaminated abrasion, with local contusional damage to skin or muscle, moderately severe fracture configuration.
- *CIII*: high energy; extensive skin contusion or crushing or muscle destruction, severe fracture, compartment syndrome.

Signs

- Swelling: loss of wrinkles and palpable landmarks indicate moderate to severe swelling.
- Fracture blisters: represent dermoepidermal cleavage injury. If blood-filled, the epidermis is not viable; hence, avoid incising (risk of exposed metalwork and infection).
- Abrasions, contusions.
- High-energy fracture pattern.

Management

- Closed reduction and splinting (or spanning external fixation).
- Pneumatic foot/hand pumps.
- Cold compression (e.g. cool/ice packs).
- Elevation.
- Non-adherent dressings for blisters.
- Delay surgery until soft tissues settled (may require 1–3 weeks).
- Careful soft tissue handling, large skin bridges.
- Minimally invasive techniques.

Compartment syndrome (see ⟳ Compartment syndrome, pp. 84–85) may be considered the most significant sequela of soft tissue injury. Remember that an open wound does not preclude compartment syndrome.

Sprains

A sprain is an injury to the ligaments around a joint. This commonly occurs at the ankle joint.

Some, or all, fibres of the ligament may rupture, producing a varying degree of joint instability. A ligament that appears grossly intact may have been stretched beyond its elastic range, causing permanent plastic deformation; it is now functionally incompetent.

History
- Timing and mechanism of injury.
- Position of joint during injury (e.g. inversion/eversion of the ankle).
- Location of pain.
- Ability to weight-bear after injury.
- Previous functional ability and history of injuries.

Examination
- Examine joint for evidence of swelling, bruising, and haemarthrosis.
- Palpate for bone or soft tissue tenderness; feel for fracture crepitus.
- Examine for, and document, neurovascular status.
- Assess range of joint movement, and compare with contralateral side.
- Assess stability of joint by performing appropriate special tests.

Investigations
- Plain radiograph to exclude fracture. USS or MRI to assess for rupture.

Management
Non-operative management is usually successful.
- RICE: rest, ice, compression bandage, elevation; avoid sports, etc.
- Analgesia, supports (e.g. walking boot for ankle sprains, Futuro splint for wrist).
- Longer term: bracing, physiotherapy.
- Surgery: a ligament sprain associated with ongoing, symptomatic functional incompetence may require repair or advancement (e.g. Brostrom lateral ankle ligament advancement).

Slings and casts

Slings

This is a bandage to support the weight of the arm against gravity.
• *Broad arm sling*: traditionally made from a triangular bandage, although more modern, supportive fabric designs are available (e.g. Polysling) that are more comfortable. Supports the forearm and elbow; useful in treatment of shoulder injuries, particularly ACJ disruption and clavicular fractures, as it supports the weight of the arm and thus elevates the point of the elbow and shoulder.
• *Collar and cuff*: allows the weight of the arm to act as traction force; useful in non-operative management of humeral shaft and neck fractures (alternative to a 'U-slab' or 'hanging cast').

Casts

A cast is a rigid dressing that immobilizes and protects a body part.

Casts may be used as temporary splints (e.g. for pain relief and wound protection post-operatively) or as definitive management for fractures. Follow the principles of 3-point moulding to maintain correction of a reduced fracture. Pay attention to the cast (a/b ratio, i.e. cast width in lateral view divided by the posteroanterior (PA) view), padding (x/y ratio, i.e. padding thickness under moulded cast in the plane of maximum deformity correction on lateral divided by maximum interosseous distance on PA), and Canterbury (total of cast and padding indices) indices (Fig. 3.1). Reduced fractures held with a cast index of >0.8, a padding index of >0.3, and/or a combined Canterbury index of >1.1 (i.e. more circular, overpadded casts)

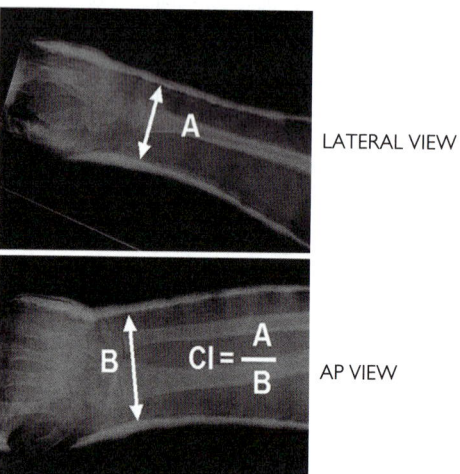

LATERAL VIEW

AP VIEW

$$CI = \frac{A}{B}$$

Fig. 3.1 Cast index is radiographically defined as the ratio of the total lateral and PA width of the inner aspect of the cast (i.e. A/B).

are at greater risk of displacement due to loss of the 3-point fixation, so they should be watched carefully.

Techniques of cast application are best learnt with the technicians in your local plaster room; they will be delighted to see you!

Cast materials

- Plaster of Paris (POP) rolls (e.g. Cellona™, Gypsona™): consist of fabric weave coated with POP (calcium sulfate hemihydrate). They are cheap and readily available, but are relatively more opaque to X-rays and susceptible to damage if exposed to moisture. Use if require a moulded plaster after manipulation of a fracture (e.g. 3-point moulding for distal radius fractures) or for backslabs (immobilization using POP encircling ~70% of the circumference of the limb) to allow for acute swelling of the injured limb.
- Synthetics (e.g. Scotchcast™—consists of knitted fibreglass; Delta-Cast™ Conformable—polyester): both are impregnated with polyurethane resin. They are lighter, more radiolucent, and resistant to degradation by moisture. Disadvantages: allow less expansion for swelling after fresh fracture, harder to mould. Use over the top of POP to reinforce and enable weight-bearing (e.g. stable ankle fractures) or use alone.

Examples

- Ankle/tibia: 4-inch POP × 3–4 rolls; 3-inch Stockinette: length cut to allow excess beyond toes and above knee; 4-inch wool. Two people (at least). Flex the knee to relax posterior calf muscles. Ensure the ankle is plantigrade (neutral dorsiflexion/plantar flexion).
- Wrist/forearm/elbow: 3-inch POP × 2–4 rolls; 2-inch Stockinette. 2- to 3-inch wool. One to two people. Do not take forearm/wrist plasters beyond the MCPJ (should be able to flex fingers, and ensure thumb/elbow are free, with no sharp POP edges rubbing).

Further reading

Charnley J. *The Closed Treatment of Common Fractures*. Baltimore, MD: Williams and Wilkins, 1968.

Iltar S, Alemdaroğlu KB, Say F, Aydoğan NH. The value of the three-point index in predicting redisplacement of diaphyseal fractures of the forearm in children. *Bone and Joint Journal*. 2013;**95**(4):563–7.

Splintage and traction

Splintage

A splint is a device used to either immobilize a joint or fracture (*static*) or allow protected movement (*dynamic*). For example, a well-moulded above-knee cast for a tibial shaft fracture maintains length and alignment by hydrostatic soft tissue pressure and 3-point moulding against the deformity; including the joint above controls rotation (*static* splint). A *dynamic* finger splint after flexor tendon repair uses elastic bands to hold the finger passively flexed but permits active extension to preserve joint motion.

Functional bracing is a technique that allows motion and loading in a controlled manner to facilitate healing. Conversion of the above-knee cast described above to a patella–tendon bearing or Sarmiento cast permits weight-bearing across the fracture, encouraging axial micromotion to stimulate healing. Another example is a humeral brace, which allows upper arm soft tissue tension to maintain alignment.

Traction

This relies on the phenomenon of creep (see ➲ Chapter 6). Longitudinal force applies constant load across a fracture and its soft tissue envelope, enabling it to progressively deform with time; this corrects shortening and angulation, together with rotation, if correctly applied. Traction as a definitive treatment (e.g. for paediatric supracondylar elbow or femoral fractures) is far less popular than historically due to the long associated in-patient stay, but it remains an effective temporary means of immobilization and analgesia prior to definitive treatment:

- *Skin traction:* longitudinal tapes (adhesive or non-adhesive) bandaged along the length of the injured limb to which weights are attached; requires careful and regular skin checks for blistering and breakdown
- *Skeletal traction:* via a pin (Steinmann—smooth, or Denham—threaded) through bone; allows more weight and causes fewer soft tissue problems, but beware applying traction across a joint in the zone of injury (e.g. proximal tibial pin for femoral shaft fracture). Also stay extracapsular with pin to prevent risk of seeding the joint with contamination.

Eponymous traction types could be the subject of an entire, if somewhat historical, handbook, but popular examples include:

- *Thomas splint:* fixed traction against a padded ring in the patient's groin; used pre-hospital to temporarily splint femoral fractures
- *Gallows traction:* for babies/infants with femoral fractures; skin traction attached to overhead bar (hips flexed near 90°), pelvis just lifted off bed, nappy area free for ease
- *Hamilton Russell traction:* for paediatric femoral shaft fracture (older age group than with Gallows); balanced traction with the knee supported by slings, resulting in net vector of pull along femur axis.

Further reading

Sarmiento A, Zagorski JB, Zych GA, Latta LL, Capps CA. Functional bracing for the treatment of fractures of the humeral diaphysis. *Journal of Bone and Joint Surgery*. 2000;**82**(4):478.

Injections and aspirations

Indications

- *Therapeutic:* used to treat inflammation within joints or soft tissues (e.g. tendons) to improve pain. Often pain relief is temporary in OA.
- *Diagnostic:* used to localize pain source by performing targeting injection into a specific joint or region. Aspirate synovial fluid for diagnosis (crystal/non-crystal arthropathy vs septic arthritis).

Site-specific aspiration techniques

First, the correct patient, site, and side should be confirmed. Drawing appropriate landmarks on the skin with a sterile marker can help. All injections/aspirations should be performed with sterile gloves and under strict aseptic technique. A green (18G) needle is often standard. Longer needles may be helpful for some joints (e.g. shoulder, hip). A grey (16G) or orange (14G) cannula may help, for comfort, if aspirating massive knee haemarthroses (smaller needles may get blocked). *Do not aspirate joint replacements outside the sterile environment of theatre.* Send samples in a universal container (e.g. sterile urine pot) and blood culture bottles; a bedside urine dipstick can also be used to check for elevated leucocyte esterase (LE), which can suggest infection (e.g. prosthetic joint infection). Ask the lab for urgent Gram staining, microscopy and crystals, and subsequent microscopy, culture, and sensitivity (MC&S). If you suspect septic arthritis, keep the patient nil by mouth; if they are haemodynamically stable and not septic, then ideally do not start antibiotics until samples are sent. State if atypical infections (e.g. tuberculosis (TB)) are suspected, as extended cultures/alternative tests may be required. Label the specimen accordingly if the patient/sample is high risk (e.g. human immunodeficiency virus (HIV) +ve). In select cases, alpha defensin or leucocyte esterase assays can help to diagnose periprosthetic infections. Some technical tips include the following (Fig. 3.2):

- *Shoulder (glenohumeral joint):* palpate the outer inferior edge of the acromion from behind. Thumb width below and medial to this is a 'soft spot'; pass the needle through this, towards the coracoid (palpate anteriorly with the index or middle finger of the free hand). For the subacromial space, enter from the same spot, but aim anterolaterally, 'under the bone' (inferior acromial edge); alternatively, a lateral approach may be performed to the subacromial space. For the ACJ, palpate medially from the lateral border of the acromion and use a smaller needle/volume (max. 1mL usually).
- *Elbow:* palpate for soft spot in triangle formed by radial head (felt by rotating forearm, with elbow flexed 90°), lateral epicondyle, and lateral border of the olecranon. Enter joint at centre of this triangle.
- *Wrist:* palpate for Lister's tubercle on dorsal distal radius. Just distal to this is soft spot (flex/extend wrist to find). Aim dorsal–distal to palmar–proximal (i.e. needle passing proximally) to account for volar tilt of distal radius.
- *Hip:* under X-ray guidance in theatre, by using contrast to confirm intra-articular position. Long needle, entry point either anterolateral or more lateral, and advancing medially along femoral neck.
- *Knee:* patient supine, knee extended. Needle is passed into joint, either between patella and femur (from under superolateral pole of patella) or from inferolateral soft spot (arthroscopy camera portal).

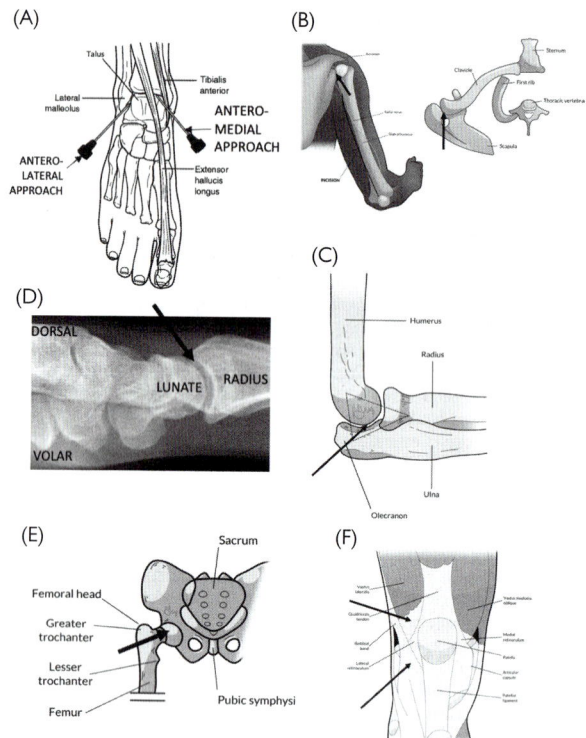

Fig. 3.2 Approaches to aspiration of joints.

- *Ankle:* plantar flex/dorsiflex foot and palpate level of joint. Enter joint between tibialis anterior and medial malleolus (soft spot).

Local anaesthetic (LA) (e.g. 10mL of 0.25% bupivacaine) ± steroid (e.g. 40mg triamcinolone) for shoulder/hip/knee. Smaller volumes (e.g. 3–5mL of 1% lidocaine ± steroid) for wrist/elbow, with even smaller volumes (0.25 - 1ml) for smaller hand joints.

Further reading
(See also ● Chapter 2.)
Crawley M. Techniques of joint aspiration. *British Journal of Hospital Medicine.* 1974;**11**:747–55.

Fractures in the elderly

Low-energy fractures occur in the elderly because of skeletal fragility; peak bone mass is achieved at the end of skeletal maturation and consolidation in early adulthood, after which there is a steady decline in bone density that is more marked in women. Since peak bone mass can no longer be influenced in the elderly, efforts to reduce fracture risk must focus on falls prevention strategies and optimization of bone mass by dietary and pharmacological manipulation of bone turnover.

Around 500,000 fractures occur each year in elderly people in the UK. The cost of providing healthcare, social care, and support for these patients is estimated at £4.4 billion for the National Health Service (NHS) per year. Commonest are fractures of the hip, vertebrae, proximal humerus, and distal radius.

Over 3 million people aged over 65 fall every year in the UK. Many elderly fracture patients have complex medical problems. Those requiring operative fracture fixation should be managed as a collaborative approach among pre-hospital services, EDs, orthopaedic surgery, and anaesthetic and orthogeriatric clinicians in a frailty-specific pathway.

Post-operative care should include identification of risk factors for, and secondary prevention of, further fractures.

Those with fragility fractures seen in the outpatient clinic setting should be referred to a local fracture liaison service.

Secondary prevention strategies

- Patient awareness and education.
- Promotion of active lifestyle.
- Falls assessment.
- Bone health review (including a DEXA scan).
- Nutritional assessment.
- Calcium and vitamin D supplementation ± bisphosphonates according to FRAX® (without a BMD score) or QFracture® results.
- Home assessment for evaluation of risk.

Other specialty involvement

- *Fracture liaison service:*
  - Should be present in all hospitals, to identify and treat patients >50 years of age with a fragility fracture.
- *Physiotherapy:*
  - Liaise closely throughout; 'motion is the lotion', particularly in this group. Post-operative instructions as to what can and cannot be done must be clear; this is the responsibility of the operating surgeon.
- *Occupational therapy:*
  - Inform early during admission if discharge home likely to be problematic due to reduced mobility and function post-operatively.
- *Acute medical team:*
  - If patient becomes acutely medically unwell during admission
  - For medical stabilization and optimization prior to surgery
  - Patient with complex medical comorbidities likely to be affected by operation.

- *Anaesthetist:*
  - Once decision has been made to manage fracture surgically
  - Seek early review if the patient has had previous adverse reactions to anaesthetic or is complex and high risk.
- *Orthogeriatrician:*
  - Should see all elderly patients admitted to the orthopaedic ward with fragility femur fractures in paricular within 72h of injury
  - Manage day-to-day medical conditions and make recommendations for further investigations and management
  - Will typically provide a holistic view of patient care, which is so important but that can often be lost in an acute environment.
- *GP:*
  - Should be informed of all admissions
  - On discharge, all patients with suspected osteoporotic fractures should be referred to their GP for assessment ± treatment (secondary prevention) unless already initiated in hospital.

Further reading

British Orthopaedic Association. *The Care of Patients with Fragility Fracture*. London: British Orthopaedic Association, 2007.

FRAX®. The WHO fracture risk assessment tool—it can be used for people aged between 40 and 90 years, either with or without BMD values, as specified. Available from: ℔ https://frax.shef.ac.uk/FRAX/

Lord S, Sherrington C, Menz HB. *Falls in Older People: Risk Factors and Strategies for Prevention*. Cambridge: Cambridge University Press, 2001.

National Institute for Health and Care Excellence (2012). *Osteoporosis: assessing the risk of fragility fracture*. Clinical guideline [CG146]. Available from: ℔ https://www.nice.org.uk/guidance

QFracture®. This can be used for people aged between 30 and 84 years; BMD values cannot be incorporated into the risk algorithm. Available from: ℔ https://qfracture.org

Open fractures

An open fracture is any fracture that has a direct communication with the external environment. Although open fractures commonly catch the attention of the trauma team by virtue of their appearance, deformity, and subsequent pain, they are not usually life-threatening and must not take precedent over a systematic primary survey. Apart from some basic first aid measures, open fractures are more formally managed as part of the secondary survey.

Gustilo–Anderson classification

- *Type I:* wound <1cm, clean, simple fracture pattern.
- *Type II:* wound 1–10cm, without extensive soft tissue damage, moderate contamination/fracture pattern.
- *Type III:* any high-energy/complex fracture pattern (e.g. segmental, comminuted), extensive soft tissue damage/contamination (e.g. farmyard, sewage):
  - *A:* adequate soft tissue for local coverage
  - *B:* extensive soft tissue injury loss (i.e. need plastic surgeons)
  - *C:* arterial injury needing repair (i.e. need vascular surgeons).

Initial treatment (British Orthopaedic Association/British Association of Plastic Reconstructive and Aesthetic Surgeons guidance)

- Stop external haemorrhage: direct pressure; tourniquet as last resort.
- Document neurovascular status examination of the distal limb (in primary survey): loss of limb perfusion requires immediate attention.
- IV antibiotics within 1h: co-amoxiclav (1.2g) or cefuroxime (1.5g) 8-hourly. Clindamycin 600mg (penicillin-allergic).
- Check tetanus status, and administer prophylaxis if required.
- Analgesia ± sedation.
- Remove gross contaminants from wound in ED. No need to irrigate or wash out in ED.
- Photograph wound (secure/encrypted hospital camera).
- Cover wound with sterile, saline-soaked dressing and adhesive film dressing. Leave undisturbed until definitive exploration in theatre.
- Reduce and splint fracture (POP backslab).
- Repeat neurovascular examination after any intervention.
- *Plain radiographs:* two orthogonal views, including joint above and below.
- Formal wound debridement within 12h (solitary, high-energy fracture) or 24h (low energy) on daytime trauma theatre list ± external/internal fixation, dependent on contamination.
- Immediate surgical debridement if: (a) gross contamination of wound (e.g. marine, agricultural, sewage); (b) compartment syndrome; (c) neurovascular compromise.
- Definitive soft tissue coverage ± fixation within 72h of injury.
- Definitive internal fixation only when definitive soft tissue cover.

Further reading

British Association of Plastic Reconstructive and Aesthetic Surgeons (2020). *Standards for the management of open fractures*. Available from: ℘ https://www.bapras.org.uk/docs/default-source/commissioning-and-policy/standards-for-lower-limb.pdf

British Orthopaedic Association (2017). *BOAST—open fractures*. Available from: ℘ https://www.boa.ac.uk/standards-guidance/boasts.html

Eccles, Simon, and others (eds), Standards for the Management of Open Fractures (Oxford, 2020; online edn, Oxford Academic, 1 Aug. 2020), https://doi.org/10.1093/med/9780198849360.001.0001, accessed 2 Apr. 2025.

Dislocations

Complete separation of two articulating joint surfaces. *Subluxation* is a partial/incomplete dislocation where some articular contact remains. Common examples include: shoulder (glenohumeral joint), patella (patellofemoral), hip (femoroacetabular), and knee (tibiofemoral). Fracture–dislocations (e.g. ankle, tibiotalar) have an associated fracture.

Investigations

- *X-rays:* minimum two orthogonal views (e.g. AP, lateral, ± obliques); taken pre- and post-reduction; if there is significant soft tissue or neurovascular compromise then do not delay reduction for imaging.
- *CT:* occasionally needed post-reduction to assess for associated fractures or bony fragments within joint (e.g. hip dislocation with acetabular rim fracture; ankle fracture for size of posterior malleolus fragment).
- *MRI:* assesses soft tissue stabilizers (e.g. glenoid labrum after glenohumeral dislocation knee ligaments after knee dislocation).

Management

- *ATLS* approach (especially if high-energy mechanism, e.g. road traffic collision).
- *Neurovascular* examination of the limb—before and after reduction clearly document each nerve and vessel function independently.
- Examine the joint above and below.
- *Analgesia and sedation* for reduction (Entonox®, conscious sedation).
- *Reduce and splint* (e.g. POP backslab) as soon as possible.
- *Plain radiograph* to confirm reduction; CT/MRI for anatomy; CT angiography (CTA) for perfusion (e.g. following knee dislocation).
- Definitive treatment (e.g. ligament reconstruction) may be at later date.
- If irreducible in ED, will require formal anaesthesia (general) and urgent closed ± open reduction in theatre. Ex-fix if unstable (e.g. knee).

Complications

- Vascular and neurological injury.
- Recurrent dislocation (e.g. if loose total hip replacement (THR), patellofemoral joint).
- Avascular necrosis (AVN) (e.g. femoral head).
- Heterotopic ossification.
- Joint stiffness.
- Secondary OA.

Compartment syndrome

↑ pressure in a closed fascial space, causing muscle ischaemia.

Pathology

The insult occurs at the capillary bed level where ↑ pressure in the muscle compartment causes venous collapse, ↑ capillary pressure, and extravasation of fluid. As pressure rises, the venous drainage is compressed, but large arterial vessels passing through the compartment remain patent due to their high intraluminal pressures and thick walls. Muscle ischaemia progresses rapidly to necrosis, with subsequent fibrosis and disabling contractures. Long-term changes become inevitable within 4–6h into an evolved compartment syndrome, becoming irreversible after 12h. Early diagnosis and decompression are vital to avoid severe disability.

Presentation

Assessment for compartment syndrome should form a routine part of your evaluation of any significant limb injury. Lower leg and forearm compartments (e.g. following fractures) are the commonest sites affected, but the syndrome can occur anywhere where muscles are bound in fascial envelopes (e.g. gluteal, abdominal). It can also be seen with reperfusion after treatment for acute limb ischaemia or crush injuries when pressure is released and inflow restored. A tight circumferential cast, dressing, or burn may precipitate or exacerbate the condition.

The patient complains of pain, requiring ↑ amounts of strong analgesia, and resists active movement. In particular, passive muscle stretching of the affected compartment is a classic feature. The involved compartment is tensely swollen. Paraesthesiae, paralysis, pulselessness, and pallor should all be considered late signs demonstrating acute ischaemia is established. Limb neurology and perfusion should be assessed and documented, but not relied upon to form a diagnosis.

Management

Diagnosis is clinical, unless the patient is unconscious, or has an anaesthetic limb block, in which case measurement of compartment pressures is indicated. Guidelines suggest pressures within 30mmHg of diastolic pressure or >40mmHg absolute are indicative of compartment syndrome (normal resting muscle pressure 0–12mmHg).

Initial management should include splitting dressings/casts to skin, elevating, and regular review. It is sensible to plan for theatre early by ensuring nil-by-mouth status, necessary blood tests are complete, and theatre staff alerted. Failure to improve within 30min should prompt emergency fasciotomy. Adopt a low threshold to perform fasciotomy, given the severe consequences (e.g. muscle necrosis and fixed contractures) of a late decision.

Fasciotomy incisions must be full length, as the skin is itself a constricting layer. The fascial envelopes of all involved muscle compartments must be released, and the fracture, if present, stabilized. Skin wounds are left open for delayed closure or later grafting.

When the presentation or diagnosis is delayed beyond 12h, then fasciotomy may introduce infection (to necrotic tissue) or precipitate the release of myoglobin into the circulation, causing renal compromise. Under these circumstances, fasciotomy carries little chance of muscle recovery and non-operative management should be considered. Decision-making is difficult and should ideally involve two consultants.

Further reading

British Orthopaedic Association (2014). *BOAST—diagnosis and management of compartment syndrome of the limbs*. Available from: 🔗 https://www.boa.ac.uk/standards-guidance/boasts.html

Bulstrode C. Compartment syndrome. In: Bulstrode C, Buckwater J, Carr A, et al., eds. *Oxford Textbook of Orthopaedics and Trauma*. Oxford: Oxford University Press, 2002; pp. 2412–17.

Elliott KG, Johnstone AJ. Diagnosing acute compartment syndrome. *Journal of Bone and Joint Surgery. British volume*. 2003;**85**(5):625–32.

McQueen MM, Court-Brown CM. Compartment monitoring in tibial fractures: the pressure threshold for decompression. *Journal of Bone and Joint Surgery. British volume*. 1996;**78**(1):99–104.

Head injury

Includes *primary* brain injury (skull fractures, intracranial bleed, and diffuse axonal injury) and *secondary* sequelae (hypoxia, hypovolaemia, cerebral hypoperfusion, intracranial haematoma causing ↑ intracranial pressure (ICP), seizures, and infection).

Skull fractures

- Signs of base of skull fractures include bruising behind the ears (Battle sign), periorbital area (Raccoon sign), CSF rhinorrhoea, and cranial nerve dysfunction.
- May require prophylactic antibiotics and pneumococcal vaccine.

Intracranial bleeds

- *Subdural:* concave, conform to shape of brain. Commoner.
- *Epidural:* biconvex on axial CT. Lucid interval before deterioration.
- *Contusions and intracerebral haemorrhage:* very common and associated with significant neurological deficit.

Diffuse axonal injury

- Sudden acceleration/deceleration inflicts shearing forces, leading to significant axonal damage at the junction of the grey and white matter, especially in the corpus callosum and brainstem.
- Persistent low GCS scores and punctate haemorrhages on CT aid in clinical diagnosis.
- Poor prognosis.

Signs of primary brain injury

Complete neurological examination is required. Assess GCS (see ➲ Chapter 1), pupils, and limb movements during 'D' of primary survey. In children, always consider non-accidental injury (NAI).

Management

- *A:* consider definitive airway if GCS score ≤8. Protect and image (CT) C-spine (consider concomitant injury in all cases).
- *B:* avoid hypoxia (give 100% oxygen) and hyperventilation (low carbon dioxide—cerebral vasoconstriction). Give tranexamic acid 1g IV over 10min + 1g over 8h (CRASH-3 trial) within 3h of injury.
- *C:* avoid hypotension (aim for SBP 110mmHg).
- *D:* try and assess neurology before intubation.
- Imaging (CT, as per NICE guidelines). Neurosurgical referral.

Further reading

CRASH-3 trial collaborators. Effects of tranexamic acid on death, disability, vascular occlusive events and other morbidities in patients with acute traumatic brain injury (CRASH-3): a randomised, placebo-controlled trial. *The Lancet.* 2019;**394**(10210):1713–23.

National Institute for Health and Care Excellence (2014).*Head injury: assessment and early management.* Clinical guideline [CG176]. Available from: ✆ https://www.nice.org.uk/guidance

Wyatt J, Illingworth R, Clancy M, *et al. Oxford Handbook of Accident and Emergency Medicine,* 2nd edn. Oxford: Oxford University Press, 2003.

Burns

Majority thermal, also chemical and electrical. Damage depends on temperature and duration of burning. Three categories:

- *Superficial (first degree):* erythema, pain (e.g. sunburn). Not included in total burn surface area (TBSA; Fig. 3.3)
- *Superficial and deep partial thickness (second degree):* superficial are painful and moist, and blanch to touch; deep do not blanch, are less painful
- *Full thickness (third degree):* dry, white, painless, leathery.

Management

Initially standard ATLS primary and secondary surveys. Seek advice from local burns unit regarding transfer of care.

- *A:* consider early intubation if signs of facial burns (singed eyebrows, nostrils), extensive body burns (>40%), hoarseness, difficulty swallowing. Do not delay.
- *B:* treat hypoxia (100% oxygen); check carboxyhaemoglobin level (>10% suggests inhalation injury); CXR as baseline and later if ventilation worsens (possible inhalation injury).
- *C:* second-/third-degree burns of >20% need fluid replacement; assess % TBSA by using the rule of nines, Lund and Browder chart, or Mersey Burns app (easier, quicker, tells you the fluid required); 2mL/kg of Hartmann's solution × % TBSA in first 24h (half given in the first 8h, the rest over 16h)—replaces Parkland formula. Children <14 years: 3mL/kg of Hartmann's/%TBSA. Adjust based upon urine output.

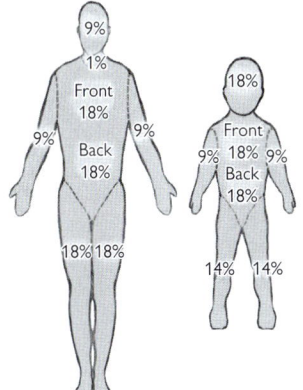

	% total **BSA**	
	Adult	**Child**
Arm	9%	9%
Head and neck	9% (head) 1% (neck)	18%
Leg	14%	18%
Anterior trunk	18%	18%
Posterior trunk	18%	18%
Genitalia	1%	—

Fig. 3.3 Burns body surface area estimate.

- *E:* burnt tissue contracts—may restrict breathing and distal circulation, or cause muscle compartment syndrome requiring emergent full-thickness escharotomy. Non-adherent dressings to burns if painful and moist. Prevent hypothermia. No need for antibiotics/antiseptics.

Chemical burns

Acids, alkalis (penetrate deeper), petroleum products. Brush off any dry powder, then copious irrigation with water for minimum 30min. Remove clothes ASAP.

Electrical burns

Deep tissue damage can occur, with skin appearing normal over deep muscle necrosis. Rhabdomyolysis causes myoglobin release and acute renal failure. As part of ATLS, push IV fluids (4mL/kg × % TBSA), aiming for large diuresis of 1–1.5mL/kg/h. Reduce once urine clear.

Chest trauma

Thoracic trauma encompasses *life-threatening* (identify in primary survey) and *potentially life-threatening* conditions (secondary survey). Mechanism of injury can be *blunt* or *penetrating*.

Life-threatening injuries

Aide-memoire—'ATOM CT':

- **A**irway obstruction: remove obvious foreign bodies, suction, reduce SCJ dislocation if the cause (towel clip on clavicle and pull), jaw thrust, and establish definitive airway.
- **T**ension pneumothorax: 'one-way valve' leak allows gas into pleural space that cannot leave. Extended FAST (eFAST) may diagnose (see ➋ Chapter 2).
  - *Signs:* respiratory distress, tachypnoea, tachycardia, hypotension, hyperresonance to percussion, unilateral breath sounds absent, tracheal deviation away from affected side, neck vein distension.
  - *Management:* immediate decompression by large-bore needle/cannula insertion into fifth intercostal space just anterior to mid-axillary line of affected side (more likely to reach pleural cavity than traditional second intercostal space/mid-clavicular line). Then insert definitive intercostal chest drain.
- **O**pen pneumothorax (sucking chest wound)—penetrating injury of chest wall. With each breath, air passes through hole rather than into the lung. Ventilation compromised→respiratory failure.
  - *Management:* cover defect with sterile dressing secured on three sides, producing flutter valve effect. Then insert a formal chest drain on same side, remote from wound. Can close wound after.
- **M**assive haemothorax—causes respiratory difficulty and haemodynamic shock.
  - *Signs:* respiratory distress, shock, dullness to percussion, ↓ air entry, 'white-out' on CXR.
  - *Management:* restore blood volume by rapid blood infusion through two large-bore cannulae. Decompress chest via chest drain (28–32Fr). If >1500mL drained immediately or continued blood loss >200mL/h, discuss with cardiothoracic surgeons (? potential thoracotomy).
- **C**ardiac tamponade: bleeding between fibrous pericardium and myocardium, impairing cardiac output. Usually penetrating injuries.
  - *Signs:* may be subtle; include shock, muffled heart sounds, and raised jugular venous pressure (JVP) (Beck's triad). FAST scan for bedside diagnosis.
  - *Management:* urgent thoracotomy (pericardiocentesis as last resort).
  - *Tracheobronchial tree injury:* rapid deceleration after blunt trauma, or penetrating injury. Most within 1 inch of carina. Laboured breathing, haemoptysis, cervical subcutaneous emphysema, tension pneumothorax, cyanosis. Continued leak after chest drain insertion (may need >1 tube). Bronchoscopy diagnostic. Need definitive airway (may be difficult, distorted anatomy). Requires prompt thoracic surgical team input.

Potentially life-threatening injuries

- *Simple pneumothorax:* usually needs decompression (chest drain). *Always* insert a drain in a patient who is to be intubated or transported via air (may become tension, especially under positive pressure ventilation).
- *Haemothorax:* insert chest drain to improve ventilation.
- *Blunt myocardial injury:*
  - *Signs:* sternal tenderness/fracture may be only sign. Hypotension, ECG changes possible (multiple ventricular ectopics, atrial fibrillation, bundle branch block, and ST changes)
  - *Management:* if sternal fractures or ECG changes, should have cardiac monitoring for 24–48h post-injury. Transthoracic echocardiogram indicated if ECG changes or raised troponin.
- *Traumatic diaphragmatic rupture:* associated with both blunt and penetrating trauma. Commoner on left side (liver protects right). May present late with respiratory compromise, pleural collection, or intestinal obstruction/strangulation. CXR (bowel loops in chest) or CT for diagnosis, though sensitivity <66%. Mandates surgical repair.
- *Flail chest/multiple rib fractures:* ≥3 ribs fractured in ≥2 places, causes segment of chest wall to move independently from thoracic cage (paradoxical respiration). CT diagnosis usually. Respiratory compromise exacerbated by pain ± underlying pulmonary contusions. Treat hypoxia, adequate analgesia (epidural/intercostal blocks), prevent secondary infection, consider rib fixation (especially polytrauma).

Chest drain insertion (large bore)

This differs from fine-bore tube insertion (Seldinger technique).
- Analgesia (± sedation if appropriate).
- Position patient's arm above head to expose area.
- Palpate fifth intercostal space (approximately at nipple level) just anterior to mid-axillary line.
- Surgically prepare and drape; infiltrate skin and deep tissues with local anaesthetic (10–20mL of 1% lidocaine). *Discard* trocar if the set has one (risk of causing serious injury).
- Make a 2–3cm transverse incision, and use needle holder to bluntly dissect over top of the inferior rib ('go above the rib below' to avoid neurovascular bundle inferior to rib).
- Clear and pierce pleura; dilate hole with needle holder, and finger-sweep to clear any adhesions.
- Clip tip of chest drain with needle holder, and use to guide tube into chest. Clamp outer end of tube to prevent contents of the chest cavity from spilling everywhere.
- Suture skin on either side of the drain. Suture drain to skin.
- Connect tube to underwater-seal apparatus at ground level; look for fogging of tube and 'swinging or bubbling' of water in the drain container to confirm expulsion of air from pleural space with respiration.
- Obtain a check CXR to identify drain tip position.

Abdominal injuries

The primary danger of abdominal injury is life-threatening haemorrhage (identified within 'C' of ATLS).

History

- *Blunt injury:* was the patient restrained in vehicle or ejected? Did an airbag deploy? Commonest is splenic injury, followed by liver. Sudden deceleration leading to flexion–distraction spinal (Chance) fractures has associated intra-abdominal injury up to 50% of the time.
- *Penetrating injury:* time of injury, type of weapon/item.
- *Force imparted:* high- or low-velocity mechanisms.

Examination

Is the patient *haemodynamically stable?* If *unstable* after attempted resuscitation, with evidence of abdominal injury, consider immediate laparotomy (need pelvic X-ray in ED or theatre; keep pelvic binder on).

- *Inspection:*
  - Penetrating injuries, bruises, seatbelt marks, evisceration
  - Blood at urethral meatus and scrotal/perineal haematoma suggest urethral injury.
- *Palpation:*
  - Localized or generalized tenderness/guarding
  - ectal examination (secondary survey): high-riding prostate (urethral injury), sphincter tone (spinal injury), gross blood (viscus perforation)
  - Gently palpate iliac wings and pubic symphysis for signs of pelvic fracture. Only perform once. Do not distract pelvis. *Apply binder* if any suspicion.

Investigations

- *CT with contrast:*
  - High specificity/sensitivity, preferred first-line imaging modality
  - Accurate at detecting free fluid/organ injury (guides laparotomy)
  - Can image from head to pelvis to identify other injuries
  - Suitable only for haemodynamically *stable* patient.
- *FAST scan* (see ➲ Chapter 2):
  - Rapid, non-invasive tool to detect abdominal free fluid, and splenic and liver injuries. Less commonly used due rapid CT access
  - Sensitivity 86–97% (significant false −ve rate); operator-dependent.
- *Angio-embolization:* instead of laparotomy to treat splenic rupture or pelvic fracture-related (arterial) bleeds (venous needs packing).

Indications for laparotomy

- Blunt abdominal trauma in haemodynamically unstable patient without another source of bleeding
- Hypotension with penetrating abdominal wound
- Bleeding from stomach, rectum, or genitourinary tract secondary to penetrating trauma
- Gunshot wounds traversing the peritoneum
- Evisceration
- Free air, retroperitoneal air, diaphragmatic injury, rupture of hollow viscus on CT

Urogenital injuries

Renal trauma is commonest (5% of trauma patients) due to side impact/seatbelts. Bladder and posterior urethra injury usually due to pelvic fractures; anterior urethra injury due to blunt trauma or 'falling astride' injury (bike handlebars, straddle).

Initial assessment

- ATLS protocol. Apply pelvic binder if any suspicion of pelvic injury.
- Inspection of external genitalia (blood at urethral meatus), perineum (bruising) ± digital rectal examination.
- Contrast CT identifies visceral injury and pelvic fractures.
- Avoid catheterization until imaging performed; however, a single gentle attempt to pass a catheter can be attempted.

Renal injuries

Signs and symptoms of renal injury

- Penetrating injury.
- Rib fractures.
- Flank pain/bruising/tenderness.
- Haematuria (visible/urine dipstick).

CT can help to stratify the severity of injury (Table 3.1).

Management

- Majority of stable patients with blunt trauma or grade 1–3 penetrating injuries→non-operative management.
- If active bleeding, but no other abdominal injury→embolization.
- Surgical exploration: grade 5 vascular injury or as part of trauma laparotomy for additional injuries.

Table 3.1 American Association for the Surgery of Trauma (AAST) Kidney Injury Scale, 2018

Grade	CT imaging criteria
I	• Subcapsular haematoma and/or parenchymal contusion without laceration
II	• Haematoma confined to Gerota's fascia • Laceration ≤1cm deep without urinary extravasation
III	• Laceration >1cm deep without urinary extravasation • Vascular injury/active bleeding contained within Gerota's fascia
IV	• Laceration into collecting system • Segmental renal vein/artery injury, active bleeding beyond Gerota's fascia, segmental/complete kidney infarction
V	• Main renal artery or vein laceration or avulsion of hilum • Devascularized kidney with bleeding • Shattered kidney (loss of parenchymal anatomy)

Bladder injuries

Types of bladder rupture

- *Extraperitoneal:* commonest. Peritoneum intact and urine escapes into the space around the bladder. Usually due to pelvic fracture.
- *Intraperitoneal:* peritoneum over bladder breached and urine escapes into peritoneal cavity. Usually sudden impact over full bladder.

Symptoms and signs

- Classic triad of: (1) suprapubic pain and tenderness; (2) difficulty or inability in passing urine; and (3) haematuria.

Investigations

- Retrograde cystography or CT cystography: extraperitoneal perforations—contrast extravasation limited to surrounding bladder. Intraperitoneal perforations—bowel loops may be outlined by contrast.

Treatment

- *Intraperitoneal:* surgical repair.
- *Extraperitoneal:* if urethral catheter is passed, leave in for 2–3 weeks until bladder is healed (+ antibiotics). If there are combined bladder and urethral injuries, then a suprapubic catheter should be placed (via an open approach), along with repair of the bladder.

Urethral injuries

Urethra in ♂ is more fixed and prone to injury than in ♀. Two levels of injury with different mechanisms:

- *Posterior* (membranous urethra): with pelvic fractures
- *Anterior* (bulbar and pendulous urethral segments): urethra compressed against pubic symphysis (kick, handlebars, straddle).

Signs and symptoms of urethral injury

- Blood at urethral meatus.
- Frank haematuria.
- Inability to pass urine.
- Perineal/scrotal bruising.
- 'High-riding' prostate.
- Unable to pass urethral catheter.

Management

- Attempt a single gentle pass of catheter, even if signs of injury.
- If bloodstained urine, requires retrograde cystography via catheter. If catheter will not pass, perform retrograde urethrography (Fig. 3.4). Will require suprapubic catheter after and possible delayed reconstruction.

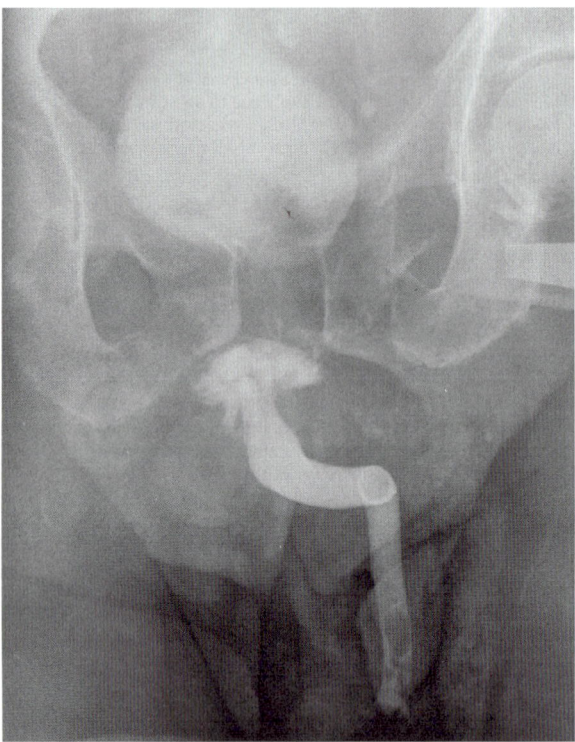

Fig. 3.4 Retrograde urethrogram showing discontinuity of the urethra.

Injuries to scrotum and testis

Blunt trauma, with crushing of the genitals, may cause testicular dislocation (rare—manually replace or perform surgical orchidopexy) or rupture (severe pain—surgical exploration + repair), or a haematocele (surgical exploration if >3 times the size of the contralateral testis).

Further reading

British Orthopaedic Association (2016). *BOAST—the management of urological trauma associated with pelvic fractures.* Available from: ℘ https://www.boa.ac.uk/standards-guidance/boasts.html

Vascular injuries

Extremity vascular injuries may be caused by fractures/dislocations or penetrating trauma (stab, bullet, blast injuries). Arterial injuries range from kinking, spasm, or intimal flap to laceration, segmental loss, and arteriovenous fistula (if the adjacent vein is injured). More commonly present with fractures around joints/dislocations (e.g. knee, supracondylar humerus in children, femoral shaft). Associated with nerve injury/compartment syndrome.

Examination

Signs of vascular injury

- Obvious deformity and active bleeding should alert one to the potential of a significant vascular injury.
- Signs of acute limb ischaemia: pain, pallor, paraesthesiae, cold/cool limb, paralysis, pulseless (use Doppler ultrasonography).
- Ankle–brachial pressure index (ABPI) ratio is systolic pressure in the ankle (for suspected lower limb vascular injury) divided by systolic pressure in the arm. If ABPI is <0.90, arteriography is generally indicated.
- If ABPI is abnormal, then consider CTA.

Management

- Treat associated life-threatening injuries (ATLS).
- Fluid-resuscitate.
- Direct pressure (pad and bandage) to external bleeding (avoid direct use of arterial clamps, which can damage vessels and nerves).
- Tourniquet as last resort (once applied, write time of application on the limb in indelible ink) to minimize duration (distal ischaemia).
- Adequate analgesia/sedation.
- Reduce and splint fracture/dislocation. Repeat neurovascular examination after this.
- Radiographic evaluation to determine extent of injury.
- If remains devascularized post-reduction, requires urgent revascularization in theatre: temporary shunt, then stabilize by using fixation—usually spanning external fixator—then definitive vascular reconstruction (e.g. vein graft) ± prophylactic fasciotomy (prevent/treat associated compartment syndrome due to reperfusion).
- CTA if time, but do not delay for this—can do on-table angiography in theatre if required.

Further reading

British Orthopaedic Association (2020). *BOAST—diagnosis and management of arterial injuries associated with extremity fractures and dislocations.* Available from: ℗ https://www.boa.ac.uk/standards-guidance/boasts.html

Oncological emergencies

Secondary (bone metastasis) are commoner than primary bone/soft tissue tumours. Common sources are: breast, lung, thyroid, renal (kidney), prostate (*aide memoire*: 'BLT' sandwich with 'KP' sauce).

Metastatic spinal cord compression

For metastatic spinal cord compression (MSCC), see ➲ pp. 648–650.

Hypercalcaemia

Occurs in 20–30% of patients with malignancy. More common with:
- Solid tumours with bone metastases (local osteolysis)
- Humoral hypercalcaemia of malignancy (tumours secrete parathyroid hormone-related peptide)
- Haematological malignancy (e.g. myeloma).

Definition
- Adjusted calcium concentration: mild, 2.6–3.0mmol/L; moderate, 3.01–3.40mmol/L; severe, >3.4mmol/L (emergency). Recognize early.

Symptoms and signs
- Nocturia, polyuria, thirst, dehydration, nausea, anorexia, constipation, depression, confusion, psychosis.

Management
- *Isotonic saline* rehydration 200mL/h (caution with renal failure in myeloma); consider urinary catheter and fluid balance monitoring.
- *Bisphosphonates* (e.g. zoledronic acid 4mg IV over 15min or pamidronate 30–90mg at 20mg/h). *Calcitonin* 4IU/kg (second line).

Pathological fracture

Consider malignancy (often metastasis) with pathological fractures. Solitary lesions without a known primary should be investigated before treatment with *bloods* (bone profile, myeloma, tumour markers), *CT* (chest/abdomen/pelvis; identify primary) ±*MRI* (soft tissue invasion), and *MDT discussion* (with specialist tumour unit—is biopsy needed?).

Once a diagnosis of bone metastasis is confirmed, treatment depends on pain, disability, size, and location. The source of the primary, patient prognosis, and anaesthetic assessment/physiological status guide management. The Mirel score helps to guide impending fracture risk (see ➲ Chapter 12).

Treatment goals are to stabilize the whole bone and allow early weight-bearing. Options include: prophylactic long bone nailing, arthroplasty, or endoprostheses (e.g. proximal femoral replacement). Consider preoperative selective angio-embolization of hypervascular metastases such as those from renal or thyroid cancer.

Further reading

Fisher CG, DiPaola CP, Ryken TC, *et al*. A novel classification system for spinal instability in neoplastic disease: an evidence-based approach and expert consensus from the Spine Oncology Study Group. *Spine*. 2010;**35**(22):E1221–9.

National Institute for Health and Care Excellence (2008). *Metastatic spinal cord compression in adults: risk assessment, diagnosis and management*. Clinical guideline [CG75]. Available from: ➲ https://www.nice.org.uk/guidance

Piccioli A, Spinelli MS, Maccauro G. Impending fracture: a difficult diagnosis. *Injury*. 2014;**45**:S138–41.

Tokuhashi Y, Matsuzaki H, Oda H, Oshima M, Ryu J. A revised scoring system for preoperative evaluation of metastatic spine tumor prognosis. *Spine*. 2005;**30**(19):2186–91.

Stab wounds

Determine site and extent (size, depth) of wounds. Assess for damage to underlying structures. Ensure haemodynamically stable (ATLS approach). Continuous pressure if active bleeding. Antibiotics/tetanus prophylaxis. Wash with normal saline. Involve other teams as needed.

Haemodynamically stable patients

- *Dress wound* temporarily (3-sided dressing if chest wound).
- *Limbs:* examine distal extremities for neurovascular involvement and functional deficit. If normal and wound small/superficial, may clean and close in ED. If abnormal features or large/contaminated wound, may need formal exploration and closure in theatre.
- *Chest/abdomen:* contrast CT imaging to assess for pneumo-/ haemothorax, organ perforation, and active bleeding. Treatment includes monitoring, chest drain, or laparotomy.

Cardiac arrest following penetrating trauma: ERT

For patients in cardiac arrest after penetrating trauma, an emergency re-suscitative thoracotomy (ERT) may be attempted in the ED if the relative skill set and equipment are available. Each ED has their own indications. In general, patients should have been alive at the scene/in hospital and had a witnessed cardiac arrest. ERT should only be attempted if the patient has been in cardiac arrest for <15min or has signs of life (e.g. reactive pupils, pulseless electrical activity). Goals are to:

- Decompress the chest cavity and control thoracic bleeding
- Relieve cardiac tamponade and perform open cardiac massage
- Divert blood towards the heart and brain.

Technique

- Bilateral thoracostomy incisions (mid-axillary line, fifth intercostal space). Join them up by using a scalpel and heavy scissors to cut through the skin, intercostals, and sternum.
- Chest wall is lifted in a clam shell technique. The pericardium is incised to relieve any tamponade; cardiac defects are sutured; any bleeding hilar vessels are clamped; the descending aorta is clamped to ↑ blood volume to the brain, and cardiac massage performed.
- The patient will be simultaneously intubated/ventilated and have fast warmed blood products infused via the massive haemorrhage protocol. Prognosis is poor.

Gunshot wounds

Generally, these cause much more internal damage than may appear on initial examination. Depends upon ballistic profile of weapon/projectile. Injuries can be *primary* (missile itself) vs *secondary* (fragmented projectiles). Shock waves cause visceral/soft tissue injury.

Management

- ATLS assessment and adequate resuscitation.
- Trauma CT imaging if stable (rather than mandatory laparotomy).
- Tetanus prophylaxis and appropriate antibiotic prophylaxis.
- *Chest:* drain usually adequate if pneumo-/haemothorax. Thoracotomy in theatre if unstable, massive haemothorax, or uncontrolled bleeding.
- *Abdomen:* may require emergency laparotomy if perforated hollow viscus, active bleeding, or unstable. If stable, no free fluid/air, normal abdominal examination, single gunshot→monitor for 24h.
- *Extremities:* treat as per any other vascular injury.
- Debride wounds of all grossly necrotic/contaminated tissue, bony fragments, and foreign material. Good idea to leave wounds open and heal by secondary intention. All lead shot (shotgun wounds) does not need removal (risk of causing more damage in retrieval).
- Look for associated injuries (e.g. cardiac involvement, diaphragmatic rupture, retroperitoneal bleeding, bladder/rectal involvement).

Further reading

Garner J, Watts S, Parry C, Bird J, Cooper G, Kirkman E. Prolonged permissive hypotensive resuscitation is associated with poor outcome in primary blast injury with controlled hemorrhage. *Annals of Surgery.* 2010;**251**(6):1131–9.

Martin MJ, Brown CV, Shatz DV, *et al.* Evaluation and management of abdominal gunshot wounds: a Western Trauma Association critical decisions algorithm. *Journal of Trauma and Acute Care Surgery.* 2019;**87**(5):1220–7.

Perioperative care

Preoperative care

The decision to operate

Doctors hold a unique place in society. We have the power to improve and sustain life; equally, our misjudged actions can cause harm and accelerate death. The public has historically put considerable faith in the inherent altruism of the medical profession, but in recent years, societal evolution has demanded change. We can no longer make decisions about our patients, without our patients. This principle is at the core of shared decision-making and fundamental to modern medical practice. But how to reconcile these ambitions with the complexity of modern medicine where interpretation of evidence and decision-making are not always straightforward, even for experts within a field? Furthermore, how to shield patients from our own bias when discussing potential treatments?

Although many patients will still defer to the expert opinion of their doctor to advise them, ultimately it is the doctor's responsibility to ensure that all our patients are as well informed as possible. This means making sure we honestly discuss the proposed treatment in a way that allows us to compare the surgical route with medical and non-operative alternatives. We need to be prepared to openly discuss the advantages and disadvantages of each option in the treatment algorithm. We must allow patients time and space to contextualize this information to their own values.

This approach requires knowledge of the natural history of disease and recovery from surgery. It also requires an appreciation of the (evidence-based) real risks that our patients undertake when they submit themselves to our care. For many, this will be straightforward, and the advantages of surgery obvious. But for those with medical multi-morbidity or frailty, with limited life expectancy, decisions may be more finely poised. The benefits of surgery may be less clearly defined, and the risks are likely to be substantially more elevated. We should also consider the risks not only to life and health, but also to independence, quality of life, and overall well-being.

To permit genuine shared decision-making, open conversations must be undertaken to ensure the patient and/or their representatives really understand. This chapter aims to provide readily accessible information about anaesthesia and potential complications, to permit an open dialogue with your patient about their risks of surgery. It also aims to provide a summary of what can be done in the perioperative period to attenuate, but not eliminate, the risks to which we expose our patients.

Organization of a preoperative clinic

Aims of preoperative assessment

The preoperative clinic should provide a suitable environment to counsel and prepare patients for elective orthopaedic surgery. The patient's physical condition and disease process can change between booking and surgery, so this serves as a useful checkpoint to review their status and consent for surgery, alongside medical risk stratification.

A standardized care pathway is a useful means of organizing and documenting the preoperative review, which usually involves a junior doctor (e.g. FY1/2 or CT), a clinic nurse, a phlebotomist, the operating surgeon (SpR/Consultant), and specialist teams (e.g. nurses, physiotherapists, occupational therapists, as appropriate).

Medical optimization

Significant medical comorbidities that are identified may require investigations and/or assessment by an anaesthetist via referral to a 'high-risk anaesthetic clinic' for preoperative risk assessment and investigations to optimize their baseline. Involvement of other specialists may also be helpful (e.g. cardiologist (echocardiography), haematologist (anaemia), respiratory physician (pulmonary function tests)), in good time prior to surgery. The likelihood of requiring blood transfusion perioperatively should be assessed. Most hospitals have protocols for guidance as to which patients to group and save and cross-match. Potential risks/hazards, such as recent transfusion in sickle-cell patients or the patient's wishes (e.g. Jehovah's Witness), must be flagged up at this stage.

Consent

Consent is a process, not a single entity, and begins at the very first outpatient clinic appointment. Patients should provide informed consent to the proposed procedure offered and therefore must gain an adequate understanding of it. Prerequisites to valid consent include capacity, the ability to retain and process information (i.e. to weigh up the indication/benefits, alternatives, risks, outcomes/rehabilitation), and the ability to communicate that information. A signed consent form alone does not serve as adequate evidence of consent. The use of skeletal models, radiographs, and actual implants or frames in the clinic is very helpful in explaining relevant concepts.

Peri- and post-operative planning

Following orthopaedic surgery, a patient's ability to ambulate and self-care may be restricted. Assessment by physiotherapists and occupational therapists allows this to be anticipated, so modifications to the home and living environment can be undertaken in advance, if necessary. Also, social networks to support the patient can be activated.

The surgeon can also avail this opportunity to plan the operation (e.g. software template of arthroplasty implants) and ensure any additional instruments, custom implants, and bone allograft/substitutes are ordered well in advance of surgery.

Consent

Respect for patient autonomy is a fundamental ethical principle; a patient with capacity is entitled to make decisions that may be deemed irrational or contrary to the views of the treating clinician, and competent patients may withdraw their consent at any time. Surgeons have an ethical and legal duty to take *informed consent* for any procedure or operation; proceeding without this would constitute an assault. Informed consent requires the provision of sufficient information for the patient to make a balanced decision regarding their treatment. The basis of consent may be implied (e.g. holding an arm out for a blood test), verbal (e.g. for clinical examination), or written (e.g. consent form).

Components of informed consent

Patient factors

- The patient must be mentally competent and able to:
  - Understand the issues involved

- • Retain information to make a rational decision
- • Communicate their wishes.
- If the patient is mentally competent and above the age for legal consent, nobody else is allowed to make decisions on their behalf; consent by proxy is not provided for in English law.
- If a language barrier exists, informed consent must be taken through an interpreter.

Information that should be given
- An explanation of the disease process, its consequences, and its prognosis.
- What the proposed treatment involves, its intended benefits, and its practical implications.
- Risks of the proposed procedure, both general (e.g. cardiovascular, anaesthetic) and specific (e.g. prosthesis dislocation).
- Alternative treatment options (including no treatment at all), with risks and benefits.
- Discussion of consent should commence at the initial outpatient clinic (and documented in the letter to the patient). Further information, such as leaflets and approved/standardized (e.g. British Orthopeadic Association (BOA), National Institute for Health and Care Excellence (NICE), specialist orthopaedic society) online resources, should be provided for patients to take away, read, and digest, with the opportunity to later return to address any queries.

Who should take consent?
- Ideally the doctor performing the actual investigation or operation
- Another doctor who is appropriately trained and qualified in the relevant procedure may also take consent.

Emergency situations
- When emergency treatment is required, and informed consent cannot be obtained (e.g. unconscious trauma patient), the legal duty of the surgeon is to act in the best interests of the patient.
- Any valid advance directive should be respected. The relatives should be consulted, and information about the patient's premorbid state sought, but the decision on whether to treat or not rests with the surgeon.
- Treatment under these circumstances should be restricted to that necessary to save life or limb.
- In complex cases (e.g. amputation, blood transfusion to a child of Jehovah's Witness parents), a second consultant opinion is prudent. Consultation with the trust's legal team to gain court orders may be required.

Children
- Any person over the age of 16 is presumed competent to make decisions and can be treated as an adult.
- Children under the age of 16 may give consent if competent to understand the issues involved (Gillick competence/Fraser guidelines); however, if such a child refuses treatment this can be over-ruled by a parent if treatment is deemed in the child's best interests. If parents refuse treatment for a child, doctors may apply for a court ruling.

Bolam and Montgomery
- *Bolam:* the Bolam test is based upon an English tort law case that governed the basis of clinical negligence cases for many years. This test states that if a doctor reaches the standard of a responsible body of medical opinion, they are not negligent.
- *Montgomery:* Bolam was rejected in the 2015 Supreme Court decision of Montgomery v Lanarkshire Health Board. The ruling went beyond Bolam to apply a far greater test to medical negligence by expecting a clinician to fully disclose *all* 'material' risks. The test of materiality was whether 'a reasonable person in the patient's position would be likely to attach significance to the risk, or the doctor is or should reasonably be aware that the particular patient would be likely to attach significance to it'.

Aide-memoire for consent: DIAPER
- *D*iagnosis explained
- *I*ndications for surgery discussed
- *A*lternatives to operation considered
- *P*rocedure explained
- *E*xpected outcome discussed
- *R*isks discussed

Further reading

Bolam v Friern Hospital Management Committee [1957] 1 WLR 582.

Gillick v West Norfolk and Wisbech Area Health Authority and Department of Health and Social Security: HL 17 Oct 1985.

Montgomery v Lanarkshire Health Board [2015] UKSC 11.

Preoperative assessment for anaesthesia

Prior to undergoing anaesthesia for surgery, patients require a formal anaesthetic preoperative assessment. This is an opportunity to identify any patient-specific issues that require optimization prior to surgery. It is also the time and place to consider potential anaesthetic techniques, to discuss anaesthetic and perioperative risk and the intended perioperative plan, and to identify any patient concerns or preferences. It also provides an opportunity to plan and organize higher levels of post-operative care for patients either undergoing major surgery or at ↑ risk of complications.

The format of preoperative assessment varies, depending on the nature of the surgery and patients' comorbidities. Broadly speaking, it is performed formally in the preoperative assessment clinic by specialist nurses and anaesthetists, or ad hoc on the wards or emergency department for emergency procedures. For elective procedures, the anaesthetist caring for the patient will additionally review the patient on the day of surgery.

History and examination

Anaesthesia can significantly disrupt normal physiology, particularly of the cardiac and respiratory systems. Medical issues can therefore affect the choice of anaesthetic and analgesic technique. A thorough preoperative systems-based history and a focused examination are vital.

- *Systems review*: pay particular attention to the respiratory and cardiovascular systems. Identify whether medical issues are well controlled. Determine the patient's ASA status (American Society of Anesthesiologists physical status classification system) (Table 4.1).
- *Functional capability*: this is key in estimating how successfully a patient will tolerate anaesthesia. Ascertain whether the patient can achieve 4 metabolic equivalents (METs) (able to climb two flights of stairs without needing to stop).
- *Drug history*: most drugs should be continued preoperatively. Omitting some medications (such as β-blockers) can cause harm. However, some drugs do specifically impact on anaesthesia:
  - Angiotensin-converting enzyme (ACE) inhibitors and angiotensin receptor blockers (ARBs) can cause profound refractory hypotension under anaesthesia; they are routinely omitted on the day of surgery.
  - Anticoagulants and most antiplatelet agents are contraindications to spinal anaesthesia and epidural placement due to the risk of spinal/epidural haematoma. Preoperative planning for perioperative cessation or bridging is important.
  - VTE prophylaxis is also a contraindication to neuraxial anaesthesia, unless sufficient time following drug administration has elapsed; this time varies, depending on agent and dose. Typically, VTE prophylaxis given >12h before neuraxial anaesthesia is acceptable.
- *Anaesthetic history*: identify any prior issues or family history of problems with anaesthesia. This should identify common issues such as post-operative nausea and vomiting, difficult venous access, and rarer, but life-threatening or hereditary, issues (e.g. malignant hyperthermia, suxamethonium apnoea).
- *Airway assessment*: review mouth opening, neck extension, dentition, and abnormal facial/neck anatomy to predict ease of managing the

Table 4.1 American Society of Anesthesiologists physical status classification system

ASA 1	A normal healthy patient
ASA 2	Mild systemic disease
ASA 3	Severe systemic disease
ASA 4	Severe systemic disease—constant threat to life
ASA 5	Moribund, not expected to live without operation

patient's airway. A history of a previous *difficult airway* should prompt a review of past anaesthetic charts to understand the problems encountered and solutions used.
- *Aspiration risk:* uncontrolled reflux, hiatus hernia, obesity, or impaired gastric emptying may alter the anaesthetic technique employed, irrespective of preoperative starvation time. Patients with a raised BMI or pregnancy are usually given ranitidine or a proton pump inhibitor (PPI) to take on the day before surgery.
- *Baseline observations:* patient's weight and height dictate anaesthetic dosing; baseline BP guides intraoperative BP management.

Investigations

Investigations carried out preoperatively guide anaesthetic technique and inform perioperative risk. The choice of investigations is dependent on both the operative severity and patients' specific considerations.
- *Full blood count (FBC):* all major surgery, or ASA >2 undergoing any operation other than minor surgery.
- *Urea and electrolytes (U&Es):* all major surgery; ASA >2 undergoing any surgery; risk of acute kidney injury (AKI).
- *Clotting:* all intermediate or more severe surgery when a patient has a history of chronic liver disease (CLD); taking anticoagulants.
- *Glycated haemoglobin (HbA1c):* all patients with diabetes.
- *Group and save:* varies by institution, but generally for all major surgery or where the predicted blood loss is >500mL. For surgery with expected major blood loss, or for patients with rare antibodies, anticipatory *cross-matching* of blood may be required.
- *ECG:* all major surgery, ASA >2, patients with cardiovascular, renal, or diabetes complications; patients >65 years old with no ECG within 12 months.
- *N-terminal pro-B-type natriuretic peptide (NT-proBNP):* may be useful in selected patients with symptoms or signs consistent with possible cardiac failure, to exclude significant congestive cardiac failure (CCF).
- *Echocardiography:* rarely indicated unless evidence of undiagnosed structural/valvular heart disease, cardiovascular/respiratory symptoms, or change in clinical status in known disease.
- *Cardiopulmonary exercise testing (CPET):* this provides dynamic measurement of cardiorespiratory function and the effects of exercise

on patient physiology. It informs the risk of complications in patients undergoing major surgery.
- Most important physiological CPET parameter is anaerobic threshold (AT).
- This is an indicator of the combined efficiency of the lungs, heart, and circulation.
- AT closely correlates with an elevated risk of perioperative mortality. AT <11mLkg^{-1}min^{-1} indicates a substantially elevated risk of perioperative mortality.
- AT <11 should prompt careful review of the appropriateness of planned surgery. Where surgery proceeds, despite such an adverse risk profile, planned post-operative intensive care admission should strongly be considered.
- *Risk assessment and prediction:* this should be formally calculated for every patient to inform shared decision-making and plan perioperative care. A number of tools can be used to calculate perioperative risk and are freely available to access, including P-POSSUM (Portsmouth-Physiologic and Operative Severity Score for the Study of Mortality and Morbidity), SORT (Surgical Outcome Risk Tool), and ACS NSQIP (American College of Surgeons National Surgical Quality Improvement Program). The more sophisticated tools provide information on functional outcomes; this may be helpful for frail, older patients.

Any subspecialty expert input or investigations (such as cardiac catheterization or pulmonary function tests) may require deferral of surgery. In elective patients, any disease process which is poorly controlled (such as diabetes or hypertension) is usually referred back to the patient's GP or to a specialist for optimization prior to listing for surgery.

Anaesthetic implications

Specific issues identified in preoperative assessment impact anaesthesia delivery; some may be amenable to optimization prior to surgery.
- *Thrombocytopenia:* risk of haematoma following regional anaesthetic techniques. Highest risk with central sites (spinal or epidural). Continuum of risk, but generally considered high risk if platelets <75,000/μL.
- *Abnormal clotting:* INR >1.4 is generally considered a contraindication to neuraxial anaesthetic techniques.
- *Cardiac pathology:* severe aortic/mitral stenosis is a relative contraindication to neuraxial anaesthetic techniques due to reduction in systemic vascular resistance (SVR). Any significant valvular pathology, ventricular failure, or significant pulmonary hypertension will require an arterial line for intraoperative monitoring.
- *Significant organ dysfunction:* renal or liver failure will alter the drugs used during anaesthesia and post-operative analgesia. Significant cardiac or respiratory dysfunction may favour regional anaesthetic techniques over general anaesthesia. A post-operative ICU bed may be required, depending on the severity of organ dysfunction and operative severity.

- *Predicted difficult airway:* after reviewing prior anaesthetic charts, where available, the anaesthetist will make an airway plan, which may include videolaryngoscopy or awake fibreoptic intubation.
- *Surgical position:* patients requiring anything other than supine or lateral positioning normally require a change in anaesthetic technique and equipment. Patients should be consented for the risks of positioning (such as eye issues from proning).

Specific perioperative issues

Cardiovascular disease

Patients with pre-existing cardiac disease are less able to withstand the physiological challenges of volume shifts, blood loss, and ↑ myocardial oxygen demand during surgery. They are therefore at substantially elevated risk of perioperative myocardial ischaemia, heart failure, and mortality. Conditions associated with elevated perioperative cardiac risk include ischaemic heart disease (IHD), CCF, stroke, peripheral vascular disease (PVD), diabetes, chronic kidney disease (CKD), older age, impaired functional status, obesity, and atrial fibrillation (AF). Preoperative assessment of patients with cardiovascular disease aims to:

- Assess perioperative cardiovascular risk
- Optimize the condition of the patient prior to surgery
- Plan the type of operation and anaesthesia
- Plan post-operative monitoring and care.

Risk assessment

Symptoms and functional ability are central to risk assessment. Ask the following:

- Exercise tolerance on flat ground; chest pain or dyspnoea?
- Can the patient exercise to METS 4 or higher (climb two flights of stairs without stopping) (Table 4.2)?
- Peripheral oedema, orthopnoea, paroxysmal nocturnal dyspnoea, palpitations, uncontrolled hypertension
- Pacemakers (or other implanted devices): these can cause problems with monopolar or bipolar diathermy. Find out: type, manufacturer, when the battery was last checked, what happens if it stops working (pacemaker-dependent?).

Examination

- Is the patient in a state of cardiac decompensation?
- Assess pulse: rate, rhythm; check BP. Look for evidence of peripheral oedema, elevated JVP, and displaced apex.
- Auscultate for murmurs, crepitations, and/or wheeze.

Table 4.2 MET scale

MET scale	Activity level
1	Basal metabolic rate at rest
2	Walking slowly
3	Walking at average pace; light gardening
4	Climbing stairs to second floor
5	Mowing lawn or brisk walking
6	Moving heavy objects
7	Swimming
8	Running

Investigations
- ECG: if risk factors/symptoms of cardiac disease.
- CXR: if features of CCF on examination.
- NT-proBNP: if suspected CCF, to identify those needing echocardiography.
- Echocardiography: if suspected valvular lesion or left ventricular failure (LVF).
- Holter monitoring: if suspected arrhythmia.
- Stress imaging.

Patients symptomatic of cardiac disease at exercise tolerance METS <4 may benefit from further pharmacological stress testing (myocardial perfusion scanning or dobutamine stress echocardiography). This provides prognostic information, but it is currently unclear if reperfusion prior to surgery improves outcomes. Discussion on a case-by-case basis is advised with cardiology. Most cardiologists will aim to reperfuse reversible ischaemia prior to elective orthopaedic surgery if:
- The left mainstem is heavily occluded
- Large-volume left ventricular (LV) ischaemia
- High-volume multifocal ischaemic territory
- Exercise-induced LV dilatation
- Surgery can be deferred until the mandatory period of dual anti-platelet therapy (DAPT) has expired (typically 6 months).

Specific cardiac conditions

Ischaemic heart disease
- Patients with IHD are likely to benefit long-term from β-blockade. However, the role of β-blockers in the perioperative period is controversial. They should not be routinely commenced within 2 weeks of surgery unless for symptomatic control of angina or AF.
- Patients on β-blockers should continue through the perioperative period, including on the day of surgery.
- It is reasonable to withhold ACE inhibitors (ACEIs) and ARBs on the day of surgery to reduce the risk of hypotension. In the context of established CCF, continued use may be beneficial.

General principles
Where symptomatic IHD is known (or identified via stress imaging) preoperatively:
- When revascularization is not undertaken before surgery, patients with proven IHD should all be treated medically with aspirin, β-blockade, statin, and ACEI/ARB therapy prior to surgery.
- In patients who have never undergone percutaneous coronary intervention (PCI), aspirin may be safely stopped for 5–7 days before planned surgery (if bleeding risk is considered high).
- In patients who have previously undergone coronary angioplasty, suspension of antiplatelets is less safe. These patients have ↑ rates of perioperative myocardial ischaemia if all antiplatelet therapy is stopped. Careful consideration must be given to timing of planned surgery. Collaborative decision-making with cardiology is advised.

- Wherever possible, delay elective surgery 6 months after PCI (or 2 weeks after balloon angioplasty).
- In an emergency, where surgery cannot be delayed and the patient takes DAPT, consider platelet transfusion.
- Urgent surgery (e.g. cancer) at elevated risk can be conducted at 1–3 months after PCI, but risks of in-stent thrombosis are higher during this period and will ↑ substantially if DAPT is stopped for surgery.
- In these circumstances, it is possible to operate on DAPT (at ↑ bleeding risk) if the surgical site permits adequate control of surgical bleeding (not ocular, spinal, or neurosurgery).
- If unable to operate on DAPT, and surgery cannot be delayed, operate without stopping aspirin and aim to stop second antiplatelet for a minimum duration before surgery (clopidogrel 5 days; prasugrel 7 days; ticagrelor 3 days).
- Reinstate second antiplatelet as soon as the surgical team is satisfied with haemostasis. Reload clopidogrel.

Valvular heart disease

Where valvular heart disease is severe, consideration should be given to correction of the primary cardiac disorder before embarking on elective orthopaedic surgery. However, in the context of trauma, this is rarely possible. Where severe mitral or aortic valve disease is present, specific anaesthetic interventions may be needed to ensure maintained preload, afterload, heart rate, and contractility. Intraoperative anaesthesia is highly challenging; preoperative anaesthetic review is essential.

Heart failure

Patients with known heart failure are prone to decompensation with high rates of mortality in the perioperative period. Perioperative management should focus on ensuring preoperative optimization of heart failure to reduce risks of surgery. Meticulous fluid balance must be maintained intraoperatively and post-operatively. Specific measures preoperatively include the following:

- Optimization of heart failure: may require preoperative uptitration of diuretic, β-blockade, ACEI ± spironolactone ±SGLT2i, cardiac rehabilitation. Seek medical advice.
- Cardiac drugs should all be continued in the perioperative period and on the day of surgery, with the exception of ACEIs or ARBs, which may be withheld on the day of surgery if hypotension is anticipated intraoperatively.
- Patients with restrictive or obstructive cardiomyopathy must be discussed with cardiology and anaesthetics preoperatively.

Aims of intraoperative and post-operative management

- Monitor cardiac function.
- Carefully evaluate the patient for signs of volume overload.
- Avoid excess IV fluid administration.
- Maintain euvolaemia, with diuretic treatment of pulmonary oedema.
- In cases of severe CCF, this may require planned critical care admission and medical support in the perioperative period.
- Long-term cardiac medications should be reinitiated as soon as the patient is haemodynamically stable.

Arrhythmias

Patients with a history of arrhythmia are at elevated risk during the perioperative period, especially if their medication is suspended.
- Anti-arrhythmic medication should be continued throughout the perioperative period, including on the morning of surgery.
- Maintain electrolyte concentrations (potassium (K^+) >4, magnesium (Mg^{2+}) >1.0) during the perioperative period.

Pacemakers and implanted defibrillators

These are subject to electromagnetic interference from diathermy above the umbilicus—this is hazardous if the patient is pacing-dependent or has an implantable cardioverter–defibrillator (ICD) *in situ* (which may fire).
- Ensure battery check within 3 months of planned surgery.
- Liaise with local pacing service: ICDs will need deactivation at start of surgery; permanent pacemakers (PPMs) may need reprogramming.
- In emergency surgery, a magnet can be placed over the PPM/ICD to disable cardioversion and initiate asynchronous pacing.
- Where possible, use bipolar diathermy (not monopolar).
- Remove magnet or arrange reprogramming immediately after completion of surgery (before leaving theatre) to revert to normal pacing/cardioversion settings.

Hypertension

Severe uncontrolled hypertension is associated with adverse outcomes from surgery. Diastolic BP (>110mmHg) appears to be most prognostic, but other data show systolic BP >200mmHg are also adverse markers.
- Preoperatively, BP should be controlled to below 160/100mmHg.
- Elective surgery should be postponed if BP is not controlled.
- Withdrawal of antihypertensives can cause rebound hypertension. Antihypertensives (excluding ACEIs/ARBs) should therefore be continued in the perioperative period, including on the morning of surgery.

Other cardiac conditions

Rare, but important conditions, including congenital heart disease, pulmonary hypertension, and hypertrophic or restrictive cardiomyopathy, may have important implications for anaesthesia. Escalate to cardiology and anaesthetic teams preoperatively.

Elevated troponin and post-operative myocardial injury

This term describes cardiac injury characterized by elevated troponin without symptoms or ECG changes consistent with myocardial infarction, and without a clear non-cardiac source. It is believed to represent cardiac damage due to the inflammatory response to surgery (or hypotension), rather than due to coronary atheromatous plaque disruption typical of myocardial infarction. Although less well understood, it carries an adverse prognosis, with perioperative mortality proportional to troponin rise. Treatment with aspirin and statin is recommended by some authorities, although the benefit (and hence the role of routinely measuring perioperative troponin) is unclear.

Respiratory disease

Chronic respiratory disease is often progressive and may limit cardio-respiratory reserve; this influences the rehabilitation potential following surgery. Patients with advanced disease may also have limited life expectancy. Careful consideration of these factors should therefore be undertaken before planned surgery to ensure patients at high risk of complications are likely to gain meaningful benefit from planned surgery. In patients with chronic respiratory disease, various factors predict pulmonary complications:

* *Patient factors:* age, chronic obstructive pulmonary disease (COPD), CCF, ASA status >2, pulmonary hypertension, impaired functional status, albumin <35g/L, and resting hypoxia
* *Surgical factors:* long operating time, patient positioning, and type of anaesthesia.

Risk assessment

* Current functional ability: 'how far can you walk before getting breathless?', 'can you climb two flights of stairs or more without stopping to rest?'
* Use of home oxygen and nebulizers.
* Previous admissions to hospital with respiratory problems, in particular if non-invasive ventilation (NIV), intensive therapy unit (ITU), or intubation.
* Examine the patient for signs of disease severity: cyanosis, use of accessory muscles, pursed lip breathing, chest wall deformities, crepitations, wheeze, cor pulmonale.
* Pulse oximetry to assess baseline hypoxia.
* CXR should be performed in the presence of respiratory disease/smoking when undergoing significant surgery.
* Pulmonary function tests may have a role in assessing unexplained dyspnoea and for guiding optimization of COPD/asthma.
* Consider serum bicarbonate level and ABG sampling in selected patients considered likely to have chronic type 2 respiratory failure.
* Use the ARISCAT tool to predict risk of pulmonary complications after surgery.
* If obese, think about obstructive sleep apnoea (OSA) and screen with STOP-BANG tool.

General measures

Preoperative

* Anaesthetic review: consider regional and spinal anaesthesia.
* Smoking cessation.
* Teach deep breathing exercises and/or incentive spirometry use before surgery.
* Chest physiotherapy review; consider using the I COUGH pulmonary care programme.
* Treat any current infections; prophylactic antibiotics in bronchiectasis.
* Consider planned critical care admission in severe disease.
* Pulmonary rehabilitation referral where available; consider prehabilitation.

Post-operative
- Ensure proactive multimodal analgesia to facilitate deep breathing, coughing, and pain-free movement after surgery.
- Early mobilization.
- Monitor patients on opiates post-operatively for respiratory depression.
- Chest physiotherapy.
- Nutrition: dietician referral, supplements.

Specific respiratory issues

Smoking
With smoking cessation, best results are seen by stopping 8 weeks before surgery. However, some benefits may be observed even by stopping 1 week before surgery.

Chronic obstructive pulmonary disease and asthma
- Optimize COPD and asthma treatment: bronchodilators, inhaled steroids, as per British Thoracic Society (BTS) guidelines.
- Plan stress-dose steroids for any patient taking >20mg prednisolone (or equivalent, for >3 weeks in a 6-month period).
- Controlled oxygen therapy may be indicated in patients with COPD who retain carbon dioxide.
- Restart regular inhalers and oral medication promptly.

Obstructive sleep apnoea
OSA is becoming increasingly important with rising obesity, and ↑ the risk of respiratory complications 4-fold.
- In obese patients, think about OSA and screen with the STOP-BANG tool.
- In elective surgery, refer high-risk screened patients to a sleep clinic for preoperative diagnosis and optimization.
- Patients using NIV should bring their continuous positive airway pressure (CPAP) machine to hospital and expect to use in the perioperative period.
- Anaesthetic review: may benefit from regional anaesthesia, avoidance of long-acting opiates/sedatives and/or short-acting general anaesthesia. Neuromuscular blocking agents (NMBAs) should be reversed.
- Extended recovery may be required, with careful monitoring for post-operative ventilatory failure.

Pulmonary hypertension
In patients with severe pulmonary hypertension, and in particular, right ventricular dysfunction, anaesthetic agents of induction can cause haemo-dynamic instability, severe hypoxia, and circulatory collapse. Specialist anaesthetic techniques and expertise are required. Preoperative anaesthetic review is essential.

The post-operative breathless patient
A recommended management algorithm is shown in Table 4.3.

Table 4.3 Recommended management algorithm for the post-operative breathless patient

History	Symptoms: SOB, chest pain, sputum, fever, orthopnoea, palpitations, leg swelling
	Observations: NEWS score, hypoxia, hypercapnia
	Type of surgery: how long ago? Complications? Have they received VTE prophylaxis?
	What has happened post-operatively: fluid charts (volume overload?) Urine output? Drug chart: anything suspended (e.g. diuretics?) Sedatives? Opiates? PCA?
	Past medical history: COPD, asthma, OSA, obesity, ILD, bronchiectasis, CCF, IHD, PE, DVT. What are they predisposed to?
Examination	Wheeze, crepitations, reduced air entry, dullness, JVP, fever, oedema
Differential diagnosis	Pneumonia (community/hospital-acquired)
	PE (or fat embolus)
	COPD/asthma exacerbation
	Acute heart failure
	Hypoventilation, especially if opiates or sedating drugs
	ARDS, especially if sepsis or major trauma
Investigation	Consider: bloods (CRP/FBC), CXR, ECG, ABG
	CTPA if PE possible
	NT-proBNP may help to rule out heart failure
Immediate management	A–E approach. Give oxygen if hypoxic—monitor dose of oxygen in patients with COPD, as high levels can reduce the respiratory drive
	Antibiotics for hospital-acquired pneumonia
	Diuresis for heart failure
	If suspected PE, carefully consider full anticoagulation (with low-molecular weight heparin), pending further investigation. If <48h after surgery, the bleeding risk may be high. Discuss with senior surgeon
	Seek medical support

ABG, arterial blood gas; ARDS, acute respiratory distress syndrome; CCF, congestive cardiac failure; COPD, chronic obstructive pulmonary disease; CRP, C-reactive protein; CTPA, computed tomography pulmonary angiography; CXR, chest X-ray; DVT, deep vein thrombosis; FBC, full blood count; IHD, ischaemic heart disease; ILD, interstitial lung disease; JVP, jugular venous pressure; NT-proBNP, N-terminal pro-B type natriuretic peptide; OSA, obstructive sleep apnoea; PCA, patient-controlled analgesia; PE, pulmonary embolism; SOB, shortness of breath; VTE, venous thromboembolism.

Haematological issues

Anaemia

- Anaemia is associated with significant perioperative morbidity and mortality. Transfusion of blood products can be lifesaving; however, it is also potentially hazardous (and expensive).

- Where surgery cannot be delayed, preoperative transfusion can be considered to ensure haemoglobin (Hb) >70g/L. Where massive transfusion is required in the context of trauma, transfusion thresholds have a limited role.
- In stable anaemic patients, Hb should be maintained >70g/L in the perioperative period. This threshold ↑ to >80g/L in patients with cardiac disease. Transfusion may be acceptable if Hb <100g/L in patients who are *symptomatic* with established cardiac or respiratory disease, especially if recent myocardial ischaemia.
- However, wherever possible, perioperative management of anaemia should follow the principles of *patient blood management*. This essentially mandates that all efforts should be made to maintain Hb, minimize blood loss, and optimize physiology without resorting to transfusion of blood products.
- *Preoperative assessment:*
  - Hb check at least 4 weeks preoperatively.
  - Where anaemia is found, aim to identify and treat the cause before planned surgery. Check ferritin, iron studies, B12, folate, thyroid-stimulating hormone (TSH), liver function tests (LFTs), U&Es, FBC, and blood film.
  - Iron deficiency is very common. Perform coeliac screen, and consider the need for investigation of blood loss. This may require a delay or an onward referral and a delay to planned surgery.
  - Correct iron, B12, or folate deficiency. Oral iron may be suitable if 4- to 6-week interval to surgery. Where less time is available, IV iron is preferred. This will have maximal effect at 6–8 weeks but may have some effect at 2–4 weeks. The IV route is preferred if oral iron is poorly absorbed or tolerated.
  - Erythropoietin (EPO) is usually considered in CKD stage 4/5. It may also reduce transfusion in patients with anaemia of chronic disease (baseline Hb <120g/L) and functional iron deficiency where potential surgical blood loss is >500mL.
- *Intraoperative measures:*
  - Maintenance of euvolaemia and normothermia, cell salvage, acute normovolaemic haemodilution, surgical haemostatic measures. Tranexamic acid use has reduced transfusion rates considerably.
- *Post-operative measures:*
  - Cell salvage; correct iron deficiency IV; consider EPO in anaemia of chronic disease.
  - Transfuse if Hb <70g/L or signs of tissue hypoperfusion. Patients with cardiorespiratory disease or frailty may benefit from less restrictive threshold if rehabilitation is impaired by fatigue, chest pain, or dyspnoea.

Patients refusing blood transfusion

Some individuals may refuse transfusion of blood products for religious reasons (e.g. Jehovah's Witnesses), whereas others may refuse transfusion due to concerns regarding transfusion safety. Where patients refuse transfusion, careful consideration must be given to ensure that the patient is adequately informed, while respecting their autonomy and right to refuse transfusion. Shared decision-making is essential, and what products a patient will accept may vary from individual to individual. It is therefore important that all options are discussed and explored preoperatively. Clear discussion and documentation should take place before surgery to contingency plan for life-threatening haemorrhage. In some situations, advance directives may be advisable.

Thrombocytopenia

Thrombocytopenia is associated with an ↑ risk of haemorrhage. Where the aetiology is unknown, planned surgery may require a delay for investigation and management. All cases of significant thrombocytopenia should be discussed with haematology.

- Platelet transfusion may be required perioperatively if platelets <50 in major surgery (or <100 in spinal, ocular, or neurosurgical procedures). Platelet counts of 30–50 might be acceptable for minor procedures.
- In immune-mediated thrombocytopenia, preoperative steroid or immunoglobulin may be indicated to augment platelet count. Discuss with haematology.

Other disorders of haemostasis

These include haemophilia, von Willebrand disease, and congenital or acquired clotting factor deficiencies. Perioperative management and correction of these deficiencies can be complex and must be co-managed with haematology.

Anticoagulation

The bleeding risks of trauma and orthopaedic surgery can be substantial. It is therefore almost always necessary to suspend anticoagulants in the perioperative period. Haematology advice is recommended.

- In emergencies where bleeding is life-threatening, reversal of anticoagulant effect is advised. Discuss with haematology.
  - In the context of warfarin, this is likely to require vitamin K and prothrombin complex concentrate.
  - In the context of direct oral anticoagulant (DOAC) use, this may involve specific monoclonal therapy and/or prothrombin complex concentrate.
- In planned surgery, the risks of anticoagulant suspension must be balanced against the risks of bleeding. Patients with metallic heart valves, inherited thrombophilia, VTE (<3 months), and high-risk AF (CHADS2 score 5–6) are at greatest risk of thrombotic complications.
- In these cases where surgery cannot be delayed or where the risk will not change, these patients may benefit from anticoagulant bridging with low-molecular weight heparin (LMWH) after their anticoagulant has been stopped.
- Lower-risk patients do not require bridging, which can ↑ the risks of intraoperative bleeding.
- Patients receiving DOACs with normal renal function should stop their anticoagulant 48–72h before orthopaedic surgery.
- Patients with impaired renal function (creatinine clearance (CrCl) <50mL/min) should stop DOACs 3–5 days before surgery.
- Warfarin should be suspended 5 days before surgery.
- Where anticoagulation bridging is required, treatment-dose LMWH should be prescribed after the anticoagulant has been suspended, at 3 days before surgery. The last dose should be given 24h before surgery.

- Anticoagulants should be restarted 48h after surgery, assuming satisfactory haemostasis.

Antiplatelet agents

As with anticoagulants, the risk of cessation must be balanced with the risk of continued therapy. Cessation of antiplatelets is associated with an ↑ risk of vascular events. However, it may also ↑ bleeding.

- In most cases, aspirin can be continued through the perioperative period, with a minimal risk of excess bleeding. Exceptions to this include spinal, ocular, and neurosurgery where full cessation of antiplatelet effects is advised preoperatively.
- In patients taking clopidogrel for transient ischaemic attack (TIA) or CVA, preoperative conversion to aspirin 7 days before surgery can be considered where the risks of perioperative stroke are considered high.
- In the context of IHD, see ➲ Cardiovascular disease, pp. 108–111. Discussion with cardiology is recommended in patients with established IHD prior to suspension of any antiplatelet treatment, given the risks of perioperative cardiac ischaemia.
- In IHD patients who have never required coronary revascularization, suspension of aspirin 5–7 days before surgery is reasonable.
- Patients taking dual antiplatelets (i.e. coronary procedure or event <1 year) must be discussed with cardiology prior to suspension of any antiplatelet treatment. Where surgery cannot be delayed, suspension of clopidogrel, ticagrelor, or prasugrel 3–7 days before surgery may be acceptable for the perioperative period. Aspirin is usually continued in this context.
- In emergency surgery complicated by haemorrhage where preoperative suspension of antiplatelet treatment has not been possible, platelet transfusion can be considered (although this has not been shown to improve outcomes).

Venous thromboembolism prophylaxis

Patients undergoing orthopaedic surgery (especially THR, total knee replacement (TKR), fracture of neck of femur) are at high risk of developing post-operative VTE. Where no bleeding contraindication exists, chemical prophylaxis is usually indicated.

- Early mobilization should be encouraged in all patients (unless contraindicated).
- In patients at very high bleeding risk (e.g. polytrauma), mechanical prophylaxis with intermittent pneumatic devices or TEDS should be deployed. Inferior vena cava (IVC) filters can be considered in selected cases. Chemical prophylaxis is likely to be indicated, as these patients are at high risk of VTE. We tend to delay administration 24–48h in patients at high risk of bleeding in whom haemorrhage would be difficult to control or have catastrophic complications (e.g. brain/spinal injury).
- Prophylaxis with LMWH is the typical form of chemoprophylaxis (e.g. enoxaparin 40mg once daily (OD), tinzaparin 3500U OD, dalteparin 5000U OD).
- Dose adjustment or replacement with unfractionated heparin (5000U twice daily (BD)) may be needed in the context of either renal impairment (CrCl <20mL/min) or extremes of body weight.
- Heparins should be given no less than 12h before surgery and started 6–12h afterwards.

- Emerging evidence (and NICE 2018 guidance) also supports the use of DOACs (rivaroxaban or apixaban) or oral aspirin as an alternative to LMWH, particularly after elective THR/TKR.
- After THR, fracture of neck of femur, or TKR, VTE prophylaxis should be continued for a minimum of 10–14 days, and up to 38 days after THR (e.g. 10 days of LMWH, followed by 28 days of aspirin 75/150mg orally).

Renal disease

Chronic kidney disease

Patients with CKD, and in particular those with end-stage renal failure (ESRF) (on haemodialysis), are at high risk of perioperative mortality and morbidity. This is due to cardiac comorbidity, haemodynamic instability, bleeding complications, and fluid and electrolyte imbalance. Patients are also at ↑ risk of perioperative AKI.

- Preservation of existing renal function is paramount. Ensure euvolaemia and maintenance of BP during surgery to prevent prerenal injury.
- Optimize anaemia preoperatively. Correct iron deficiency. Consider IV iron and EPO.
- Consider cardiovascular comorbidity, and evaluate/optimize accordingly.
- Perioperative prescribing must account for reduced estimated glomerular filtration rate (eGFR) (especially VTE/opiates/antibiotics).
- Preoperative anaesthetic review to consider the technique and plan multimodal analgesia.

End-stage renal failure on renal replacement therapy

- Patients should be co-managed with nephrology and/or perioperative medical support.
- Surgery should ideally be performed with the patient at their dry weight. If dialysis is performed on the day of surgery, attention should be paid to anticoagulant use—heparin-free dialysis is likely to reduce haemorrhagic complications.
- Typically, dialysis should be performed on the day before planned surgery.
- K⁺ should be <5.5 for planned surgery, and <6.0 for emergency surgery.
- Patients should have a post-operative measurement of K⁺ level, as certain anaesthetic agents can cause an efflux of K⁺ into the circulation.
- ACEIs and ARBs should be stopped for 2 days before surgery to reduce perioperative haemodynamic instability. Where diuretics are still used (where there is some residual renal function), these should also be discontinued.
- Dialysis access should be meticulously protected through the perioperative period and only used for dialysis (arteriovenous (AV) fistula; tunnelled line).

Transplant patients

- Perioperative care must be conducted in collaboration with the patient's transplant team.
- Maintain immunosuppressants throughout the perioperative period.
- In patients taking steroids with a suppressed adrenal axis, care must be taken to prescribe appropriate stress-dose steroid (see ➋

Endocrinology, pp. 131–135 for more detail on adrenal insufficiency). Usually this is managed by double-dose steroid for 48h (or parenteral equivalent), with reversion to normal dose after 48h.
- Remember the patient is immunosuppressed. Low threshold for antimicrobial treatment if potential infective complications.
- Early escalation to medical and transplant team in the event of complications.
- Avoid erythromycin and clarithromycin in patients taking ciclosporin or tacrolimus.
- Skin staples may need to be kept in for 2–3 times longer than normal due to impaired skin integrity.

The post-operative oliguric patient: an approach

Table 4.4 shows the approach to the post-operative oliguric patient.

Table 4.4 Approach to the post-operative oliguric patient

History	Symptoms: do they have specific symptoms? Pain? Visible blood loss? Most oliguric patients will be unwell without primary renal problems. The most important thing to consider is post-operative blood loss and sepsis
	Observations: early warning (e.g. MEWS/NEWS) score, BP, pulse, oxygen saturation, RR
	Type of surgery? How long ago? Complications? Look at anaesthetic charts—was the patient hypotensive for a long time in theatre?
	What has happened post-operatively? Fluid balance (input/output) charts—how much intake has the patient received? What is their UO?
	Drug chart: any nephrotoxic drugs (e.g. NSAIDs), diuretics, ACEIs?
	Past medical history: COPD, asthma, OSA, obesity, ILD, bronchiectasis, CCF, IHD, PE, DVT. What is the patient predisposed to?
Examination	*Key question: is the patient wet (hypervolaemic), dry (hypovolaemic), or euvolaemic?*
	Observation (early warning score) clues: low BP, tachycardia, high RR, and low UO indicate the patient is probably underperfusing their kidneys
	Assess peripheries: are they cool and shut down? Mottled? Are peripheral blood vessels visible on the hand? Is the urine dark and concentrated? If so, the patient is probably dry
	JVP (and external jugular): can you see it? If not, the patient is probably dry
	Peripheral oedema: common after major surgery (including localized, e.g. lower leg swelling after TKR) when albumin often drops and fluid collects in third spaces. Patients with oedema can still be intravascularly deplete and therefore physiologically 'dry'. Do not set too much store by modest peripheral oedema, unless the JVP is elevated. Remain vigilant for VTE

(Continued)

Table 4.4 (Contd.)

Differential diagnosis	Prerenal: commonest. Post-operative patients have often lost blood and insensible fluids before and during surgery. They are usually dry and need fluid
	Renal: less common, except when drugs are responsible. Look at the drug chart. Stop anything that could be contributing. Intrinsic renal disease can occur, especially if recognition of oliguria or hypotension is delayed
	Post-renal: this is common. Retention of urine or blocked catheters are usually responsible, but sometimes urological disease can cause hydronephrosis
Investigation	Bedside bladder scan: is the patient in retention?
	Urine dip: look for proteinuria/haematuria, indicating intrinsic renal disease
	Bloods: U&Es, CRP, FBC, calcium group, LFTs
	VBG: base excess and lactate. Sepsis? Acidosis?
	USS of kidneys: to rule out hydronephrosis
	CXR: may help to tell if patient is volume-overloaded
Immediate management	Check patient not in retention of urine if not catheterized. Bedside bladder scan
	Likely to need catheter. If already catheterized, check catheter not blocked. Flush
	Decide volume status. Is the patient wet, dry, or euvolaemic? If not sure, get senior help
	Unless in pulmonary oedema, consider fluid challenge (e.g. 250mL of crystalloid) and monitor response at 1h. May need multiple challenges and background IV fluid
	If sepsis possible, take blood cultures and administer antibiotics within 1h (as per local guidelines)
	Escalate if hypotensive or septic to senior colleague
	Review drug chart. Stop anything that might be nephrotoxic (commonly ACEIs, ARBs, diuretics, NSAIDs). Review dosing—what needs changing with reduced eGFR? VTE? Antibiotics? Get pharmacy help
	Seek medical support

ACEI, angiotensin-converting enzyme inhibitor; ARB, angiotensin receptor blocker; BP, blood pressure; CCF, congestive cardiac failure; COPD, chronic obstructive pulmonary disease; CXR, chest X-ray; DVT, deep vein thrombosis; eGFR, estimated glomerular filtration rate; IHD, ischaemic heart disease; ILD, interstitial lung disease; JVP, jugular venous pressure; NSAID, non-steroidal anti-inflammatory drug; OSA, obstructive sleep apnoea; PE, pulmonary embolism; RR, respiratory rate; TKR, total knee replacement; UO, urine output; USS, ultrasound scan; VBG, venous blood gas; VTE, venous thromboembolism.

Gastrointestinal disease

Chronic liver disease

Hepatobiliary disorders can present a number of anaesthetic and medical challenges in the perioperative period. Surgical risk is particularly high in alcohol-induced liver disease; however, other aetiologies also carry a substantial risk profile. Perioperative mortality in advanced CLD may reach

80% in Child–Pugh C cirrhosis. However, a significant number of patients with CLD have no known diagnosis. In patients with underlying risk factors for liver disease, the diagnosis of cirrhosis should be contemplated perioperatively.
- Look for peripheral stigmata of CLD, including: jaundice, spider naevi, encephalopathic tremor, gynaecomastia, leuconychia, anaemia, raised JVP, caput medusae, ascites, and hepatomegaly.
- Where cirrhosis is suspected, request an USS of the liver or Fibroscan.
- If confirmed, delay planned surgery and refer to hepatology where possible.

In cases of known CLD, surgery should only be undertaken after careful consideration of risks and benefits; the decision to operate is likely to involve the surgeon, anaesthetist, and hepatologist. CLD patients may have a number of problems to address prior to surgery:
- Portal hypertension: oesophageal varices and risk of GI haemorrhage
- Impaired synthesis of clotting factors leading to coagulopathy
- Electrolyte abnormalities, including dilutional hyponatraemia
- Risk of hepatic encephalopathy
- Nutritional deficit.

Risk assessment
- Clinical examination: is liver disease compensated or decompensated?
- Calculate a Child–Pugh Score (Tables 4.5 and 4.6).
  - This requires clinical examination to determine the presence of encephalopathy and ascites.
  - Laboratory results required for risk assessment also include bilirubin, albumin, and clotting profile.

Table 4.5 Child–Pugh classification of cirrhosis severity

	1 point	2 points	3 points
Ascites	Absent	Slight	Moderate
Bilirubin (µmol/L)	<34.2	34.2–51.3	>51.3
Albumin (g/L)	>35	28–35	<28
INR	<1.7	1.7–2.3	>2.3
PT (sec > control)	<4	4–6	>6
Encephalopathy	None	Grades 1–2	Grades 3–4

INR, international normalized ratio; PT, prothrombin time.

Table 4.6 Child–Pugh status and associated perioperative mortality

Child–Pugh score	Child–Pugh status	Perioperative mortality (%)
5–6	A	10
7–9	B	17
10–15	C	63

Perioperative management
- Involve a hepatologist, and aim for medical co-management of the patient through surgical admission.
- Correct coagulopathy with 10mg vitamin K IV before surgery. Do not use blood products routinely.
- Ensure platelet counts are >50,000/µL before surgery (>100,000 for spinal procedures).
- If ascites is present, correct volume status with spironolactone.
- Prescribe gastric protection to prevent peptic ulceration and upper GI bleeding.
- Correct nutritional deficits: prescribe dietary supplements and multivitamins. Nasogastric (NG) feeding may be required; non-bleeding varices are not a contraindication to NG tube (NGT) insertion.
- Anaesthetic review.
- Avoid hepatotoxic medications (including halothane, sedatives, opiates, and NMBAs).
- Maintain perioperative euvolaemia: avoid salt and volume overload (will exacerbate ascites).
- Circulatory volume expansion may require redistribution of fluid from third spaces. Consider 20% human albumin solution (HAS) (e.g. three times daily (TDS)) in the perioperative period.
- Ensure bowels open at least daily: prescribe lactulose 20mL TDS.

Alcohol misuse
Harmful alcohol consumption is under-recognized in patients admitted with trauma or for elective surgery. It is associated with ↑ perioperative complications.
  Preoperative assessment and recognition may improve outcomes by:
- Reducing preoperative alcohol use
- Aiding in prevention or early detection and treatment of alcohol withdrawal
- Allowing early diagnosis and management of perioperative complications of alcohol use.

Perioperative management
- Reduce alcohol consumption before surgery; aim for preoperative abstinence.
- Consider referral to alcohol cessation service prior to surgery.
- On admission, use Clinical Institute Withdrawal Assessment for Alcohol (CIWA) to monitor for alcohol withdrawal.
- In patients with heavy alcohol consumption, consider prophylaxis with chlordiazepoxide 20–40mg four times daily (QDS). Wean progressively over 2–3 days, according to local protocol. Treat detoxification as per local protocol. Dosing depends on symptom severity but would typically commence at 20–40mg chlordiazepoxide QDS.
- Monitor for medical complications of surgery; treat promptly.

Nutrition
Both trauma and surgery result in physiological stress with a resultant catabolic state. Malnourished patients have poor clinical outcomes, including a 4-fold risk of mortality, ↑ risk of complications, ↑ length of stay, and higher readmission rates.

Perioperative management
- All patients undergoing surgery should be screened for malnutrition by using the Malnutrition Universal Screening Tool (MUST)—this can be performed by any healthcare professional.
- If concerns regarding malnutrition are identified during screening, dietician input is required.
- The patient may need preoperative nutritional support; this can range from supplements (e.g. Fortisip®) to parenteral nutrition.
- In the case of non-urgent surgery, surgery may need to be delayed to allow nutritional optimization.

Electrolyte disturbance
Individual Trusts will have their own guidelines for electrolyte replacement. Table 4.7 provides a guide.

Neurological disease

Parkinson's disease
Parkinson's disease (PD) is a common multisystem neurological disorder. The key clinical features of PD include tremor, rigidity, and bradykinesia, as well as a whole host of motor and non-motor symptoms. PD is associated with ↑ perioperative mortality, as well as with a number of complications, including falls, aspiration pneumonia, delirium, VTE, and ↑ length of stay.

Perioperative management
- Involve specialists in movement disorders early.
- Operate first on the list, where possible, to avoid disruption to medication doses.

Avoiding missed medication doses
- Anti-Parkinsonian medication should *NOT* be withheld or missed; can be taken with sips of water on morning of surgery and should be taken ASAP after surgery.
- Missed doses will result in 'off'-state of rigidity and freezing.
- Complications include swallowing impairment, aspiration, immobility and functional decompensation, falls and fractures, and Parkinsonism–hyperpyrexia syndrome (PHS).
- *Management*:
  - If anticipating missed doses of PD medications, impaired swallowing, or non-functioning digestive tract (e.g. ileus/bowel obstruction), consider an alternative route (i.e transdermal).
  - Where possible, use enteric route (e.g. Madopar® dispersible via NGT.
  - Alternatives include rotigotine transdermal patch.
  - Use *PDMedCalc* for converting oral PD medications to other routes.

Delirium
- Patients with PD may have underlying cognitive impairment and will therefore be at risk of perioperative delirium.
- See ◐ Delirium, pp. 129–131 for details on diagnosis and management.

Table 4.7 Electrolyte replacement guide

Electrolyte	Level (mmol/L)	Route	Supplement	Daily dose	Provides per 24h	Comment
Potassium	2.5–3.5	PO/NG	Sando-K®	Two tablets TDS	72mmol K^+	Adjust dose accordingly if known renal impairment
		PO/NG	Kay-Cee-L®	15mL TDS	45mmol K^+	Adjust dose accordingly if known renal impairment
	<2.5	IV	Premixed bag (40mmol KCl in 1L of 0.9% saline or 5% glucose)	40mmol K^+ in 1L of IV fluid	40mmol K^+	40mmol K^+ must be given over at least 4h Concentrations of >40mmol/L only in ITU via central line
Phosphate	0.65–0.8	PO/NG	Phosphate Sandoz®	One tablet BD	32mmol PO_4^{3-} 40mmol Na^+ 6mmol K^+	Can use potassium phosphate (17.42% oral solution) if required ↑K^+ or ↓Na^+ input—unlicensed, discuss with pharmacy
	0.5–0.64	PO/NG	Phosphate Sandoz®	Two tablets BD	64mmol PO_4^{3-} 80mmol Na^+ 12mmol K^+	
	0.32–0.5	PO/NG	Phosphate Sandoz®	Two tablets TDS	96mmol PO_4^{3-} 120mmol Na^+ 18mmol K^+	
	<0.32	IV	Phosphate Polyfusor® (50mmol in 500mL)	100mL	10mmol PO_4^{3-} 2mmol K^+ 16mmol Na^+	Can use potassium acid phosphate injection 13.6% if ↓Na^+ input required—unlicensed, controlled drug, must be given in HDU environment

Magnesium	0.5–0.66	PO/NG	Magnesium aspartate	1–2 sachets per day	10mmol Mg^{2+} per sachet	
	<0.5	IV	Magnesium sulfate	20mmol Mg^{2+} in at least 50mL of 5% glucose or 0.9% saline over 24h	10mmol Mg^{2+} per 5mL of magnesium sulfate	Maximum rate 0.6mmol Mg^{2+}/min. Maximum 40mmol Mg^{2+}/24h Monitor BP, RR, ECG, tendon reflexes, renal function, and Mg^{2+}, Ca^{2+}, and K$^+$ levels

PO, orally; NG, nasogastric; K$^+$, potassium; KCl, potassium chloride; ITU, intensive therapy unit; BD, twice daily; PO$_4$$^{3-}$, phosphate; Na$^+$, sodium; TDS, three times daily; HDU, high dependency unit; Mg^{2+}, magnesium; RR, respiratory rate; Ca^{2+}, calcium.

Swallowing impairment
- Common in PD patients due to bradykinesia and rigidity of the pharyngeal musculature.
- This may be exacerbated by missed medication doses, other medications, or dysphagia resulting from intubation.
- Complications include aspiration pneumonia and impaired nutrition.
- *Management*:
  - Ensure no missed medication doses.
  - Early speech and language therapy (SLT) review if concerns.
  - Simple measures to minimize risk of aspiration: ensure sitting upright while eating and drinking, etc.

Constipation and post-operative ileus
- PD patients can be prone to constipation and ileus due to underlying autonomic dysfunction. This is likely to be exacerbated in surgical patients receiving opiate analgesia.
- Complications include poor absorption of PD medications and delirium.
- *Management*:
  - Ensure regular laxatives are prescribed, especially in those patients on regular opiates.
  - Stool chart to monitor bowels.

Pulmonary complications
- PD patients can have rigidity and bradykinesia of the respiratory muscles, as well as pharyngeal dysfunction and excess salivation. These patients may therefore have compromised baseline respiratory function and reserve.
- *Management*:
  - Ensure no missed medication doses.
  - Aim to sit out of bed and mobilize ASAP post-operatively.
  - Chest physiotherapy input if concerns.

Functional decompensation
- PD patients are at risk of functional decline in hospital.
- Complications include ↑ length of stay and ↑ care level at discharge.
- *Management*:
  - Early physiotherapy and occupational therapy review
  - Early, proactive discharge planning involving MDT and family
  - Timely and appropriate management of risks mentioned above.

Other medication advice
- Certain medications are contraindicated in PD patients, mainly due to dopamine antagonism—these drugs can cause acute worsening of Parkinsonism.
- These include: haloperidol, metoclopramide, prochlorperazine, and typical antipsychotics.

Stroke

The incidence of perioperative stroke in non-cardiac surgery is 0.1–0.6%. Although rare, it is associated with up to an 8-fold ↑ in mortality. Preventative strategies are therefore important. Risk factors for perioperative stroke include: age, previous stroke/TIA, renal impairment, AF, and valvular disease.

Timing of surgery
- Surgery within 6–9 months of stroke is associated with ↑ risk of perioperative mortality, stroke, and cardiac events. The risk declines over time following stroke but is likely to remain elevated indefinitely.
- Delay elective surgery for at least 6–9 months post-stroke/TIA, if possible.
- Emergency surgery is unlikely to be delayed. The risk of perioperative stroke should form part of the consent process.

Continuation of antiplatelets/anticoagulation
- The decision to stop or continue antiplatelets requires careful balancing of the risks of thromboembolic complications associated with cessation, versus the risk of surgical bleeding if they are continued. This must be conducted on a case-by-case basis depending on patient risk factors and nature of surgery.
- Where surgically possible, guidelines advise:
  - *Aspirin monotherapy:* if a patient is high risk for perioperative stroke (e.g. stroke within preceding 3 months), then aim to continue aspirin.
  - *Clopidogrel monotherapy:* if high-risk patient, switch to aspirin 10 days before surgery and continue aspirin through the perioperative period. Generally required to be off clopidogrel for 7 days prior to surgery to minimize bleeding.
  - *Anticoagulation for AF:* if high-risk/stroke within previous 3 months, then may need to consider anticoagulation bridging (refer to local hospital policy).

Dementia
Around 850,000 people in the UK live with dementia; this is estimated to ↑ to 1 million by 2025. The prevalence of dementia in hip fracture patients is around 20%; the prevalence of mild cognitive impairment in older elective joint replacement patients is around 20%.

Surgical patients with dementia have higher rates of:
- Post-operative medical complications, including delirium, pneumonia, stroke, and AKI
- Long-term cognitive deterioration triggered by surgery
- ↑ length of stay
- Discharge to a care home
- Readmission.

Perioperative management
Given the adverse risk profile, the decision to proceed with surgery in patients with dementia must be carefully weighed up. Patients with dementia commonly (but not always) lack mental capacity to consent to surgery. In this situation, a shared decision-making process must occur, involving the patient, treating MDT, next of kin, and/or lasting power of attorney (LPA) for health and welfare (where available).

The first step is to assess mental capacity to consent to surgery (see ➲ Consent, pp. 101–103) This can be challenging in patients with dementia. In the context of trauma or acute illness, delirium may exacerbate cognitive deficits of dementia. A patient with dementia should not be assumed to lack capacity. Where there is doubt or concern, assistance with assessment and decision-making should be sought (e.g. from geriatric medicine, old age psychiatry, or dementia specialist nurse).

In a patient who lacks capacity, important things to consider include:
- A patient's expressed wishes when previously deemed to have capacity
- Advance directive
- Involving a patient's LPA for health and welfare.

If a patient has none of the above, the next of kin should be consulted to help determine their best interests.

Remember to consider the impact of ongoing medications and their interaction in the perioperative period (Table 4.8).

Pain assessment and management
- Pain management can prove challenging, as patients with advanced dementia can find it difficult to articulate pain due to problems with memory and communication.
- A number of valid and reliable self-report measures are available and can be used, even when moderate dementia exists. The Numerical

Table 4.8 Medication considerations during the perioperative period

Medication	Interaction	Advice
AChEIs Acetylcholinesterase inhibitors (e.g. donepezil, rivastigmine, galantamine)	Interacts with muscle relaxants in anaesthesia	Case-by-case risk vs benefit discussion (e.g. potential for worsening cognitive function if AChEI stopped vs risk of interference if neuromuscular blockade during anaesthesia)
NMDA receptor antagonists (e.g. memantine)	↑ CNS toxicity of ketamine, ↑ side effects of anticholinergic and dopaminergics	Care with choice of anaesthetic agents
SSRIs (e.g. citalopram)	↑ risk of serotonin syndrome and enhanced effects of opiates and induction agents	Avoid fentanyl, tramadol, and ondansetron
Antipsychotics (e.g. quetiapine, risperidone)	Enhanced risk of vasodilatation and hypotension with anaesthetics	Care with choice of anaesthetic agents; risk vs benefit discussion (e.g. risk of worsening BPSD with stopping, risk of intraoperative hypotension if continued)

AChEI, acetylcholinesterase inhibitor; BPSD, behavioural and psychological symptoms of dementia; CNS, central nervous system; NMDA, *N*-methyl-D-aspartate; SSRI, selective serotonin reuptake inhibitor.

Rating Scale or verbal descriptors can be used with people who have mild to moderate cognitive impairment. For people with severe cognitive impairment, Pain Assessment in Advanced Dementia (PAINAD) and Doloplus-2 are recommended.

- The Abbey Pain Scale is widely used throughout the UK.

Delirium

Delirium is an acute confusional state, usually with a fluctuating course, characterized by disturbed consciousness and impaired cognitive function or perception. It is common and present in up to 40% of patients sustaining a fractured neck of femur. It is associated with substantially ↑ morbidity and mortality, and ↑ length of hospital stay.

Causes—'PINCH ME'

- Pain.
- Infection.
- Nutrition.
- Constipation.
- Hydration.
- Medication and alcohol.
- Environment.

Detection and assessment

- 4AT tool: the 4 As test (Arousal, Attention, Abbreviated Mental Test 4, Acute change).

Management

- Identify and treat medical causes of delirium.
- Optimize the environment; orientation—ensure patients have their glasses and hearing aids; reduce noise; ensure optimal lighting.
- Ensure good sleep hygiene.
- Explain the diagnosis to patients and family; encourage involvement of family in care.
- Prevent complications: immobility, falls, pressure sores, dehydration, and malnourishment.
- Treat agitation and distress by using non-pharmacological means wherever possible.
- Promote cognitive engagement, mobilization, and other rehabilitation strategies.
- Consider specialist referral if not recovering.

Pharmacological treatment

- Routine use of sedation in the treatment of delirium is not recommended, as this is associated with ↑ mortality.
- Sedation can be justified in patients with intractable distress, or where the safety of themselves or others is compromised—seek expert advice from geriatric medicine/old age psychiatry.
- Haloperidol is contraindicated in patients with PD or Lewy body dementia; short-acting benzodiazepines (e.g. lorazepam) should be used in this context where absolutely necessary.

Epilepsy

Patients with epilepsy are at ↑ risk of seizures in the perioperative period. The commonest risk factor for perioperative seizure is poor preoperative seizure control. Others include alcohol withdrawal, subtherapeutic anticonvulsant levels, missed medications, and sleep deprivation.

Perioperative management

Patients with epilepsy should have their antiepileptic drugs (AEDs) continued perioperatively, ideally orally on the morning of surgery with sips of water. If the oral route is not possible, AEDs can be given parenterally/IV (Table 4.9).

Myasthenia gravis

Myasthenia gravis (MG) is an autoimmune disorder of the neuromuscular junction that results in weakness of skeletal muscle; it can result in respiratory muscle compromise and bulbar symptoms.

MG patients react unpredictably to a number of anaesthetic agents, namely NMBAs, due to the disease and acetylcholinesterases used to treat it.

Perioperative management

Preoperative

• Anaesthetic review to determine the need for post-operative critical care and modification of anaesthetic technique (e.g. avoidance of NBMAs).

Table 4.9 Alternative routes of administration of various drugs

Tablet	Other preparations	Dose conversion	Notes
Carbamazepine	Liquid for NG PR suppository (max. 7 days)	1:1 total daily dose 100mg = 125mg suppository	Liquid/PR available for IR only; if on MR preparation, split total daily dose into BD/TDS
Levetiracetam	Liquid/crushable tablets with water for NG IV	1:1 1:1	
Sodium valproate	Liquid/crushable tablets for NG IV	1:1 1:1	
Phenytoin	Liquid for NG IV	Discuss with pharmacy 1:1	Poorly absorbed in conjunction with NG feeding ECG monitoring needed
Lamotrigine	Nil	n/a	Discuss with neurology if multiple doses will be missed

NG, nasogastric; PR, per rectum; IR, immediate release; MR, modified release; BD, twice daily; TDS, three times daily.

- In elective surgery, obtain preoperative pulmonary function tests to include forced vital capacity (FVC) as baseline for perioperative monitoring.
- Vital capacity of <2 to 2.9L may be a risk factor for crisis and need for post-operative ventilation on ITU.

At surgery
- Ensure close liaison with neurology and/or perioperative medicine team throughout admission.
- Continue pyridostigmine up to, and including, the morning of surgery.
- Ideally, operate first on the list.
- Meticulous post-operative monitoring of vital capacity; assess for bulbar weakness, change in phonation, and aspiration.
- If on steroid, double-dose perioperatively for 48h to accommodate stress response (if taking >10mg prednisolone daily).
- Continue immunomodulatory therapy through perioperative period.
- If oral route not possible in the perioperative period, then oral pyridostigmine can be converted to IV neostigmine—discuss with neurology and pharmacy.
- Avoid medications which may precipitate myasthenic crisis (e.g. aminoglycosides, clindamycin, fluoroquinolones, vancomycin, β-blockers, magnesium).

Endocrinology
Diabetes mellitus
Diabetes affects 10–15% of the surgical population. These patients have higher complication and mortality rates, and ↑ length of inpatient stay.

Perioperative management
The guidelines below are based on the Joint British Diabetes Societies (JBDS) for inpatient care guidelines.

Planning for surgery
- Early preoperative assessment is important to establish a perioperative diabetes management strategy.
- If HbA1c >69mmol/mol, consider referral to diabetes team for optimization.
- Aim for day-of-surgery admission where possible.
- Prioritize on the theatre list; aim for short starvation periods (i.e. only one meal missed, allowing avoidance of variable-rate insulin infusion (VRII)).
- Ensure all patients are prescribed emergency treatment for hypoglycaemia on their drug chart (i.e. Glucogel® and 20% glucose). Rapid-acting insulin should also be prescribed for hyperglycaemia.
- Ensure usual diabetes medications are prescribed with the appropriate adjustments (see local/national guidance, including NICE guidance).
- Be aware of coexisting PVD or neuropathy, which are contraindications to TEDS.

Perioperative blood sugar monitoring
- Capillary blood glucose (CBG) levels should be monitored at least hourly during the procedure and in the immediate post-operative period.

- Target should be 6–10mmol/L (up to 12mmol/L may be appropriate in certain patients)
- Ensure early referral to diabetes or perioperative medicine team if unable to maintain CBG within this range.

Management of perioperative hyperglycaemia
- If blood glucose >12mmol/L, need to check capillary ketones.
- If capillary blood ketones are >3mmol/L (or urinary ketones > +++), then need urgent blood gas to check pH.
  - If acidotic, then manage as per diabetic ketoacidosis (DKA) protocol and contact diabetes specialist/perioperative medicine team in normal hours or the on-call medical team if out of hours.
  - If pH normal, then likely appropriate to manage with VRII; contact diabetes specialist/perioperative medicine team in normal hours or the on-call medical team if out of hours.
- If capillary ketones <3mmol/L, give subcutaneous rapid-acting insulin analogue.
  - Type 1 diabetes: where possible, take advice from the patient about the number of units normally required to correct high CBG.
  - Type 2 diabetes: JBDS for Inpatient Care Group (JBDS-IP) guidelines recommend giving 0.1U/kg.
  - Recheck CBG an hour later to ensure it is falling.
  - Repeat the subcutaneous insulin dose after 2h if CBG still >12mmol/L (consider ↑ the dose if the response is inadequate).
  - Recheck blood glucose after 1h—if not falling, consider VRII.

Stress hyperglycaemia
- Hyperglycaemia may occur in patients not known previously to be diabetic.
- These patients are still at high risk of post-operative morbidity and mortality—need to manage in the same way as if known diabetes.
- If CBGs normalize, patient should have glucose tolerance test or fasting blood glucose in primary care 6 weeks later.
- If CBGs remain elevated once acute episode has resolved, diabetes can be diagnosed without formal testing.

Management of perioperative hypoglycaemia
- If CBG is 4–6mmol/L and the patient is symptomatic: consider giving 50–100mL of 10% glucose IV stat and repeat CBG after 10min.
- If CBG is <4mmol/L: give 100mL of 20% glucose (i.e. 400mL/h by using an infusion pump) and repeat the CBG after 10min.
- Persistent hypoglycaemia is a medical emergency—discuss urgently with the diabetic specialist team or on-call medical team.

Use of variable-rate insulin infusion
- Previously known as a 'sliding scale'.
- VRII involves infusing a constant rate of glucose-containing fluid as substrate, while infusing insulin at a variable rate.
- Indications for VRII include:
  - Patient with type 1 diabetes with a starvation period of >1 missed meal or who have not received background insulin

- Patient with type 2 diabetes with a starvation period of >1 missed meal or who develop hyperglycaemia (CBG >12mmol/L)
- Patients with poorly controlled diabetes (e.g. HbA1c >69mmol/mol)
- Likely needed in the majority of emergency surgery patients.
- Long-acting insulin analogues (e.g. Levemir®, Lantus®, Tresiba®) should be continued at 80% of the usual dose.
- Short- and intermediate-acting insulins should be held while the patient is on VRII.
- Each organization will have its own specific proforma for prescription, monitoring, and dose adjustment of VRII. Use it.
- There are generally three rates of VRII: standard, reduced, and ↑. Which one to use depends on how many units of insulin a patient takes per day.
- Initial insulin infusion rate is determined by CBG prior to commencement.
- Fluids are required to run alongside the VRII to supply a steady state of substrate and sodium, thereby preventing hypoglycaemia. Guidelines advocate the use of 0.45% saline with 5% glucose and 0.15% potassium chloride (KCl) as the first-choice solution.

Thyroid disease

Routine preoperative thyroid function testing is not recommended for patients with no history of thyroid disease or concerning signs or symptoms. In patients with known thyroid disease on treatment, TSH should be included in the preoperative assessment if it has not been checked in the past 6 months. Euthyroid patients do not need any special consideration prior to surgery.

Perioperative management

Hypothyroidism

- *Subclinical/mild* (largely asymptomatic; elevated TSH, normal serum free thyroxine (T4)):
  - No need to delay surgery.
- *Moderate* (signs and symptoms of overt hypothyroidism; elevated TSH, low free T4):
  - *Elective:* delay until euthyroid
  - *Urgent:* proceed with surgery, accepting the risk of possible minor perioperative complications (e.g. hypotension, hyponatraemia, postoperative ileus, neuropsychiatric).
- *Severe* (very low free T4—e.g. <0.5ng/dL):
  - *Elective:* delay until euthyroid.
- *Urgent:* if surgery must be performed, begin treatment of hypothyroidism as soon as possible. Discuss with endocrinology (likely to need triiodothyronine (T3) and T4 to rapidly normalize thyroid function and prevent myxoedema coma) and ITU (likely to need level 2 care post-operatively).

Hyperthyroidism

- *Subclinical hyperthyroidism* (suppressed TSH, with normal free T4 and T3):

- Reasonable to proceed with elective or urgent surgery
- If no contraindications, consider commencing preoperative β-blocker (e.g. 25–50mg atenolol) in older patients/younger patients with a history of arrhythmia, then wean to stop after surgery.
- *Overt hyperthyroidism* (suppressed TSH, with elevated free T4 and/or T3):
  - Surgery in patients with untreated or poorly controlled hyperthyroidism can precipitate decompensation with thyroid storm—life-threatening
  - *Elective surgery:* delay until patient euthyroid
  - *Urgent surgery:* discuss with endocrinology, and initiate treatment as soon as possible.
    ○ *β-blockers:* start atenolol 25–50mg and titrate as necessary to aim for heart rate <80. Continue until thyroid disease under control.
    ○ *Thionamides* (e.g. propylthiouracil (PTU), carbimazole): used in Graves' disease, toxic adenoma, and toxic multinodular goitre. Block new thyroid hormone synthesis but does not affect release of preformed hormone from the thyroid; therefore, takes a few days to have effect on systemic hormone levels.
    ○ *Iodine:* potassium iodide solution blocks release of T4 and T3 from the thyroid. Used in Graves' disease, toxic adenoma, and toxic multinodular goitre. In toxic adenoma and toxic multinodular goitre, it must be used in conjunction with thionamide; otherwise it can exacerbate hyperthyroidism.

Medications for thyroid disease
- *Thyroxine:*
  - T4 therapy has a long half-life; it can be safely omitted on the morning of surgery.
  - Patients only need parenteral thyroxine if oral intake is not possible for 5–7 days.
  - Can be given IV or intramuscularly (IM) at 80% of normal oral dose—discuss with endocrinology.
- *Thionamides:*
  - PR route possible if patient is unable to take oral medication for longer than 1–2 days; discuss with pharmacy and endocrinology.

Adrenal suppression
The two major categories of adrenal suppression include:
- *Primary:* due to diseases of the adrenal gland
- *Secondary:* due to hypothalamic–pituitary causes:
  - Those taking long-term steroids for other medical conditions (e.g. rheumatological or respiratory disease) can develop secondary adrenal suppression.
  - Prednisolone doses of ≥5mg per day (across all routes) for ≥1 month can result in suppression of the hypothalamic–pituitary–adrenal (HPA) axis.

During times of physiological stress (e.g. infection, trauma, surgery), patients with adrenal suppression are at risk of adrenal crisis due to inability to produce sufficient physiological cortisol. Insufficient cortisol production leads to loss of vasomotor tone and α-adrenergic receptor responses to noradrenaline. Progressive loss of vasomotor tone leads to orthostatic hypotension, followed by supine hypotension and then shock. Adrenal crisis is a medical emergency and can be fatal if not rapidly corrected.

Signs and symptoms of impending adrenal crisis
- Malaise, reduced conscious level, new confusion.
- Orthostatic hypotension, followed by supine hypotension.
- Hyponatraemia, hypoglycaemia.
- Raised CRP (but limited value in the post-operative period as usually elevated after major surgery).
- Persistent fever.

An impending adrenal crisis can be mistakenly treated as post-operative sepsis with antibiotics. Steroid supplementation should *not* be reduced or withdrawn while the patient is febrile.

Perioperative management of patients with adrenal insufficiency
- Hydrocortisone 100mg IV should be given at induction of anaesthesia.
- This should be followed by 50mg hydrocortisone QDS IV (or less pragmatically, a continuous IV infusion of hydrocortisone 200mg/24h) until the patient can take oral medication.
- Once able to take medication orally, patients should take double their usual glucocorticoid dose.
- This double dose should then be reduced back down to their normal pre-surgical dose, in most cases within 48h after surgery if recovery is uncomplicated.

Immunosuppressive agents

Common indications for immunosuppressant therapy include rheumatological disease, IBD, and organ transplant. Local and national protocols vary regarding whether (and for how long) these need to be withheld preoperatively (Table 4.10). Studies are ongoing to evaluate the impact of these agents on post-operative outcomes.

Corticosteroids

For advice about perioperative management of patients taking long-term steroid therapy, see Endocrinology, pp. 131–135 for more details on adrenal suppression.

Perioperative glucocorticoid therapy may cause a number of complications:
- Impaired wound healing
- ↑ risk of wound infection
- ↑ friability of skin leading to pressure damage, damage due to sutures, etc.
- ↑ risk of gastric ulceration and GI bleeding
- Hyperglycaemia
- Fluid retention.

If a patient is on high-dose steroid in the elective setting, it may be appropriate to discuss with the patient's rheumatologist preoperatively. In some circumstances, it may be possible to safely taper the steroid dose prior to surgery to reduce associated risks.

Table 4.10 Perioperative management

Drug	Recommendation
Non-biologic DMARDs: Methotrexate Hydroxychloroquine Azathioprine	Can usually continue Consider stopping if the patient develops a significant infection or acute illness
Leflunomide	Consider withholding one dosing interval before surgery
Anti-TNF: Adalimumab Infliximab Etanercept	Consider withholding one dosing interval before surgery
Other biologics: Abatacept Rituximab Tocilizumab	Consider withholding one dosing interval before surgery
Anti-rejection drugs: Tacrolimus Sirolimus Mycophenolate mofetil Or ANY medication used for anti-rejection purposes	*Always* continue

Frailty

Frailty is a physiological state in which multiple body systems progressively lose their in-built reserves, making a person vulnerable to external stressors and adverse outcome. It is estimated that 10% of individuals aged ≥65 years are frail; this rises to 50% of adults aged >85 years.

Frailty and outcomes

In older people hospitalized with acute illness, frailty is associated with higher rates of:

- Mortality
- Morbidity
- Delirium
- Adverse functional outcomes; institutionalization
- Readmission.

Co-management of frail patients between orthopaedic and geriatric medicine teams is associated with significantly improved outcomes, including reduced length of stay, time to surgery, mortality, and morbidity.

Assessing frailty

The Clinical Frailty Scale (CFS) is the most commonly used tool for measuring frailty. It is reproducible and can be applied at the bedside without any biochemical or physiological parameters. It ranges from 1 to 9 as follows, as shown in Table 4.11.

Table 4.11 Clinical Frailty Scale

1	Very fit	Very active and fit, exercises regularly.
2	Well	No active disease, but not as fit as 1
3	Managing well	Underlying disease, but symptoms well controlled
4	Very mild frailty	Independent, but evidence of slowing up or disease symptoms that limit activity
5	Mild frailty	Need assistance with higher-order IADLs (e.g. finances, transport, heavy housework)
6	Moderate frailty	Need assistance with all outdoor activities. Indoors they often need help with basic housework, climbing the stairs, bathing
7	Severe frailty	Completely dependent for all personal care, but relatively physically stable
8	Very severe frailty	Completely dependent for all personal care, approaching the end of life
9	Terminally ill	Life expectancy <6 months, but otherwise not frail

Analgesia in the frail older patient

Although frail patients may be at higher risk of complications of analgesia, this risk must be balanced against the substantial risks of inadequate analgesia. Remember that pain is often underappreciated in frail older patients who may not articulate their symptoms adequately. Furthermore, uncontrolled pain is a common cause of delirium, failure to rehabilitate, ↑ length of stay, and nosocomial infection in the older trauma patient. Always aim to treat dynamic pain (i.e. with movement). Failure to do so will prevent mobilization and recovery, so do not be fooled by pain control that is adequate just at rest. Follow the analgesia ladder (Box 4.1).

Paracetamol
- First-line analgesia.
- Good efficacy and safety profile; minimal cautions and absolute contraindications.
- Dose reduced if eGFR <30, liver disease, or weight <50kg.

Non-steroidal anti-inflammatory drugs
- NSAIDs and COX-2 inhibitors should be used with *caution* in older people: they can have significant adverse GI, renal, and cardiovascular effects.
- The lowest dose should be used, for the shortest duration.
- Should be co-prescribed with a PPI in older people with frailty.

Opiates
- Weak opiates are problematic: they have a significant side effect profile and do not allow uptitration for breakthrough with the same agent.
- Tramadol is highly delirogenic and poorly tolerated by older adults.

> **Box 4.1 Analgesic ladder in frail trauma patients**
>
> For frail trauma patients with moderate to severe pain, consider the following starting analgesia regime:
> - 1g paracetamol QDS regularly
> - Morphine sulfate solution 2.5mg QDS regularly, plus 2.5–5mg 4-hourly PRN.
>   - This is the opiate dose equivalent to 15mg codeine QDS.
>   - Uptitrate morphine sulfate solution as needed, depending on PRN doses needed and patient/nursing/physiotherapy feedback.
> - If eGFR <30: start with oxycodone dose equivalent: 1.25mg QDS regularly, plus 1.25–2.5mg 4-hourly PRN.
> - If CKD stage 5, consider hydromorphone or fentanyl. Discuss with pain team.
> - Macrogol 1 sachet BD/senna 7.5–15mg OD.
> - PRN antiemetic (check local guidelines).
>   - Ondansetron is very constipating, so to avoid if possible.
>   - Remember metoclopramide, haloperidol, etc. are contraindicated in patients with Parkinson's disease/Lewy body dementia.

- Thirty per cent of the population are unable to metabolize codeine to active metabolites, rendering it useless in approximately one-third of patients.
- Low-dose strong opiates should therefore be considered as starting agents in patients with moderate and severe acute pain in the setting or surgery or trauma.
- Patients should be carefully monitored for adverse effects of opiates (e.g. constipation, nausea and vomiting, sedation, delirium).
- Always co-prescribe regular laxatives/PRN antiemetic and naloxone.
- Daily review is required to assess the therapeutic benefit and adverse effects.
- Aim to de-escalate opiates as soon as possible.

Treatment escalation and advance care planning

In frail patients, it is important to ensure that discussions surrounding advance care planning (ACP) and treatment escalation form part of wider patient assessment and management.

The ACP process aims to create a summary of personalized recommendations for a person's clinical care in a future emergency in which they do not have capacity to make or express choices. Such emergencies may include death or cardiac arrest (Do Not Attempt Cardio-Pulmonary Resuscitation (DNA CPR)) but are not limited to those events. The process is intended to respect both patient preferences and clinical judgement.

Evidence shows that frail patients (CFS >4) are unlikely to survive to hospital discharge following an in-hospital cardiac arrest. Frailty is also associated with ↑ inpatient mortality and long-term mortality among older patients on intensive care units (ICUs). These factors will influence clinical decision-making and determine the ceiling of care (e.g. whether cardiopulmonary resuscitation (CPR) or escalation to ICU is appropriate).

Intraoperative care

Anaesthetic considerations on the day of surgery

General principles apply to all patients on the day of surgery, with complex or emergency patients requiring consideration of additional factors.

Preoperative

- *Ensure patients are adequately fasted.* Clear liquids encouraged prior to elective surgery, with most centres additionally allowing 50mL of water hourly while awaiting elective surgery ('sip till send'). Fasting ('nil by mouth' (NBM)) is required for all patients undergoing either general or regional anaesthesia for:
  - 6h for solid foods
  - 2h for clear liquids (including squash, black tea, or coffee) and carbohydrate-rich preoperative drinks.
- *Medication review:* ensure that instructions to omit key medications have been followed (e.g. anticoagulants, ACEIs). Patients can still take normal medications with a sip of water while NBM.
- *Emergency patients undergoing major surgery:* ensure fluid resuscitation prior to theatre if needed; check group and save and cross-match completed; ensure active warming if hypothermic before theatre.
- *Pregnancy test:* for women of childbearing age, this is usually indicated, particularly if intraoperative fluoroscopy is required (see local guidelines).

Intraoperative

- *Positioning:* careful positioning to avoid pressure areas (particularly the abdomen and ♂ genitalia/♀ breasts in prone patients, e.g. spinal surgery) and peripheral nerve injury (most vulnerable nerves are the ulnar nerve, common peroneal nerve, and brachial plexus).
- *Blood loss:* consider cell salvage if major blood loss expected (e.g. revision surgery, spinal surgery). Confirm the location of any cross-matched blood. Consider tranexamic acid use.
- *Body temperature:* perioperative hypothermia (temperature <36.0°C) is a significant problem, particularly in trauma, low BMI, or older patients. It is a risk factor for surgical site infection, coagulopathy, ↑ transfusion requirements, and adverse cardiac events. Forced-air warmer should be used for all patients whose anaesthetic time is >30min, and any fluids used should be warmed.
- *Antibiotic prophylaxis:* given at induction for most procedures before tourniquet inflated, or after infective samples taken. This is one of the most important ways to reduce deep infection in arthroplasty surgery. One to two further post-operative doses may be needed following longer procedures (see local guidelines).
- *Tourniquets:* inflate to around 100mmHg above systolic BP (250mmHg upper limb and 300mmHg lower limb are often used). Maximum inflation time is usually around 1.5h (upper limb) and 2h (lower limb), after which a period of reperfusion (around 10min) is needed to avoid injury (muscle, nerve, skin, or vasculature). Inflation is associated with pain (can be after 10–15min) and rising BP and HR. On deflation, reperfusion occurs, with a drop in temperature, BP, and pH, and an

↑ in carbon dioxide. Contraindicated in sickle-cell disease, as it will precipitate a crisis.

- *Thromboprophylaxis:* ensure graduated compression stockings (unless contraindicated, e.g. PVD, severe neuropathy) and intermittent pneumatic device or foot pumps.
- *Cementing:* often associated with hypotension—must communicate with the anaesthetist prior to cementing or reaming. Bone cement implantation syndrome is a rare emergency caused by fat embolization as a result of high intramedullary pressures developing during (femoral) canal preparation and cement insertion/pressurization; presents with hypotension, hypoxia, and loss of consciousness (if awake), and can lead to death.
- *Venous air embolism:* an emergency where air is entrained into the vascular system, causing cardiovascular collapse. Most likely when the operative site is above the level of the heart and when surgery is performed in the sitting position (e.g. shoulder surgery). Immediate management is supportive, along with flooding the operative field with saline to prevent further entrainment.

Post-operative

- *Analgesia:* appropriate analgesia is extremely important in the immediate post-operative period. It ensures patient comfort, and facilitates physiotherapy and enhanced recovery; it reduces the likelihood of developing chronic pain (see ➲ Analgesia, pp. 145–148).
- *Fluid management:* most patients are able to eat and drink as soon as they are recovered from anaesthesia; ongoing IV fluids are not usually required. Maintenance fluids may be required in patients who are unable to resume normal intake, but slow infusions of IV fluid over several days should normally be avoided. Boluses of fluid in response to hypotension (e.g. bleeding, sepsis) should be given after an ABCDE assessment of the patient, with response to the fluid bolus assessed.
- *Oxygen:* patients who have undergone general anaesthesia normally require oxygen post-operatively. Oxygen should be titrated to achieve patient-specific goals; for the majority of patients, this is 94–98% saturations, or 88–92% for those at risk of hypercapnic respiratory failure. Overoxygenating can cause harm and so should be avoided.
- *Thromboprophylaxis:* patients undergoing orthopaedic procedures are at higher risk of post-operative VTE; all patients should have a VTE risk assessment on admission. Thromboprophylaxis should be as per NICE/local guidelines and can be mechanical (compression stockings or foot pump devices) and pharmacological (anticoagulants). Patients at risk of significant post-operative bleeding or with additional injuries (polytrauma) may have post-operative pharmacological prophylaxis delayed, with the decision reviewed at 24–48h; mechanical prophylaxis should be continued during this time.
- *Nausea and vomiting:* prompt treatment is important to ease symptoms and prevent subsequent related problems (e.g. dehydration, reduced absorption of drugs). Treatment should include antiemetics (Table 4.12), IV fluids if dehydrated, reducing opiate intake by using multimodal analgesia, and treating any exacerbating factors (e.g. constipation). Laxatives are commonly prescribed for post-operative patients in

Table 4.12 Commonly used antiemetics

Antiemetic	Dose (mg)	Administration	Doses per day
Ondansetron	4	PO/IV	TDS (maximum 16mg per day)
Cyclizine	50	PO/IM/IV	TDS
Metoclopramide	10	PO/IV	TDS
Droperidol	0.625–1.25	IV	QDS
Prochlorperazine	5–10	PO	BD/TDS
	12.5mg	IM	OD followed by oral dose
	3–6mg	Buccal	BD

PO, orally; IV, intravenous; TDS, three times daily; IM, intramuscular; QDS, four times daily; BD, twice daily; OD, once daily.

whom pain, alongside constipating (opiate) analgesics, can lead to ileus. The IV or buccal route is most effective for patients with persistent vomiting, to ensure absorption.

Mode of anaesthesia

Anaesthesia for surgery can be provided in several ways; these can be broadly grouped into general, regional, and local anaesthesia. The choice of anaesthesia depends on the operation being performed, patient comorbidities, and patient preference. All, except local anaesthesia, are normally administered by an anaesthetist.

General anaesthesia

General principles

- The patient is rendered unconscious by using anaesthetic drugs for the duration of the operation. These act on the CNS and are given either IV or by inhalation.
- The airway is maintained after induction of anaesthesia either by using a supraglottic airway device (such as a laryngeal mask airway (LMA)) or by endotracheal intubation; rarely, the airway is manually held open ('bag-and-mask' ventilation ± supraglottic adjuncts such as a Guedel).
- The patient either breathes spontaneously or is ventilated for the duration of the operation.

Specific considerations

- Physiological effects of general anaesthesia include hypotension (from a reduction in SVR) and reduced cardiac output (from negative inotropy). These are managed with vasopressors and fluid therapy intraoperatively. Anaesthesia also affects the respiratory system by creating changes in lung ventilation and perfusion.
- These physiological changes are tolerated and managed safely for most patients. However, for patients with significant respiratory or

cardiovascular comorbidities, it may be that avoidance of general anaesthesia by using regional techniques is preferable.

- Induction and emergence from general anaesthesia are the most critical moments where significant problems can arise; the anaesthetic team should not be interrupted during these times.
- General anaesthesia can be combined with regional anaesthetic techniques in some circumstances.

Regional anaesthesia

General principles

- Regional anaesthesia can be differentiated further into neuraxial blocks (spinal and epidural anaesthesia) and peripheral nerve blocks.
- Regional techniques are increasingly popular, as they can provide post-operative analgesia and mitigate the risks of general anaesthesia for higher-risk patients, while reducing anaesthetic recovery time.
- They are contraindicated in patients with abnormal coagulation or overlying infection at the site of injection, or if the patient refuses.

Specific considerations

- The smallest needle should be used for injection of local anaesthetic where possible—25G for initial infiltration.
- Inject slowly to avoid discomfort.
- Always aspirate to confirm the needle tip is not in a vessel prior to injecting.
- Safe doses are drug-specific and calculated by using the patient's body weight.
- *Local anaesthetic toxicity* can result from overdosing local anaesthetic beyond the safe volume or from inadvertent intravascular injection causing cardio- and neurotoxicity; this is an emergency.
  - *Symptoms and signs:* perioral tingling, tinnitus, a sense of impending doom, arrhythmias, seizures, or even cardiac arrest.
  - *Management:* any local anaesthetic being infused should be stopped; administer Intralipid® to which the on-call anaesthetist will have access.

Neuraxial blocks

General principles

- Include both spinal and epidural anaesthesia, and can be used to anaesthetize for lower limb surgery.
- Spinal anaesthesia involves a one-off dose of local anaesthetic (with/without an opiate) into the subarachnoid space.
  - Local anaesthetic causes a dense sensory and motor block of rapid onset (<10min).
  - Level of the block achieved depends on the volume of anaesthetic injected, but is always administered below L2 level to avoid spinal cord damage.
- Epidural anaesthesia involves catheter insertion and infusion of local anaesthetic into the epidural potential space.
  - Local anaesthetic (usually with opiates) is infused into the epidural space, causing sensory loss, normally with retention of motor function, over 30min.

- Level of the block is dependent on the insertion site of the epidural and the volume of the infusion administered, and the density of the block by the strength of local anaesthetic used.
- Epidurals are most commonly used for intra- and post-operative analgesia, and are rarely used as the primary mode of anaesthesia.
- Spinal and epidural anaesthesia can be used in combination, usually for longer procedures.

Specific considerations

- Spinal anaesthesia can maintain operative conditions for up to 2h; shorter-acting agents can be used for day-case surgery to facilitate more rapid return of function.
- Epidural anaesthesia can be maintained for longer periods of time via ongoing infusion.
- All neuraxial techniques block sympathetic nerve fibres, causing hypotension from reduced SVR; this is more pronounced with spinal anaesthesia, and is managed with vasopressors and fluid therapy intraoperatively.
- Neuraxial techniques have an ↑ likelihood of causing urinary retention, particularly if opiates are added to the local anaesthetic mixture.
- *Complications:* CSF leak from dural puncture, nerve damage, or, very rarely, haematoma or abscess (emergency—causes compression of the spinal cord or nerve roots, or cauda equina, leading to complete or progressive motor and sensory block below the site of insertion. More likely with epidurals. Without prompt treatment, this can lead to permanent paralysis—contact the on-call anaesthetist urgently if suspected).

Peripheral nerve blocks

General principles

- Nerve plexuses or individual peripheral nerves supplying the surgical site are blocked by using local anaesthetic under US guidance.
- Depending on the surgical site, this may involve blocking more than one nerve to achieve satisfactory anaesthesia.
- Resulting motor and sensory block evolves over 10–20min.
- Blocks can be used as the sole method of anaesthesia, in combination with general anaesthesia or sedation, or to provide intra- and post-operative analgesia.

Specific considerations

- Length of block depends on the local anaesthetic used; nerve sheath catheters can be inserted at the time of the block to facilitate local anaesthetic infusion to provide post-operative analgesia for >24h.
- Blocks should not be performed normally in patients at risk of compartment syndrome due to masking of clinical signs.
- Some blocks can cause specific side effects (e.g. interscalene brachial plexus block can also block the phrenic nerve on that side, causing shortness of breath from diaphragmatic paresis).

Local anaesthesia

General principles
- Use of local anaesthetic to anaesthetize limited wounds or surgical areas.
- Direct infiltration into the tissue at the site of surgery.
- Useful for minor procedures.

Specific considerations
- Useful for a range of procedures and can be performed by surgical team.
- Able to deliver outside of theatre environment.
- Anaesthetic used dictates length of block; addition of adrenaline ↑ the duration of the block (reduced systemic absorption) and the safe total amount that can be given, as well as reduces surgical bleeding. Adrenaline-containing solution should not be used near end arteries (such as in the finger) due to the risk of terminal ischaemia.
- Local anaesthetics do not work well in infected tissue due to lower pH reducing the amount of unionized molecules.

'WALANT' ('Wide Awake Local Anaesthesia No Tourniquet')
- Increasingly popular technique for hand and upper limb surgery.
- Utilizes lidocaine with adrenaline to create a bloodless field.
- Adrenaline known to be safe in peripheries despite historic myths of it causing terminal ischaemia.
- Learning curve, but is cheaper and safer than other types (e.g. regional block, general anaesthesia), with quicker recovery. Also allows motor function to be maintained to test function intraoperatively (e.g. tendon repair).

Common local anaesthetic agents
Table 4.13 shows common local anaesthetic agents.

Table 4.13 Common local anaesthetic agents

Lidocaine	Onset: few minutes Duration of action: 30–60min Available strengths: 1%, 2%
Bupivacaine	Onset: 6–10min Duration of action: 2+ hours Available strengths: 1.25, 2.5, and 5mg/mL solutions Levobupivacaine most commonly used (except for spinal) as better safety profile
Ropivacaine	• Onset: 6–10min • Duration of action: up to 6+ hours • Available strengths: 2, 7.5, and 10mg/mL solutions
EMLA	• Mixture of 2.5% prilocaine and 2.5% lidocaine • Used for topical anaesthesia prior to cannulation or injection (children) • Takes at least 1h to work, thick layer needed

Analgesia

Appropriate analgesia is extremely important in the immediate post-operative period, as well as later in the surgical journey. It ensures patient comfort, facilitates physiotherapy, enhances recovery, reduces the physiological stress response to surgery, and improves outcomes, while also reducing the likelihood of developing chronic pain.

Analgesia should be bespoke to each individual patient, depending on the surgical procedure performed or injury sustained, the patient's pre-existing analgesia, and any organ dysfunction, but there are general principles to guide prescribing.

Pharmacological treatment

Once pain has been assessed, prescribing is normally based on the WHO analgesia ladder (originally described for use in cancer pain, but widely adopted for acute pain) (Table 4.14). See local guidelines—if pain is severe (i.e. limiting activity and preventing independence), then do not just start with mild pain prescription, but give multimodal analgesia appropriate to the stage of pain.

Table 4.14 World Health Organization analgesic ladder

Mild pain—step 1	Moderate pain—step 2	Severe pain—step 3
Paracetamol ± NSAID	Step 1 + weak opiate	Step 1 + strong opiate
Paracetamol	Codeine	Oral morphine
Ibuprofen	Dihydrocodeine	Oral oxycodone
Naproxen	Tramadol	IV opiates—local guidelines

- Avoid NSAIDs in older patients or those with impaired renal function. Consider a short, limited course, with gastric protection (e.g. PPI), if absolutely necessary.
- Some drugs are contraindicated or require reduced doses in renal failure and liver failure, or in frail older persons. Always consider these factors prior to prescribing, and check in the *British National Formulary* (*BNF*) if unsure.
- IV opiates require the patient to be monitored, as they are at ↑ risk of opiate toxicity and respiratory depression; it is not always possible to give them on a normal surgical ward for this reason (may require monitored bays, e.g. in ED—see local guidelines).
- Opiates have predictable side effects/complications; pre-emptively prescribe additional medications such as antiemetics, laxatives, and naloxone.
- *Patient-controlled analgesia (PCA)*: this is a pump device that delivers a bolus of opiate IV when the patient presses a button connected to the device. This is used for the management of severe pain with ongoing opiate requirements.
  - PCA can be used with morphine, oxycodone, or fentanyl (fentanyl used for patients with severe renal impairment).

- The usual programming is a 1mg bolus (morphine) with each button press, with a 5min lock-out before another dose can be administered. The lock-out duration and bolus size can be changed for patients with higher opiate requirement (e.g. chronic pain).
- A background infusion, in addition to patient-controlled boluses, can be set up; this is not routine and is used only for specific patients when indicated.
- For patients unable to press a button (e.g. severe arthritis, small children), alternative methods include an adapted button controlled by blowing into the device; alternatively, a nurse caring for the patient presses the button after assessing the latter's pain (nurse-controlled analgesia (NCA)).
- PCAs are managed and reviewed by the acute pain team, and normally arranged by the anaesthetic team (see local guidelines).

Adjunct pharmacological treatment
- *Nitrous oxide:* inhaled drug, useful for short-acting analgesia such as manipulation under anaesthesia (MUA) of a fracture. Can be delivered in the ED or on the ward. Penthrox® preparations are also available in some UK centres.
- *Ketamine:* NMDA receptor antagonist that can be given as an infusion for difficult-to-control pain. Not commonly used post-operatively and given under direction of anaesthetist/pain team. More commonly used in the paediatric ED environment to provide analgesia prior to fracture manipulation.
- *Anticonvulsants:* amitriptyline, gabapentin, and pregabalin are used not for their anticonvulsant properties, but as adjuncts in neuropathic (e.g. spinal radiculopathy) and post-operative pain.

Interventional treatment
This encompasses use of regional techniques and local anaesthetic infusions specifically for the management of pain. Patients with in-dwelling devices normally require care on specific specialist wards and should remain under the care of the pain team.

Epidurals can provide analgesia for the chest (thoracic epidural) and lower limb/pelvis (lumbar epidural). Local anaesthetic (normally with fentanyl) is infused via an epidural catheter. Attention to post-operative anticoagulation, including VTE prophylaxis, is paramount for patients with epidurals—for example, the epidural catheter should not be removed until 12h after a prophylactic dose of enoxaparin, and a dose should not be given until 4h after removal.

Common epidural problems
- *One-sided analgesia:* tilting the patient onto the side that does not have adequate analgesia can help the spread of the local anaesthetic to this.
- *Inadequate pain relief:* most commonly pain felt above or below the level of the epidural block; sometimes specific segments can be missed in the middle. Increasing the rate of the epidural infusion can ↑ the height of the block.
- *Inability to pass urine:* patient will require urinary catheterization.
- *Catheter disconnected from pump:* the catheter is a potential route of infection to the CNS and should never just be reconnected. The on-call

anaesthetist/pain team should be contacted—depending on the site of the disconnection, they may be able to restart the epidural or it will need removing and alternative analgesia initiated.

- *Hypotension:* caused by blockade of the autonomic nerves, causing peripheral vasodilatation. The first step is normally to give fluid boluses, although hypotension can be refractory, requiring admission to the high dependency unit (HDU)/ITU for vasopressors.
- *Itching:* normally a side effect of the opioid (usually fentanyl) in the epidural infusion. Initially prescribe ondansetron 4mg (if clinically safe to do so). If remains severe, the pain team may consider changing to an opioid-free infusion.
- *Additional analgesia:* it is normal for patients to take additional analgesia in combination with their epidural such as paracetamol, NSAIDs, and tramadol. Opioids such as morphine PCA, oxycodone, and morphine sulfate solution are normally withheld until the epidural is removed.

Nerve blocks can be placed pre- and post-operatively, to provide analgesia.
- Examples include fascia iliaca block for a fractured neck of femur, and erector spinae block for multiple rib fractures.

Nerve sheath catheters can be placed at the time of placement to provide ongoing analgesia via a local anaesthetic infusion; these should be placed under US guidance; patients should be reviewed regularly by the pain team. Most commonly, the local anaesthetic is delivered by a prefilled fixed-rate delivery device that infuses over 24–72h. These devices can also be used to deliver local anaesthetic into a joint or wound area.

Additional considerations

- *Post-operative pain:* immediate stronger post-operative analgesia to be given in recovery will be prescribed by the anaesthetist, but regular analgesia for the ward should also be prescribed before the patient leaves recovery. Transfer to the post-operative ward should normally be delayed until pain is well controlled.
- Patients who have undergone regional techniques may not develop pain until several hours after their surgery as the local anaesthetic wears off.
- *Breastfeeding:* codeine should not be used by breastfeeding women following concerns of excessive sedation in some infants. Opioid-sparing analgesia is preferable, although opiates are safe to use with caution—the infant should be observed for signs of abnormal drowsiness and respiratory depression, especially if the woman is also showing signs of sedation.
- *Chronic pain:* generally, normal pain medications should be continued (if no contraindications), with additional analgesia added to cover operative pain; these patients may need ↑ opiate doses perioperatively as they are not opiate-naïve. Acute-on-chronic pain can be difficult to manage and should be discussed with the pain term early.
- *Enhanced recovery after surgery (ERAS) pathways:* most relevant to hip and knee arthroplasty surgery; these 'rapid recovery' pathways involve a multimodal and coordinated clinical care approach, delivered by an MDT. Goals are to reduce post-operative complications and length of stay, while improving patient satisfaction and recovery. Optimizing analgesia to encourage early mobilization and rehabilitation is key;

pathways differ across units but can be divided broadly into *preoperative* (nutrition, physiotherapy/education, anaemia/medical optimization, pre-warming, oral analgesia), *intraoperative* (regional anaesthesia, short-acting sedative hypnotic agents, normothermia, normovolaemia, blood conservation, antibiotic prophylaxis), and *post-operative* (multimodal opioid-sparing analgesia, early mobilization, early oral intake, nausea prophylaxis).

Sedation

Providing sedation for a procedure outside of the operating theatre involves administering medications to achieve minimal to moderate sedation where no interventions are required to maintain a patent airway and spontaneous ventilation is adequate. Anything further than minimal sedation should only be carried out by those trained with sedation and/or anaesthetic competencies (anaesthetists or trained ED physicians) in an area with appropriate monitoring and resuscitation equipment.

- Minimal sedation with Entonox® or Penthrox® requires oxygen saturation monitoring and can be carried out by one immediate life support (ILS)-trained individual.
- Deeper sedation requires full monitoring, including capnography, along with full resuscitation equipment.
- Fasting is not mandated for minimal or moderate sedation where verbal contact is maintained.

Post-operative care

Perioperative ward round

When reviewing a patient on the ward round in the post-operative period, it helps to have a structure to follow to ensure you do not miss any important points (Table 4.15).

Table 4.15 Perioperative ward round algorithm

Check observations and ask about any symptoms	
Targeted examination	Should be guided by the injury/operation and any symptoms the patient reports
Pain	Ensure adequate analgesia
	Escalate analgesia as per WHO analgesia ladder
	Investigate any pain that seems disproportionate or is not explained by known injuries or surgery
Drug chart review	Do any of the patient's regular medications need to be held or adjusted in the perioperative period (e.g. anticoagulation, antiplatelets, antihypertensives, insulin and oral hypoglycaemics, etc.)?
	Important to review nephrotoxic medications in the event of AKI
Delirium screen	4AT as quick and easy screen
	Good practice in all patients aged 65 and over
	If evidence of delirium, look for, and manage, causes (see ➲ Delirium, pp. 129–131)
	Review drug chart for possible causes. Consider drug and alcohol withdrawal
Bowels	Ensure bowels opening regularly
	Regular opiates cause constipation—ensure laxatives prescribed
Bladder	Monitor urine output as marker of hydration
	Monitor for urinary retention
	If catheterized, aim TWOC ASAP—catheters risk restricted mobility, falls, infection, and delirium. Removal of a urinary catheter can promote enhanced recovery and early rehabilitation
Fluid balance	Especially important in patients with known cardiac or renal impairment
Capillary blood glucose (CBG)	Any issues with hypo- or hyperglycaemia must be managed appropriately (see ➲ Endocrinology, pp. 131–135)
Wound check	Any evidence of infection or bleeding?
	Consider when stitches or clips should be removed
VTE prophylaxis	Ensure on appropriate treatment (see ➲ Haematological issues, pp. 114–120)
	Make sure you have checked the weight; monitor renal function and platelet count. Review if these have changed

(Continued)

Table 4.15 (Contd.)

Check observations and ask about any symptoms	
Pressure areas	Ensure being checked and skin chart being completed; this is usually completed by nursing staff
Mobility and weight-bearing status	Important to encourage early mobilization, especially in frail patients at risk of functional decline and worsening sarcopenia
	Do not let inadequate pain control become a barrier to rehabilitation. Uptitrate analgesia if this is a problem
	Make sure weight-bearing status is made clear. This will impact on physiotherapy and OT assessment
Falls assessment	If injury occurred as a result of fall, identify factors precipitating falls (e.g. syncope, poor balance, postural hypotension)—falls in frail older patients will often be multifactorial
	Can any contributory factors be modified? Review drug chart
Bone health assessment	In older patients who have sustained a fragility fracture, check for risk factors for osteoporosis.
	Check Vitamin D level and replace if deplete as per local guidelines.
	Consult with an Orthogeriatrican with regards to investigating with DEXA/starting osteoporosis treatment.
	First line treatment anti-osteoporisis treatment is IV zoledronic acid**, in those with no contra-indication (most common contra-indications include CrCl <30, previous atypical femoral fracture, or previous osteonecrosis of the jaw). In those who are vitamin D deplete, rapid loading with vitamin D is required prior to administration of IV zoledronic acid.
Discharge planning and rehabilitation	Declare patients medically fit for discharge as soon as no medical or surgical issues mandate continued admission to hospital. This allows nursing and therapy teams to focus on discharge planning
	Ensure early physiotherapy and OT input in frail older patients
	Important to consider the likely discharge pathway on admission to avoid prolonged post-operative length of stay.

**reference = Antony Johansen, Opinder Sahota, Frances Dockery, Alison J Black, Alasdair M J MacLullich, M Kassim Javaid, Emer Ahern, Celia L Gregson, Call to action: a five nations consensus on the use of intravenous zoledronate after hip fracture, Age and Ageing, Volume 52, Issue 9, September 2023, afad172, https://doi.org/10.1093/ageing/afad172.

WHO, World Health Organization; AKI, acute kidney injury; TWOC, trial without catheter; CBG, capillary blood glucose; VTE, venous thromboembolism; OT, occupational therapy; DEXA, dual-energy X-ray absorptiometry.

Rehabilitation

Physiotherapy

Physiotherapy is a healthcare profession that helps to restore movement and function when someone is affected by injury, illness, or disability. It is a science-based profession and takes a 'whole person' approach to health and well-being, which includes the patient's general lifestyle.

For many patients who present in the elective or trauma orthopaedic department, physiotherapy is often required as the first line of treatment. Physiotherapists are autonomous practitioners and will take a pragmatic approach to fully assess the patient's problems and assist in rehabilitating and restoring function and reducing pain accordingly.

Rehabilitation involves a multidisciplinary approach to enable and support individuals to recover or adjust, to achieve their full potential, and to live as full and active lives as possible following an injury. Research shows early rehabilitation can improve mobility and activity levels, shorten the length of stay in hospital or off work, and greatly improve the quality of life.

A physiotherapist will:
- Complete a detailed subjective and objective assessment of the nature and extent of the injury
- Facilitate patients to set SMART (Specific, Measurable, Attainable, Realistic and Time-related) goals. Creating goals will direct a rehabilitation intervention towards a specific outcome meaningful to the individual, which can result in greater compliance and satisfaction during rehabilitation
- Review and update goals regularly with the patient. This can help to evaluate the progress of patient recovery and the success of the treatment intervention.

There are multiple treatment interventions widely used.

Education and advice

Giving general advice to improve the patient's health and well-being, and managing expectations and false beliefs are an important part of treatment.

Exercise

- Joint ROM exercises.
- Graded strengthening exercise programme to improve muscle strength.
- Balance, stability, and plyometric exercises for higher-level rehabilitation returning to sport.

Manual techniques

Methods include joint mobilization, joint manipulation, massage and soft tissue techniques, and minimal energy techniques (METs).

Hydrotherapy

- The warmth of water at 33–36°C allows muscles to relax and eases the pain of stiff joints, helping to exercise.
- The buoyancy of water can facilitate movement, ↑ joint ROM.
- The resistance of water can be used to strengthen muscles.

Cryotherapy

Ice/cold can be used to reduce pain and swelling by superficial vasoconstriction.

Transcutaneous electrical nerve stimulation

Transcutaneous electrical nerve stimulation (TENS) can be used for pain control and promotion of healing: sensory TENS (high rate) for acute-phase or post-operative pain; motor TENS (low rate) for subacute/chronic pain.

Functional electrical stimulation

Functional electrical stimulation (FES) is a technique that uses low-energy electrical pulses to artificially stimulate muscle contraction in a patient who has sustained an injury to the central nervous system.

Ultrasound

US heats deep tissues by high-frequency sound waves, stimulating blood circulation and cell activity and thus aiming to reduce pain and speed up the healing process.

Acupuncture

May be a useful modality to provide pain relief and assist in injury rehabilitation. There is some positive evidence for acupuncture, but NICE only recommends considering it for chronic tension-type headaches and migraines.

Upper limb

Shoulder

Patients in pain often develop poor patterns of movement and lose the ability to take their arm through the full range of motion. Joints can become stiff or limited by pain. Many shoulder conditions, such as subacromial impingement, rotator cuff tendinopathies, rotator cuff tears (partial and full thickness, degenerative, and traumatic), instability (especially secondary to hypermobility), and frozen shoulder/adhesive capsulitis require physiotherapy as the first line of treatment. In many cases, physiotherapy can resolve the problem. Referral to secondary care generally should not be considered prior to a patient engaging in a course of physiotherapy. Most patients requiring physiotherapy need to engage in an exercise-based approach, which requires compliance. If the patient has poor beliefs that exercises will not address their problem, then this generally affects their outcome. Be mindful of negative language, over-medicalization, and use of 'structural damage' terminology.

Elbow

The commonest elbow conditions that present are lateral or medial epicondylitis. These conditions are often difficult to treat and require a prolonged course of physiotherapy exercises to address. Other elbow disorders that physiotherapy can help with include biceps tendinopathy, mild instabilities (especially related to hypermobility), and low-grade ligament sprains (MCL/LCL). Physiotherapy is essential to treat/prevent post-traumatic stiffness. Again, the approach will be mainly exercise-based and require engagement and compliance.

Hand and wrist

Hand conditions that physiotherapy can help with include De Quervain's tenosynovitis, generalized OA/RA, post-injury, joint stiffness, and mild instabilities. Physiotherapists work closely with occupational therapists, who can provide scar management, splinting to support, offload, rest, or stretch contractures, and functional advice. Hand therapy has evolved as its own subspecialty, comprising a hybrid of physio and occupational therapy techniques.

Lower limb

Hip

Commonly treated hip conditions include OA, greater trochanteric pain syndrome, gluteal/proximal hamstring/adductor tendinopathies, femoral acetabular impingement syndrome, labral tears, psoas tendinopathies, and groin conditions. Physiotherapists will assess to help aid in diagnosis and formulate a progressive treatment plan accordingly.

Knee

Knee conditions that physiotherapy can help with include OA, ligament strains (ACL/PCL/MCL/LCL), patella/quadriceps tendinopathies, meniscal injuries/degenerative changes, fat pad impingement, and patellofemoral pain syndrome. Again, a progressive treatment plan will be formulated to help reduce pain and restore function.

Foot and ankle

Foot and ankle conditions include OA, ligament sprains, plantar fasciopathy, Achilles/tibialis posterior tendinopathy, and ankle instability. Strengthening, stretching, and balance work are often key factors in foot and ankle rehabilitation.

Examples of rehabilitation programmes

Example 1 (upper limb)

A 45-year-old ♀ with subacromial impingement pain. Presents with insidious-onset upper arm pain, with a painful arc on overhead movement.

The key aims of physiotherapy are to:
- Correct any scapula dysrhythmia
- Regain fluid overhead movement, with good muscle patterning
- Strengthen the rotator cuff
- Rehabilitate functional strength/endurance.

Example 2 (upper limb)

A 36-year-old ♂ manual worker with lateral epicondylosis.

The key aims of physiotherapy are to:
- Reduce pain and offload the tendon with splinting (an epi-clasp splint is helpful if a medial glide on the tendon reduces pain-free grip strength)
- Strengthen the wrist extensors (isometrically if pain levels high, progress to eccentric and concentric loading as able)
- Strengthen the rotator cuff (stabilize throughout the kinetic chain)
- Progress to functional loading and restore normality as able.

Example 3 (upper limb)

A 65-year-old ♀ with first carpometacarpal joint (CMCJ) OA.

The key aims of physiotherapy are to:
- Rest/settle down pain with use of a splint—off-the-shelf thumb spicas often help or can be custom-made by occupational therapists
- Strengthen pinch, grip, and globally around the wrist and forearm
- Advise and educate on activity modification to reduce load through painful area.

Example 4 (lower limb)

A 26-year-old patient following an ACL reconstruction whose goal is to return playing football.

The key aims of physiotherapy are to:
- Reduce swelling to enable full ROM, with particular focus on knee extension equal to that of the non-operative knee
- To facilitate muscle activity with focus on good quadriceps control (open-chain knee exercises are not recommended due to the risk of damage to the graft)
- Promote early weight-bearing and issue of walking aids as indicated (check post-operative plan as can vary among different surgeons)
- Graded exercise programme to ensure similar muscle strength and neuromuscular control of knee flexors and extensors on both the operated and non-operated limbs
- Progress to dynamic control, power, and endurance exercises
- Return to sport.

Example 5 (lower limb)

A 77-year old with bilateral OA of the hips whose goal is to improve standing up from a chair unassisted.

- Complete a full subjective and objective assessment of the lumbar spine and lower limbs, including neurological assessment.
- Set SMART goals with the patient.
- Education and advise about OA management.
- ROM exercises to improve hip joint flexibility and motion.
- Commence strengthening exercises, targeting specific muscle groups in order to sit-to-stand from a chair.
- Add resistance to progress strengthening exercises further (i.e. Theraband or weights).
- Assess sit to stand and modify as required (i.e. assess with aids or adjust height of chair, so that the patient's goal is achievable).

Example 6 (spine)

A 40-year-old taxi driver with chronic low back pain who wants to return to work.

- Complete a full subjective and objective assessment, including neurological assessment. Look out for yellow and red flags.
- Set SMART goals.
- Education is vital! Advise patient to stay as active as possible and continue ADLs, as prolonged periods of rest can worsen symptoms. Adults are advised to do 150-min exercise a week.
- Postural re-education—avoiding prolonged periods in one position.
- ROM exercises to reduce joint stiffness and improve ROM.
- Manual techniques, if indicated; however, this should be in conjunction with an exercise programme and not be an isolated treatment.
- Core-strengthening exercises—strong evidence to support group exercise classes such as Pilates or yoga can be helpful in managing back pain.
- Advise on how to manage 'flare-ups': analgesia, non-steroidal anti-inflammatory drugs (NSAIDs), use of heat/cold to manage pain, modification of exercises, avoiding to sit for long periods, manual handling advice, and signposting to services if patient needing psychological support or weight management.
- Return to work—encourage patient to modify their job if indicated (i.e. only complete short journeys initially, take regular breaks to change position, and optimize use of lumbar supports to avoid aggravating postures).

Orthotics and prosthetics

Orthosis

- An externally applied device used to control the motion of a body segment to:
  - compensate for muscle weakness
  - control an unstable joint
  - reduce a dynamic deformity to its fixed component.
- Named with respect to anatomy (e.g. ankle–foot orthosis (AFO), knee–ankle–foot orthosis (KAFO)) or to function (e.g. hip abduction spinal orthosis (HASO)). Less commonly named after people or places (e.g. Boston brace, a thoracolumbar spinal orthosis).
- *Leaf spring AFO*—allows dorsiflexion in stance and prevents foot drop in swing.
- *Hinged AFO*—as leaf spring, but better ankle varus/valgus control.
- *Ground reaction AFO (GRAFO)*—used for 'crouch gait' (weak plantar flexors); blocks excess ankle dorsiflexion in stance, so ground reaction force moves in front of the knee and passively extends it.

Prosthesis

A device that replaces a missing limb or body segment.

A prosthetist, as part of your MDT, will assess:
- Premorbid function (vocational and recreational)
- Cognitive state
- Expected function post-operatively.

Preferred levels of amputation for prosthetic fitting (always discuss with the prosthetist where possible) are 1 inch per foot of height below the knee joint (below-knee amputation) and 15cm above the medial joint line (above-knee). Following amputation, a preparatory prosthesis may be fitted; the definitive one requires a well-healed, stable stump.

Prosthetic elements
- Socket with a means of suspension.
- Shank (body) ± an articulation.
- Terminal device (e.g. solid ankle cushioned heel (SACH)), dynamic response (better force absorption).

Indications for amputation and prosthesis

Mnemonic PAT TIN:
- Peripheral vascular disease
- Anomaly (congenital)
- Trauma
- Tumour
- Infection
- Nerve injury

Further reading

Bodeau VS (2002). *Lower limb prosthetics*. Available from: ℘ www.emedicine.com

Colbum J, Ibbotson V. Amputation. In: Turner A, Foster M, Johnson S, eds. *Occupational Therapy and Physical Dysfunction: Principles, Skills and Practice*, 4th edn. London: Churchill Livingstone, 1997.

Walking aids

- Provide an extension of the upper extremities to help transmit body weight and provide support for a patient. Patients need upper limb strength, coordination, and proper hand function. Indications are to:
  - Improve balance
  - Redistribute forces across or unload a weight-bearing limb
  - Provide tactile feedback in patients lacking proprioception.

Walking stick

- Consists of handle, shaft, end piece, and ferrule (rubber bit on the end).
- Can be made of wood or aluminium—latter lighter and height-adjustable.
- Types include:
  - Single point or C-stick—basic cane with a single point at base
  - Functional grip stick—better grip and more comfortable than C-stick to hold
  - Quad stick—has four legs at base. Provides additional support but may slow patient down.
- Size walking stick from tip to level of greater trochanter, with patient upright.
- Hold on **opposite** side to affected hip (reduces joint reaction force in contralateral hip) and on same side for affected knee.

Crutches

- Better stability than stick, as there are two points of contact with body.
- With crutch placed 5–8cm lateral to the foot, the hand piece height should produce 30° elbow flexion, with wrist in maximal extension and fingers in a fist.
- Often used bilaterally.
- Made of aluminium, height-adjustable.
- Transfer 40–50% of patient's body weight (non-axillary; axillary crutches transfer more but can cause nerve palsies due to pressure).
- Hands are free to perform tasks.

Crutch gaits

- *Four-point:*
  - Left crutch, right foot, right crutch, left foot
  - Always three points of contact with ground
  - Used for ataxic gaits.
- *Three-point* (non-weight-bearing):
  - Both crutches down with weaker limb, followed by stronger, unaffected limb
  - Used for lower limb fractures/amputations.
- *Two-point:*
  - Left crutch and right foot, then right crutch and left foot
  - Faster than 4-point gait
  - Reduced weight-bearing in both legs
  - Used for bilateral weakness or ataxia.
- *Swing-through gait:* for patients with good upper limb and abdominal muscle strength.

Frames and walkers

- Provide maximum support.
- Slower for patient.
- May encourage bad posture.
- Limited use outside home.

Standard pick-up walker

- Requires upper extremity strength to pick up walker and place forward.

Rolling walker (wheeled)

- For patients with poor coordination and upper body strength (e.g. Kaye walker for child with cerebral palsy).
- *Others:* forearm support walkers (for patients with forearm deformities) and stair-climbing walkers.

Aids to daily living

Many patients require additional help on discharge from hospital with ADLs: mobility, self-care, communication, and ability to use environmental hardware. Assessment is undertaken by occupational therapists and physiotherapists, who may prescribe several assistive devices.

Problems and solutions

Mobility

(See ➲ Chapter 5, Walking aids, pp. 159–160.)

Self-care: dressing, feeding, toileting, bathing, and grooming

Problems faced by orthopaedic patients include:
- Limited hand movement and loss of fine motor control:
  - Eating: built-up utensils, universal cuff with utensil hold
  - Dressing: button hook, zipper hook, Velcro closure, sock aid, long shoe horn, elastic shoelaces
  - Bathing: long-handled sponges, wash mitts
  - Grooming: built-up combs and brushes, electric toothbrush, electric razors with customized handles
- Loss of function in one hand:
  - Plate guards and rocker knife to aid eating
- Impaired coordination and tremor:
  - Weighted utensils to provide accuracy of movements
- Impaired range of motion of shoulder/proximal weakness:
  - Reachers to open cupboards and pick up objects
- Impaired mobility for toileting:
  - Raises for toilet seat, bars around toilet, commodes
- Impaired mobility for bathing:
  - Tub transfer benches, hand-held showers, grab rails on bath/shower, shower chairs.

Communication
- Difficulty with holding pens: built-up pens.
- Difficulty with typing: typing stick.
- Impaired vision to read: large-print book/magnifying glasses, talking clocks/watches.
- Difficulty with using telephone: push-button dialling, voice-activated/speaker phones.
- Difficulty with calling for help: buzzers requiring minimal pressure, community alarm connected to local emergency services.

Environmental hardware
- Keys, light switches, doors, and windows can also be modified for ease of use.

Occupational therapy referral necessary
- Dressing aids.
- Toileting/bathing aids.
- Home adaptations (grab rails, ramp access, stair rail, etc.); home assessment required by an occupational therapist—should be discussed with them.
- Feeding aids.
- Wheelchairs.

Physiotherapy referral necessary

- Walking aids (sticks, crutches, walking frames); physiotherapist assessment required to prescribe appropriate equipment. Proper instruction important; not uncommon for various items to be used incorrectly and therefore inefficiently.

Specialist services required

- *Prosthetic limbs:* specialist field, needs suitable assessment and multidisciplinary approach to prescribe and train in the most appropriate prosthesis. Regional services exist and should be consulted early; when amputation is considered, advice from rehabilitation consultant is essential from the outset.
- *Orthotics:* referrals can be made for specially adapted footwear (e.g. shoe raises in leg length discrepancy, custom-made shoes). Seek advice from the orthotist in each situation, if necessary.

Long-term management of head injury

Head injury has a major impact on the patient, their family, and society as a whole. Careful assessment, setting achievable goals, and involvement of an MDT will aid in achieving the ultimate goal of community reintegration, but this may take many years. The goals of neurorehabilitation are to prevent and minimize complications, and to maximize recovery and function.

Issues in neurorehabilitation and some solutions

Medical problems

- Nutrition:
  - Build up to full oral intake once gag reflex and swallowing have been assessed to be present and safe.
  - Involve dieticians to ensure adequate calorific intake.
  - Patient's ability for oral intake may be compromised and/or unsafe. Enteral feeding via nasogastric tube or percutaneous gastrostomy/jejunostomy may be preferable.
- Neuroendocrine complications:
  - Reduced antidiuretic hormone (ADH) secretion (from posterior pituitary) causing diabetes insipidus; severe water loss and hypernatraemia. May require synthetic vasopressin (DDAVP).
  - Conversely, may be ↑ secretion of ADH; syndrome of inappropriate ADH secretion (SIADH) causing hyponatraemia.
  - Cerebral salt wasting syndrome; loss of both sodium and water in the urine, with loss of circulating volume and hyponatraemia.
  - Sodium imbalances may affect conscious level and may precipitate seizures.
- Seizures secondary to underlying brain injury:
  - Treated with long-term carbamazepine or sodium valproate. Benzodiazepines and phenytoin are reserved for acute treatment of seizures or status epilepticus.
- Pulmonary complications:
  - ↑ risk of pneumonia secondary to immobility, inability to clear secretions, and aspiration due to impaired gag reflex.
  - Chest physiotherapy invaluable in rehabilitation.
  - Tracheostomies for long-term ventilation prior to rehabilitation; consult intensive care/outreach team before any decision to wean.
- Bowel and bladder dysfunction:
  - Depending on the severity of brain injury, there may be loss of voluntary control, which should be assessed by continence nurse and appropriate specialists.
- Musculoskeletal injuries:
  - Fix long bone fractures early, where possible, to facilitate care and rehabilitation. Consider prophylaxis for heterotopic ossification (oral indometacin). Regular and early physiotherapy to prevent joint contracture. Antispasmodics, such as baclofen, may be required for spasticity, alongside use of Botox (botulinum toxin) to help relax soft tissue contractures as a precursor to soft tissue surgical releases.

Cognitive and behavioural problems

- Cognitive state: may be assessed by using tools such as the Wechsler Adult Intelligence Scale; incorporates memory and learning, attention, verbal and perceptual abilities, reasoning, and organizational ability.

- *Mood:*
  - Patients and families prone to depression.
- *Behavioural problems:*
  - Personality changes, aggressive behaviour, and anxiety
  - Family distress: address this to optimize rehabilitation following discharge of patient into community.
- *Deterioration in sexual relationships:*
  - Should be discussed and referred as appropriate.

Social problems

Occupational therapists will assess level of function and needs of patient:

- Assessment of level of disability by using scales such as the Barthel Index or Disability Rating Scale
- Assessment of ability to perform ADLs and providing aids if required
- Prevocational assessment and training
- Gentle reintroduction into household activities
- Supported work programmes
- Community reintegration—there may be a need for transitional living arrangements prior to reintegration.

Community services

Intermediate care

Recommended for patients requiring further therapeutic intervention out of the acute setting. Facilitates short-term focused rehabilitation therapy in medically stable patients with appropriate healthcare professionals: occupational therapy, physiotherapy, and speech and language therapy. Decision to refer based on multidisciplinary assessment:

- *Domiciliary (home-based):* patient safe to return home but needs further therapy
- *Inpatient:* usually based in nursing or residential homes according to a goal-focused rehabilitation programme
- *Community hospital:* referrals generated by ward team while in acute hospital or by GP in primary care. Patient remains under care of own GP who has local 'admission rights'. Places cannot be provisionally booked, and a post-operative assessment is required.

Social services care packages

Local social worker or care manager organizes appropriate package of care, based on multidisciplinary assessment ± individual case conference, to address particular needs (e.g. washing, dressing, feeding) (healthcare assistant).

Other community services

Red Cross

- Medical equipment loans not covered by the NHS (e.g. wheelchairs for outdoor use).

Age Concern

- Arranging delivery of shopping.
- Carer support.
- Telephone support for isolated or vulnerable individuals.

Home-from-hospital schemes

- Support visits after discharge from hospital.

Chapter 6

Basic sciences

Healing in musculoskeletal tissues

Stages of tissue healing

In general, healing in musculoskeletal tissues follows four phases:
- Haematoma
- Inflammation
- Repair
- Remodelling.

Healing occurs best in well-vascularized tissues, with haemorrhage from surrounding tissues and the injured structure. Some musculoskeletal tissues (e.g. meniscus, articular cartilage) have less capacity for healing than others due to their limited blood supply, particularly in adults.

Haematoma (minutes)

Bleeding secondary to trauma activates the clotting cascade, with a primary platelet plug and secondary clotting and fibrin. Platelets release inflammatory mediators, stimulating the next phase.

Inflammation (hours)

Phagocytosis of non-viable and necrotic tissue occurs. Further inflammatory mediator and cytokine release attracts mesenchymal stem cells to migrate to the injured area, and to proliferate and differentiate.

Repair (weeks)

Granulation tissue is replaced by tissue-specific matrix. Pluripotent mesenchymal cells differentiate into tissue-specific cells and create material close to the original tissue.

Remodelling (months)

Disorganized repair tissue is optimized to tissue approaching pre-injury structure and function.

Further reading

Broughton G 2nd, Janis JE, Attinger CE. Wound healing: an overview. *Plastic and Reconstructive Surgery.* 2006;**117**(7S):1e-S–32e-S.
Bulstrode C, Wilson-MacDonald J, Eastwood DM, *et al.* (eds). *Oxford Textbook of Trauma and Orthopaedics.* Oxford: Oxford University Press, 2011.

Bone

Bone is a specialized connective tissue, comprising cells (10%) that sit within a matrix (90%). The matrix is composed of an inorganic (60%) component that resists compression, and an organic (40%) component that resists tension (Fig. 6.1).

Functions

- Calcium and phosphate reservoir (99% of total body calcium in bone).
- Haematopoietic (marrow—erythrocytes, leucocytes, platelets).
- Mechanical support (skeleton—protect organs, muscle attachments).

Types

Bone can be classified either *anatomically* (long, flat) or based upon its *structure* at a macroscopic (cortical, cancellous) or microscopic level (woven or immature, lamellar or mature) (Fig. 6.2).

Composition

Matrix
- *Inorganic:* primarily calcium hydroxyapatite ($Ca_{10}(PO_4)_6(OH)_2$).
- *Organic:* 90% type I collagen. Also proteoglycans, non-collagenous matrix proteins, and growth factors/cytokines.

Cells
- *Osteoclasts:* multinucleated cells from macrophage/monocyte line. Resorb bone in Howship's lacunae. Lead cutting cones—primary healing/remodelling.
- *Osteoblasts:* from mesenchymal stem cells, produce osteoid (bone matrix) in response to bone morphogenetic protein (BMP), growth factor, and cytokines.
- *Osteocytes:* osteoblasts trapped by calcified matrix (90% of all cells in bone).
- *Bone-lining cells:* inactive osteoblasts, can be recruited if needed.

Blood supply

Bone receives 5–10% of cardiac output. In adults, three supply systems are interconnected. In children, the metaphyseal–epiphyseal system separates once the ossific nucleus appears, until the growth plate fuses.
- *Nutrient artery* (endosteal, high pressure): inner two-thirds of cortex.
- *Metaphyseal–epiphyseal system:* metaphysis, physis, and epiphysis.
- *Periosteal system* (low pressure): outer third of cortex.

In children, the periosteal system is dominant to allow circumferential growth. Interconnection between systems allows each to become dominant if the other is damaged. Normal flow direction is inside to out (centrifugal) but can become outside to in (centripetal) with injury.

Bone growth

Occurs by two mechanisms:
- *Intramembranous ossification:* ↑ the diameter of bones and completely forms cranial and facial bones, as well as part of clavicle. Mesenchyme-derived cells develop sites of ossification without cartilage precursor.

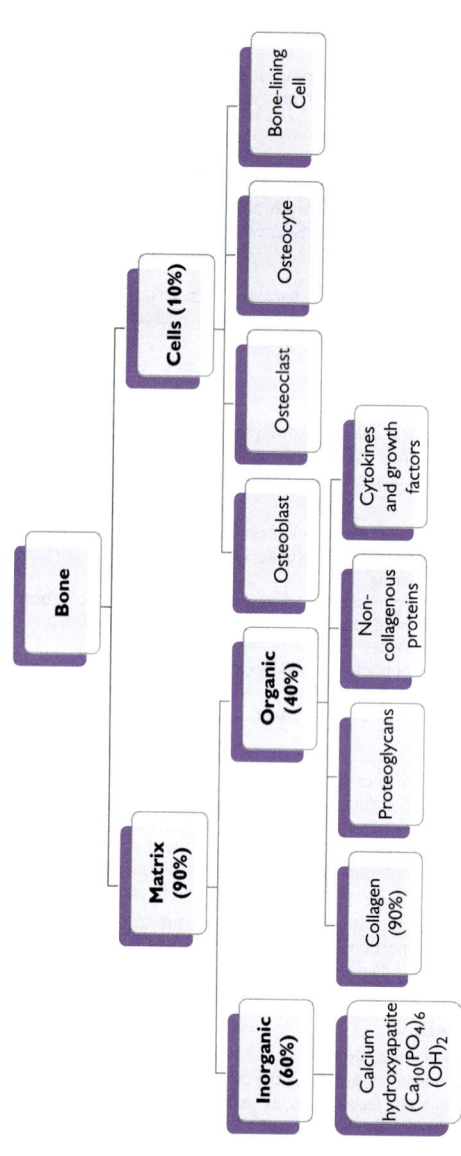

Fig. 6.1 Compostion of bone.

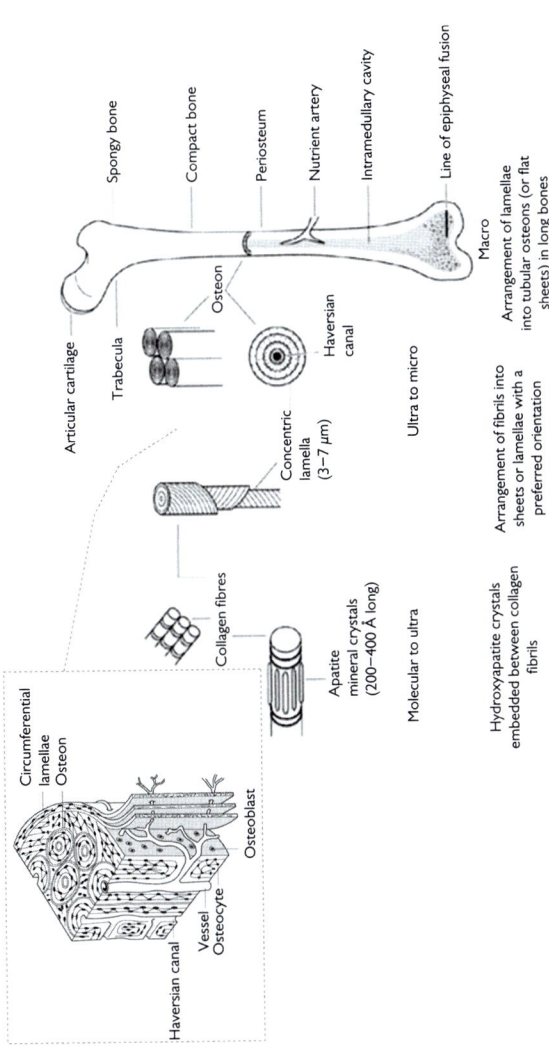

Fig. 6.2 Microscopic to macroscopic structure of bone.

- *Endochondral ossification:* all other skeletal growth. Primary ossification centres develop in long bones (all present by 12 weeks of gestation). Secondary centres appear at extremities at variable times after birth (exception in distal femur—secondary centre present at birth).

The physis

The physis is between the secondary (epiphyseal) ossification centre and the metaphysis, and responsible for longitudinal bone growth. It has several zones (from epiphysis to metaphysis) (Fig. 6.3):
- Reserve (or germinal)
- Proliferative (zone of growth)
- Hypertrophic (zone of transformation and calcification).

Significant nutrients required for longitudinal bone growth are held in the *reserve zone*. Physeal chondrocytes multiply in the proliferative zone and then ↑ in volume, principally by fluid swelling, preparing around them a matrix scaffold. Within the *hypertrophic zone*, chondrocytes prepare the matrix for calcification, and their eventual apoptosis further releases calcium, allowing full calcification of the matrix. Vascular loops from the metaphysis then invade this newly calcified matrix, and osteogenesis with remodelling begins to eventually create new laminar bone. Around the physis lies the

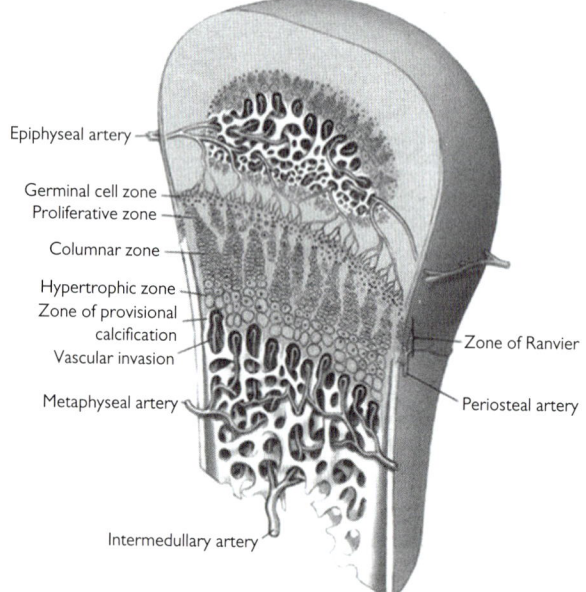

Epiphyseal artery

Germinal cell zone
Proliferative zone

Columnar zone

Hypertrophic zone
Zone of provisional calcification
Vascular invasion

Zone of Ranvier

Metaphyseal artery

Periosteal artery

Intermedullary artery

Fig. 6.3 Structure of the physis (growth plate).

perichondral ring of LaCroix, a membranous structure that provides vascular supply, as well as structural stability to the physis.

Biomechanics and response to injury are determined by:
- The strength and attachment of local ligaments
- The perichondral ring
- The shape of the physis
- Whether the fracture plane crosses the reserve zone.

In Salter–Harris I or II injuries, the reserve zone is not crossed, whereas it is in type III and IV injuries. The smooth capital femoral physis is less resistant to shear or torsion than the 'W'-shaped distal femoral physis, making the former more prone to a Salter–Harris I or II injury (e.g. slipped capital femoral epiphysis (SCFE)). On the other hand, a distal femoral fracture (also a high-energy injury) indicates greater disruption (i.e. the fracture crosses the undulating physis in multiple locations). A Salter–Harris fracture here is less likely to have a benign outcome, despite adequate reduction, as the perichondral ring is uniquely vulnerable to injury and predisposes to eccentric physeal arrest and can lead to rapid accumulation of secondary angular deformity.

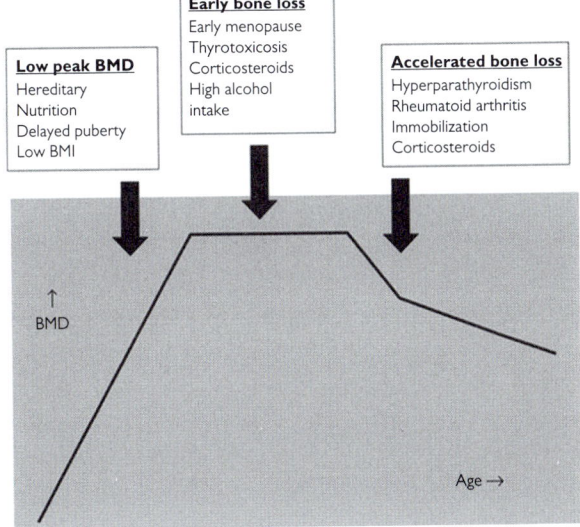

Fig. 6.4 Changes in bone mineral density with age.

Changes with ageing and osteoporosis

Peak bone mass is reached between the ages of 25 and 30 years. After the age of 40 years, bone mass ↓ with ageing; this differs in men and women due to the impact of the menopause (Fig. 6.4).

Further reading

Buckwater JA, Glimcher MJ, Cooper RR, Recker R. Bone biology: I. Structure, blood supply, cells matrix and mineralization. *Instructional Course Lecture*. 1996;45:371–86.

Fractures

Types of fractures

Always consider the mechanism of injury with any injury, as this guides management. In children, *always* consider whether the story fits—is this NAI? Children have more elastic bone with a thicker periosteum; hence, they sustain different injury patterns to adults.

- *Single-force trauma* (generally a higher-energy force): can be direct (e.g. transverse fracture) or indirect (e.g. spiral fracture/avulsion).
- *Repetitive force:* stress fractures (e.g. metatarsal).
- *Avulsion:* pull-off of bone fragment by tendon/ligament (children).
- *Impaction:* such as axial loading with fall from height (e.g. spinal or calcaneal fractures).

Different mechanisms impart different forces, resulting in fractures:
- Compression
- Tension
- Bending
- Torsional.

The fracture type/pattern is based upon the:
- Position of the limb/body
- Load applied
- Rate of loading
- Direction of force
- Bone properties (e.g. shape, quality, paediatric vs adult)
- Soft tissue forces.

Describing fractures

Fractures can be described in different ways:
- Anatomical location:
  - Which bone
  - Which region of the bone—proximal/middle/distal third; diaphyseal/metaphyseal/epiphyseal
  - Intra-articular vs extra-articular
- *Complete vs incomplete:* e.g. buckle vs greenstick in children
- *Open vs closed:* 'soft tissue injury with a broken bone beneath'
- *Simple vs comminuted:* segmental, butterfly fragment
- *Pathological:* is there an underlying lytic lesion/cancer?
- *With bone loss:* is there comminution? Is it a high-velocity injury?
- *Degree of displacement:* undisplaced vs minimally vs significantly
- *Type of displacement:* translation, angulation, rotation.

Further reading

Brinker MR. *Review of Orthopaedic Trauma*. Philadelphia, PA: WB Saunders, 2001.

Fracture healing

A series of steps that aim to restore bone to its pre-injury state. The mode of healing depends on the strain (Perren's strain theory): with <2% strain, *primary* bone healing can occur (no callus); with between 2% and 10% strain, *secondary* healing occurs (callus). In environments with higher strain or in-adequate stability, fibrous/granulation tissue forms (leading to non-union). The most important factors affecting healing are stability and bone blood supply. Head injury can ↑ osteogenic response, resulting in bone formation in soft tissues (heterotopic ossification). Nicotine ↑ healing time/non-union risk, and ↓ the strength of callus formed.

Primary bone healing

- Requires absolute stability with anatomical reduction and interfragmentary compression→healing without callus.
- Minimal activity for the first few days, then new blood vessels grow into the fracture gaps. Mesenchymal stem cells differentiate to osteoblasts, laying down lamellar bone in small gaps and woven in larger gaps.
- *Cutting cones:* osteoclasts tunnel across, creating a path for blood vessels/osteoblasts to follow (as in remodelling phase in secondary healing) (Fig. 6.5).

Secondary bone healing

The healing process produces soft callus, which is converted to hard callus (usually within 1–4 months), then remodelled. Four classic stages include (Fig. 6.6):

- *Haematoma (hours):* bleeding from fracture site and soft tissues
- *Inflammation (days):* haematopoietic cells secrete growth factors. Fibroblasts, mesenchymal and osteoprogenitor cells→granulation tissue
- *Repair (days to weeks):* soft callus forms within first 2–4 weeks. Type of healing depends on fracture stability and fixation, with amount of callus inversely proportional to the extent of immobilization. Relative stability allows controlled motion at fracture site under load. Movement stimulates healing: (1) either via primary cortical healing (intramembranous ossification—multipotent cells in periosteum differentiate to osteoprogenitor cells and produce periosteal bony callus, without cartilage formation); (2) or via endochondral ossification (fibrocartilage-bridging callus forms, calcifies, and is replaced by osteoid/woven bone)
- *Remodelling (weeks to months):* starts in middle of repair phase, continues several years after fracture has clinically healed. Bone attempts to regain normal configuration and shape, based on stresses applied (*Wolff's law*). Woven bone (disorganized) replaced by stronger lamellar bone (organized). Healing complete when marrow space repopulates. Expected speed of healing is different for different bones (e.g. a metacarpal usually takes 4–6 weeks to heal, and the tibia 3–4 months).

Remodelling

Various observations and principles exist, although this remains a poorly understood process:

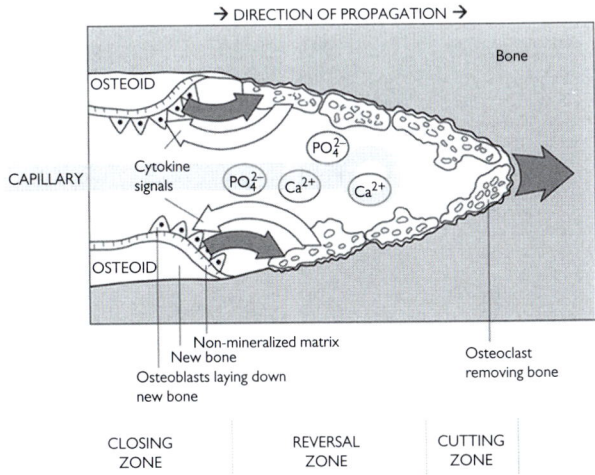

Fig. 6.5 Primary bone healing—cutting cone.

- *Wolff's law (1892):* bone will respond based on the stress or demand placed on it (i.e. the physical environment), explaining 'form follows function'. Bone formation and density are directly proportional to the applied load.
- *Hueter–Volkmann's law (1862):* the physis responds to load; hence, growth can be inhibited by mechanical compression and accelerated by tension. Blount's disease is an example where growth is inhibited due to excessive forces applied on the medial proximal tibial physis.
- *Angular remodelling:* influenced by age (younger patients do better, as there is time to correct), location of deformity (injury close to physis improves outcomes), and orientation (in plane of movement of adjacent joint improves outcome).

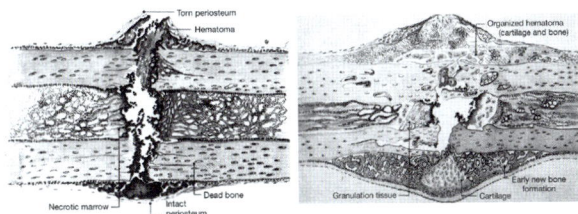

Fig. 6.6 Early phases of secondary bone healing.

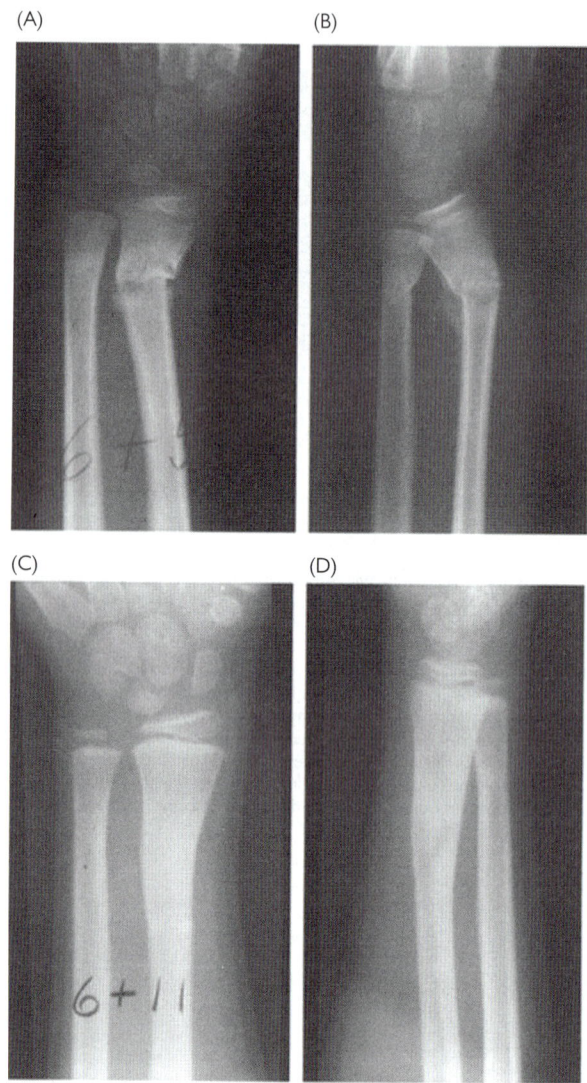

Fig. 6.7 Paediatric distal radius and ulnar fractures remodelling over 6 months.

- *Rotational correction:* very limited scope for correction of any rotational deformity.
- *Translational correction:* side-to-side displacement remodels very well, especially in prepubertal bone where 100% displacement may be entirely remodelled in 1–2 years (so 'bayonet apposition' acceptable if alignment and rotation corrected).
- *Length correction:* following fracture, overgrowth occurs due to physeal hyperstimulation by a variety of factors, but probably mainly vascular. Peaks at 3 months and complete by 18 months. Effects are minimal in the upper limb but can produce 5–20mm ↑ in length in the lower limb, most noticeable in the femur.

Fig. 6.7 demonstrates the remodelling potential in the paediatric skeleton shown in the natural healing and resolution of deformity following a proximal humerus fracture.

Further reading
Ramachandran M, ed. *Basic Orthopaedic Sciences: The Stanmore Guide*. London: Hodder Arnold, 2006.

Fracture non-union

Non-union is defined as failure of biological union of a fracture within a time frame by which that fracture is expected to heal. ~2–5% of fractures develop non-union. Union can be defined as either clinical or radiological, or both.

- *Clinical* union is the absence of pain and movement at the fracture site.
- *Radiological* union has varying definitions (e.g. bridging on CT, or either healing of three of four cortices or complete disappearance of the fracture line on 2-view plain radiographs).

Delayed union describes slower fracture healing than expected, which may, in turn, progress to non-union. Long bone fracture non-union cannot usually be determined until 6–9 months post-injury.

Hypertrophic non-union

- Non-union secondary to *mechanical instability* at fracture site; excessive motion prevents biological union. Characterized by hypertrophic bone ends and exuberant callus formation. Radiological 'elephant's foot' appearance of bone ends. Biologically active.
- Seen classically in fractures mobilized too early or with insufficient rigidity of surgical fixation to allow union. Examples include metatarsal and metacarpal fractures, fractures treated by intramedullary nailing, or ulnar nightstick fractures treated non-operatively.
- Treatment involves improving stability of the fracture (e.g. casting/ bracing, off-loading (non-weight-bearing), and/or rigid internal or circular external fixation. It is unnecessary to bone graft these non- unions or even open the fracture gap surgically. Rapid progression to union is seen when adequately stabilized.

Atrophic non-union

- Non-union due to lack of biological activity in fracture site. Most commonly seen in high-energy/open/infected fractures, in smokers, and with use of NSAIDs. Poor nutritional status and immune compromise are important considerations in this type of non-union.
- Classic cause of failure of internal fixation. Often seen in mid-shaft humerus, clavicle, and scaphoid fractures, and internally fixed tibial shaft fractures. Bone ends are usually sclerotic or osteopenic, without evidence of callus formation, and may taper into fracture site. Can occur with aggressive periosteal stripping during internal fixation.
- Management strategies include surgical debridement of bone ends, and autologous or allogeneic bone grafting (and possible use of BMPs). Rigid compression and stability, with either traditional compression plating or circular external fixation. This allows progressive distraction of an initially compressed non-union, according to principles of distraction osteogenesis.
- Use of electric field induction has theoretical potential and some evidence to support its use in certain non-unions.

Oligotrophic non-union

- Non-union secondary to excessive fracture gap distraction, post- infection segmental defect, extruded fracture fragments, or interposed avascular comminuted fragments. Commonly seen in the tibia.

- Minimal callus formation without hypertrophic bone ends, but biological activity present. Results from inability of biological effort to cross fracture gap. Cause of failure of bridge plating osteosynthesis.
- Treatment similar to that for atrophic non-union.

Fibrous union

Synonymous with non-union. Used to describe an asymptomatic non-union, with dense fibrous tissue bridging the fracture and giving some stability. Expectant management may be applied.

Pseudoarthrosis

- End result of non-union; mobile non-union site develops synovial characteristics with membrane. May be subdivided into *stiff* (hypertrophic) or *lax* (atrophic) types. Often painless. May be the end result of multiply grafted non-union attempts or recurrent infection, and, if asymptomatic, may be desirable to accept asymptomatic pseudoarthrosis.
- Management, if symptomatic, is similar to that of atrophic non-union, with addition of full surgical excision of synovial envelope. High risk of failure with grafted rigid internal fixation osteosynthesis. Preferred management is circular external fixation, with initial compression and subsequent distraction osteogenesis.

Infected non-union

- Infection is a potent cause of non-union. The pattern may be atrophic or hypertrophic. These non-unions always have segments of non-viable bone, with bacteria living in biofilms on dead bone.
- Treatment is complex, requiring excision and sampling of all infected tissue, with reconstruction by using external fixation (Ilizarov method). Prolonged specific antibiotic treatment may be indicated with systemic and local therapy.
- Referral to a specialist centre with a MDT is recommended.

Further reading

Biasibetti A, Aloj D, Di Gregorio G, Massè A, Salomone C. Mechanical and biological treatment of long bone non-unions. *Injury*. 2005;**36**(4):S45–50.
Panagiotis M. Classification of non-union. *Injury*. 2005;**36**(4):S30–7.

Biomechanics and biomaterials

Orthopaedic surgeons need to understand some key properties and interactions of the materials that either are used as implants or are present in the body. A *biomaterial* is something applied internally to a body part in order to enhance its function such as a joint replacement or an internal fixation plate. The behaviour of biomaterials is best considered by looking at their physical properties.

Stress–strain curves

Stress is the force applied to a material per unit of cross-sectional area (units $= N/m^2 = Pa$). *Strain* is the ratio of the resultant change in length of that material to its original length (a proportion—therefore, no units). When a material is stressed to failure, a plot of stress (*y*-axis) against strain (*x*-axis) will display an elastic phase over which the two values are directly proportional. The slope of this straight line part of the graph is the *Young's modulus of elasticity* (*E*); the steeper the line, the stiffer the material (Fig. 6.8). Elastic materials return to their original shape when deforming stress is removed.

With additional stress (i.e. beyond the '*yield point*'), the material deforms permanently; this is the *plastic* phase. *Brittle* materials show little or no plastic deformation before they fracture (e.g. ceramics, bone cement), whereas ductile materials display large amounts of plastic deformation (e.g. metals).

Viscosity is the resistance of a fluid to shear. A *viscoelastic* material, such as a ligament or cartilage, combines the behaviour of an elastic solid and that of a viscous fluid. Critically, its deformation in response to load varies according to the rate of application of that load. At low strain rates, it behaves as a viscous fluid, with no elastic (all plastic) deformation; at high strain rates, it behaves as an elastic (but brittle) solid. Injury to the ACL, for example, is therefore more likely at high rates of strain.

Other important viscoelastic properties are (Fig. 6.9):
- *Stress relaxation:* with time, a viscoelastic material held at constant length shows a reduction in internal stress (the principle behind serial splintage)
- *Creep:* the material progressively deforms under constant load (explaining why traction restores length and alignment to a fractured bone)
- *Hysteresis:* loading and unloading force—displacement curves follow different paths, so although the material returns to its original shape, energy is lost to the system as heat.

Tribology

The study of lubrication and wear (Greek *Tribos* = rub). Wear is the erosion of a solid surface by interaction with another. Lubrication is the introduction of various substances between sliding surfaces to reduce wear and friction.

Three main types of lubrication
- *Fluid film:* completely separates sliding surfaces.
- *Boundary:* failure of the fluid film to completely separate the surfaces, so that friction between them is determined by the properties of both the lubricant and the surfaces.
- *Solid:* when liquid lubricants lack adequate resistance to load.

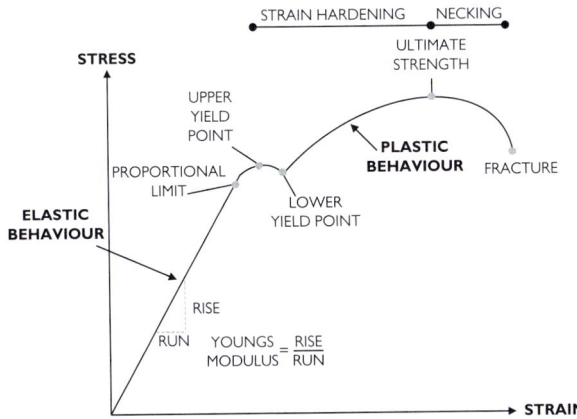

Fig. 6.8 Stress–strain curve.

Subtypes of fluid film lubrication
- Hydrodynamic: surfaces moving above a critical speed entrain fluid which separates them (*fluid film lubrication*). This is the rationale behind large-diameter bearing surfaces in hip replacement.
- Elastohydrodynamic: deformation of moving articular surfaces (e.g. cartilage, separated by a thin layer of fluid).
- Microelastohydrodynamic: as above, with deformation of surface asperities.

Other subtypes of lubrication
- *Squeeze film*: advancing joint surfaces, separated by a fluid front squeezed out between them.
- *Weeping*: fluid shifts from surfaces under load.
- *Boosted*: concentrated pool of large molecules left behind in areas under contact; solvent (water) is driven into cartilage.

Types of wear relevant to orthopaedics
- *Adhesive*: bonds form between sliding surfaces, so a thin film is stripped off one material by a harder one (e.g. metal–polyethylene bearing in hip replacement).
- *Abrasive*: surface roughness or asperities cause erosion (e.g. scratched metal bearing during implantation).
- *Fatigue-induced*: repetitive loading causes catastrophic failure by cracking and sub-surface delamination (e.g. knee replacement with thin polyethylene insert).
- *Third body wear*: small particles acting between sliding surfaces (e.g. cement particles or polyethylene debris).

Further reading
Ramachandran M, ed. *Basic Orthopaedic Sciences: The Stanmore Guide*. London: Hodder Arnold, 2006.

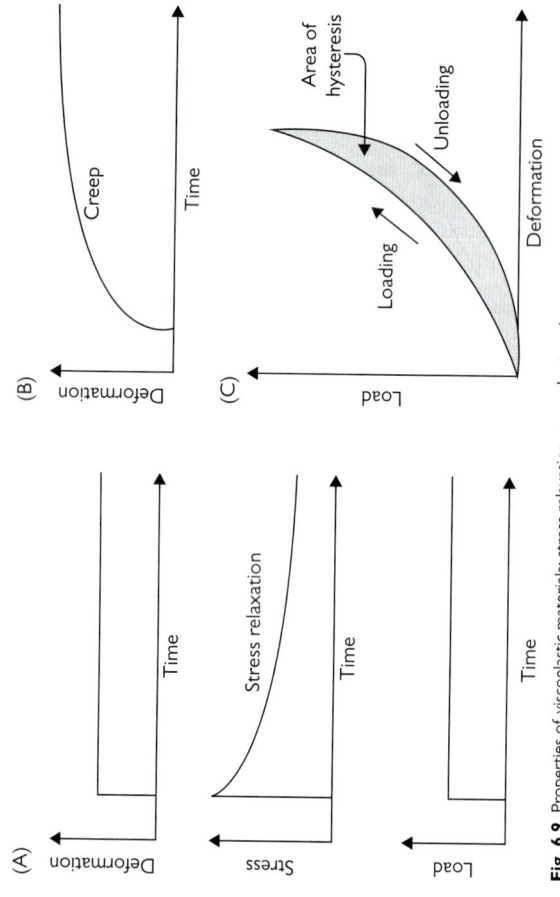

Fig. 6.9 Properties of viscoelastic materials: stress relaxation, creep, hysteresis.

Implants

These are non-living objects inserted into the body to perform a specific function and intended to potentially remain there for a significant duration. The ideal implant should be biocompatible (inert, non-immunogenic, non-toxic, non-carcinogenic), of sufficient strength, easily worked, free from corrosion, and inexpensive, and should not affect future imaging. Implants can be used to replace damaged or diseased structures, aid fracture healing, or correct deformity.

Screws

Transform rotational force into compression between two or more surfaces. Screws have a head, a shaft, and a thread (Fig. 6.10). The profile of the thread determines the pull-out strength (grip) of a screw. Bone screws, commonly made of stainless steel, are predrilled and tapped to cut a thread, although self-tapping screws are now commonplace.

Plates

Stabilize bone fragments, allowing early movement of muscles and joints. Compression at a fracture site encourages bone healing. Plate bending stiffness is predominantly related to the thickness of the plate (to the third power), as well as to the length.

Intramedullary nails

The tubular cross-section of long bones allows internal placement of a nail for stabilization after a fracture or an osteotomy, or for protection from an impending pathological fracture. Nail stiffness is proportional to the diameter (fourth power) and inversely proportional to the *working length* (greatest distance between points of bone contact or between locking screws). Locking screws primarily resist rotational deformation.

Joint replacements

Commonly made of metals (e.g. stainless steel or cobalt chrome) by casting from a mould. Joint replacements have a bearing surface where movement occurs (e.g. metal/ceramic on polyethylene for a hip replacement). Metal-on-metal and ceramic-on-ceramic bearings are alternatives with improved wear characteristics, although metal-on-metal hip implants have had issues with adverse reactions to metal debris.

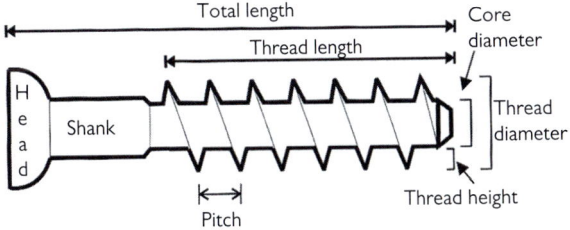

Fig. 6.10 Screw.

1	1a	Pistoning: stem within cement	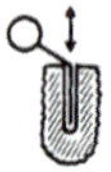
	1b	Pistoning: stem within bone	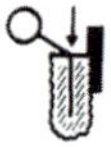
2		Medial midstem pivot	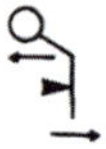
3		Calcar pivot	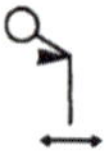
4		Bending cantilever (fatigue)	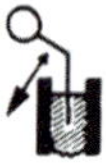

Fig. 6.11 Four modes of cemented hip replacement stem loosening. Adapted from: Gruen TA, McNeice GM, Amstutz HC. "Modes of failure" of cemented stem-type femoral components: a radiographic analysis of loosening. Clin Orthop Relat Res. 1979 Jun;(141):17-27. PMID: 477100.

Failure of implants

Implants can fail in several ways. Infection must always be excluded. *Wear* is progressive loss of material by either mechanical or chemical means; several different *modes* exist by which this can occur (e.g. two implant-bearing surfaces rubbing against each other or third body particles interposing between two articulating surfaces). In the absence of infection, this can lead to a vicious cascade, with inflammatory mediators causing progressive loss of implant and bone (osteolysis), resulting in 'aseptic loosening'.

Wear occurs by several *mechanisms* (may occur simultaneously):

- *Fatigue:* cyclical or repetitive loading of a material below its endurance limit, resulting in premature failure
- *Abrasion:* two materials with different surface properties or 'asperities' (e.g. hard on soft), causing one or both to damage each other
- *Adhesion:* bond formed between two surfaces, which can shear off material as they separate
- *Chemical means* (i.e. corrosion—a chemical reaction where material is removed from an object).

Failure of hip replacement implants

These most commonly fail by either infection (acute, <28 days postoperatively; delayed, >28 days post-operatively; delayed acute in previously uninfected prosthesis) or osteolysis (secondary to wear debris

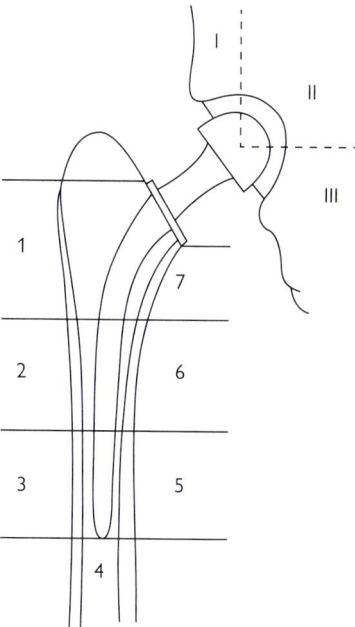

Fig. 6.12 Loss of bone can be described on radiographs, by either the Gruen zones (femoral component, 1–7) or DeLee and Charnley zones (acetabular component, I–III). Adapted from Gruen TA, McNeice GM, Amstutz HC. "Modes of failure" of cemented stem-type femoral components: a radiographic analysis of loosening. Clin Orthop Relat Res. 1979 Jun;(141):17-27. PMID: 477100 & DeLee JG, Charnley J. Radiological demarcation of cemented sockets in total hip replacement. Clin Orthop Relat Res. 1976 Nov-Dec;(121):20-32. PMID: 991504.

from articulating materials). Loosening an can be characterised by mode (Fig 6.11) and zone of bone loss (Fig 6.12).

Further reading

DeLee JG, Charnley J. Radiological demarcation of cemented sockets in total hip replacement. Clin Orthop Relat Res. 1976 Nov-Dec;(121):20-32. PMID: 991504.

Gruen TA, McNeice GM, Amstutz HC. "Modes of failure" of cemented stem-type femoral components: a radiographic analysis of loosening. Clin Orthop Relat Res. 1979 Jun;(141):17-27. PMID: 477100.

Miller M. *Review of Orthopaedics*, 9th edn. Philadelphia, PA: Saunders Elsevier (2025).

Tendon, ligament, and muscle injury

Tendon and ligament injury

Tendons are connective tissues that attach muscle to bone. Ligaments attach bone to bone. There are many similarities in the injury mechanisms, patterns, and healing between these two tissue types.

Factors associated with risk of injury

- Skeletal maturity (in children, growth plates/developing bone tend to be weaker than ligaments, so avulsions are more common).
- Pregnancy.
- Certain medications (e.g. steroids, fluoroquinolones).
- Immobilization.

Sites of injury

Insertion injury (avulsion) can occur with or without fracture:

- Mid-substance
- Musculo-tendinous junction
- Combination of both.

Mechanism of injury

The level of injury is related to the *rate* of loading and the *amount* of load. There are two main mechanisms:

- *Repetitive micro-trauma:* more common in tendons than in ligaments, as they carry higher loads. Repeated loading below the ultimate tensile strength leads to micro-tears. An inflammatory reaction is initiated in an attempt to heal, which leads to altered biomechanical properties, and can lead to calcification (seen on X-ray).
- *Macro-trauma—blunt or laceration:* blunt macro-trauma results in acute failure due to force above the ultimate tensile strength. Rupture can be partial or complete. Ligament fibres tend to rupture sequentially in different regions, rather than in one defined area.

Grading of severity

- *Grade I—mild:* some pain, no clinically detected laxity. Micro-failure of some fibres.
- *Grade II—moderate:* severe pain, some clinically detectable laxity. Partial rupture.
- *Grade III—severe:* severe pain at injury, less after. Joint unstable clinically. Most/all fibres ruptured.

Healing

Slower, more limited healing than bone (less vascularized). Phases include:

- Haematoma
- Inflammation—rapid response. Lasts from hours to a few days; debris removed and fibroblasts appear
- Repair (proliferation)—new blood vessels. Fibroblasts produce collagen matrix; inflammation ↓ over few weeks
- Remodelling—starts within weeks, can last years. Maturation, reorganization, and conversion of collagen to type I. Does not restore perfect tissue in terms of mechanical properties.

Tendon repairs

Weakest in first week (days 7–10). Most of original strength is regained by 3–4 weeks. Maximum strength by 6 months.
   Healing is affected by:

- Mobilization: controlled active movement (CAM) protocols are beneficial, and many rehabilitation regimes exist (e.g. Belfast, Kleinert, Duran)
- Method of repair: gold standard is 4–6 core strands ± epitendinous repair
- Quality of surgical repair.

Muscle injury

Injury is more common with inflammation following (especially unexpected) exercise.

Site of injury

- Muscle belly.
- Musculo-tendinous junction: weak site of muscle—tears often occur with eccentric contraction (lengthening).

Mechanism of injury

- Acute trauma (blunt).
- Laceration.
- Compartment syndrome (ischaemia).
- Crush injury.
- Denervation.

Healing

More proximal belly tears have a worse prognosis, due to a greater amount of tissue denervated. Healing occurs by dense fibrous scar tissue formation.

Further reading

Ramachandran M, ed. *Basic Orthopaedic Sciences: The Stanmore Guide*. London: Hodder Arnold, 2006.
Tang JB. Recent evolutions in flexor tendon repairs and rehabilitation. *Journal of Hand Surgery (European Volume)*. 2018;**43**(5):469–73.
Wu F, Nerlich M, Docheva D. Tendon injuries: basic science and new repair proposals. *EFORT Open Reviews*. 2017;**2**(7):332–42.

Articular cartilage

One of several forms of cartilage (fibroelastic—meniscus; fibrocartilage—tendon/ligament insertion; physeal—growth plate; elastic—trachea) (Fig. 6.13). Lines joint surfaces. Composed of extracellular matrix (type II collagen, water, and proteoglycans) and cells (chondrocytes). Nourished by synovial fluid at the surface and the underlying subchondral bone. Cartilage changes biochemically with age and in OA.

Functions
- Smoothing the articular surface.
- Joint lubrication.
- Reducing friction.
- Shock absorption.
- Distributing forces more evenly.

Characteristics
- Avascular.
- Aneural.
- Alymphatic.

Layers
- *Superficial:* highest collagen content (fibres parallel to joint), lowest proteoglycan content, progenitor cells present, flat chondrocytes.
- *Intermediate:* random collagen organization, thickest layer, round chondrocytes.
- *Deep:* perpendicular collagen, highest proteoglycan content, round chondrocytes.
- *Tidemark:* deep to basal layer, separates articular cartilage from deeper calcified cartilage.
- Subchondral bone.

Injury

Due to its avascular nature, injury to cartilage that does not also injure the underlying bone does not have the ability to heal. If the injury also affects the underlying (subchondral) bone, this can bleed, allowing some chance of healing under the correct circumstances (e.g. limited movement and weight-bearing) to allow clot formation and subsequent organization of tissue. However, if healing occurs, the tissue produced is fibrocartilage, which is biomechanically inferior to articular cartilage.

Meniscus

The knee is not the only joint with menisci. However, the menisci of the knee are most frequently treated for injury; hence, they will be discussed here. The menisci are fibrocartilaginous crescent-shaped structures made of fibroelastic cartilage (90% of dry weight is type I collagen; 70% water, proteoglycans, and glycoproteins) (Fig. 6.14). The lateral meniscus (circular) covers a larger surface area than the medial meniscus (C-shaped). A combination of radial and longitudinal (circumferential) fibres help the meniscus to expand with compression, thereby ↑ contact surface area. A discoid meniscus is a common normal variant, most commonly seen on the lateral side.

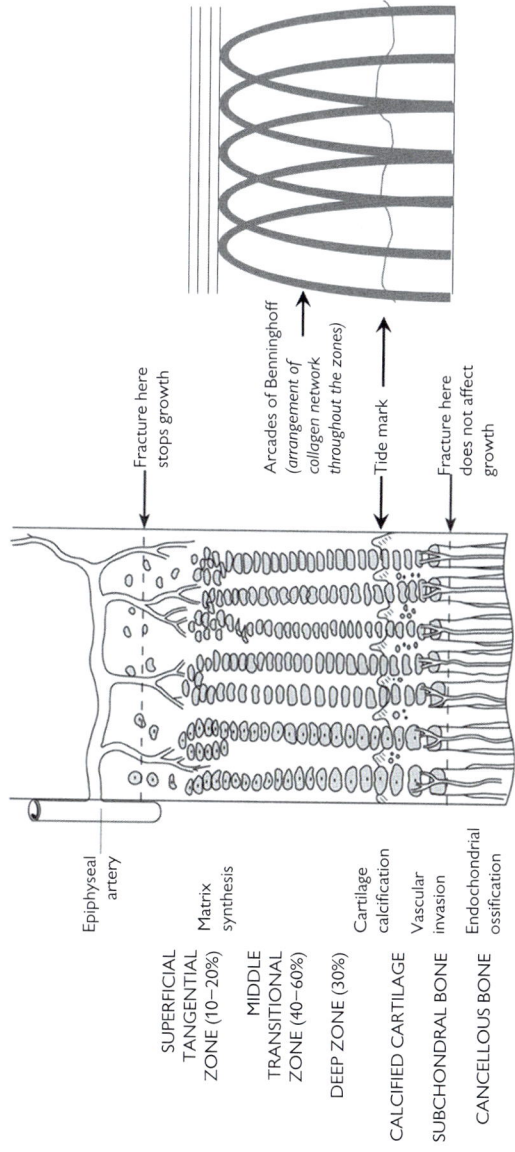

Fig. 6.13 Articular cartilage.

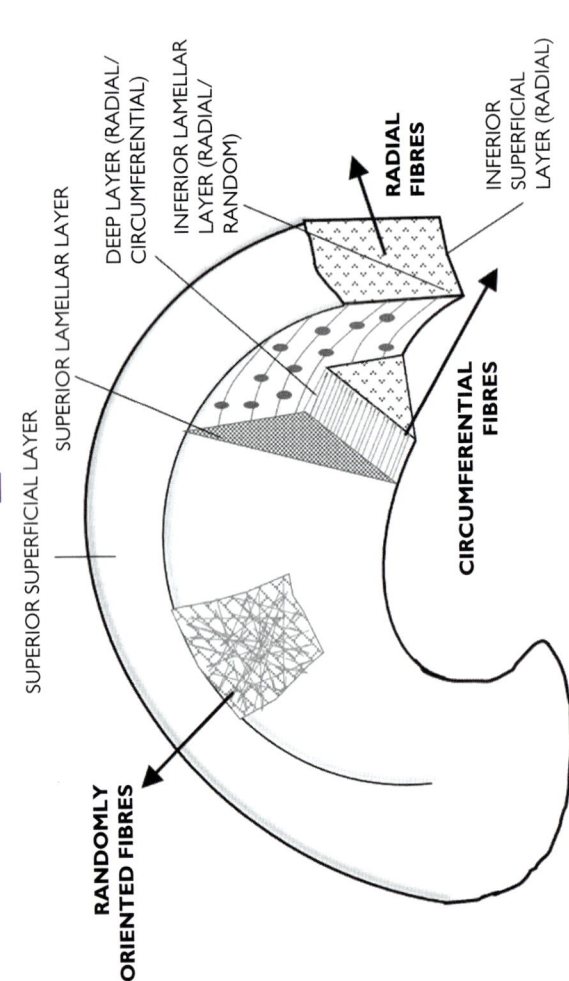

Fig. 6.14 Meniscus.

Attachments

The lateral meniscus has greater excursion on knee movement than the medial meniscus, due to attachment of the latter to the superficial MCL. Other attachments include:

- Intermeniscal (transverse) ligament: anterior link between menisci
- *Coronary ligaments:* peripheral attachments from meniscus to tibia
- *Meniscofemoral ligament:* arises from posterior horn of lateral meniscus and attaches to medial femoral condyle. Ligament of Humphrey is anterior to the PCL, and Wrisberg posterior to the PCL.

Functions

- Load transmission.
- Joint conformity.
- Synovial fluid distribution.
- AP stabilization (especially with ACL injury).
- Proprioception.
- Nutrition of chondral surfaces.

Blood supply

Lateral and medial geniculate arteries form a capillary plexus in the synovium and capsule. Blood supply only penetrates into the periphery of the meniscus in adults ('red-red' zone—outer third). This means that only peripheral tears have the potential for healing, or surgical meniscal repair, with rapid diagnosis and treatment being one of the important factors for successful treatment of repairable meniscal tears. Blood supply reaches more of the meniscus in children (red-white zone, middle third), and the amount supplied ↓ up to adulthood. The inner third (white-white zone) has a poor blood supply and hence has limited healing potential following injury.

Sutures

Sutures can be categorized due to various properties. The ideal suture material is inert (producing minimal tissue reaction), produces secure knots (that do not slip), has high tensile strength (adequate for the tissues it is required to hold), and is absorbed when the tissues have healed.

Natural vs synthetic materials
- *Natural fibres* are less commonly used in orthopaedics, perhaps with the exception of steel skin clips (staples) that are used by some surgeons for wound closure.
- *Synthetic sutures* are more commonly used, with their more predictable properties in terms of absorption and strength.

Monofilament vs braided
Monofilaments provide less surface area for organisms to settle and therefore confer a lower infection risk than their *braided* (multifilament) counterparts, although the latter are easier to handle, hold their shape, and provide greater knot security.

Absorbable vs non-absorbable
- *Absorbable sutures* are naturally degraded by enzymatic action/hydrolysis. The time required for this varies, depending upon the suture. Examples: natural (collagen-based); synthetic (Monocryl and PDS-monofilaments; Vicryl-braided).
- *Non-absorbable sutures* provide longer-term tissue support. Examples: natural (silk, steel); synthetic (Ethilon and Prolene monofilaments).

Suture size
The size of the suture affects its handling and strength. The nomenclature follows $x/0$; the larger the 'x', the smaller the suture (e.g. a 6/0 suture is finer than a 2/0 suture). Thereafter, single-digit numbers are followed (0, 1, 2, etc.), with larger numbers indicating a suture of greater diameter. In orthopaedics, larger sutures (e.g. a 1 Vicryl) are used for deeper, tougher tissues (e.g. abductor repair following total hip replacement), whereas finer sutures (e.g. 6/0 Prolene) may be used for a finger flexor tendon repair.

Needles
Sutures are attached to needles, which are required for suture handling and passage through tissues. Needles must be strong enough to pass through tough tissues, while being handled by a needle holder and without causing tissue damage. Needles can be round-bodied, cutting, or reverse cutting (Fig. 6.15). Furthermore, needles come in different sizes and shapes, based upon the proportion of a complete circle completed (e.g. 1/4 vs 1/2).

Common orthopaedic sets
The numerous instruments encountered in the operating theatre can be bewildering at first, due to the variety of sets and eponymous names, with different units often having their own nicknames to add to the mix! Major procedures require a multitude of manufacturer/procedure-specific sets. However, there are a few universal sets with which it is worth being more

POINT	SHAPE	ICON
TAPER		●
BLUNT TAPER		○
CUTTING		▲
REVERSE CUTTING		▼
TAPER CUT		◐
MICRO POINT (SPATULA CURVED)		▼

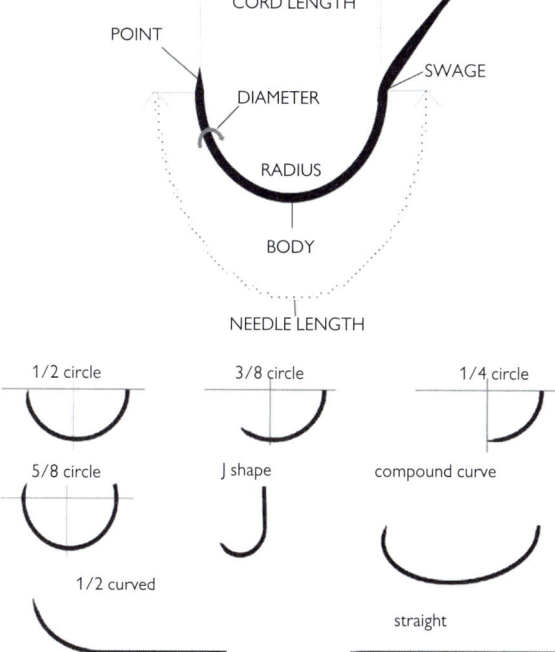

Fig. 6.15 Needle: point types, structure, and shapes.

Table 6.1 Different small-fragment screw types and measurement examples

Screw type	Cortical	Cortical	Cancellous	Locking	Locking
Thread diameter (mm)	2.7	3.5	4.0	2.7	3.5
Drill bit size (mm)	2.0	2.5	2.5	2.0	2.8
Tap size (mm)	2.7	3.5	4.0	Self-tap	Self-tap

Table 6.2 Different large-fragment screw types and measurement examples

Screw type	Cortical	Cortical	Cancellous	Locking	Locking
Thread diameter (mm)	4.5	5.5	6.5	4.0	5.0
Drill bit size (mm)	3.2	4.0	3.2	3.2	4.3
Tap size (mm)	4.5	5.5	6.5	Self-tap	Self-tap

familiar, as these are more frequently encountered. Note that the screw sizes presented may differ across implant manufacturers.

Basic orthopaedic set

This set is used in most operations, as it consists of a range of universally useful instruments. Commonly included instruments are: scalpel handles, forceps, dissection and suture scissors, small retractors, towel (drape) clamps, periosteal elevators, and osteotomes.

Small fragment set

Variations of this are used during open reduction and internal fixation of smaller bones/joints (e.g. forearm or ankle fractures), with screw sizing usually between 2.7 and 4.0mm (Table 6.1). Instruments included are: periosteal elevator, k-wires, reduction forceps, retractors, drill sleeves and bits, and plate benders.

Large fragment set

Variations of this are used during open reduction and internal fixation of larger bones/joints (e.g. femur or humerus fractures), with screw sizing usually between 4.0 and 6.5mm (Table 6.2).

The operating theatre complex

Layout of the operating room

The operating theatre should ideally be located close to other facilities such as the intensive care unit (ICU), ED, and radiology. Infection prevention remains as the priority; several zones exist, with the operating table at the heart: *outer* (wider hospital, reception), *clean* (reception → operating theatre entrance), *aseptic* (central area of the operating room where surgery takes place), and *dirty* (waste disposal) (Fig. 6.16).

Controlled factors

Temperature, humidity, light, ventilation, and (organism/particulate) filtration systems are vital to maintain the optimal environment:

- *Temperature:* usually kept at 19–20°C. Patient warming is employed (warming blankets, forced-air warming, e.g. Bair Hugger™) to prevent hypothermia. Extremes of temperature can affect patient homeostasis and the setting of polymethylmethacrylate (PMMA) cement.
- *Humidity:* 40–60% is optimal.
- *Lighting:* shadow-free lighting, at least 40,000 lux at the surgical site. Usually two satellite lights are used.
- *Ventilation:* two main types are employed—plenum and (vertical) laminar flow. The aim is to minimize colony-forming units (CFUs) of bacteria carrying particles to below established standards.
  - *Plenum* theatres have around 15–30 air changes per hour.
  - *Laminar flow* moves a single body of air through the room, with around 300 air changes per hour. They utilize a high-efficiency particulate air (HEPA) filter in the ceiling that filters particles of 0.5µm with 99.97% efficiency. The operating table, operating staff, and surgical trays must remain within the ceiling canopy (i.e. a 'room within a room').

Preventing infection

Several factors have been shown to reduce the incidence of surgical site/ deep infection and remain in common orthopaedic use, including: antibiotic-loaded cement (during arthroplasty); parenteral antibiotics (at induction of anaesthesia); skin antisepsis; and ultra-clean air systems. Skin preparation is commonly with iodophors (povidone iodine), chlorhexidine, or alcohols. While specialist wound covering drapes (e.g. Ioban) are not specifically recommended by WHO, use of iodine-impregnated drapes is permitted by NICE. NICE also provides guidance on management of post-operative wounds, including 'leaky' wounds. Appropriate surgical attire (sterile gowns, masks, gloves, and occasionally hoods/exhaust systems) also helps to protect patient and surgeon. When high-risk pathogens are present (e.g. TB, coronavirus disease 2019-COVID-19), specialist personal protective equipment (PPE) may be required to protect operating theatre personnel, including FFP3 masks or respirator hoods, alongside stringent *donning* (application of equipment) and *doffing* (careful, contamination-free removal of PPE) protocols.

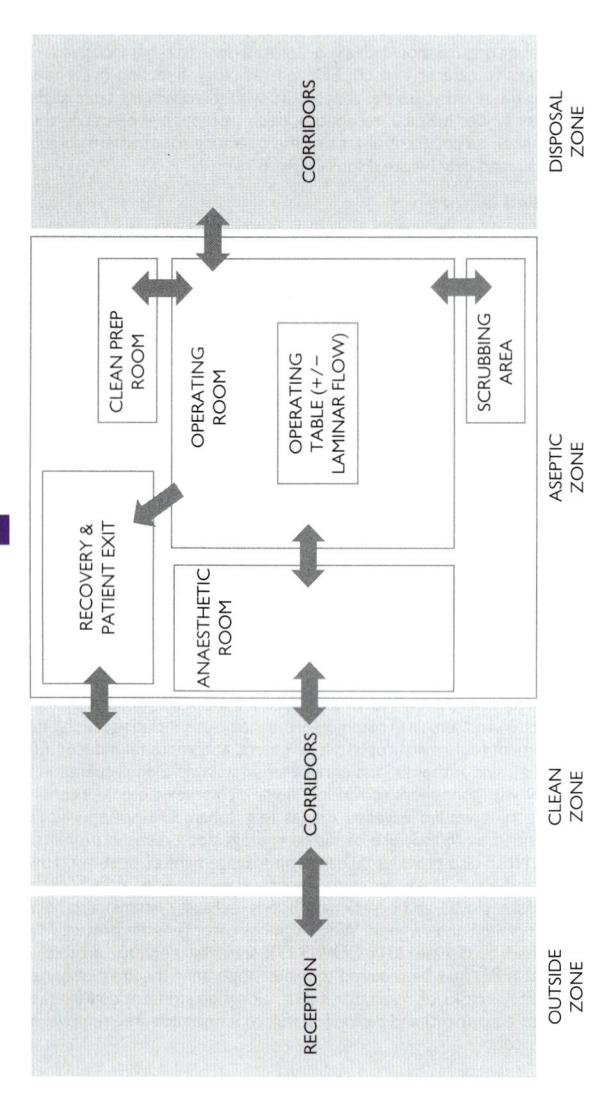

Fig. 6.16 Operating theatre complex.

List order planning and special considerations

When planning the operating list order, several factors must be considered, including:

- *Staff:* staff and surgeon experience/skill set. Need for surgical assistance. Dual consultant operating (complex cases)
- *Equipment:* type of operation and routine equipment needs (i.e. 'trays'). Specific specialist equipment. Manufacturer representatives to assist theatre team with trays
- *Patient:* age (extremes of age usually earlier to minimize nil by mouth time). Comorbidities (e.g. diabetes)—higher-risk patients usually earlier on list. Other risk factors (e.g. infectious diseases—TB, COVID-19). Allergies (e.g. latex). Clean (e.g. arthroplasty) cases generally before infected cases (e.g. abscesses)
- *Environment:* type of theatre (e.g. laminar flow for arthroplasty). Post-operative monitoring (e.g. HDU or ICU bed). Need for air changes or deep cleaning between cases.

Principles of evidence-based medicine

Adapted from Harrison J, Kulkarni K, Baguneid M, Prendergast B (eds). Oxford Handbook of Key Clinical Evidence, 2nd edn. Oxford: Oxford University Press, 2016.

Introduction to evidence-based medicine

The process of evidence-based medicine

'The practice of evidence-based medicine means integrating clinical expertise (proficiency, judgement acquired through clinical practise and use of individual patient's right, predicaments, preferences) with the best available expert evidence from systematic research.'

This definition, from Sackett's seminal paper in 1996, has been translated into five steps ('Five As': Asking, Acquiring, Appraising critically, Applying, and Accessing), designed to help clinicians find the best available expert evidence from a systematic search.

Asking

Asking the right question is key to obtaining a useful outcome from research. Refining a question into several parts by using the PICO (*Population/Patient problem, Intervention, Comparison, Outcome*) framework can help to identify useful keywords for a search to ↑ the chances of finding an appropriate answer.

Acquiring

The lower the level of evidence, the greater the risk of bias (Table 7.1). Randomizing study participants reduces bias, because confounding factors (such as age, gender, and smoking status) are evenly distributed between the intervention and control arms of the study. In other words, the only difference between the groups is whether or not they receive the intervention, as their allocation to a particular arm of the study is purely by chance. Expert opinion or clinical experience is more open to bias, although, in some cases (e.g. rare events/conditions), this may be the only evidence available.

The Grading of Recommendations, Assessment, Development, and Evaluation (GRADE) Working Group framework was developed to help guideline developers make evidence-based recommendations (Table 7.2). Its approach to assessing the quality of evidence is widely used and makes an important distinction between evidence quality and the strength of a recommendation. It also helps to highlight the importance of looking at the 'body of evidence' for a clinical question.

Table 7.1 Level of evidence

Level	Type of evidence
1a	Evidence from systematic reviews or meta-analysis of RCTs
1b	Evidence from at least one RCT
2a	Evidence from at least one controlled study without randomization
2b	Evidence from at least one other type of quasi-experimental study
3	Evidence from non-experimental descriptive studies such as comparative studies, correlation studies, and case-control studies
4	Evidence from expert committee reports or opinions and/or clinical experience of respected authorities

RCT, randomized controlled trial.

Table 7.2 A summary of GRADE's approach to rating the quality of evidence

Study design	Initial quality of body of evidence	Lower if	Higher if	Quality of body of evidence
Randomized trials	High	Risk of bias	Large effect	High ++++
		−1 Serious	+1 Large	
		−2 Very serious	+2 Very large	
		Inconsistency	Dose response	Moderate
		−1 Serious	+1 Evidence of a gradient	
		−2 Very serious		
		Indirectness	All plausible residual confounding	
		−1 Serious		
		−2 Very serious	All plausible residual confounding	
Observational studies	Low	Imprecision		Low ++
		−1 Serious	+1 Would reduce a demonstrated effect	
		−2 Very serious		
		Publication bias		Very low +
		−1 Serious	+1 Would suggest a spurious effect if no effect was observed	
		−2 Very serious		

Adapted from Balshem H, Helfand M, Schunemann HJ, et al. (2011) GRADE guidelines: 3. Rating the Quality of evidence. *J Clin Epi* **64**, 401–6.

Appraising

Critical appraisal is the process of assessing the quality of a study. A poorly conducted systematic review or randomized controlled trial (RCT) may not be worth considering, as the results may be misleading due to methodological flaws and sources of bias. Numerous checklists have been developed to help clinicians decide whether a study is valid or not (Table 7.3).

Applying

Applying embodies the true art of medicine, as it requires the 'integration of best evidence with clinical expertise, the patient's circumstances, and their personal preferences'. This step remains one of the most challenging, yet most important, steps within the evidence-based medicine (EBM) process.

Table 7.3 Common appraisal and reporting checklists

Checklist source	Study types	Location
JAMA Users' Guide Series	All	℘ www.jamaevidence.com
PRISMA	Systematic reviews	℘ www.prisma-statement.org/
GRADE	Clinical practice guidelines	℘ www.gradeworkinggroup.org
CONSORT	Randomized controlled trials	℘ https://www.equator-network.org/reporting-guidelines/consort/
STROBE	Non-randomized observational studies	℘ www.strobe-statement.org/

CONSORT, Consolidated Standards of Reporting Trials; GRADE, Grading of Recommendations Assessment, Development and Evaluation; PRISMA, Preferred Reporting Items for Systematic reviews and Meta-Analyses; STROBE, Strengthening the Reporting of Observational studies in Epidemiology.

When the appraisal of RCTs is concerned, a few key concepts are important to ensure their results are valid and suitable for application:
- *Null hypothesis and errors:* the null hypothesis is formed at the outset of a study involving a treatment vs a control, which is presumed true, unless nullified or refuted by statistical evidence. For example, when comparing a drug with placebo, the null hypothesis would be: 'the new drug is of equal efficacy to the placebo'. Statistically significant analysis of the data would then be required, in order to prove that the new drug was more effective. Two types of errors can subsequently arise:
  - *Type 1 or* α: rejecting a hypothesis that should have been accepted (false positive) (i.e. stating that a difference was observed when this was not actually the case)
  - *Type 2 or* β: accepting a hypothesis that should have been rejected (false negative) (i.e. stating that no difference was observed when, in fact, a difference was present).
- *Bias:* bias, the systematic over- or underestimation of the true effect, can be introduced at a number of stages. The main sources of bias in RCTs come either from poor randomization and/or through loss to follow-up after randomization.
- *Randomization:* the method of randomization is important in a trial. Where possible, it should be done independently, so that researchers are 'blinded' to the allocation of participants. Randomly allocating participants to treatment or control groups is a highly effective way of reducing bias, as it ensures both groups are likely to be very similar (i.e. similar baseline characteristics) to begin with. Any differences between the two groups are then most likely to be attributable to the intervention itself.
- *Blinding:* blinding participants (and/or researchers), when measuring the outcomes of interest, is a way in which studies can attempt to reduce unwanted influences of bias and improve internal validity. This can take several forms: *single-blind* (patient is unaware to which intervention

Type of bias

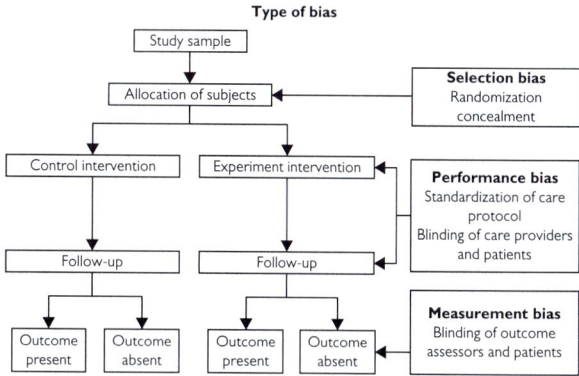

Fig. 7.1 Types of bias.

Reproduced from: Khan K, Kunz R, Kleijnen J, Antes G. (2003) Systematic reviews to support evidence-based medicine: How to review and apply findings of systematic reviews. *BJS*. 91: 3 p375. Royal Society Medicine Press, London, with permission from John Wiley and Sons.

they have been allocated); *double-blind* (both researcher (clinician) and patient are unaware to which intervention the patient has been allocated); and *triple-blind* (when the researcher, patient, and outcome assessor do not know to which intervention the patient has been allocated). There are several types of bias, some of which are shown in Fig. 7.1.

- *Follow-up:* another important factor to check is whether or not patients have been adequately followed up. In particular, this should be to ensure that there has not been a high dropout rate in one arm of the trial, compared with the other. Participants should not be swapped from one group to the other. If this does unavoidably occur for ethical or other reasons, then the analysis should consider what would have happened had they stayed in their original group ('intention-to-treat' analysis). Omitting patients who withdrew may overestimate treatment effects.

Accessing

This is a potentially useful step that requires the clinician to reflect upon the previous four steps and consider ways in which they might be improved in subsequent efforts.

Are the results of a study important?

There are a range of statistical tools available to assess quantitatively the relative importance and significance of study data. It is crucial to select the appropriate test for the particular data in a study. Although there is no single algorithm that can be applied to determine which test is best in every case, a decision tree can help. Further discussion of this is well beyond the scope of this book, but there are a number of helpful internet-based resources such as the *Handbook of Biological Statistics* (available from: ℛ www.bios tathandbook.com/testchoice.html).

Further reading

This chapter is adapted from: Kulkarni, K., Harrison, J., Baguneid, M. and Prendergast, B. eds., 2016. *Oxford Handbook of Key Clinical Evidence*. Oxford University Press.

Sackett DL, Rosenberg WM, Gray JM, Haynes RB, Richardson WS. Evidence based medicine: what it is and what it isn't. *BMJ*. 1996;312(7023):71–2.

Essentials: statistics 101

Statistical terms

The size and direction of the effect of a treatment (i.e. dichotomous data) are often reported as the 'odds ratio' (OR), 'relative risk' (RR), 'hazard ratio' (HR), or 'difference in means'. To see if there is much error around this estimate, the '95% confidence interval (CI)' can be calculated to ensure that it does not cross the null value (the point of no effect). Whether or not there is a statistically significant effect can be determined by seeing whether the 'p-value' is <0.05. We will now examine some of the key terminology in more detail.

A. Difference between group means

Used for continuous data—for example, the mean reading score in treatment group A minus the mean reading score in control group B.

B. Relative risk (RR)

This is the risk of outcome in the treatment group relative to the other (usually control) group. It is a ratio—for example, a cohort of patients taking a certain novel painkiller and still having pain after 5 days (19%) is divided by the proportion of patients in the control group with pain persisting at 5 days (25%) to give RR = 0.76. RR = 1.0 means that there is no effect of the treatment. In other words, this implies that there is no difference between treatment and control groups (i.e. the null value). If the RR is >1.0 for an adverse outcome, such as death, this generally means the effect is harmful. If the RR is <1.0, then the treatment is protective. To use our example, RR = 0.76 means that patients in the treatment group are 24% less likely to have pain at 5 days compared with controls. The further away the RR is from the null value, the greater the effect of the treatment.

Outcome and exposure status
(Table 7.4)

Table 7.4 Outcome and exposure status

	Outcome present	Outcome not present	
Exposed to treatment: treatment group	A	B	Number exposed (A + B)
Not exposed to treatment: control group	C	D	Number not exposed (C + D)
	Number with outcome (A + C)	Number without outcome (B + D)	

$$RR = \frac{\text{proportion with outcome in treatment group}}{\text{proportion with outcome in control group}}$$

$$= \frac{A/(A+B)}{C/(C+D)}$$

$$= \frac{\text{exposure event rate (EER)}}{\text{control event rate (CER)}}$$

C. Relative risk reduction (RRR)

Rather than trying to discuss the effect of a treatment as a ratio, it is often more clinically relevant to express the effect as a difference. This can be done in relative (i.e. in relation to the effect on controls) or absolute terms (which shows the actual size of the effect on that particular population). The RRR will be the same regardless of the population. It can be calculated by using the following formula:

$$RRR = \frac{(CER - EER)}{CER}$$

If we consider this for our example, the RRR would be $(25 - 19\%)/25\% = 24\%$ reduction in pain at day 5.

D. Absolute risk reduction (ARR)

In contrast to the RRR, the ARR is simply the difference between the event/outcome rate in the treatment group and that of the control group:

$$ARR = CER - EER$$

The ARR is said to be a much more clinically relevant estimate of effect because it takes into account the prevalence of an outcome in that particular population. For example, if the symptom rate at day 5 in a control population is 25%, the ARR for a study may show $25\% - 19\%$, which is a 6% reduction in pain by using a certain painkiller. However, if the study was conducted in a higher-risk population where the prevalence of pain in the control group was 50%, then the ARR would be much greater. You may recall that, in this example, the RR was 0.76, so we would expect the treatment group in this higher-risk population to have a symptom rate of around 38%. In other words, the ARR for this higher-risk population is $50\% - 38\%$, which is 12% (compared with 6% in the average-risk population).

Hopefully you can now see how important it is to consider whether you are using a *relative* or an *absolute* risk reduction. The ARR in this example shows that using antibiotics in the high-risk population will prevent many more cases than in the average-risk population. This is a point that might be very relevant when considering the trade-off between benefits and harms or the costs of treatment.

E. Number needed to treat (NNT)

This is the number of patients who need to be treated with the studied intervention in order to prevent one event. It is calculated as the inverse of the ARR:

$$NNT = \frac{1}{ARR}$$

In our hypothetical pain example, we would find that the NNT for the 'high-risk' population would be 1/0.12, or 8.33. This means that we would need to treat just over eight patients to prevent one case of persistent pain. In the 'low average risk population', the NNT would be 1/0.06, which is 16.7. In other words, in the 'average-risk' population, we need to treat 17 patients with the painkiller to prevent one case of persistent pain, but only 1/0.12, or 8, patients in the higher-risk group.

It is important to note that the NNT is only applicable when the study population is similar to the target patient population for whom the tested intervention is intended. When the treatment ↑ the risk of the harmful outcome, then the inverse of the risk difference is called the 'number needed to harm' (NNH).

F. Odds ratio (OR)

We often talk about the 'odds' of an event occurring. The 'odds'—or chance—of us winning the lottery are small. This seems obvious, but how do we measure the odds of a clinical event occurring? The OR is the ratio of the odds of a disease occurring in the presence of an exposure relative to the odds of the disease occurring in the absence of the exposure. The OR is commonly used in case-control studies.

Looking back to Table 7.4, the OR can be defined by using the following formula:

$$OR = \frac{\text{odds of disease in the presence of exposure}}{\text{odds of disease in the absence of exposure}}$$

$$= A/B \text{ divided by } C/D$$

$$= AD/BC$$

Therefore, this is the odds of the outcome in the treatment group relative to the odds of the outcome in controls. Again, an OR of 1.0 means that there is no difference between the treatment and control groups. An OR >1.0 for an adverse outcome, such as death, means ↑ risk. In some studies, the OR is a reasonable estimate of the RR, but only if the outcome is uncommon.

G. Hazard ratio (HR)

Used in survival analysis, this is the probability of a hazard at time 't' in the treatment group compared with the probability of a hazard at time 't' in the control group (i.e. the effect of a variable upon the risk of an event). Sometimes, the HR is simply referred to as the 'relative risk'.

H. 95% confidence interval (CI)

The terms outlined in this section (RR, OR, HR, and difference of the means) are all estimates of the effect of the study factor on the population in question. However, there will always be some error associated with this, particularly if there are only a small number of people participating in the study (i.e. a small sample size). The 95% CI is the range within which we are 95% confident that the true estimate of effect lies. Note, that if the 95% CI for an OR or RR value crosses 1.0 (the point of no effect), then it is possible that the true effect is none (i.e. the effect is not statistically significant).

I. p-values and statistical significance

A p-value is the probability of the observed difference being due to chance. Traditionally, if the p-value is <0.05, then the result is considered statistically significant.

J. Tools applicable to diagnostic studies

These studies investigate the ability of a particular diagnostic or screening test to detect a disorder in the sample population (Table 7.5). The performance of the test can then be evaluated.

- *Sensitivity:* the proportion of people with a disorder who are correctly diagnosed as positive by the test. The higher the sensitivity of a test, the more likely a negative result will rule out the presence of the disorder (high SeNsitivity rules *OUT* = SNOUT); few false negative results, and so fewer cases of disease are missed.
- *Specificity:* the proportion of people without the disorder who are correctly excluded as negative by the test. The higher the specificity of a test, the more likely a positive result will rule in the presence of the disorder (high SPecificity rules *IN* = SPIN); this means there are few false positive results.
- *Positive predictive value (PPV):* the proportion of people with a positive test who actually have the disorder.
- *Negative predictive value (NPV):* the proportion of people with a negative test who do not have the disorder.
- *Likelihood ratio (LR):* provides a direct estimate of how much a test result will change the odds of having a disease. The LR for a positive result (LR+) is how much the odds of the disease ↑ when a test is positive. The LR for a negative result (LR−) is how much the odds of the disease ↓ when a test is negative.

Table 7.5 Sensitivity and specificity

	Disorder present	Disorder absent
Positive test	a	b
Negative test	c	d

Sensitivity = a/(a + c)

Specificity = d/(b + d)

PPV = a/(a + b)

NPV = d/(c + d)

LR = Probability of test result in someone with the disease/probability of test result in someone without the disease

LR+ (+ve test) = sensitivity/(1 − specificity)

LR− (−ve test) = (1 − sensitivity)/specificity

Further reading

This chapter is adapted from: Kulkarni, K., Harrison, J., Baguneid, M. and Prendergast, B. eds., 2016. *Oxford Handbook of Key Clinical Evidence.* Oxford University Press.

Evidence-based medicine in practice

Translating evidence-based medicine to patient care

For some clinical questions, there are good-quality RCTs conducted across different populations, and these are often summarized in systematic reviews/meta-analysis. Clearly, if a good-quality systematic review summarizes and pools the results of several RCTs, then that source of evidence should be considered. The Cochrane database of systematic reviews is an excellent source of such evidence. If results from several trials can be pooled quantitatively (into a meta-analysis), this will provide a summary estimate of the effect of the treatment. Clinical practice guidelines are often a locally derived summary of systematically derived evidence, which has taken into account local application and health system contexts. They may also be an excellent source of evidence.

The GRADE group suggests that, when considering a recommendation to apply evidence (or not), four domains must be considered:
1. Balance between desirable and undesirable outcomes (estimated effects), with consideration of values and preferences (estimated typical) (trade-offs)
2. Confidence in the magnitude of estimates of the effect of the interventions on important outcomes (overall quality of evidence for outcomes)
3. Confidence in values and preferences and variability
4. Resource use.

Note that not every clinical condition or topic will necessarily have a simple, accurate, up-to-date, and unbiased research-based answer. As an adjunct to clinical expertise, EBM has become increasingly central to medical practice, providing the impetus for ensuring healthcare professionals remain up to date with advances.

National Joint Registry

In 1972, Sir John Charnley recommended that 'serious consideration should be given to establishing a central registry to keep a finger on the pulse of total implant surgery on a nationwide basis. Surgeons should not be permitted to perform total hip implant work (especially those involving the use of cement) unless prepared to have weekly returns made of the operations as they are performed and thereafter to have patients questioned annually by circular from the Registry'.

In 1975, the Swedish Knee Arthroplasty Registry was established, followed a year later by the Swedish Hip Arthroplasty Registry. The UK did not follow suit for a number of years, with the first regional registries not established until the early 1990s (the Trent Regional Arthroplasty Study and the North West Arthroplasty Register). It was not until 1998, when a hazard notice regarding a higher-than-expected incidence of femoral component loosening of the 3M Capital Hip was issued by the Medical Devices Agency, that there was impetus for a national registry to detect failing implants at an earlier stage. The National Joint Registry (NJR) of England and Wales was subsequently established in 2002, with data collection commencing from April 2003. Initially confined to hip and knee arthroplasty, the NJR started to collect information on elbow and shoulder replacements from 2012.

NJR outputs are divided into 'open/public access' (e.g. NJR annual report, public surgeon/hospital profile) and 'secure/restricted access' (e.g. consultant-level report) (available from: ℘ https://reports.njrcentre.org.uk). The annual report presents an overview and analysis of submitted data. Implants and bearings are listed as both brands and constructs, allowing variations (e.g. different hip stem/socket combinations) to be assessed. Hospital outcomes include revision rates over the entire period covered by the NJR, as well as over the previous 5 years, mean improvement in patient-reported outcome measure (PROM) scores (e.g. Oxford Hip or Knee Scores), compared with the national average gain, the EQ-5D, and the EQ-VAS. Thermometer plots demonstrate whether the performance by the hospital is within the expected range, or better or worse than expected. Consultant reports display activity subdivided by fixation, bearing, and, for hips, use of Orthopaedic Data Evaluation Panel (ODEP)-rated components.

Other registries

An increasing number of registries are emerging for other orthopaedic conditions, procedures, and specialties, known as the Trauma and Orthopaedic Unifying Structure (TORUS). These include the British Spine Registry (BSR), UK National Ligament Registry (NLR), UK Knee Osteotomy Registry (UKKOR), Non-Arthroplasty Hip Registry (NAHR), Bone and Joint Infection Register, British Orthopaedic Foot and Ankle Society (BOFAS) Registry, UK National Hand Registry, and British Limb Reconstruction Society Registry (BLRS).

Orthopaedic Data Evaluation Panel

This organization was established in 2002 to implement NICE guidance on benchmarking primary hip implants. Hip resurfacing followed in 2004, knees in 2014, and shoulders in 2017. Prior to its inception, there was limited audit of outcomes of joint replacement. With data submitted biannually for each joint, manufacturers now use ODEP to benchmark prostheses at regular time points (3, 5, 7, 10, and, since 2018, 13 years) against agreed standards. Note that hip hemiarthroplasty or revision implants are not rated. In 2011, 'Beyond Compliance' was developed to plug the gap between the granting of a CE mark and ODEP 3 ratings. Note that manufacturers will also publish extensive research and educational materials relating to their implants; appraise these critically with potential bias in mind.
- ODEP: ℘ www.odep.org.uk
- 'Beyond Compliance': ℘ www.beyondcompliance.org.uk

National Hip Fracture Database

This was established in 2007 between the British Geriatrics Society (BGS) and the BOA. The National Hip Fracture Database (NHFD) is designed to facilitate improvements in quality and cost-effectiveness of hip fracture care through auditing the care of patients with hip fractures against six evidence-based standards set out in the BOA/BGS Blue Book on the care of patients with fragility fractures. Individual unit performance can be compared against

national data. The NHFD publishes an annual report summarizing performance and trends across the country.
- NHFD: ✌ www.nhfd.co.uk

Guidelines

For most clinicians, it can be difficult to appraise the masses of published
evidence and readily translate this to direct patient care. This is where
guidelines come in; while not always universally agreed as the *only* 'right'
way to do things, they do present a useful means of standardizing care.
Ultimately, this makes compliance with national standards a medico-legally
robust means of clinical practice that serves to minimize negative/un-
wanted variations. There are numerous established sources of guidance
to guide EBM-based clinical practice. Some key resources (primarily UK-
focused) include the following.

British Orthopaedic Association

As the national representative body of UK trauma and orthopaedics, the
BOA publishes standards and guidance, primarily through BOA Standards
for Trauma and Orthopaedics (BOASTs) summary documents on aspects
of care, 'Blue Books' (more detailed guidance), commissioning guides, and
associated guidelines (together with other subspecialty organizations).
BOASTs are trauma-focused short standards documents that encompass
topics ranging from distal radius to ankle fractures.
- BOA: ✌ www.boa.ac.uk

Getting It Right First Time

An important NHS improvement programme to be aware of (that has now
expanded beyond trauma and orthopaedics) is Getting It Right First Time
(GIRFT). GIRFT's mission statement is to tackle variations in the way in
which services are delivered across the NHS. By sharing best practice and
standardizing care pathways across trusts, GIRFT's goal is to improve care
and patient outcomes, as well as to deliver cost and resource savings.
- GIRFT: ✌ https://gettingitrightfirsttime.co.uk/

National Institute for Health and Care Excellence

NICE has a wealth of national guidelines, encompassing a range of conditions spanning both elective orthopaedics and trauma, and other relevant
topics (e.g. VTE, perioperative glycaemic control in diabetic patients).
- NICE: ✌ www.nice.org.uk/

Subspecialty organizations

Each orthopaedic subspecialty has a representative organization that pro-
duces its own guidelines, as well as collaborative guidelines with other
bodies (e.g. BOA, NICE). These include:
- British Elbow and Shoulder Society (BESS)
- British Society for Surgery of the Hand (BSSH)
- British Association of Spine Surgeons (BASS)
- British Hip Society (BHS)
- British Association for Surgery of the Knee (BASK)
- British Orthopaedic Foot and Ankle Society (BOFAS)
- British Society for Children's Orthopaedic Surgery (BSCOS).

AO Foundation

Arbeitsgemeinschaft für Osteosynthesefragen (AO) is a long-established (1950s) not-for-profit organization that was formed to conduct research on bone healing (particularly the influence of the mechanical environment). AO produces extremely useful online guides and courses. The AO Principles and Advances courses have provided the foundation of trauma fixation techniques for surgeons worldwide for many years. While the AO Trauma section is perhaps the most well known, other wings exist (e.g. AO Spine, AO Recon).

• AO: ✍ www.aofoundation.org/

Other organizations

Multiple other national and subspecialty orthopaedic representative bodies release guidance similarly to the BOA. Examples include:

• Trauma Audit and Research Network (TARN): organizes and collates data on the UK Major Trauma Network
• Orthopaedic Trauma Association (OTA)
• American Academy of Orthopaedic Surgeons (AAOS): the North American BOA (✍ www.aaos.org)

Further reading

Balshem H, Helfand M, Schunemann HJ, *et al.* GRADE guidelines: 3. Rating the quality of evidence. *Journal of Clinical Epidemiology*. 2011;**64**:401–6.

Porter M, Armstrong R, Howard P, Porteous M, Wilkinson JM. Orthopaedic registries—the UK view (National Joint Registry): impact on practice. *EFORT Open Reviews*. 2019;**4**(6):377–90.

Outcomes assessment and tariffs

The success of orthopaedic interventions has traditionally been assessed through clinician-reported indicators such as post-operative complications, rates of reoperation, and radiological measures. However, there has remained a growing emphasis on measuring PROMs to monitor the effects of an intervention treatment or service over a period of time. PROMs have increasingly become incorporated into clinical practice and NJRs.

Patient-reported outcome measures

PROMs are validated tools that can be used to assess the quality of care delivered to patients from their perspective. Through a questionnaire format, PROMs can help to objectively calculate the health gains after healthcare interventions using pre- and post-intervention surveys containing questions on symptoms, function, and other facets of health quality. PROMS can evaluate both *general* health and *specific* procedures/aspects of health:

- *General outcome measures:* aim to assess all dimensions of health-related quality of life (QoL) through largely self-administered questionnaires. Examples include the Short Form 36 (SF-36) item health survey and the EuroQol Groups' five dimensions (EQ-5D).
- *Disease/joint-specific measures:* these are more responsive than generic QoL measures and allow comparison of different operative and non-operative treatment options for a particular pathology or anatomical site. They typically combine physician-assessed parameters, functional scores, and the patient's perception of their symptoms, to derive an overall score. Examples include:
  - Hands: Disabilities of the Arm, Shoulder, and Hand (DASH) score
  - Shoulders: Oxford Shoulder Instability Score (OSIS)
  - Spine: the Oswestry Disability Index
  - Hips: Oxford Hip Score
  - Knees: Oxford Knee Score
  - Foot and ankle: Manchester–Oxford Foot Questionnaire
  - Disease-specific: Western Ontario and McMaster Universities Osteoarthritis Index (WOMAC) for assessment of lower limb OA.

Choosing the most appropriate outcome measure requires careful consideration of multiple factors, including its reliability, validity, and responsiveness, in peer-reviewed testing compared with previously accepted gold standards. Statistically significant improvement in outcome measure scores may not translate into patient- or clinician-perceived improvement. The minimum clinically important difference (MCID) is the smallest change in score that patients perceive beneficial. Clinicians may also choose to examine different aspects of the patient's function through a combination of instruments, as together they provide more information than one questionnaire alone.

Outcomes can be used to determine the efficacy of interventions, as well as to guide decision-making. PROMs are often proprietary/copyrighted, although most tools are available online. Examples include:

- NJR patient decision support tool for joint replacement (available from: ℘ https://jointcalc.shef.ac.uk/)
- Orthopaedic Scores (available from: ℘ www.orthopaedicscore.com).

Best Practice Tariff

Tariffs are a means of financially incentivizing better clinical care. They exist throughout healthcare, and trauma and orthopaedics is no exception. Essentially, they divide payment for care provision into a base payment, with additional payment only provided if certain conditions are met.

Patients with a fractured neck of femur have complex care needs; while the hip fracture requires operative intervention, the trigger for a fall is often related to a deterioration in their underlying health. For this reason, their management is truly multidisciplinary, encompassing orthopaedic surgeons, orthogeriatricians, anaesthetists, physiotherapists, and occupational therapists. As a result, there are nationally agreed standards to which all Trusts must adhere, with payments incentivized based upon compliance. In conjunction with the NHFD, several standards of care must be met to claim the full tariff for each patient treated, including:

• Being clerked on the correct integrated care pathway
• Having an operation within 36h of ED admission
• An orthogeriatric review (by ST3+ or higher) within 72h of ED admission
• Falls assessment
• Preoperative AMTS
• Post-operative AMTS
• Bone protection prescribed (or valid reason for omission).

As a result of Best Practice Tariff (BPT) being applied to the care of these patients, there has been an improvement in mortality for this patient cohort.

Further reading

Ashby E, Grocott MP, Haddad FS. Outcome measures for orthopaedic interventions on the hip. *Journal of Bone and Joint Surgery. British volume.* 2008;90(5):545–9.

Chapter 8

Global orthopaedics

Introduction

The *Lancet* Commission on Global Surgery estimated over 18 million deaths per year from surgically treatable conditions. This is four times the number due to HIV, malaria, and TB combined. Most cases are trauma-related, predominantly in low- and middle-income countries (LMICs), affecting the young.

It is easy when working in the NHS to take it for granted. Yet 5 billion of the world's 7 billion people do not have access to surgery that is affordable, safe, and locally available. Global orthopaedics, as a branch of global surgery, is concerned with understanding this massive inequity, and collaboration with colleagues around the world in working to address it.

Getting involved with global orthopaedics calls for humility and openness, but is an opportunity to learn about pathology and new skills, to share some of your training, and to make lifelong professional friendships. This chapter provides an introduction to some of the key issues to consider.

Why bother getting involved?

There are several potential benefits to host countries or institutions:
- Providing direct care can have significant short-term benefits for the communities you serve, especially during emergencies
- Teaching and training can have a longer-term impact on capacity building and improving the health systems of LMICs
- Fostering of long-term networks at personal and institutional levels—continuing professional development for individuals; institutional support in terms of skills/capacity transfer
- Targeted support driven by specific needs analysis to avoid inappropriate donations and support.

In addition, there are several benefits to the NHS:
- Working in small MDTs helps to renew interest in service integration, commissioning, and teamwork
- Opportunity to experience a diverse range of pathology and cultures
- Corporate NHS will benefit from its international linkages and skills transfer as a responsible global/corporate citizen
- NHS staff with global linkages and knowledge will bring knowledge that is beneficial to NHS
- Opportunity to attract overseas trainees for targeted short training visits/opportunities
- Opportunity to attract funds for collaborative research and projects with institutions from LMICs
- Built-in flexible time for NHS consultants to provide support for LMIC visits (e.g. shared appointments for consultants).

Finally, there are numerous benefits to you as an individual clinician:
- Challenging working environments provide healthcare professionals with the opportunity to test resourcefulness and resilience. Volunteers often return with greater clinical, leadership, and educational skills
- Often improves work satisfaction and has a positive impact on personal and professional development

- Opportunity to develop long-lasting personal networks and friendships with colleagues from LMICs
- Opportunity for an academic career as visiting lectureships and external examining/accreditation of educational programmes
- Opportunities for research collaborations.

Important planning considerations

There are myriad opportunities for overseas work as medical students, junior doctors, and beyond. It is important to understand who, or what, a given project is looking for and carefully consider whether you are the right fit. While many prospective volunteers are well intentioned, one must understand the potential for the unintended negative impact that volunteerism can have.

Long-term projects are often of greater benefit to the volunteer and host alike. It takes time to understand the community with which you are working, to adapt to their needs, and to learn how to gain the skills required to meet those needs. While it is more challenging to make the same impact on shorter trips, it is possible, provided the aims and scope are realistic and well planned.

Ask yourself the following questions before considering overseas work:
- What are the needs and expectations of the host country/institution?
- What can I offer?
- For how long can I go?
- What do I want to do?
- What do I expect to get out of it?
- What will happen when I come back?
- When is the best time to undertake such visits in relation to the stage of personal career development? As a junior or senior trainee? As an early or senior consultant?
- If a trainee, how will the time out affect the training period towards a certificate of completion of specialist training (CCST)?
- What skills do I have that can be transferred?
- Is my own training in LMICs more paramount than the skills I will transfer—especially so for those in training?
- Who are the beneficiaries in LMICs? Health workers? Institutions? Patients?
- Legal issues (e.g. registration formalities).
- Health insurance/travel insurance/occupational health issues.
- Logistics (e.g. accommodation, local transportation).
- What medical indemnity is available for work in LMICs? Does the host country offer medical indemnity for short-term visitors?

Dos and don'ts

When visiting an LMIC, it is importance to stick to a few basic rules. This is by no means a comprehensive list (Table 8.1).

Table 8.1 Dos and don'ts of working abroad

Do	Don't
Adhere to a strict code of conduct for overseas work, including local laws in the country. Below is a list of suitable resources: • Universal Declaration of Human Rights • Humanitarian Charter • Accountability Charter of international non-governmental organizations (INGOs) • Code of conduct of International Federation of Red Cross and Red Crescent Societies (IFRC) • World Orthopaedic Concern UK (WOC-UK) code of conduct	Don't behave in a way that is unprofessional or unlawful
Be mindful and respectful of local cultural or religious practices	Don't behave in a way that may be culturally insensitive
Ask what your host centre would like from you regarding training (e.g. a course, lectures, specialist opinion on cases)	Don't make the mistake of thinking that the way you have been taught is the only way, or even the best way
Remember your aim is to enable your overseas counterparts through teaching and training, not to practise your own surgical skills on their patients	Don't take training opportunities away from local trainees or consultants
Plan your trips meticulously with your hosts and your team to ensure you make the most of the time you are in country If planning regular trips to the same centre, consider a memorandum of understanding (MOU) to manage expectations	Don't expect to make a plan of action when in country
Always consult the Foreign Office website ahead of your trip Talk to your hosts at the centre you are visiting about the safety of the trip Ensure you have a safe exit strategy, should you need it	Don't proceed with your trip if it is unsafe to go

How to get involved

There are many organizations working in the global health arena. They have well-established project aims and governance structures, and will often have funding available for trips. Working as part of an organization will enable you to clarify the objectives of a mission and will reduce your personal risk significantly. Here is a short list of specific organizations involved with global orthopaedics work:

- World Orthopaedic Concern UK (WOC-UK) is a UK-based charity and specialist society of the BOA. It has links with projects across the globe, including short- and long-term projects for junior and senior trainees and consultants. Funding through fellowships and bursaries are available. Website: ℘ https://wocuk.org
- King's Global Health Partnerships connect UK and African health professionals, providing training, mentoring, and hands-on support, and undertake collaborative research to inform policy and practice. Website: ℘ https://www.kcl.ac.uk/kghp
- COSECSA Oxford Orthopaedic Link (COOL) is a multi-country partnership programme between Nuffield Department of Orthopaedics, Rheumatology and Musculoskeletal Sciences (NDORMS), University of Oxford, and the College of Surgeons of East Central and Southern Africa (COSECSA). Covering a region of 14 countries in sub-Saharan Africa, COSECSA fosters postgraduate education in surgery and provides surgical training throughout East, Central, and Southern Africa. Website: ℘ https://www.ndorms.ox.ac.uk/research/research-groups/global-surgery
- NIHR Global Health Research Unit on Global Surgery aims to improve surgical outcomes through collaborative surgical and clinical research. Website: ℘https://www.globalsurgeryunit.org
- The GlobalSurg Collaborative conducts collaborative international research through global networks: Website: ℘https://globalsurg.org/who-we-are/

Safety considerations

Concerns regarding personal safety can pose a significant barrier to working in LMICs. While the risks can never be totally mitigated, plenty of advice is available. Trainees wishing to visit an LMIC should gather as much information as possible and then plan for all eventualities.

The travel advice section on the UK Foreign Office website (available from: ℅ www.gov.uk/foreign-travel-advice) provides a wealth of up-to-date information on 225 countries and territories, ranging from the risk of violence to recent dangerous weather systems and what vaccinations you might need. Other resources can be accessed from organizations listed below:

- International Committee of the Red Cross. Available from: ℅ https://shop.icrc.org/safe-manuel-de-securite-pour-les-humanitaires-print-fr-1.html
- Tropical Health and Education Trust. Available from: ℅ www.thet.org/wp-content/uploads/2017/09/HPS-Duty-of-Care-Toolkit.pdf
- Médecins Sans Frontières. Available from: ℅ www.medicalguidelines.msf.org

Indemnity (medico-legal cover)

NHS indemnity provided through a UK employer will not cover work done overseas, including for voluntary or charitable bodies. It is strongly recommended that supplementary insurance with one of the medical defence bodies or other personal indemnity insurance is obtained for work in LMICs.

Further guidance can be found on the British Medical Association (BMA) website (⊛ https://www.bma.org.uk/advice-and-support/career-progression/working-abroad/working-abroad-as-a-doctor-key-considerations).

Funding

Travelling fellowships, bursaries, or grants are available from a number of sources and for varying amounts. This can help with the financial barrier associated with overseas work. Below is a list of travelling grants currently available:

- Royal College of Surgeons of England. Available from:
  ✆ https://www.rcseng.ac.uk/about-the-rcs/international-affairs/grants-and-fellowships/
- Royal College of Surgeons of Edinburgh. Available from: ✆ www.rcsed.ac.uk/professional-support-development-resources/grants-jobs-and-placements/research-travel-and-award-opportunities/grants
- Royal College of Surgeons in Ireland. Available from: ✆ https://www.rcsi.com/surgery/training/fellowship-opportunities/rcsi-travel-grants
- British Orthopaedic Association. Available from: ✆ www.boa.ac.uk/learning-and-events/fellowships-awards.html
- British Orthopaedic Trainees Association. Available from: ✆ www.bota.org.uk
- World Orthopaedic Concern UK. Available from: ✆ https://wocuk.org
- British Orthopaedic Foot and Ankle Society. Available from: ✆ www.bofas.org.uk/clinician/fellowships/travelling-fellowships
- British Society For Surgery of the Hand. Available from: ✆ https://www.bssh.ac.uk/professionals/fellowships.aspx

Further reading

British Medical Association. *Volunteering abroad*. Available from: ✆ www.bma.org.uk/advice-and-support/career-progression/working-abroad/working-abroad-as-a-doctor-key-considerations

Meara JG, Leather AJ, Hagander L, et al. Global Surgery 2030: evidence and solutions for achieving health, welfare, and economic development. *The Lancet*. 2015;**386**(9993):569–624.

Yeomans D, Le G, Pandit H, Lavy C. Is overseas volunteering beneficial to the NHS? The analysis of volunteers' responses to a feedback questionnaire following experiences in low-income and middle-income countries. *BMJ Open*. 2017;**7**(10):e017517.

Part 2

Anatomy and surgical approaches

Chapter 9

Anatomy

Head and neck anatomy

Skull

The frontal, parietal, and occipital bones make up the cranial vault; between these are the coronal, sagittal, and lambdoid sutures (Fig. 9.1) The skull base is made up of the sphenoid, the petrous part of the temporal and occipital bones. The cranium houses the brain, its meningeal coverings, and the CSF in which the brain is suspended.

Skeleton of the cervical spine

The cervical vertebrae are specialized in several ways:
- There is no vertebral body to C1. Instead, there is a narrow anterior arch, behind which lies the odontoid process of C2 (the dens), which is stabilized by the alar and cruciate and transverse ligaments.
- C2–C6: bifid spinous processes provide attachments for the ligamentum nuchae; the foramen transversarium transmits the vertebral arteries bilaterally. The lateral masses articulate through facet joints with the vertebra above and below. The vertebral bodies have a small upward projection on each side (the uncus), which articulates with the inferior aspect of the vertebral body above (the uncovertebral joint).
- C7: has a large spinous process ('vertebra prominens'); the foramen transversarium does not transmit the vertebral artery at this level.

Cervical fascia

Beneath the skin are the superficial fascia and platysma muscle. The deep cervical fascia encases the major structures of the neck:
- Deep investing layer (the most superficial part, which splits to encase the sternocleidomastoid and trapezius muscles)
- Pretracheal layer (which splits to encase the thyroid gland)
- Prevertebral layer (which covers the prevertebral muscles, the cervical plexus, and trunks of the brachial plexus)
- Carotid sheath (which contains the carotid arteries, internal jugular vein, vagus nerve, and ansa cervicalis—the cervical sympathetic trunk lies just posterior, on top of the prevertebral fascia).

Triangles of the neck

The main landmark is the sternocleidomastoid muscle, which demarcates the anterior and posterior triangles (Fig. 9.2).

The posterior triangle (between the sternomastoid, clavicle, and trapezius) contains:
- *Muscles:* scalenes, levator scapulae, inferior belly of omohyoid
- *Vasculature:* external jugular vein, occipital and transverse cervical arteries, and, at the inferior margin, subclavian and suprascapular vessels
- *Nerves:* accessory nerve, cervical plexus, brachial plexus, phrenic nerve
- *Lymphatics:* lymph nodes (and at the inferior margin on the left side lies the thoracic duct).

The anterior triangle (between the sternomastoid, mandible, and midline) contains:
- *Midline structures:* thyroid and parathyroid glands, hyoid bone, trachea and larynx, oesophagus, and pharynx
- *Muscles:* suprahyoid muscles, infrahyoid ('strap') muscles, omohyoid

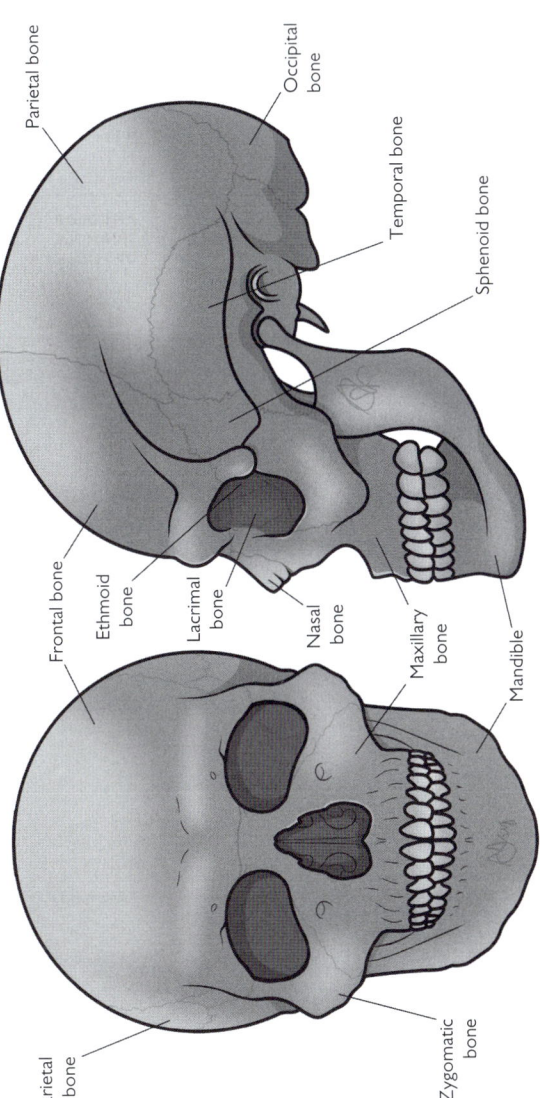

Fig. 9.1 Skull skeletal anatomy.
Illustrated by Aqua Asif and Ayaan Asif.

(A)

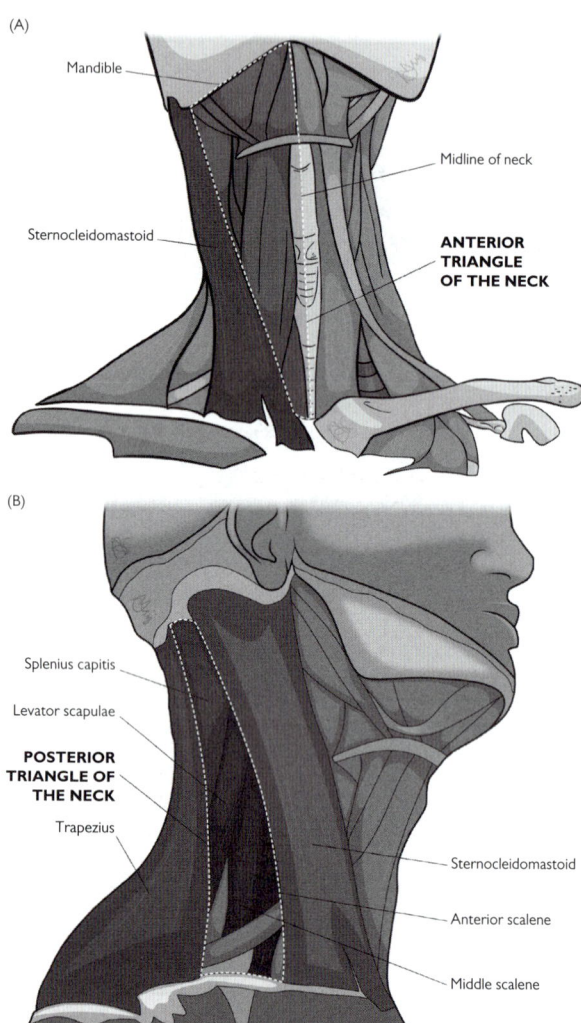

Mandible

Midline of neck

Sternocleidomastoid

ANTERIOR TRIANGLE OF THE NECK

(B)

Splenius capitis

Levator scapulae

POSTERIOR TRIANGLE OF THE NECK

Trapezius

Sternocleidomastoid

Anterior scalene

Middle scalene

Fig. 9.2 Anterior (A) and posterior (B) triangles of the neck.
Illustrated by Aqua Asif and Ayaan Asif.

- *Vasculature:* common carotid with bifurcation into internal carotid and external carotid (and branches). Internal jugular vein (and branches)
- *Nerves:* hypoglossal and branches of glossopharyngeal and vagus nerves.

NB the carotid sheath lies under cover of the sternocleidomastoid and is therefore not included in the contents of the triangles of the neck.

Recurrent laryngeal nerve

This ascends in the tracheo-oesophageal groove and is at risk during anterior cervical surgery. A left-sided approach is said to be safer with regard to nerve injury. On the right side, the nerve is occasionally non-recurrent.

Spinal anatomy

The spine comprises the vertebrae, neural tissue (spinal cord and spinal nerves) and their coverings, intervertebral discs, ligaments, and muscles (Fig. 9.3). The vertebrae are stacked in a column, which is straight when viewed in the coronal plane. There are physiological curvatures in the sagittal plane: cervical lordosis, thoracic kyphosis, lumbar lordosis. However, these curves are normally balanced, so that the head is centred over the pelvis when viewed in both the sagittal and coronal planes.

Vertebrae

There are seven cervical, 12 thoracic, and five lumbar vertebrae, a sacrum composed of five fused vertebrae, and a rudimentary coccyx. The main bulk is anterior (vertebral body), with an arch extending posteriorly to form the vertebral canal containing the neural elements. The arch comprises the pedicles (continuous with the body) and the inferiorly sloping laminae more posteriorly, which meet in the midline to form the spinous process. Below each pedicle, a spinal nerve root is transmitted via the intervertebral foramen. Superior and inferior articular processes from adjacent vertebrae articulate to form the facet joints. Transverse processes are large in the lumbar spine, and smaller in the thoracic and cervical regions.

Neural elements and coverings

The spinal cord is continuous with the brainstem at the foramen magnum of the skull and runs caudally to L1 where it terminates as the conus medullaris. It is covered with the dura mater, continuous with that of the brain. Outside of the dura is the epidural space; within it is the neural tissue bathed in CSF in the subarachnoid (spinal) space. Paired nerve roots branch off the spinal cord and exit through the intervertebral foramina. The nerve roots for segments below L1 are contained within the dural sac as the cauda equina.

Intervertebral discs

Secondary cartilaginous joints (symphyses) between vertebral bodies, composed of a fibrous ring (annulus fibrosus) and a gelatinous centre (nucleus pulposus). The annulus is made up of lamellae that are predominantly type I collagen. The fibres of one lamella run at an angle of 30° to its immediate neighbour. The nucleus contains proteoglycans that are strongly hydrophilic.

Ligaments

There are three ligaments that run the length of the spine—all in the midline:
• Anterior longitudinal ligament—anterior to vertebral bodies
• Posterior longitudinal ligament—immediately posterior to vertebral bodies
• Supraspinous ligament—between the tips of the spinous processes.

Shorter ligaments—consistent paired ligaments between each vertebra:
• Interspinous ligament—between spinous processes
• Intertransverse ligament—between transverse processes
• Ligamentum flavum (yellow ligament)—between laminae.

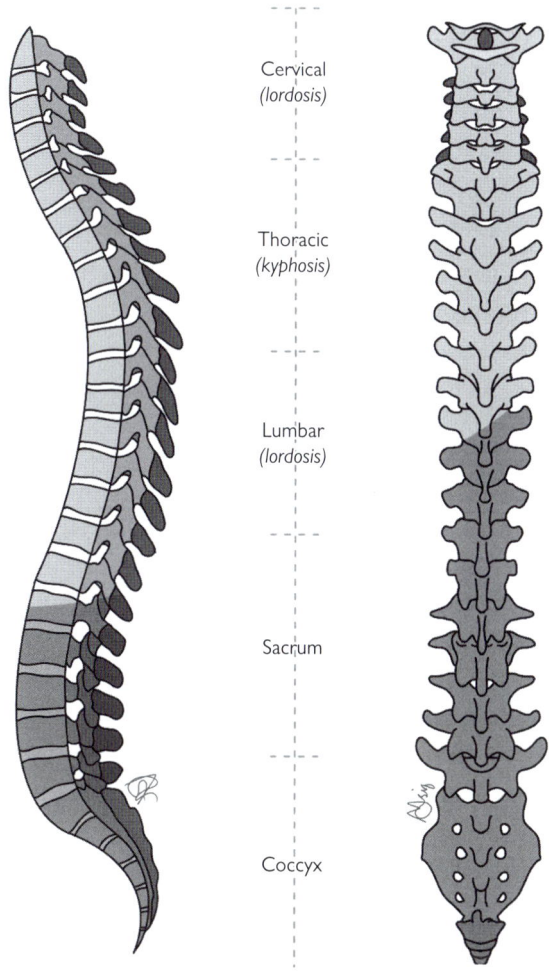

Cervical
(lordosis)

Thoracic
(kyphosis)

Lumbar
(lordosis)

Sacrum

Coccyx

Fig. 9.3 Anatomy of the spine.
Illustrated by Aqua Asif and Ayaan Asif.

Muscles

Spinal movement is brought about by many different muscles, including those distant from the spine itself (e.g. rectus abdominis). The paraspinal musculature is composed of both flexors and extensors.

- The flexors are situated anterior to vertebral bodies—longus colli from T4 to the skull base; in the lumbar spine, the psoas major acts as a powerful flexor.
- Extensors—divided into superficial, intermediate, and deep muscle groups, all supplied by posterior primary rami of the spinal nerves:
  - Superficial—the erector spinae muscle group: iliocostalis, longissimus, and spinalis
  - Intermediate—the transversospinalis group: multifidus, levator costarum, and the semispinalis capitis, cervicis, and thoracis
  - Deep—intertransversalis, interspinalis, and rotatores.

Anatomy of the shoulder girdle

The upper limb, shoulder girdle, arm, forearm, wrist, and hand are attached to the body by one bone—the clavicle—and muscles (Fig. 9.4).

Embryology

The upper limb bud appears at 24 days, formed from the ectoderm and mesoderm from C5 to T1. Longitudinal growth is governed by the apical ectodermal ridge and the post-axial border (ulnar side) defined by the zone of polarizing activity.

Biomechanics

Sternoclavicular joint

The proximal end of the clavicle articulates with the sternum. The SCJ is a synovial joint with an intervening fibrocartilage disc; involved in elevating the arm >90°, depression of the shoulder, protraction/retraction, and rotational GHJ movement.

Clavicle

Stabilizes the upper limb to the axial skeleton. Muscle attachments include the sternocleidomastoid, pectoralis major (clavicular head), and subclavius. Anterior and posterior divisions of the brachial plexus pass deep to it, as do the subclavian vessels.

Acromioclavicular joint

The distal end of the clavicle articulates with the acromion of the scapula. The ACJ is a synovial joint with an intervening fibrocartilage disc. It allows a small amount of rotation of the shoulder girdle on the long axis of the clavicle. It is stabilized by intrinsic (acromioclavicular) and extrinsic (coracoclavicular) ligaments.

Scapula

Parts of the scapula are the: body, spine, acromion, neck, and glenoid fossa. The rotator cuff muscles arise from the posterior (supraspinatus, infraspinatus, and teres minor) and anterior (subscapularis) aspects of the body. Muscle attachments to, or those crossing, the scapula stabilize it to the thorax (rhomboid major and minor, pectoralis minor, levator scapulae, serratus anterior, latissimus dorsi, and trapezius). The deltoid muscle arises from the spine of the scapula and acromion, in addition to the clavicle. It gives the shoulder its rounded shape. The coracoid is palpable just medial to the GHJ line and distal to the ACJ. It serves as origin or insertion point for three muscles (pectoralis minor, coracobrachialis, short head of the biceps) and three ligaments (coracoclavicular, coracohumeral, coracoacromial). The brachial plexus and subclavian vessels are immediately medial to the coracoid.

Proximal humerus

The proximal humerus consists of an articular surface, which meets the shaft at the anatomical neck; the surgical neck, which is more distal; the greater tubercle (the supraspinatus, infraspinatus, and teres minor muscles attach here), the lesser tubercle (the subscapularis attaches here), and the intertubercular groove (the long head of the biceps tendon runs through this groove).

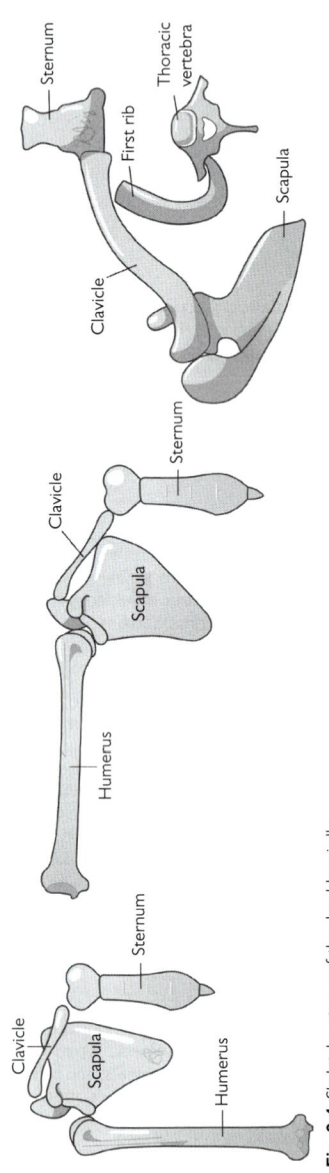

Fig. 9.4 Skeletal anatomy of the shoulder girdle.

Illustrated by Aqua Asif and Ayaan Asif.

Glenohumeral joint

Rotation occurs around the humeral head. Due to a large lever arm, lifting even small masses can create large forces within the GHJ, making it equivalent to a weight-bearing joint. Only a third of the humeral head is in contact with the glenoid. Stability is enhanced by static constraints (capsule, ligaments, labrum, negative intra-articular pressure, surface adhesion) and dynamic constraints (muscles).

During movement at the GHJ, the stabilizers of the shoulder keep the humeral head opposed to the glenoid surface:

- Abduction—deltoid (axillary nerve) and supraspinatus (suprascapular nerve)
- Adduction—latissimus dorsi (thoracodorsal nerve), pectoralis major (medial and lateral pectoral nerves), and cuff muscles, except supraspinatus
- Flexion—deltoid (axillary nerve), biceps (musculocutaneous nerve), and pectoralis major (lateral pectoral nerve)
- Extension—latissimus dorsi (thoracodorsal nerve), deltoid (axillary nerve), and triceps (radial nerve)
- External rotation—supraspinatus, infraspinatus (suprascapular nerve), and teres minor (axillary nerve)
- Internal rotation—subscapularis (subscapular nerves), pectoralis major (medial and lateral pectoral nerves), and teres major (lower subscapular nerve).

Blood supply of humeral head

- Anterior and posterior circumflex humeral arteries from the third part of the axillary artery anastomose around the neck of the humerus.
- Intramedullary supply from the humerus.

Blood supply can be disrupted with an anatomical neck fracture and may result in osteonecrosis.

Anatomy of the elbow

Biomechanics

The elbow (Fig. 9.5) can be thought of in terms of the:

- Humeroulnar joint (HUJ)—the trochlea of the humerus articulates with the trochlea notch of the ulna
- Radiocapitellar joint (RCJ)—the capitellum of the humerus articulates with the radial head
- Proximal radioulnar joint (PRUJ)—the proximal radius articulates with the ulna.

With the elbow extended, there is valgus angulation called the carrying angle. Greater in women than in men (15° vs 10°). The biceps and brachialis act to flex the elbow at a mechanical disadvantage due to the lever arm effect of the forearm. The ulnar collateral ligaments stabilize the elbow medially, and the radial collateral ligaments stabilize the joint laterally.

Ossification centres

Useful to estimate the age of a child. They appear in the following order (approximate age)—aide-memoire 'CRITOL': Capitellum (1 year), Radial head (3 years), medial (Internal) epicondyle (5 years), Trochlea (7 years), Olecranon (9 years), and Lateral epicondyle (11 years).

Surface landmarks

Bony landmarks

- Lateral epicondyle of the humerus—from the anterior surface arise the extensor tendons of the forearm and hand.
- Medial epicondyle—forearm and hand flexors arise from here.
- Olecranon of the ulna—posteriorly provide insertion for triceps.

With the elbow flexed to 90°, these three points above form an isosceles triangle. With the elbow fully extended, they line up in the transverse plane.

Anterior structures

From medial to lateral, the following structures cross in front of the elbow: (1) flexors of the wrist and hand; (2) median nerve; (3) brachial artery; (4) biceps tendon; (5) lateral cutaneous nerve of the forearm (terminal sensory branch of the musculocutaneous nerve); (6) brachialis tendon; (7) radial nerve (posterior interosseous and superficial branches); (8) brachioradialis; and (9) common extensors. The ulnar nerve passes behind the medial epicondyle in a groove.

Elbow joint

Stabilized by static and dynamic constraints.

Static

- Capsule.
- Ligaments—medially, the anterior band of the medial collateral ligament is the most important restraint to valgus force. Laterally, the lateral ulnar collateral ligament is important, and loss may result in posterolateral instability. The radial head is constrained by the annular ligament and provides further valgus stability in extension.

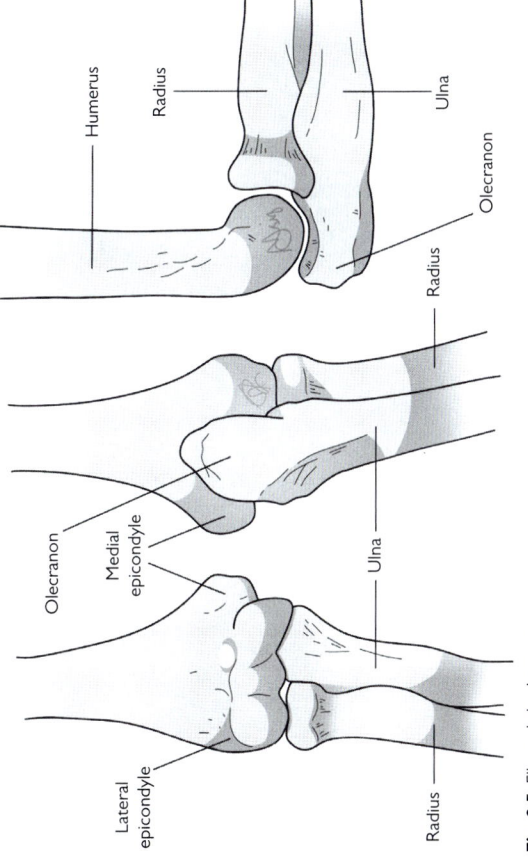

Fig. 9.5 Elbow skeletal anatomy.
Illustrated by Aqua Asif and Ayaan Asif.

- Bony architecture—stability provided by congruency. Fractures of the radial head may contribute to valgus instability.

Dynamic
- Common flexor origin.
- Common extensor origin.
- Instability may occur if these are avulsed traumatically.
- The anconeus may help to limit posterior subluxation of the radial head.

Anatomy of the forearm

Flexors in the forearm

Muscles controlling elbow movements include (Fig. 9.6):
- Biceps—flexion and supination
- Brachialis—flexion
- Triceps—extension
- Pronator teres—flexion and pronation.

These can be thought of in three layers, from superficial to deep:
- Superficial (lateral to medial)—pronator teres, flexor carpi radialis (FCR), palmaris longus (PL), and flexor carpi ulnaris (FCU)
- Middle layer—FDS
- Deep layer (proximal to distal)—FDP, FPL, and pronator quadratus (PQ).

Extensors in the forearm

In addition to the brachioradialis and supinator, the extensor compartment includes the following muscles:
- Extensor carpi radialis longus (ECRL) and brevis (ECRB)—supplied by the radial nerve, although ECRB is occasionally supplied by the posterior interosseous nerve (PIN)
- Extensor digitorum (ED), extensor carpi ulnaris (ECU), extensor indicis (EI), EDM, and extensor pollicis longus (EPL), which are supplied by the PIN.

Course of major nerves

- Radial nerve—formed from the posterior cord of the brachial plexus. Passes through the triangular interval bounded by the long head of the triceps, the humeral shaft, and the teres major. Then it winds around the back of the humerus in the spiral groove to pierce the lateral intermuscular septum. It enters the forearm anterior to the lateral epicondyle, passes between the brachialis and brachioradialis, and splits to form the PIN and superficial branch. The PIN pierces two heads of the supinator and travels in the extensor compartment, terminating at the wrist. The superficial branch travels deep to the brachioradialis.
- Median nerve—from the medial and lateral cords of the plexus. Accompanies the brachial artery in the arm, crosses the antecubital fossa, then passes between the two heads of the pronator teres. In the forearm, it lies deep to the FDS before entering the carpal tunnel, superficial to the flexor tendons. The AIN is given off at the elbow and accompanies the equivalent artery.
- Ulnar nerve—from the medial cord of the plexus. Passes from anterior to posterior through the medial intermuscular septum, then behind the medial epicondyle. It then passes between the two heads of the FCU into the forearm where a dorsal branch is given off before the nerve enters Guyon's canal.

Range of movements of the elbow

Flexion is from −5° to 150°. Pronation 80° and supination 90°.

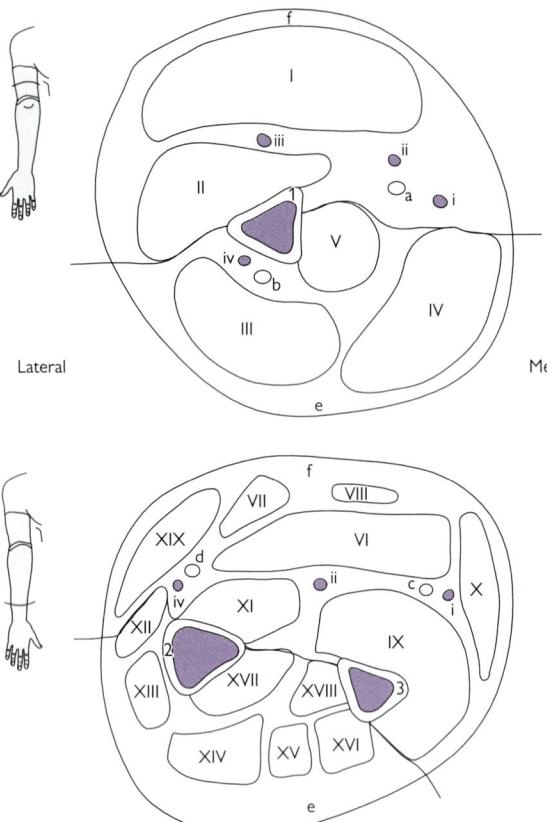

Fig. 9.6 Upper limb—transverse sections. 1, humerus; 2, radius; 3, ulna. I, biceps; II, brachialis; III, lateral head of triceps; IV, long head of triceps; V, medial head of triceps; VI, flexor digitorum superficialis; VII, flexor carpi radialis; VIII, palmaris longus; IX, flexor digitorum profundus; X, flexor carpi ulnaris; XI, flexor pollicis longus; XII, extensor carpi radialis longus; XIII, extensor carpi radialis brevis; XIV, extensor digitorum communis; XV, extensor digiti minimi; XVI, extensor carpi ulnaris; XVII, abductor pollicis longus; XVIII, extensor pollicis longus; XIX, brachioradialis. a, brachial artery; b, deep brachial artery; c, ulnar artery; d, radial artery; e, extensor compartment; f, flexor compartment. i, ulnar nerve; ii, median nerve; iii, musculocutaneous nerve; iv, superficial branch of radial nerve.

Illustrated by Aqua Asif and Ayaan Asif.

Anatomy of the wrist

The wrist (Fig. 9.7) is composed of eight carpal bones, arranged in two rows. From radial to ulnar:
- Proximal row: scaphoid, lunate, triquetrum, pisiform
- Distal row: trapezium, trapezoid, capitate, hamate.

There are six dorsal and two volar compartments that contain tendons to the hand.

Biomechanics

Interosseous ligaments (e.g. scapholunate ligament) are vital in guiding movements of the carpal bones relative to each other. The action of particular muscles on joint movement depends on whether the tendon passes in front of (flexion) or behind (extension) the centre of rotation of that joint, not on the position of the muscle. Forearm pronation and supination occur by rotation of the radius around the fixed ulna.

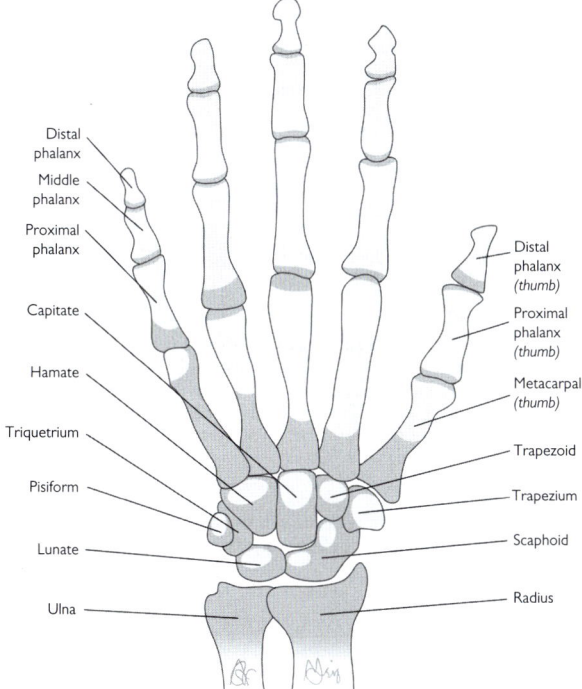

Fig. 9.7 Bony anatomy of the hand and wrist.

Illustrated by Aqua Asif and Ayaan Asif.

Carpal ossification

Appearance of the ossification centres of the carpal bones (approximate age in years) is useful to estimate a child's age: capitate (1 year); hamate (2 years); triquetrum (3 years); lunate (4 years); scaphoid (5 years); and trapezium and trapezoid (5–6 years). The pisiform (9 years) is a sesamoid bone within the tendon of the FCU.

Bony landmarks

- *Anatomical snuffbox:* this is the concavity formed with extension of the thumb, between the EPL and the extensor pollicis brevis (EPB). Within this space can be palpated the radial artery overlying the radial styloid and scaphoid waist.
- *Lister's tubercle:* this is a bony prominence on the dorsum of the distal radius. The tendon of the EPL passes around the ulnar border, using it as a pulley.
- *Ulnar head* (distal end; radial head proximal): this sits slightly dorsally relative to the distal radius.

Extensor compartments of the wrist

(Fig. 9.8)

The extensor tendons at the distal radius/ulna run deep to the extensor retinaculum in six distinct compartments. From radial to ulnar, these are:

- First—APL and EPB
- Second—ECRL and ECRB
- Third—EPL
- Fourth—EI and ED
- Fifth—EDM
- Sixth—ECU.

Where two extensor tendons act on a finger (EI and EDM), the ED tendon is located on the radial side.

Carpal tunnel

A fibro-osseous tunnel whose boundaries are the carpal bones, with the transverse carpal ligament (TCL) forming the roof (Fig. 9.9). The TCL is attached to the hamate and pisiform and the scaphoid tubercle. It contains the tendons of FDS and FDP within synovial sheaths, the tendon of FPL, and the median nerve. The motor branch of the median nerve to the thenar muscles may pass through the TCL.

Guyon's canal

The canal lies between the pisiform and the hook of hamate. The floor is the TCL, with the roof being the volar carpal ligament (VCL). It contains the ulnar nerve and artery.

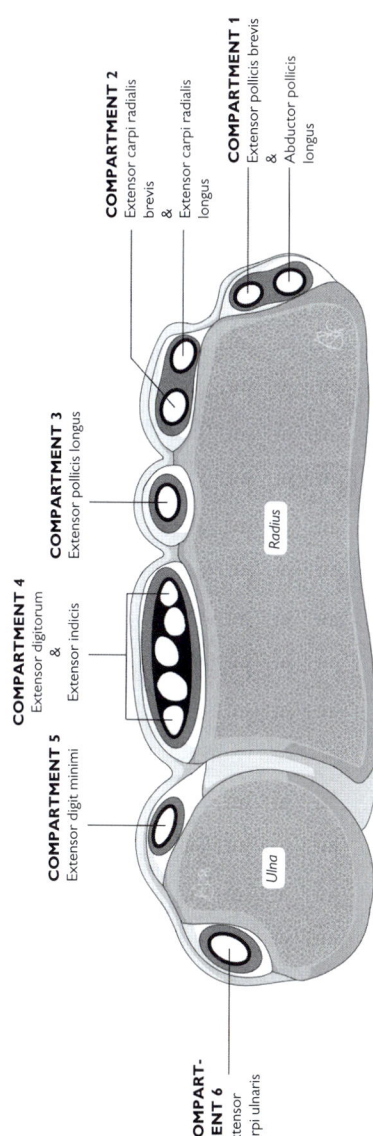

Fig. 9.8 Extensor compartments of the wrist.
Illustrated by Aqua Asif and Ayaan Asif.

COMPARTMENT 1
Extensor pollicis brevis
&
Abductor pollicis longus

COMPARTMENT 2
Extensor carpi radialis brevis
&
Extensor carpi radialis longus

COMPARTMENT 3
Extensor pollicis longus

COMPARTMENT 4
Extensor digitorum
&
Extensor indicis

COMPARTMENT 5
Extensor digiti minimi

COMPARTMENT 6
Extensor carpi ulnaris

Radius

Ulna

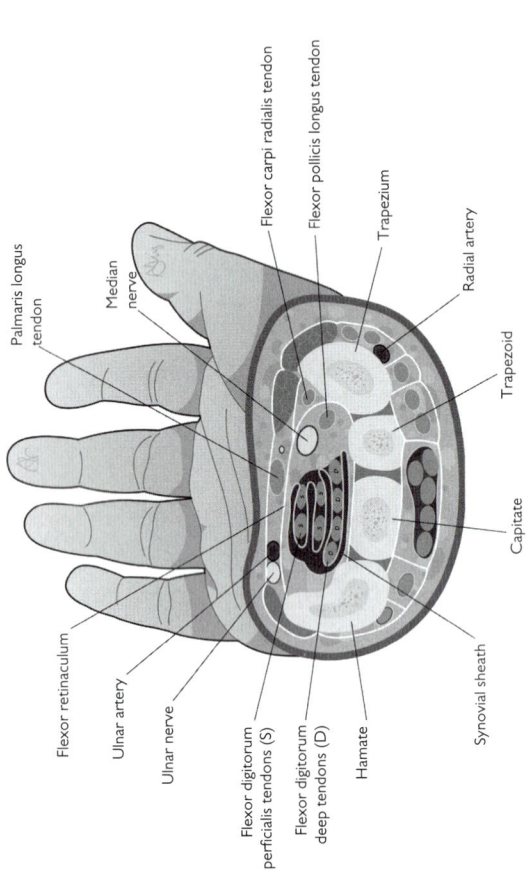

Fig. 9.9 Cross-section of the wrist at the carpal tunnel.
Illustrated by Aqua Asif and Ayaan Asif.

Anatomy of the hand

The hand is composed of five metacarpals and 14 phalanges (Fig. 9.7). The bony architecture is complex. It can be divided into the:
- *Volar (palmar) aspect:* contains muscles, flexor tendons, and digital nerves
- *Dorsal aspect:* contains muscles and extensor tendons/mechanisms.

Flexor zones

(Fig. 9.10)
- *Zone 1:* distal to FDS insertion (fingertips to middle of middle phalanx; includes the FDP tendon only).
- *Zone 2:* between zone 1 and distal palmar skin crease. Termed 'no man's land', as contains both FDS and FDP within their flexor sheath; hence, repairs are prone to adhesions and difficult to rehabilitate.

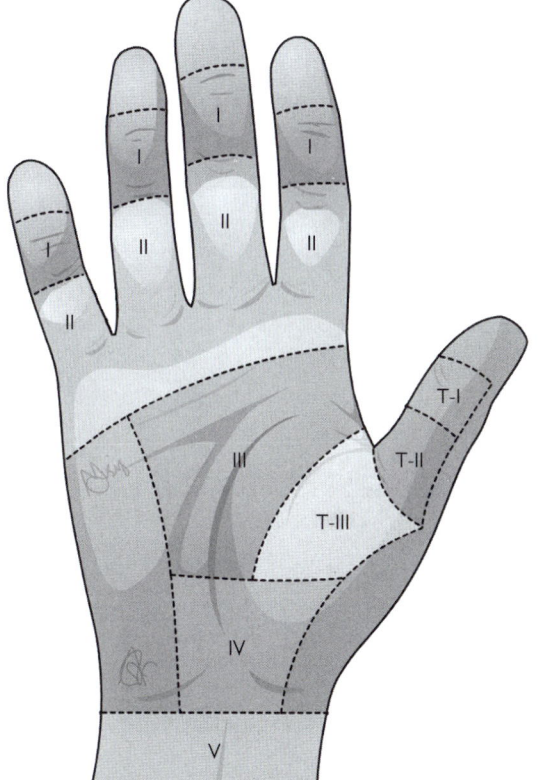

Fig. 9.10 Flexor zones of the hand.
Illustrated by Aqua Asif and Ayaan Asif.

- *Zone 3:* distal palmar skin crease to start of carpal tunnel.
- *Zone 4:* within carpal tunnel.
- *Zone 5:* proximal to carpal tunnel.

For the thumb, there are four zones, with T-1 distal to the IPJ, T-2 distal to the MCPJ, T-3 being the thenar eminence, and T-4 within the carpal tunnel.

Extensor zones
(Fig. 9.11)
- *Zone 1:* DIPJ.
- *Zone 2:* middle phalanx.

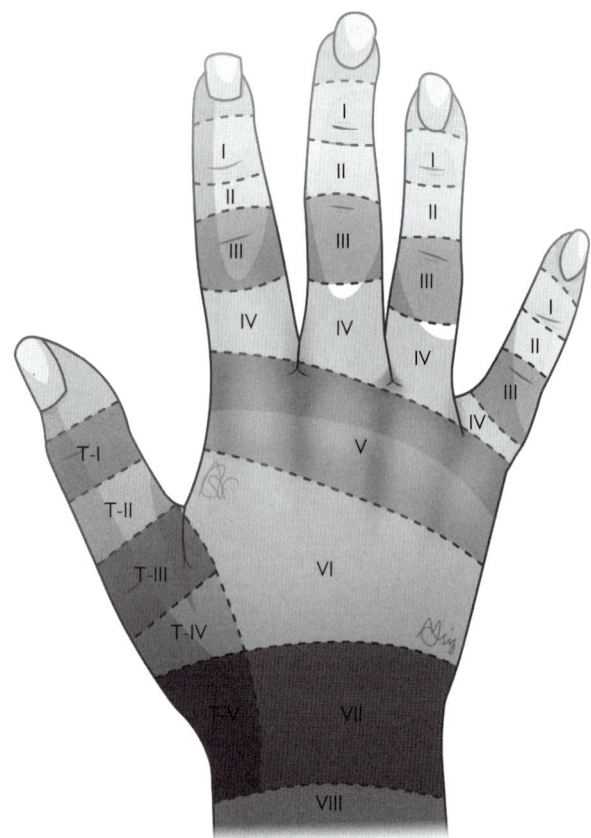

Fig. 9.11 Extensor zones of the hand.
Illustrated by Aqua Asif and Ayaan Asif.

- *Zone 3*: proximal interphalangeal joint (PIPJ).
- *Zone 4*: proximal phalanx.
- *Zone 5*: MCPJ.
- *Zone 6*: metacarpals/carpals (dorsum of hand).
- *Zone 7*: over wrist joint (extensor retinaculum).
- *Zone 8*: distal forearm (proximal to wrist crease).

For the thumb, there are five zones, with T-1 at the IPJ, T-2 the proximal phalanx, T-3 the MCPJ, T-4 the metacarpal, and T-5 under the extensor retinaculum at the wrist.

Innervation of the hand

Median nerve
- *Sensory:* palmar skin of radial three-and-a-half digits.
- *Motor:* aide-memoire 'LOAF'—Lateral two lumbricals, Opponens pollicis, Abductor pollicis brevis, Flexor pollicis brevis.

Ulnar nerve
- *Sensory:* ulnar one-and-a-half digits.
- *Motor:* remaining intrinsic muscles of the hand (i.e. those intrinsic muscles not innervated by the median nerve).

Radial nerve
- *Sensory:* remaining dorsal skin, particularly over the first dorsal webspace/anatomical snuffbox.
- *Motor:* finger and wrist extensors.

Movements of the fingers

The complexity of movements depends on the fine balance between the intrinsic muscles of the hand and the more powerful extrinsic muscles from the forearm which act on the hand.

Movements of joints of fingers
- *MCPJs:* Flexion—intrinsics. Extension—ED. Abduction—dorsal interossei. Adduction—palmar interossei.
- *PIPJs and DIPJs:* Extension—intrinsics. Flexion—PIPJ by FDS, DIPJ by FDP.
- *Movements of joints of the thumb:* Flexion at MCPJ is by flexor pollicis brevis (FPB), and at IPJ is by FPL. Extension at MCPJ is by EPB, and at IPJ by EPL. Other movements are provided by the thenar muscles. The axis of thumb movement is rotated by 90°.

Pelvic girdle

Bones

The pelvic girdle is composed of two innominate bones and the sacrum. Each innominate bone comprises three united bones: the ischium, ilium, and pubis. These meet in the cup-shaped acetabulum and unite here by calcification of the triradiate cartilage after puberty.

The orientation of the pelvis in the upright adult is such that the ASIS and symphysis pubis lie in the same coronal plane.

Joints and ligaments

Viewed from above, the pelvis makes an obvious ring structure, and strong connecting joints form the articulations between its individual component bones. Supporting ligaments further strengthen the complex.

- *Sacroiliac joint:* strong synovial joint, which allows very little motion. The joint is surrounded by a strong posterior ligament complex and weaker anterior ligaments.
- *Pubic symphysis:* connects the two sides of the pelvis anteriorly.
- *Sacrococcygeal joint:* a symphysis which allows flexion and extension.
- *Sacrospinous and sacrotuberous ligaments:* help to form the greater and lesser sciatic foramen. The former transmits the sciatic nerve and piriformis muscle, and the latter the short external rotators of the hip.

Muscles

The pelvic girdle is an important site of origin and insertion (on both its internal and external surfaces) of muscles governing hip and truncal stability. The pelvic floor is a muscular sheet intrinsic to the pelvis, on which lie the pelvic viscera. Integrity (or otherwise) of this is an important factor predicting haemorrhage in pelvic fractures.

Nerves

- The *lumbar plexus* is formed in the psoas muscle, from the anterior rami of L1–L4 nerve roots. Important branches are the lateral femoral cutaneous, femoral, and obturator nerves.
- The *sacral plexus* is formed from the anterior rami of L4–S4 and is found in the pelvis, on the piriformis muscle, anterior to the sacrum. It gives rise to the sciatic nerve, superior and inferior gluteal nerves, posterior cutaneous nerve of the thigh, pudendal nerve, pelvic splanchnic nerves, and individually named branches to the quadratus femoris, obturator internus, and piriformis.

Vessels

- *External iliac arteries:* transit the pelvis for supply to the lower limbs.
- *Internal iliac arteries:* the main supply to the pelvic viscera and gluteal region. The largest branch—the superior gluteal artery—exits the pelvis via the greater sciatic foramen to supply the buttock.
- *Pelvic veins:* are numerous and form large plexuses, which eventually become confluent and drain into the internal iliac veins, but communication also exists to the vertebral venous plexuses.

Anatomy of the lower limb: thigh, knee, and leg

Accounts for up to 20% of body weight. On standing, the body's centre of gravity passes behind the axis of hip movement, anterior to the knee and ankle (Fig. 9.12).

Thigh

Anterior thigh

The flexor compartment containing the femoral nerve and vessels. The quadriceps femoris comprises the rectus femoris, vastus medialis, vastus lateralis, and vastus intermedialis. All converge into the quadriceps tendon, which attaches to the patella and is continuous with the patellar ligament. Action—flexion of the hip and extension of the knee. Sartorius.

- *Femoral triangle:* boundaries: inguinal ligament, medial sartorius, and medial border of the adductor longus. Contains the femoral nerve, artery, vein, and canal containing lymph nodes/fat. Vein, artery, and nerve (medial to lateral). The *profunda femoris* artery is the largest branch—important in blood supply to the hip joint.
- *Greater saphenous vein:* pierces the fascia lata, 4cm inferolateral to the pubic tubercle, to enter the femoral vein.

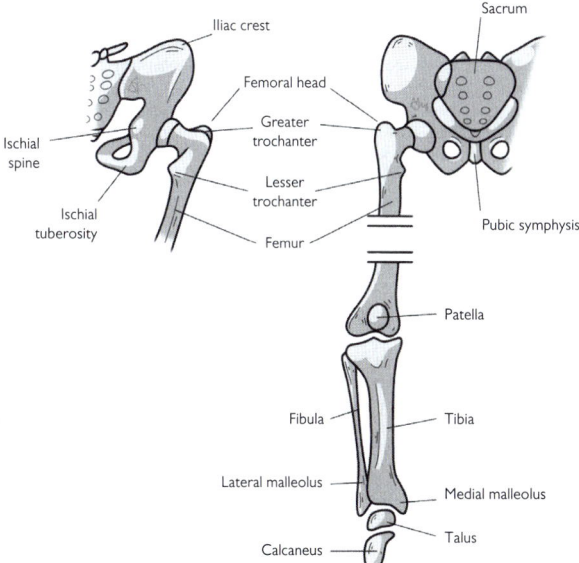

Fig. 9.12 Anatomy of the lower limb.
Illustrated by Aqua Asif and Ayaan Asif.

Medial thigh

Adductor compartment—gracilis, adductor longus, and adductor brevis deeper. These muscles arise from the pubic rami. The adductor magnus is the deepest adductor and arises from the ischial tuberosity. *Nerve supply:* obturator nerve, except adductor magnus which is partly innervated by the sciatic nerve inferiorly. The *adductor hiatus* is where the femoral artery passes en route to the popliteal fossa.

Posterior thigh

Extensor compartment.

- *Gluteal muscles:* the gluteus maximus (hip extensor) forms the bulk and is supplied by the inferior gluteal nerve. The gluteus medius and minimus (hip abductors) converge on the greater trochanter of the femur and are supplied by the superior gluteal nerve.
- *Piriformis muscle:* only the superior gluteal nerve and vessels enter from the pelvis above it, and all else below. The *sciatic nerve* enters below to the piriformis, deep to the hamstrings, and divides at the upper end of the popliteal fossa into the tibial and common peroneal nerves. The piriformis, along with the obturator internus, quadratus femoris, and tensor fasciae latae, contribute to lateral rotation.
- *Hamstrings:* the semitendinosus, semimembranosus, and biceps femoris span the hip and knee (supplied by the sciatic nerve). They arise from the ischial tuberosity. Action—hip extension and knee flexion.

Knee

Tibiofemoral and patellofemoral joints. Supported by collateral and cruciate ligaments. Synovial hinge joint—capsule replaced anteriorly by the patella complex.

- *Ligaments: LCL*—lateral epicondyle of femur to anterolateral head of fibula; resists varus. *MCL*—medial epicondyle of femur (near adductor tubercle) to inferior to medial condyle of tibia; resists valgus strain. *ACL*—front of upper tibia to inside of lateral condyle of femur; resists anterior displacement of tibia on femur. *PCL*—posterior tibia to medial condyle of femur; resists posterior displacement.
- *Menisci:* C-shaped cartilaginous structures. Medial meniscus is attached to the MCL; less mobile and more prone to injury. The lateral meniscus has fewer attachments.
- *Bursae:* suprapatellar, prepatellar, intrapatella, semimembranosus, subsartorial.
- *Movements:* flexion—hamstrings, gastrocnemius, popliteus. Extension—quadriceps femoris. Medial rotation of tibia—semimembranosus and semitendinosus. Lateral rotation—biceps femoris.
- *Popliteal fossa:* diamond-shaped. Boundaries—biceps femoris (common peroneal nerve behind and lateral), semimembranosus, lateral head of gastrocnemius, plantaris, and medial gastrocnemius. Structures—tibial nerve, popliteal vein, popliteal artery (superficial to deep). The tibial nerve runs between the heads of the gastrocnemius, deep to the

soleus—supplies all calf muscles, dividing into the medial and lateral plantar nerves. The common peroneal nerve winds around the neck of the fibula, and divides into the superficial peroneal nerve (sensory/peronei) and deep peroneal nerve (extensor muscles/first webspace skin).

Leg

Compartments of the leg
- *Anterior:* tibialis anterior, extensor digitorum longus, extensor hallucis longus, extensor digitorum brevis, extensor hallucis brevis.
- *Posterior:*
  - *Superficial:* soleus and gastrocnemius
  - *Deep:* flexor hallucis longus, tibialis posterior, flexor digitorum longus.
- *Lateral:* peroneus brevis and peroneus longus.

Fig. 9.13 shows the transverse cross-sectional anatomy of the lower leg.

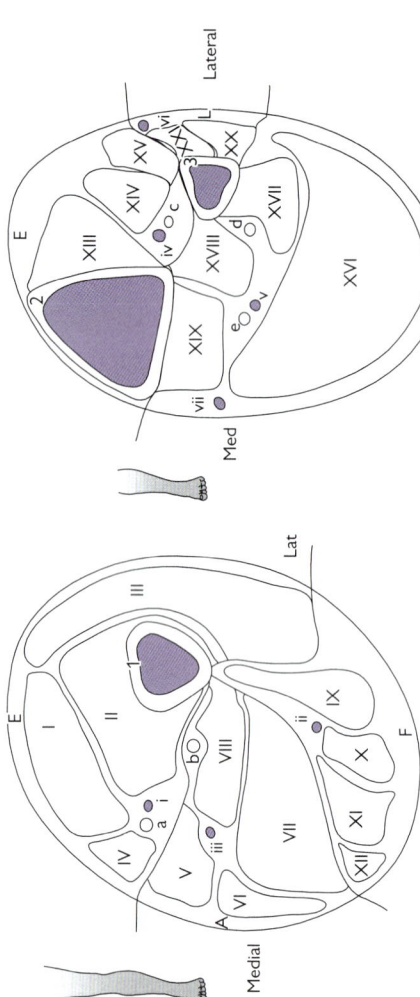

Fig. 9.13 Lower limb—transverse sections. 1, femur; 2, tibia; 3, fibula. I, rectus femoris; II, vastus medialis; III, vastus lateralis; IV, sartorius; V, adductor longus; VI, gracilis; VII, adductor magnus; VIII, adductor brevis; IX, gluteus maximus; X, biceps femoris; XI, semitendinosus; XII, semimembranosus; XIII, tibialis anterior; XIV, extensor hallucis longus; XV, extensor digitorum; XVI, soleus; XVII, flexor hallucis longus; XVIII, tibialis posterior; XIX, flexor digitorum longus; XX, peroneus longus; XXI, peroneus brevis. a, femoral artery; b, profunda femoral artery; c, anterior tibial artery; d, peroneal artery; e, posterior tibial artery; i, femoral nerve; ii, sciatic nerve; iii, obturator nerve; iv, deep peroneal nerve; v, tibial nerve; vi, superficial tibial nerve; vii, saphenous nerve.
Illustrated by Aqsa Asif and Ayaan Asif.

Anatomy of the lower limb: ankle and foot

Ankle

This joint is formed by the distal tibia and fibula and the talus (Fig. 9.14). It has a capsule that is reinforced by the medial deltoid ligament and lateral ligamentous complex, comprising the anterior and posterior talofibular and calcaneofibular ligaments.

Structures entering the foot posterior to the medial malleolus, from medial to lateral, the tibialis posterior, flexor digitorum longus, tibial nerve, posterior tibial artery, and flexor hallucis longus.

Movements

- *Dorsiflexion:* tibialis anterior, extensor hallucis longus, extensor digitorum longus, and peroneus tertius.
- *Plantar flexion:* gastrocnemius, soleus, tibialis posterior, flexor hallucis longus, flexor digitorum longus, peroneus longus, and peroneus brevis.

Stability

- *Bony mortise:* talus stabilized between tibia and fibula.
- *Ligamentous complexes:* the deltoid ligament stabilizes the ankle medially, preventing abduction, and the lateral ligament complex prevents adduction. Rotatory stability is conferred by alignment of the talus in the mortise and the collateral and syndesmosis ligaments. The syndesmosis consists of the anterior and posterior tibiofibular and interosseous ligaments.

Foot

Fig. 9.14 shows the anatomy of the foot.

Hindfoot

The bones of the hindfoot are the calcaneus and talus.

Subtalar joint

The talocalcaneal joint allows supination and pronation of the hindfoot. There are three articular facets between the talus and the calcaneus: anterior, middle, and posterior. The most important ligaments are the interosseous ligament in the sinus tarsi canal and the medial ligament (deep portion of the deltoid ligament). The calcaneofibular ligament stabilizes the subtalar joint laterally.

Midfoot

The bones of the midfoot are the navicular, the cuboid, and three cuneiforms.

Mid-tarsal joints (talonavicular and calcaneocuboid)

These movements are primarily those of:

- Inversion—tibialis anterior, tibialis posterior
- Eversion—peroneus longus and brevis.

Stability

The bifurcate ligament, consisting of the plantar calcaneonavicular (spring) ligament and calcaneocuboid ligament, contributes to stability of the joints

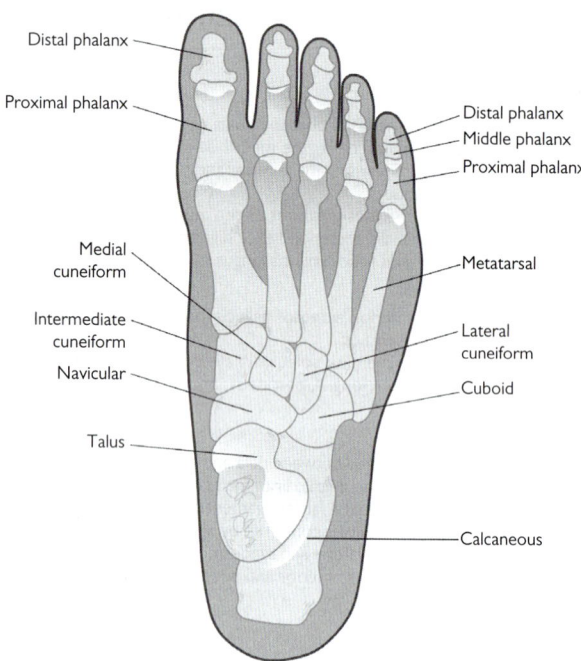

Fig. 9.14 Anatomy of the foot.

Illustrated by Aqua Asif and Ayaan Asif.

between the hindfoot and the midfoot. The spring ligament is situated between the sustentaculum tali of the calcaneus and the navicular. The talonavicular joint is a ball-and-socket type joint that allows gliding and rotatory movements. The calcaneocuboid joint is saddle-shaped and allows some abduction and adduction. Stability is conferred by the shape of the joint and the long and short plantar ligaments.

Forefoot

The bones of the forefoot are the metatarsals and phalanges.

Tarsometatarsal, metatarsophalangeal, and interphalangeal joints
Movements
The forefoot can be flexed and extended, and there is a small amount of adduction, abduction, and circumduction.

Stability
The tarsometatarsal joints are stabilized by the dorsal, plantar, and interosseous ligaments. The second and third metatarsals are attached to their

respective cuneiforms by strong ligaments limiting movements at these joints, whereas the first, fourth, and fifth metatarsals are more mobile. The metatarsophalangeal joints are condylar joints that allow flexion, extension, and some abduction, adduction, and circumduction, whereas the IPJs are hinge joints and only allow flexion and extension. The metatarsophalangeal joints and IPJs are stabilized by their capsules and collateral and plantar ligaments.

The plantar aponeurosis arises from the medial and lateral tubercles of the calcaneus, divides into five slips, one for each toe, and fuses with the fibrous flexor sheaths and metatarsophalangeal joint capsules. It contributes to stability of the longitudinal arch of the foot.

Sole of the foot muscle layers
Aide-memoire—'ALADIN' (sic):
- *First layer:* Abductor hallucis, abductor digiti minimi, flexor digitorum brevis
- *Second layer:* Lumbricals, quadratus plantae
- *Third layer:* ADductor hallucis, flexor hallucis brevis, flexor digiti minimi brevis
- *Fourth layer:* dorsal and plantar INterossei.

Innervation of the foot

Sensory
- *Dorsum:* superficial and deep fibular nerves.
- *Sole:* medial plantar nerve (medial three-and-a-half toes and medial sole) and lateral plantar nerve (lateral sole and lateral one-and-a-half toes).
- *Medial side of foot as far as the metatarsal head:* saphenous nerve.
- *Heel:* calcaneal branches of the tibial and sural nerves.

Motor
The medial plantar nerve supplies the abductor hallucis, flexor digitorum brevis, and flexor hallucis brevis, and the first lumbrical muscle. The lateral plantar nerve supplies all the other muscles of the sole.

Nervous system

The nervous system is categorized anatomically into:
- Central nervous system (CNS)—brain and spinal cord
- Peripheral nervous system—all other neural tissue.

It can also be categorized functionally into:
- Somatic nervous system—under conscious control
- Autonomic nervous system.

Somatic nervous system

The cerebrum consists of two cerebral hemispheres, which comprise grey matter (cell bodies), white matter (axons), and CSF-filled lateral ventricles. The surface folds (sulci) and prominences (gyri) create a consistent surface map of various functional centres. The central sulcus lies between the precentral and post-central gyri, which control motor and sensory function, respectively. The axons which connect these centres to their target skin and muscle locations mostly cross in the brainstem or spinal cord, such that the left motor and sensory functions of the body are controlled mostly by the right side of the brain, and vice versa.

Damage to the motor part of the CNS manifests itself clinically as an UMN dysfunction, whereas damage to the motor part of the peripheral nervous system manifests itself as LMN dysfunction.

Autonomic nervous system

The autonomic nervous system controls smooth and cardiac muscles, as well as glandular function. It is not under voluntary control. It consists of the sympathetic and parasympathetic nervous systems.

Sympathetic nervous system

Preganglionic fibres are located between T1 and L2, and synapse in paravertebral ganglia by using the neurotransmitter acetylcholine. Postganglionic axons then distribute to glands or body walls by using noradrenaline at the axonal endplate. Sympathetic innervation of the skin and blood vessels uses acetylcholine at the endplate.

Parasympathetic nervous system

The parasympathetic nervous system does not innervate the skin or extremities. Preganglionic fibres are located in the brainstem in cranial nerve nuclei and from S2–S4. The vagus nerve contains parasympathetic nerves, which supply the respiratory tract, heart, and gastrointestinal (GI) organs. The S2–S4 preganglionic axons supply the pelvic organs. The splenic flexure of the large bowel divides vagus-supplied organs from those innervated by the sacral parasympathetic nerves.

Vascular system

Arterial system

Major arteries are often given different names as they pass anatomical landmarks, as described in the examples below.

Upper limb

- The subclavian artery changes name to the axillary artery in the axilla at the outer border of the first rib.
- The axillary artery changes name to the brachial artery at the teres major muscle border.
- The brachial artery keeps its name until it bifurcates into the radial and ulnar arteries at the elbow.

Lower limb

- The external iliac artery changes name to the femoral artery at the inguinal ligament in the groin.
- The femoral artery changes name to the popliteal artery when it leaves the adductor hiatus in the distal thigh to enter the popliteal fossa.
- The popliteal artery keeps its name until it bifurcates into the anterior and posterior tibial arteries at the soleus.
- The anterior tibial artery changes name to the dorsalis pedis after it emerges from under the extensor retinaculum at the ankle.

Venous system

The venous system is anatomically divided into the:
- Superficial venous system
- Deep venous system.

In the lower limb, the short and long saphenous veins constitute the superficial venous system, whereas the femoral vein and its tributaries constitute the deep venous system.

The external vein is renamed as the femoral iliac vein when it crosses the inguinal ligament, and is renamed as the popliteal vein when it enters the popliteal fossa. The popliteal vein receives tributaries from the anterior and posterior tibial veins and the short saphenous vein. These three veins constitute the deep veins of the calf (the 'calf pump').

Venous flow is maintained by one-way valve systems and muscle contractions, which squeeze deoxygenated blood towards the heart. The superficial venous and deep venous systems communicate via perforating veins, which are also valved. Competent valves prevent blood from flowing from deep to superficial veins; incompetent valves do not prevent this, resulting in expanded or varicose veins.

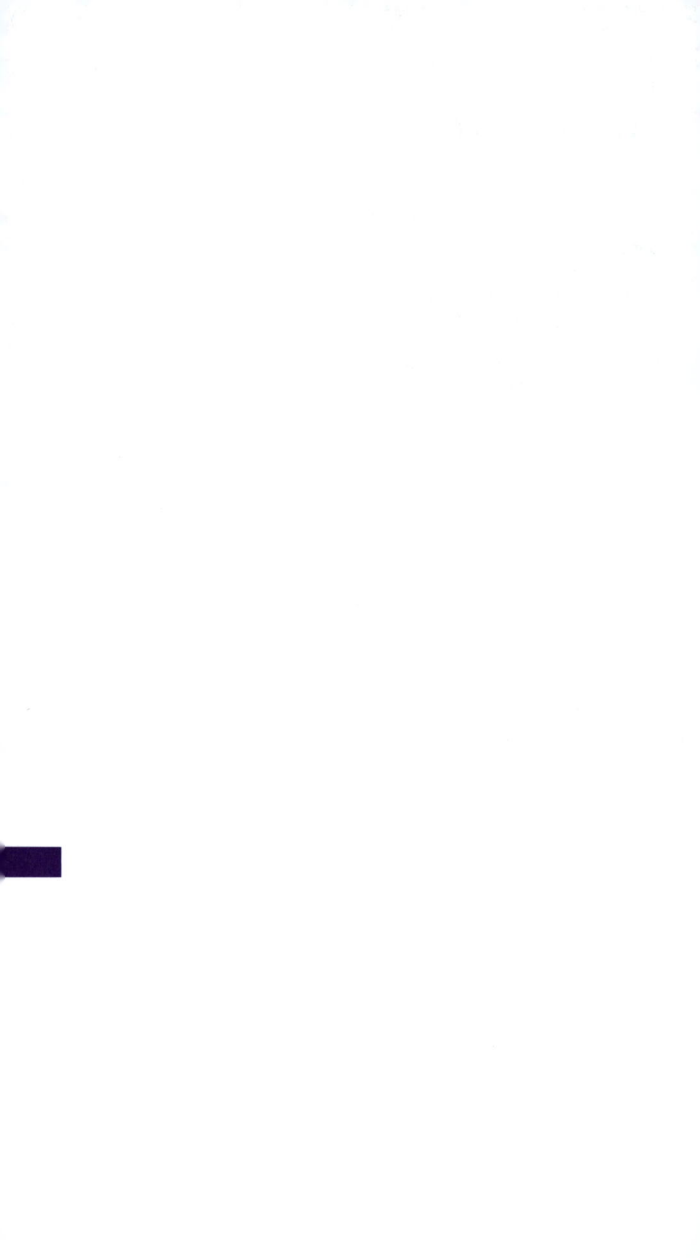

Surgical approaches and principles

Surgical principles

The practice of orthopaedic surgery has benefited enormously in the last hundred years or so with advances in anaesthesia, infection prevention, medical imaging, and surgical technology. Modern orthopaedics have seen innovation and refinement of joint replacement and arthroscopic reconstructive surgery, and management has been guided much more on scientific evidence than in the past. Today, every aspect of the surgical journey and management is reviewed, with regular updates and modifications made accordingly to improve patient care. National registries have improved care with the application of large data.

What is involved? Putting patients first

Generally, orthopaedic surgery results in good patient outcomes. Surgery primarily focuses on pain relief and functional improvement. However, as with any surgery, complications can occur, which can be severely detrimental to the patient. Poor results can also have a knock-on economic cost. Prior to operating on a patient, it is imperative that all non-operative measures have been explored. Furthermore, any intervention carried out must have a strong evidence base for being effective.

Multidisciplinary teamworking is especially important to optimize outcomes. This involves an array of team members, including: sports medicine physicians, pain specialists, nurse specialists, administrative staff, physiotherapists, orthotists, and occupational therapists. A good outcome from any orthopaedic intervention is a team effort.

Good surgeons know how to cut; great surgeons know when to cut

Shared decision-making is essential for patient satisfaction. Informed consent is an important part of the patient's decision to proceed with surgery. Recently, the consent process has been an evolving practice, with more weight given to ensure the patient is equipped with the full facts, and detailed options wholly discussed, for them to weigh up and make informed decisions. Although often rare, adverse outcomes affect patients differently and, in some cases, are sufficient enough to not proceed with surgery.

The difference between an efficient and a slow surgeon is knowledge of anatomy

Specific surgeries can take time to acquire a complete understanding and the operative technique. Preparation is important to optimize the outcome, as well as to improve learning. Therefore, it is recommended to read up on the procedure before assisting or undertaking the surgery. Knowing the anatomy, approach, objectives, and structures at risk is vital in being able to achieve a satisfactory outcome from a surgical procedure. Once the patient is in the operating theatre, attention should be paid to everything—from the patient set-up, maintenance of sterility, soft tissue handling, and wound closure to post-operative care.

Preoperative planning

It is important to ensure that a patient is medically fit for surgery and any medical factors have been optimized. The patient should be appropriately consented, preferably via a preadmission clinic with a senior surgical presence. The patient should also be marked according to the side being operated on, and checks carried out on the ward and in theatre.

Good outcomes often require a good preoperative plan. Preoperative planning includes preparing and coordinating team members (such the assistant, anaesthetist, scrub support, radiographer, etc.), ensuring the appropriate setting is available (e.g. theatre with laminar flow for joint arthroplasty) and that all necessary materials and equipment are available (e.g. range of implant sizes, saws, reamers, etc.). Orthopaedics is a highly technical specialty, and trainees are often taught to plan for all eventualities, to expect problems and intraoperative difficulties, and to consider options to overcome them. This forward thinking is vital to trying and reducing stress levels, which, in turn, will help a surgeon to remain focused. All surgeries are pre-empted with a WHO checklist at the start of the day to ensure additional plans and equipment that may become necessary should be communicated early and clearly to the team.

Below are some examples of common planning techniques used in orthopaedics and trauma.

Hip arthroplasty

Templating with appropriate radiographs prior to surgery enables:
- Determination of leg length for equalization
- Selection of correct cup size and position
- Planning of femoral neck cut and sizing/position of the femoral stem
- Ensuring availability of all potential implants.

Trauma

Planning reconstruction and placement of screws/plates (manufacturer templates available) can be done through tracing fracture fragments on overlays of radiographs. Equipment availability should be checked, and anything special ordered in. Additionally, simple measures should be taken, such as making sure the image intensifier is available for cases as required.

It is important to be familiar with the local system of external fixation for emergency surgery of open fractures and those with significant vascular injury.

Limb deformity correction

Planning of limb deformity correction is vital and should always be performed preoperatively. The type of correction will sometimes dictate what fixation method will be used. Software packages are now available to assist with 3D planning on-screen with digital imaging systems and use of CT or MRI modalities.

Aim to identify the site(s), level, and magnitude of the deformity to plan corrective osteotomy(ies). Steps include:
- Drawing the mechanical axis of the leg (select a long leg AP film, and draw a line from the centre of the femoral head to the centre of the

ankle joint). The line should pass through the centre of the knee joint if there is no mechanical axis deviation.
• Adding in the anatomical axis (along the diaphysis of the bone) for the femur and tibia, and measuring and comparing the angle they form with the joints. If these are different from the normal side or expected normal values, there is deformity in the bone.
• Analysing where the axes pass relative to the joints within that bone (which should be collinear), with the intersection marking the level of the deformity. The angle of intersection is the magnitude of the deformity.

Fig. 10.1 highlights the relevant lower leg angles.

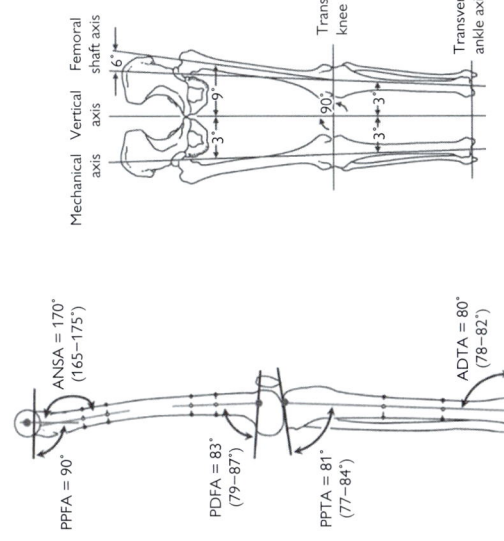

Fig. 10.1 Relevant lower leg angles.

Principles of wound care

Phases of wound healing (some overlap) include:
- Inflammation (0–5 days)
- Proliferation (3–14 days)
- Maturation (7 days to 1 year).

Clean wounds

Surgical incisions are closed with sutures (dissolvable or non-dissolvable) or staples, and skin edges are everted. Careful deeper layer closure can reduce tension on superficial layers. Minimize skin tension (can add Steri-Strips™); keep wounds clean and dry, and apply pressure on the area. Suture sizes depend on the size and location of the wound: face 5-0/6-0; hand 4-0; and limb 3-0. Suture removal should be timed by site: face, 5–7 days; limbs, 10–14 days; and trunk, 10 days.

Contaminated wounds

Foreign material should be removed and area surrounding thoroughly debrided, ideally facilitated with preoperative radiographs or USS. The wound should be washed out entirely with diluted chlorhexidine in saline. The wound can be left open or lightly packed. Tetanus status should be checked and antibiotics administered tailored to likely contaminants.

If the wound is small, community re-dressing and healing by secondary intention may be appropriate. A second look at 48–72h ± for further debridement and irrigation should be planned if the wound was heavily contaminated, large or at risk of significant complications. If clean at the relook, the skin edges may be opposed with tensionless interrupted sutures.

Infected wounds

Deep infected wounds commonly require debridement, irrigation, and sampling for microbiology prior to starting antibiotics. Leave the wound open, unless over a joint or a prosthesis, and plan a second-look procedure at 48–72h. If the infection is acute and involves a prosthesis, then perform debridement, antibiotics, and implant retention (DAIR) to exchange modular components (e.g. polyethylene insert in knee replacement).

General

Meticulous hand hygiene should be employed by all staff treating the patient, and everyone must wear appropriate PPE. Educate patients on the importance of good wound care. Factors which optimize patient wound healing include:
- Controlling blood sugar levels and encouraging good nutrition
- Smoking cessation
- Elevating the limb to reduce swelling
- Supplemental oxygen as required
- Completing an appropriate antibiotic course.

Surgical approaches: cervical spine

Anterior approach to the cervical spine

- *Indication:* spinal fracture fixation/stabilization; anterior cervical discectomy and fusion (ACDF).
- *Position:* supine with extension of the head and turned to opposing side of the approach. Caution with airway protection by the anaesthetist.
- *Incision:* an oblique skin crease incision is made at the correct vertebral level (should be confirmed with intraoperative fluoroscopy to check spinal level) from the midline to the anterior border of the sternocleidomastoid.
- *Dissection:* superficially, the incision is through the fascia over the platysma. The platysma is incised or split with fingers in the line of the fibres. Identify the sternocleidomastoid and retract it laterally, while the sternohyoid and sternothyroid muscles are retracted medially. Palpate the carotid pulse and retract the carotid sheath laterally. Medial to the carotid sheath, the pretracheal fascia is incised to reveal the longus colli muscles and the anterior longitudinal ligament. These are split from the midline and retracted laterally to reveal the anterior surface of the vertebral body (Fig. 10.2).
- *Risks:* the recurrent laryngeal nerve (right side is more vulnerable; left side runs in the tracheo-oesophageal groove), sympathetic chain, and thoracic duct (on the left). The cervical sympathetic chain sits on the lateral border of the longus colli. The superior and inferior thyroid arteries are beneath the pretracheal fascia.

Posterior approach to the cervical spine

- *Indication:* spinal fracture fixation/stabilization; posterior cervical laminectomy; discectomy; fusion; tumour surgery.
- *Position:* prone, often with flexion of the neck and use of a Halo rest and taping of the shoulders down in an inferior direction (to prevent the shoulders from getting in the way of imaging).
- *Incision:* longitudinal midline over the spinous process.
- *Dissection:* superficially, the incision is through the deep cervical fascia to then identify the nuchal ligament. Divide the ligament in the midline down to the spinous process. Dissection occurs subperiosteally and laterally, elevating and retracting the paraspinal muscles. Dissection continues to reveal the lamina (laminectomy can be performed here to access the spinal canal), lateral mass, and encapsulated facet joint.
- *Risks:* awareness and protection of the greater occipital nerve at C2 level. Innervation to the posterior cervical muscles running lateral to the facet joints—caution with dissection here. Superiorly, the vertebral artery is at risk, anterior to the lateral mass at C1/C2. The spinal canal is also increasingly nearer as the dissection deepens, so caution should be maintained.

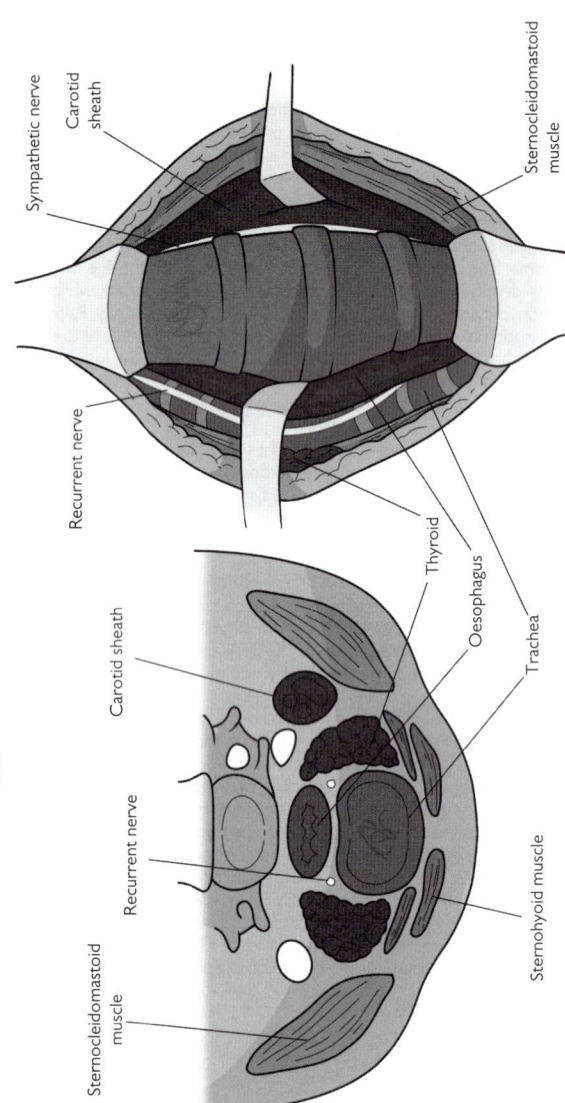

Fig. 10.2 Anterior cervical approach.

Surgical approaches: lumbar spine

Posterior approach to the lumbar spine

- *Indication:* decompression surgery from L3 to S1, and discectomies at L4/5; fusion; spinal fracture fixation/stabilization; tumour surgery.
- *Position:* prone, with slight forward flexion. Caution with airway protection by the anaesthetist when the patient is being turned over.
- *Incision:* confirm the correct vertebral level with an image intensifier. Images are saved with a metal marker identifying the operated level for medico-legal purposes. Midline longitudinal incision over the spinous processes.
- *Dissection:* continue through the lumbodorsal fascia. The paraspinal muscles are innervated segmentally, and therefore, the approach to the spine is on an internervous plane. Preserve the interspinous ligaments between the spinous processes. With use of a Cobb elevator, detach the paraspinous muscles subperiosteally and laterally (or bilaterally) until the lamina and facet joint capsule are seen. Then dissection is anterior to the transverse process, as needed. With care, excise the ligamentum flavum with fine rongeurs until the lamina insertion is reached. Perform laminectomy to enter the spinal canal. Epidural fat should be visible, and under this, following careful blunt dissection, the blue-white appearance of the dura mater that surrounds the spinal cord. Puncture of this will lead to CSF leak. Any CSF leaks must be sealed with adhesive patches and sealants.
- *Risks:* dissection lateral to the facet joint can result in injury to segmental vessels—the articular branches. Exiting nerve roots run deep to transverse processes, but throughout dissection, caution should be taken to avoid injury. Dural tears can occur during deep dissection around the spinal canal.

Anterior approaches to the lumbar spine

There are two main anterior approaches to the lumbar spine: transperitoneal and retroperitoneal.

Transperitoneal approach

- *Indication:* anterior spinal decompression; spinal fusion; tumour surgery/biopsy; total disc replacement.
- *Position:* supine and in the Trendelenburg position on table to help move the abdominal contents superiorly.
- *Incision:* longitudinal midline incision from umbilicus to pubic symphysis.
- *Dissection:* develop the internervous plane between the two recti. The incision is deepened to expose the peritoneum, which is carefully incised. Use large abdominal retractors to carefully retract the bowel and bladder, sweeping them out of the midline to reveal the posterior peritoneum. Incise this at the level of the sacral promontory, found by palpation. Ligate the median sacral artery, and divide to allow dissection down to the anterior longitudinal ligament and vertebral body or the L5/S1 disc space.
- *Risks:* injury to the superior hypogastric plexus that overlies the L5 lumbar vertebrae. Damage to this can result in retrograde ejaculation and impotence. Peritoneal contents—bowel, bladder, and ureter injury.

Median sacral artery injury. Injury to the aorta/inferior vena cava can have devastating/fatal consequences. For this reason, a combined surgical team of general surgeon/spinal surgeon is normal.

Retroperitoneal approach

- *Indication:* access to L1 to the sacrum; anterior spinal decompression; fracture fixation/stabilization; abscess (psoas) drainage; deformity correction; spinal fusion; tumour surgery/biopsy; total disc replacement.
- *Position:* lateral position, usually right side down. It is preferable to approach from the left, as it is easier to mobilize the aorta than the vena cava.
- *Incision:* correlation with preoperative imaging for the number of ribs. An oblique incision is made by extending from the border of the 12th rib to the lateral border of the rectus abdominis muscle.
- *Dissection:* divide the muscles of the anterior abdominal wall (external/internal oblique and transversus abdominis), in line with the incision. Divide the transversalis fascia and take care with the division of this, as it provides access to the retroperitoneal space. Blunt dissection between the retroperitoneal fat and the psoas fascia follows, with careful retraction of the peritoneal cavity towards the midline. This reveals the psoas major with the overlying genitofemoral nerve. Ligate the segmental vessels and mobilize the aorta, retracted at the level of the vertebra required. Frequently, the sympathetic chain also needs mobilization for access.
- *Risks:* the sympathetic chain, which lies between the vertebral body and the psoas major, can be damaged. The ureter can also be damaged, as it lies on the psoas fascia over the transverse processes. The genitofemoral nerve lies anterior to the surface of the psoas muscle. Segmental arteries and veins are at risk when mobilizing the aorta. The superior hypogastric plexus can be injured, particularly at L4–S1 levels. Spinal nerve root injury may occur closer to the spinal canal and cause cauda equina.

Surgical approaches: shoulder

Anterior approach (deltopectoral)

- *Indication:* proximal humerus fracture fixation; shoulder replacement; open glenohumeral stabilization; infection (open washout).
- *Position:* beach chair position (45° reclined), arm draped free. Head turned away from the shoulder.
- *Incision:* 10–15cm incision, from the surface marking of the coracoid process to the deltoid insertion on the humerus/axilla.
- *Dissection:* through subcutaneous fat, the deltopectoral fascia is visible. It is important to identify the groove and internervous plane between the deltoid muscle (innervated by the axillary nerve) and the pectoralis major (innervated by the pectoral nerves). Isolate and retract the cephalic vein in this interval (usually it is taken laterally, and retracted with the deltoid, as most tributaries drain here). Develop the deltopectoral groove, and identify the conjoint tendon (short head of the biceps and coracobrachialis). Retract this medially (protecting the underlying musculocutaneous nerve). Dissection through the fascia lateral to the conjoint tendon will reveal the anterior aspect of the shoulder joint, which is covered by the subscapularis (with overlying bursa). Externally rotate the shoulder to put stretch onto the subscapularis, and then divide the tendon at its insertion on the lesser tuberosity (insert stay sutures for later repair). The underlying capsule is often dissected off with the subscapularis, to then enable exposure of the GHJ.
- *Risks:* the musculocutaneous nerve (5–8cm below the coracoid) and brachial plexus, the axillary nerve passes posteriorly under the lower border of the subscapularis tendon, accompanied by the leash of humeral circumflex vessels which can be injured. The cephalic vein can be injured, but is easy to visualize and should be protected.

Superolateral approach to the shoulder

- *Indication:* rotator cuff repairs; acromion fractures; ACJ excision or reconstruction; open acromioplasty.
- *Position:* beach chair position (as above).
- *Incision:* 5cm oblique incision from the anterolateral corner of the acromion to the inferior border of the coracoid.
- *Dissection:* incise the deltoid fascia. The deltoid is split and elevated subperiosteally from the anterolateral aspect of the acromion (raphe) and ACJ. The coracoacromial ligament and subacromial bursa become visible. Internal rotation of the shoulder allows optimal visualization of the supraspinatus tendon.
- *Risks:* care with dissection and retraction to prevent suprascapular nerve injury close to the supraspinatus. Acromial branch of the thoracoacromial artery. Medial aspect of the coracoacromial ligament.

Lateral (deltoid-splitting) approach to the shoulder

- *Indication:* rotator cuff repair; proximal humerus fracture fixation.
- *Position:* beach chair position (as per previous).
- *Incision:* from the lateral edge of the acromion, 5cm distally down the lateral aspect of the arm.

- *Dissection:* split the deltoid in line of its fibres, no more than 5cm, with a stay suture at the 5cm apex to prevent split propagation. Elevate the deltoid subperiosteally to ensure a satisfactory view of the subacromial space or humerus, as needed. The subacromial bursa is then visible (often thickened), covering the superior aspect of the rotator cuff (supraspinatus predominantly and infraspinatus).
- *Risks:* the axillary nerve is at risk with distal deltoid muscle splitting that is larger than 5cm, as it winds—posterior to anterior—around the humeral neck in the deltoid musculature. It is adherent to the deep surface of the deltoid, therefore caution with muscle splitting further.

Shoulder arthroscopy portals

- *Position:* beach chair position (as per previous), or lateral decubitus position with arm traction (weights from a drip stand attached to the table to help distract the joint).
- *Incision:* small, 1cm incision with a small blade: (1) posterior portal— 2cm inferior and 1cm medial to the posterolateral corner of the acromion in the palpable 'soft spot'; aim a blunt trocar anteriorly towards the coracoid to access the GHJ, withdraw, and aim superiorly under the acromion for the subacromial bursa; (2) anterior portal— lateral to the coracoid process and anterior to the ACJ through the rotator interval; under direct view from the camera, a needle is used prior to skin incision for location; (3) lateral portal—1–2cm distal to the lateral edge of the acromion, inserted through the deltoid. Portal positions are demonstrated in Fig. 10.3.

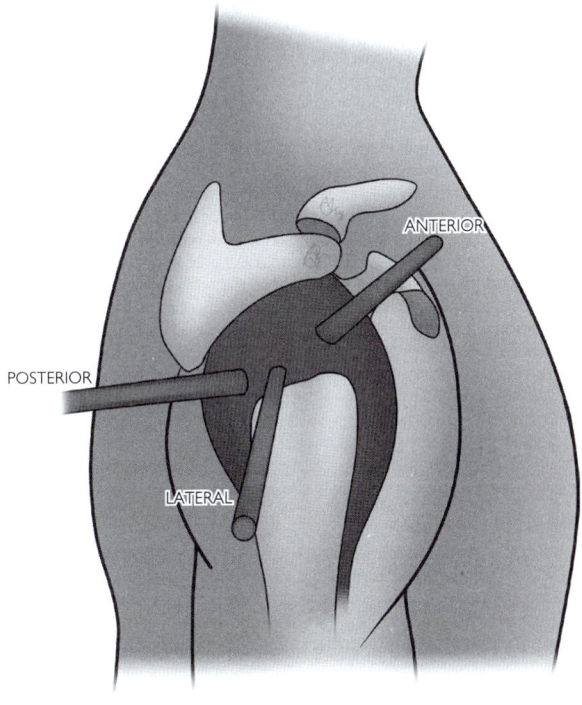

Fig. 10.3 Common portal positions for shoulder arthroscopy.

Di Giacomo G, Costantini A. Arthroscopic shoulder surgery anatomy: Basic to advanced portal placement. *Operative Techniques in Sports Medicine*. 2004 Apr 1;**12**(2):64–74.

Surgical approaches: arm

Anterior approach

- *Indication:* humeral fracture fixation; infection; tumour surgery.
- *Position:* supine, with the arm abducted on an armboard.
- *Incision:* this approach continues from the lower end of the extensile deltopectoral approach (mentioned previously). Continue down the lateral border of the biceps, 8–12cm incision (shown in Fig. 10.4).
- *Dissection:* proximally, dissect the deltopectoral groove, as for the anterior approach to the shoulder; expose the humeral shaft by incising the periosteum, lateral to the pectoralis major insertion. Distally, incise the deep fascia, lateral to the biceps; identify the brachialis, and separate the medial two-thirds (musculocutaneous nerve supply) from the lateral third (radial nerve) to expose the humeral shaft distally. In practice, exploring the interval between the biceps and the brachialis is reasonable if care is taken to protect the musculocutaneous nerve (which lies on the brachialis, with the terminal sensory branch of the lateral cutaneous nerve of the forearm).
- *Risks:* the musculocutaneous nerve during more proximal dissection. The radial nerve should be identified before brachialis dissection to avoid injury. It is at risk in the middle third posteriorly and in the distal third laterally as it exits the spiral groove. The anterior circumflex humeral artery is more at risk in proximal exposure.

Posterior approach

- *Indication:* humeral fracture fixation; radial nerve exploration.
- *Position:* lateral decubitus or prone, arm over a well-padded gutter attachment.
- *Incision:* longitudinal incision, starting 8cm distal to the acromion and extending down to the olecranon fossa (shown in Fig. 10.5).

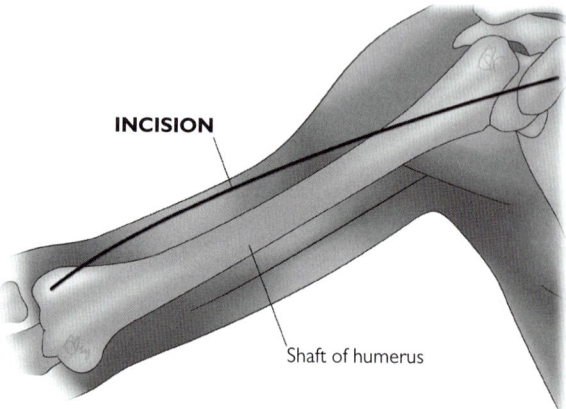

INCISION

Shaft of humerus

Fig. 10.4 Anterior approach to the arm.

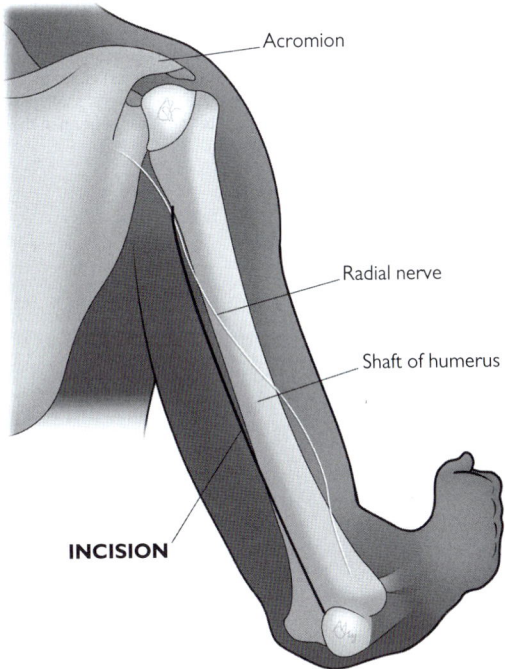

Fig. 10.5 Posterior approach to the arm.

- *Dissection:* split fascia in line with the skin incision. Identify the long and lateral heads of the triceps. Dissect in the plane between these two heads. Deep to these is the medial head, below which is the spiral groove of the humerus—the marker for the radial nerve and profunda brachii artery. Identify and protect these, then split the medial head to expose the humerus. Ensure the head is elevated subperiosteally to avoid damage to the ulnar nerve medially.
- *Risks:* the radial nerve is at risk during deep dissection, as is the profunda brachii artery. The ulnar nerve is at risk more distally and medially, particularly during medial head elevation.

Lateral approach to the distal humerus
- *Indication:* fracture fixation (lateral condyle fractures typically); lateral epicondylitis (tennis elbow) release.
- *Position:* supine, with the arm across the patient's chest.
- *Incision:* straight incision over the lateral supracondylar ridge.

- *Dissection:* incise the fascia in line with the skin incision. Then dissect the intermuscular plane between the triceps and brachioradialis (both supplied by the radial nerve). The common extensor origin (extensor carpi radialis longus and extensor carpi radialis brevis) can then be divided and elevated posteriorly to expose the humeral shaft.
- *Risks:* radial nerve (pierces the lateral intermuscular septum in the distal third of the arm—do not extend above).

Surgical approaches: elbow

Lateral approach (Kocher's)

- *Indication:* radial head fracture fixation/excision or replacement; lateral humeral column fixation; capitellum fracture fixation; coronoid fracture fixation; LCL repair/reconstruction.
- *Position:* supine with armboard or arm on the patient's chest, forearm pronated to protect the PIN.
- *Incision:* curved, off the lateral epicondyle, extending distally over the radial head (shown in Fig. 10.6).
- *Dissection:* incise the underlying fascia in line with skin incision. Identify the plane between the ECU and anconeus underneath, then split proximal fibres of the supinator along the posterior cortex of the radial head. Perform a longitudinal incision through the elbow joint capsule to reveal the joint and radial head.
- *Risks:* PIN if incision is taken too far distally (beyond the annular ligament) or from retractors and with supinator dissection. Minimize posterior dissection to preserve vascularity of the capitellum. Caution with the radial nerve more anteriorly.

Posterior approach

- *Indication:* distal humerus fracture fixation; olecranon fracture fixation; infection (open washout); elbow replacement.

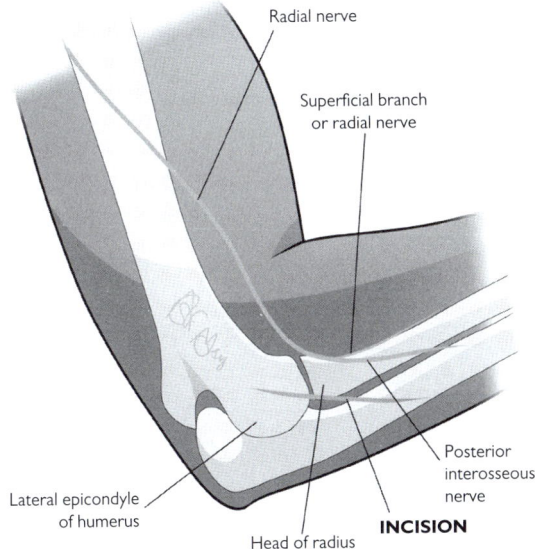

Fig. 10.6 Lateral (Kocher's) approach to the elbow.

- *Position:* lateral decubitus and arm hanging over a bolster or prone (intubated) with forearm hanging over the end of an armboard.
- *Incision:* longitudinal incision centred over the olecranon, can curve the incision laterally around the olecranon tip.
- *Dissection:* develop full-thickness skin flaps. Dissect and protect the ulnar nerve medially. Following this, depending on surgery, split the triceps or perform an osteotomy of the olecranon to elevate the triceps in order to expose the distal humerus or enter the joint.
- *Risks:* ulnar nerve on the medial aspect, radial nerve above the lateral border of the distal third of the humerus. The median nerve and brachial artery run together along the anterior aspect of the elbow joint.

Anterior approach to the cubital fossa

- *Indication:* distal biceps tendon repair; median or radial nerve and vessel repair; supracondylar fracture with injury to the brachial artery (remember distal fasciotomy); infection; fracture fixation (rare).
- *Position:* supine, arm extended on an armboard.
- *Incision:* longitudinal, with a gentle 'S' curve over the anterior aspect of the elbow. Ensure the distal limb of the 'S' is lateral, and the proximal limb medial. For distal biceps repair, the distal aspect of this incision is used and the anterior elbow crease is not passed.
- *Dissection:* identify and protect the lateral cutaneous nerve of the forearm between the biceps and brachialis. Then incise the (lacertus fibrosus) bicipital aponeurosis—caution with the brachial artery (with vein and median nerve medially), as it is directly underneath. The radial nerve crosses in front of the elbow joint between the brachialis and brachioradialis.
- *Risks:* lateral cutaneous nerve of the forearm, brachial artery, median nerve, PIN, and radial nerve as mentioned above.

Surgical approaches: forearm

Volar approach to the radius (Henry's)

- *Indication:* radial shaft fracture fixation; infection; tumour surgery; osteotomy procedures.
- *Position:* supine with an armboard, forearm supinated.
- *Incision:* longitudinal incision along a line from just lateral to the biceps's tendon proximally and to the radial styloid distally (demonstrated in Fig. 10.7). Any part of this line is utilized, dependent on what procedure is being performed.
- *Dissection:* incise the deep fascia in line with the skin; split into thirds, depending on the point of pathology. (1) *Proximal third*—beware of large veins that traverse this region. Develop a plane between the pronator teres and brachioradialis; fully supinate the forearm to displace the PIN radially and bring the supinator anterior (demonstrated in Fig. 10.8). Incise the supinator along its insertion, and dissect subperiosteally and laterally. (2) *Middle third*—pronate the forearm to bring the insertion of the pronator teres into view, then along the radial aspect of the radius, detach the pronator teres insertion from the bone and retract medially. (3) *Distal third*—supinate the arm and dissect between the flexor carpi radialis and flexor pollicis longus; detach the pronator quadratus, retracting towards the ulna.
- *Risks:* PIN in proximal third—it pierces the supinator to enter the posterior compartment of the forearm. Take care with the median nerve and radial artery to avoid injury during dissection and with retraction. Distal third incision/dissection can encounter superficial radial nerve branches.

Dorsal approach to the radius (Thompson)

- *Indication:* fixation of radius; osteotomy procedures; infection; tumour surgery.
- *Position:* supine with an armboard, forearm pronated.
- *Incision:* along a line from anterior and distal to the lateral epicondyle, proximally, to Lister's tubercle at the wrist.
- *Dissection:* (1) *Proximal third*—incise the fascia in line with the skin interval between the ECRB and extensor digitorum communis to reveal the supinator. Dissect the insertion of the supinator, and lift the supinator off subperiosteally to expose the bone. (2) *Middle third*—identify the abductor pollicis longus (APL) and EPB, and make an incision along the superior and inferior borders of the APL and EPB, and retract off the bone to expose the radius. (3) *Distal third*—undermine the APL and EPB tendons medially to identify a plane between the EPL and ECRB; separate both, and it will reveal the lateral border of the radius.
- *Risks:* PIN preservation is the key to this approach. Posterior interosseous artery, particularly in the proximal third.

Approach to the ulna

- *Indication:* ulnar fracture fixation; ulnar osteotomies.
- *Position:* supine, with arm pronated across the chest.
- *Incision:* incision along the subcutaneous border of the ulna.

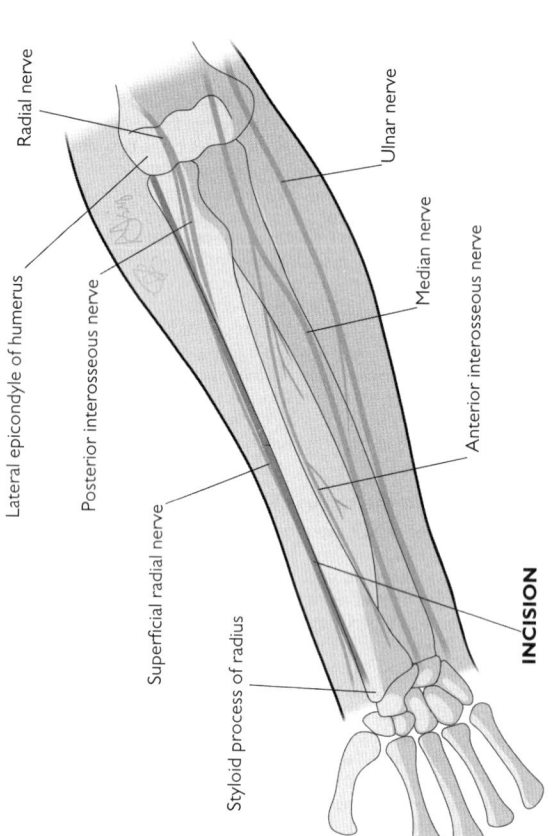

Radial nerve

Ulnar nerve

Median nerve

Lateral epicondyle of humerus

Anterior interosseous nerve

Posterior interosseous nerve

Superficial radial nerve

Styloid process of radius

INCISION

Fig. 10.7 Volar approach (Henry's) to the forearm.

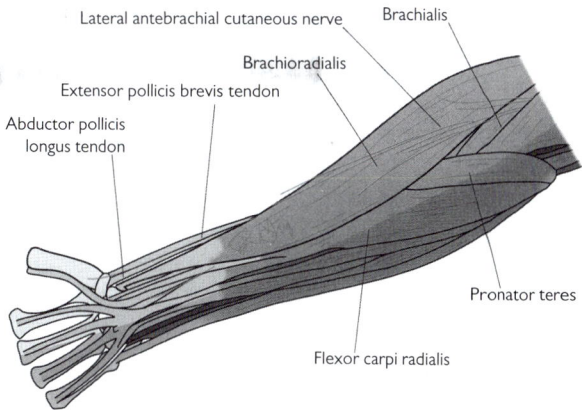

Lateral antebrachial cutaneous nerve

Brachialis

Brachioradialis

Extensor pollicis brevis tendon

Abductor pollicis longus tendon

Pronator teres

Flexor carpi radialis

Fig. 10.8 Deeper plane of dissection for Henry's approach.

- *Dissection:* continue through the internervous plane between the ECU (PIN) and FCU (ulnar nerve). Some fibres of the muscle may require elevation in the middle third.
- *Risks:* ulnar nerve and ulnar artery at risk during dissection of the FCU.

Surgical approaches: wrist and hand

Volar approach to the carpal tunnel

- *Indication:* carpal tunnel decompression of the median nerve; flexor tenosynovectomy; infection; tendon repair.
- *Position:* supine, armboard, forearm supinated.
- *Incision:* longitudinal incision, most distal at the intersection of Kaplan's cardinal line (oblique line drawn from the apex of the interdigital fold between the thumb and index finger to the hook of the hamate) and another line extending from the radial border of the ring finger up to the wrist crease (demonstrated in Fig. 10.9).
- *Dissection:* careful dissection of the superficial fat and palmar fascia; be aware and avoid the palmar cutaneous branch of the median nerve. Expose and incise the transverse carpal ligament (flexor retinaculum), based on the ulnar side to protect the motor branch of the median

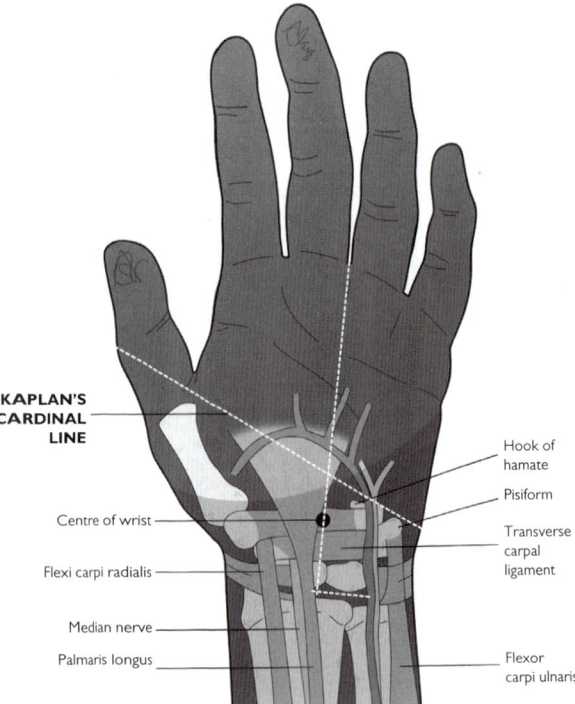

KAPLAN'S CARDINAL LINE

Hook of hamate

Pisiform

Centre of wrist

Transverse carpal ligament

Flexi carpi radialis

Median nerve

Palmaris longus

Flexor carpi ulnaris

Fig. 10.9 Markings and structures for carpal tunnel decompression.

nerve (course displays several anatomical variants). Ensure protection of the median nerve when releasing proximally and distally.
- *Risks:* superficial palmar arch, palmar cutaneous branch of the median nerve, motor branch of the median nerve, median nerve proper.

Volar approach to the distal radius (FCR)
- *Indication:* distal radius fracture fixation; tendon repair; infection.
- *Position:* supine, armboard, forearm supinated.
- *Incision:* longitudinal over tendon of the FCR.
- *Dissection:* incise the FCR tendon sheath; retract it medially, and the radial artery laterally. Through the FCR bed is the pronator quadratus; detach from its radial insertion, and reflect medially to access the distal radius and radiocarpal joint (including the proximal pole of the scaphoid).
- *Risks:* median nerve and palmar cutaneous branch, radial artery (nearby throughout); care with dissection and retraction.

Dorsal approach to the distal radius
- *Indication:* tendon repair or transfer; tenosynovectomy; fracture fixation; wrist fusion; carpal fracture fixation; decompression of De Quervain's sheath.
- *Position:* supine, armboard, forearm pronated.
- *Incision:* 8cm longitudinal incision, midway between radial and ulnar styloid processes, in the line of the third metacarpal.
- *Dissection:* sharp dissection through superficial fat to expose the extensor retinaculum; lift as an ulnar-based flap. Dissect down between the third and fourth dorsal compartments to expose the dorsal aspect of the distal radius.
- *Risks:* superficial radial nerve, dorsal cutaneous branches, extensor tendon damage, interosseous ligament damage.

Approach to the flexor tendons
- *Indication:* flexor tendon repair and digital nerve repair; Dupuytren's contracture release; infection drainage (flexor sheath infections).
- *Position:* supine, armboard with a 'lead hand' to hold the fingers extended.
- *Incision:* Brunner's incision; zigzag in the fingers between the flexion creases and extend onto the palm as necessary (demonstrated in Fig. 10.10).
- *Dissection:* develop full-thickness flaps and reflect to expose the flexor tendon sheaths.
- *Risks:* neurovascular bundles at the lateral border of flexor sheaths, separated from the volar subcutaneous flap by a thin layer of fibrous tissue.

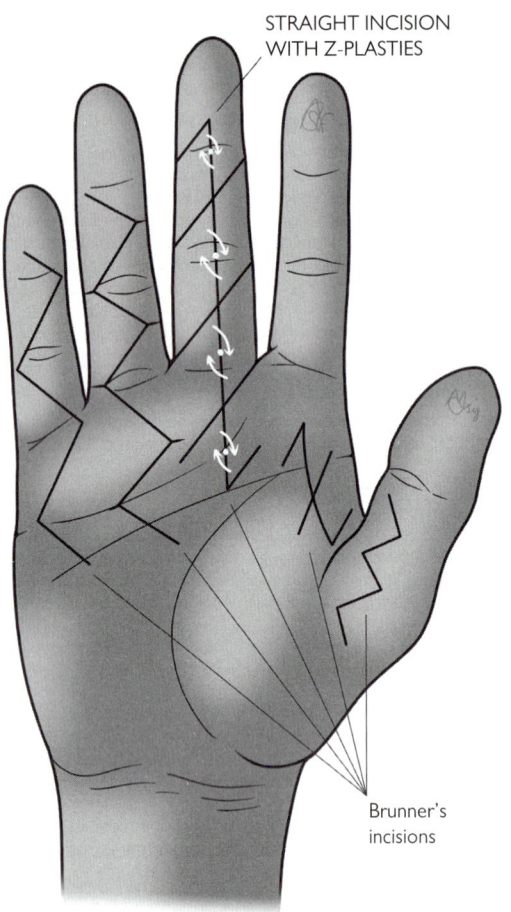

STRAIGHT INCISION
WITH Z-PLASTIES

Brunner's
incisions

Fig. 10.10 Brunner's incisions for approach to the fingers and palm.

Surgical approaches: hip and femur

There are several commonly utilized approaches to the hip (Fig. 10.11).

Lateral approach (multiple variations and eponyms)

- *Indication:* hip replacement; hip hemiarthroplasty; femoral neck fracture fixation; gluteal tendon surgery.
- *Position:* lateral (commonly) or supine with a sandbag under the affected side.
- *Incision:* a direct lateral longitudinal incision, centred over the greater trochanter, with the incision based two-thirds proximal to the trochanter to one-third distal.
- *Dissection:* sharp dissection through subcutaneous tissue to the fascia. Incise the fascia lata in line with the incision, and incise the trochanteric bursa to define the gluteus medius tendinous insertion onto the greater trochanter. Detach its anterior half to two-thirds, leaving a cuff of tendon to repair, and continue distally into the origin of the vastus lateralis to expose the neck and proximal femur. Externally rotate the hip, and incise the underlying gluteus minimus to expose the thick capsule of the hip joint. Incise the hip capsule and, if required, dislocate the femoral head with flexion, external rotation, and adduction.
- *Risks:* the superior gluteal nerve between the gluteus minimus and medius is 3–5cm above the greater trochanter; care required when splitting the muscle. Damage to this muscle can result in Trendelenburg gait.

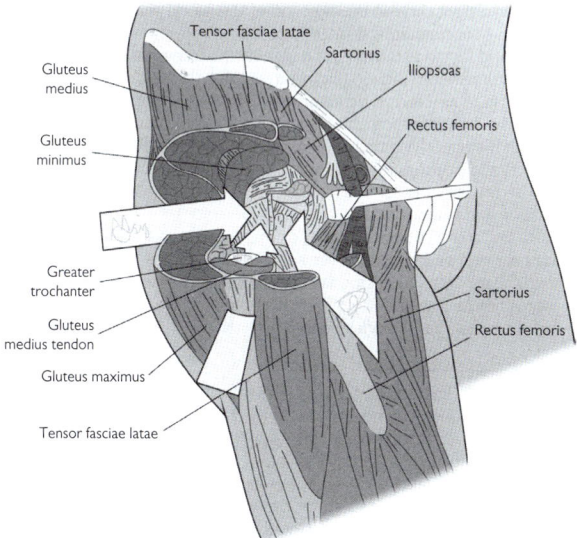

Fig. 10.11 Intervals used in anterior, anterolateral, and posterior approaches to the hip.

Posterior approach

- *Indication:* hip replacement; hip hemiarthroplasty; open reduction of posterior hip dislocations; posterior wall and column acetabular open reduction and internal fixation (ORIF).
- *Position:* lateral.
- *Incision:* curved incision, with the apex centred at the posterior aspect of the greater trochanter to continue down the shaft of the femur.
- *Dissection:* dissect subcutaneous tissue in line with the incision, taking care not to deviate posteriorly (sciatic nerve at risk). Incise the fascia lata laterally, and proximally split the gluteus maximus in the line of its fibres (beware of bleeding from avulsed small vessels). Sweep away the bursa, and identify the short external rotators (piriformis, obturator internus, and gemelli). Place a stay suture in the piriformis and obturator internus for later repair; internally rotate the hip, and detach close to the femoral insertion. Reflect backwards to protect the sciatic nerve, and expose the capsule. Incise the hip capsule and, if required, dislocate the femoral head with flexion, internal rotation, and adduction.
- *Risks:* the sciatic nerve lies in the fat on the short external rotators—to protect, reflect these back with a stay suture.

Anterior approach (Smith-Petersen)

- *Indication:* hip replacement; native septic hip washout; open reduction of a hip dislocation; pelvic osteotomies; hip fusion.
- *Position:* supine.
- *Incision:* inferior aspect of the iliac crest, just below the ASIS, extending distally in a slight curve in the direction of the lateral aspect of the patella.
- *Dissection:* subcutaneous dissection to the underlying fascia of the tensor and sartorius muscles, and identify the plane between these two muscles. Incise the fascia in this intermuscular plane on the medial side of the TFL. The TFL can be detached from the iliac crest if necessary. Ligate the ascending branch of the lateral femoral circumflex artery. Detach the underlying rectus femoris from its origin. Retract the rectus femoris and iliopsoas medially, and the gluteus medius laterally, to expose the hip capsule. The hip joint can be dislocated with external rotation and extension.
- *Risks:* the lateral cutaneous nerve of the thigh—usually lies alongside the sartorius, so identify and retract medially with the muscle. Damage to this can lead to paraesthesiae to the lateral thigh or meralgia paraesthetica. The ascending branch of the medial circumflex artery lies distally in the TFL/sartorius interval.

Lateral approach to the femur

- *Indication:* hip fracture fixation (e.g. dynamic hip screw (DHS)); excision of infected bone or tumour; osteotomy procedures.
- *Position:* supine. The patient is usually positioned on a fracture table.
- *Incision:* longitudinal, following the line of the femoral shaft.
- *Dissection:* subcutaneous dissection—split the fascia lata, split the vastus lateralis muscle in line of its fibres, or lift anteriorly and dissect off the lateral intermuscular septum to reveal the femoral shaft.
- *Risks:* arterial perforators in the lateral intermuscular septum.

Surgical approaches: knee and tibia/fibula

Medial parapatellar approach to knee

- *Indication:* knee replacement; arthrotomy; open ligament or cartilage procedures.
- *Position:* supine.
- *Incision:* longitudinal, just medial to the midline from the superior patella to the tibial tubercle (demonstrated in Fig. 10.12).
- *Dissection:* dissect to expose the quadriceps tendon. Incise the tendon in the midline, and manoeuvre towards the medial border of the patella and patellar tendon. Evert the patella and flex the knee 90° to expose joint.
- *Risks:* the superior lateral genicular artery is at risk during retinacular release. Injury may be missed if the procedure is performed under tourniquet.

Knee arthroscopy portals

- *Indication:* meniscal surgery; cruciate ligament reconstruction; loose body removal; cartilage procedures; knee washout.

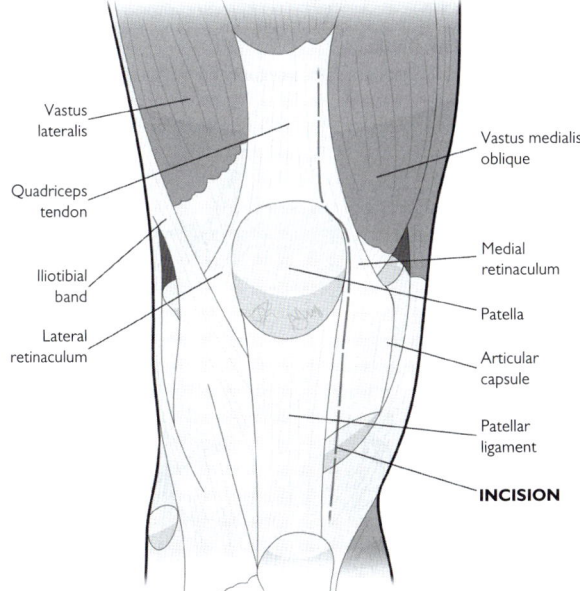

Fig. 10.12 Medial parapatellar approach.

- *Position:* supine. Allow space for the knee to flex over the side of the operating table to facilitate valgus stressing.
- *Incision:* with the knee in flexion, identify the soft spot between the inferolateral border of the patella and the lateral femoral condyle. Insert a small blade through the capsule (cutting the edge away from the meniscus), then insert the trocar and sweep up into the suprapatellar pouch, with the knee going into extension. Flex the knee again over the side of the table, and apply a valgus force; insert the arthroscope, and view the medial compartment. Insert a white needle into this compartment under direct vision through the medial soft spot (adjust according to the desired angle for anticipated procedure), and follow with the blade and probe (demonstrated in Fig. 10.13).

Anterior approach to the tibia

- *Indication:* fracture fixation; excision of infected bone or tumour; osteotomy procedures.
- *Position:* supine.
- *Incision:* longitudinal, 1cm lateral to the anterior border of the tibia.
- *Dissection:* raise skin flaps to expose the subcutaneous border of the tibia, protecting the long saphenous vein, which lies medially. Elevate or detach the origin of the tibialis anterior muscle to expose the lateral surface of the bone.
- *Risks:* the long saphenous vein may be injured, as it runs up the medial side of the calf.

Approach to the fibula

- *Indication:* fracture fixation; osteotomy procedures; fibular resection; harvest for vascularized graft.
- *Position:* supine, with sandbag under the ipsilateral buttock.

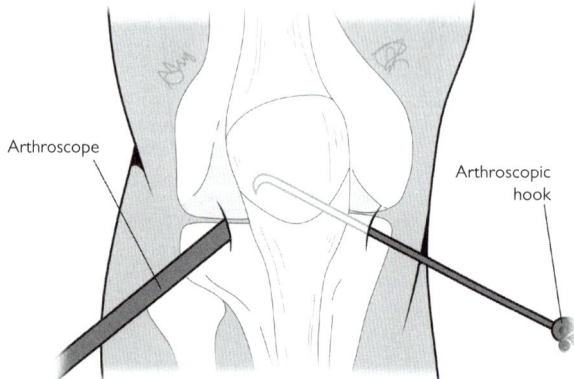

Arthroscope

Arthroscopic hook

Fig. 10.13 Arthroscopy portal placement.

- *Incision:* longitudinal, from the lateral malleolus to the fibular head, slightly posterior to the fibular shaft.
- *Dissection:* develop a plane between the peronei (peroneal compartment) and soleus (posterior compartment). Make an incision in the periosteum of the fibula, and expose the bone subperiosteally.
- *Risks:* the common peroneal nerve, which runs behind the biceps femoris tendon to wind around the neck of the fibula. Identify the nerve under the tendon, and carefully retract forward by releasing the fibres of the peroneus longus that cover it on the fibular neck. The superficial peroneal nerve is vulnerable to injury at the distal third of the leg.

Surgical approaches: ankle

Approach to the medial malleolus

- *Indication:* fracture fixation; osteotomy to expose the tibiotalar joint.
- *Position:* supine.
- *Incision:* curvilinear (distal limb curved anteriorly) over the medial malleolus.
- *Dissection:* dissect directly onto the bone to expose the malleolus. The deltoid ligament fans out below and can be split to expose the joint capsule (ensure repair later). The medial malleolus may buttonhole through the deltoid ligament as the talus displaces; if so, retrieve the ligament out of the medial gutter and repair with everting sutures.
- *Risks:* identify and protect the long saphenous vein and saphenous nerve in the superficial fat anteriorly.

Approach to the lateral malleolus

- *Indication:* fracture fixation.
- *Position:* supine, sandbag under the ipsilateral buttock.
- *Incision:* longitudinal, directly over the bone, or slightly posterior.
- *Dissection:* dissect through superficial tissue to expose the bone.
- *Risks:* the short saphenous vein and sural nerve posteriorly on dissection. The superficial peroneal nerve may cross from posterior to anterior at the proximal end of the incision.

Posterolateral approach to the ankle

- *Indication:* fracture fixation; Achilles' tendon and peroneal tendon reconstruction and lengthening; arthrodesis of the posterior facet of the subtalar joint.
- *Position:* prone, lateral, or supine, with support under the ipsilateral hip or hip flexed and internally rotated to allow for access. Position depends on procedures being performed and the surgeon/anaesthetist's preference.
- *Incision:* midway between the tendoachilles and posterior border of the fibula.
- *Dissection:* dissect down to the lateral or posterolateral fibula, and access the fibula with posterior retraction of the peroneus longus and brevis muscles. Retract the peroneus longus and brevis muscles, and identify the interval between the flexor hallucis longus (FHL) and peroneal tendons. Elevate the FHL off the posterior tibia. Retract the FHL medially to access the posterior malleolus (demonstrated in Fig. 10.14).
- *Risks:* take care not to release the posterior inferior tibiofibular ligament, which can lead to instability. The superficial peroneal nerve is at risk proximally, and the sural nerve and short saphenous vein distally.

Posteromedial approach to the ankle

- *Indication:* posterior malleolar or triplane fracture fixation; clubfoot open release; tendon repair, lengthening, or transfer.
- *Position:* supine, with hip flexed and externally rotated, or prone.
- *Incision:* midway between the Achilles tendon and posterior border of the medial malleolus.

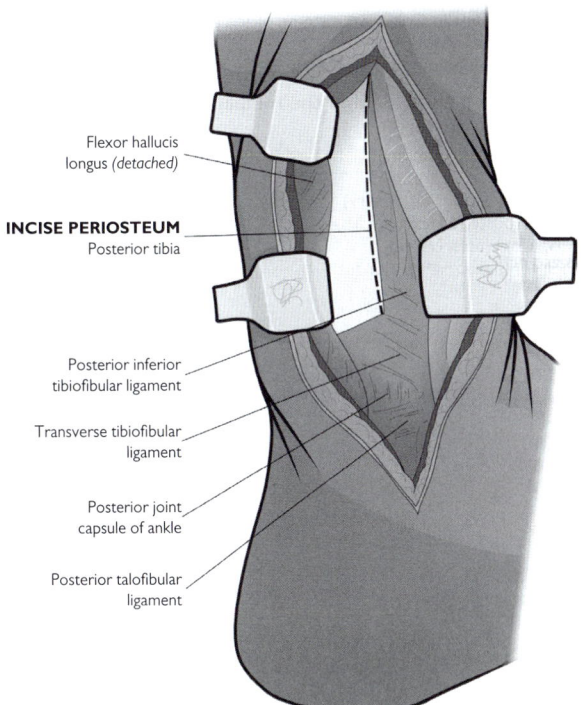

Flexor hallucis longus *(detached)*

INCISE PERIOSTEUM
Posterior tibia

Posterior inferior tibiofibular ligament

Transverse tibiofibular ligament

Posterior joint capsule of ankle

Posterior talofibular ligament

Fig. 10.14 Posterolateral approach to the ankle.

- *Dissection:* dissect to, and incise, the flexor retinaculum. Identify the FHL, the only muscle that still has fibres at this level, and retract medially or laterally to expose the joint capsule.
- *Risks:* the posterior tibial nerve and artery in front of the FHL—identify and protect.

Anterior approach to the ankle joint
- *Indication:* fracture fixation; arthrotomy; arthrodesis; total ankle arthroplasty.
- *Position:* supine.
- *Incision:* longitudinal, midway between both malleoli.
- *Dissection:* dissect to, and incise, the extensor retinaculum in the interval between the extensor hallucis longus (EHL) and extensor digitorum longus (EDL). Take care to preserve the branches of the superficial

peroneal nerve. Mobilize and retract the neurovascular bundle medially with the EHL. Incise the periosteum of the distal tibia and capsule to expose the joint.
- *Risks:* the deep peroneal nerve and anterior tibial artery.

Structures passing behind the medial malleolus from anterior to posterior
- *Tom* (*Tibialis* posterior)
- *Dick* (flexor *Digitorum*)
- *And* (posterior tibial *Artery*)
- *Very* (posterior tibial *Vein*)
- *Naughty* (tibial *Nerve*)
- *Harry* (flexor *Hallucis* longus)

Surgical approaches: foot

Dorsomedial approach to the first metatarsophalangeal joint

- *Indication:* hallux valgus correction; first MTPJ arthrodesis; cheilectomy; excision procedures.
- *Position:* supine.
- *Incision:* medial and parallel to the EHL, over the first MTPJ, preserving superficial sensory nerve branches.
- *Dissection:* incise the fascia and retract the EHL laterally to expose the joint via a capsulotomy.
- *Risks:* damage to the tendon of the EHL on the lateral aspect of the wound.

Lateral approach to the os calcis

- *Indication:* calcaneal fracture fixation.
- *Position:* supine, sandbag under the ipsilateral buttock.
- *Incision:* an L-shaped incision—the posterior arm of the incision is made midway between the fibula and Achilles tendon, and the horizontal arm passes in line with the fifth metatarsal base just above the specialized weight-bearing skin of the sole.
- *Dissection:* mobilize skin flaps, careful to avoid the sural nerve and short saphenous vein, and incise the fascia to expose the peroneal tendons. Incise the sheath of the peroneus longus, and retract the peroneal tendons anteriorly over the lateral malleolus. Locate the posterior talocalcaneal joint capsule, and incise it transversely. To access the lateral surface of the calcaneus, dissect subperiosteally and elevate the tissues inferiorly (demonstrated in Fig. 10.15).
- *Risks:* skin necrosis—minimize soft tissue stripping; make skin flaps as thick as possible, and mobilize them very gently. The sural nerve can be damaged laterally.

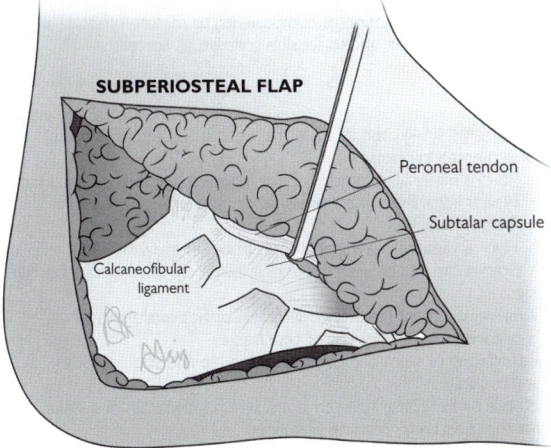

Fig. 10.15 Lateral approach to the os calcis.

Arthroplasty

Surgical reconstruction or replacement of a malformed or degenerated joint.

A brief history

The earliest arthroplasties involved excision of the articulating surface. The first recorded attempt at a hip replacement occurred in Germany in 1891. Professor Gluck used ivory to replace the femoral head in patients whose hip joint had been destroyed by TB. Subsequently, surgeons experimented with various forms of interposition arthroplasty, by using a variety of tissues and materials.

After early-twentieth century attempts at joint transplantation with cadaveric articulations, prosthetic joint replacement began in the 1930s. Smith-Petersen invented the first mould arthroplasty by using glass, followed by cobalt chrome interposition cups. However, it was not until Sir John Charnley—considered the father of modern THR—developed the Charnley low-friction hip arthroplasty in the early 1960s before very good outcomes were achieved. Now there is barely a joint in the body for which a prosthetic articulation has not been designed.

Indications

Pain resistant to conservative treatment. Function is often improved by restoration of joint motion and muscle lever arms.

Cautions

- Young or active patients due to ↑ demand in terms of load and longevity; neurological imbalance predisposing to instability; any pre-existing mobility predisposing into infection.

General considerations

- Biomechanics.
- Preoperative computer-generated X-ray templating to anticipate correct size and orientation of components, to restore offset, to equalize leg lengths, and to tension soft tissues correctly—all overlapping factors.
- Materials.
- Fixation:
  - Cement (PMMA) used as a filler between bone and prosthesis
  - Uncemented implants:
    - Porous materials promoting bony ingrowth for biological fixation
    - Needs initial fixation by 'press-fit' or interference, while biological fixation achieved
    - Hydroxyapatite coating promotes bony on-growth
    - Screws can also be used for initial stability (e.g. uncemented hip cup).
- Design:
  - Total replacement (both joint surfaces) or hemiarthroplasty
  - Hinge with varying degrees of constraint
  - Resurfacing or stemmed components in hip and shoulder arthroplasty
  - Mobile or fixed-bearing knee joints, which may retain or substitute for the (posterior) cruciate ligaments.

Long-term considerations

- *Infection:* a serious and potentially life-threatening complication, which can sometimes be resolved if confirmed early and before the formation of the 'biofilm' with a DAIR approach. Established infection will need to be treated with one- or two-stage revision surgery.
- *Loosening:* septic or aseptic.
- *Implant failure and subsidence:* corrosion, fracture, excessive wear of articulation.
- *Dislocation.*

Total hip replacement

THR gives reliable pain relief and improved function in OA and inflammatory arthritis. Across 20 developed countries, hip replacement surgery is projected to rise from 1.8 million hip replacements per year in 2015 to 2.8 million per year in 2050. Current survival rates for hip arthroplasty are in the region of 89% at 15 years, 70% at 20 years, and 58% at 25 years.

Indications

The primary indication is pain, along with loss of function. Symptoms include pain in the groin, often radiating down the thigh to the knee. Occasionally, pain from the hip can be predominantly felt in the knee. Night pain, use of a walking aid, difficulty with ADLs, and maximal analgesia are good indications that a hip replacement may be effective. In younger, active patients, revision surgery is more likely.

Choice of implant

Stemmed hip replacement has long-term data available in NJRs. Variations include cemented/uncemented fixation of implants to bone, with a combination of metal, polyethylene, and ceramic bearing options. An implant with a proven registry survival should be selected. Surface replacements use a large head and metal-on-metal articulation and may be selected for treatment of younger, active patients. Surface replacements conserve femoral bone, but not acetabular bone. There is a risk of femoral neck fracture. (THR types are demonstrated in Fig. 10.16.)

(A)   (B)

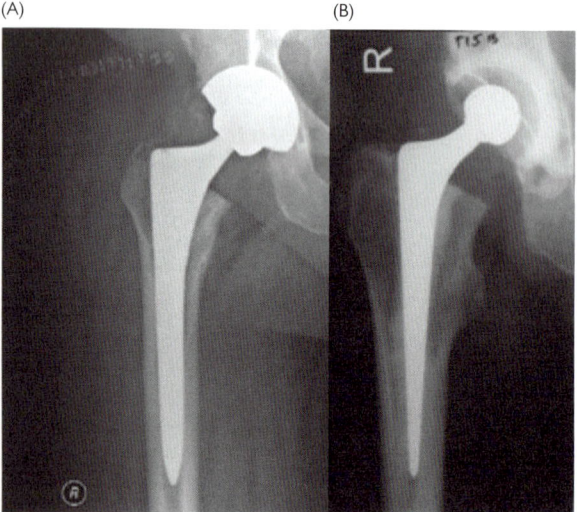

Fig. 10.16 Radiograph of total hip replacement. Uncemented (A) and cemented (B).

Risks associated with primary hip replacement

- Infection (surgical site, 2–3%; deep infection, 1%).
- Dislocation (1–2%).
- Aseptic loosening (osteolysis secondary to polyethylene wear particles).
- Leg length discrepancy.
- Periprosthetic fracture (higher risk with press-fit stemmed implants).
- Nerve or vessel damage.
- DVT, PE.
- Death (0.65% at 90 days).

Total knee replacement

The development of the modern TKR in the early 1970s was an important milestone in orthopaedic surgery. TKR now joins THR as a successful treatment modality for a painful and stiff knee. More recently, unicompartmental or partial knee replacements have been developed and are gaining in popularity for treatment of isolated medial, lateral, or patella–femoral compartment arthritis, offering a quicker recovery time due to its less invasive nature.

As with hip replacements, internationally, the number of knee replacements is projected to ↑ from 184 per 100,000 population to 275 per 100,000 population and it is expected that this figure will ↑ 4-fold by 2030.

Indications

Pain is the primary indication for knee arthroplasty. Symptoms can include stiffness and functional limitation. Moderate or severe knee pain at rest or at night, lasting knee inflammation and swelling, varus or valgus deformity, and maximal analgesia used are signs of severity of symptoms and that a knee replacement may be effective. Fractures around the distal femur and proximal tibia are more modern indications of arthroplasty treatment options—the main benefit being immediate full weight-bearing.

Total knee replacement design

Designs can be split broadly into two categories: (1) unconstrained (posterior cruciate retaining (CR; demonstrated in Fig. 10.17) where the ACL is removed, but the PCL is conserved or posterior cruciate sacrificing (PS) where both the ACL and PCL are removed); and (2) constrained (hinged, non-hinged). Unconstrained designs allow femoral rollback where there is posterior translation of the femur with progressive flexion. Constrained designs are important in the setting of ligamentous laxity and severe bone loss.

Risks associated with primary knee replacement

- Infection (0.5–2%).
- VTE (1%).
- Aseptic loosening.
- Stiffness.
- Unexplained ongoing pain (4%).
- Periprosthetic fracture.
- Nerve or vessel damage.
- Death (0.4% at 90 days).

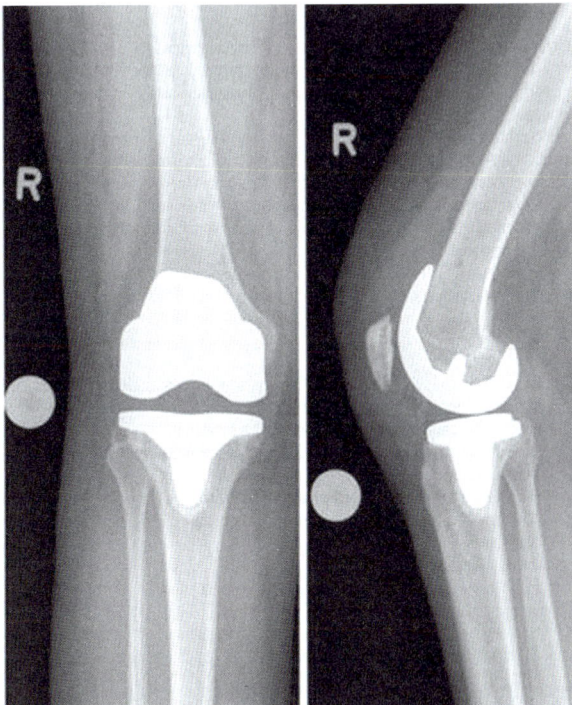

Fig. 10.17 Radiograph showing cruciate retaining (CR) total knee replacement (anteroposterior and lateral views).

Arthroscopy

Arthroscopy has become one of the great advances in orthopaedic surgery. It is used for both diagnostic and therapeutic purposes. Arthroscopy is used for multiple different joints and forms the basis of a number of reconstructive procedures.

Procedures include ACL reconstruction and surgery for anterior shoulder instability. Arthroscopy enables visualization of more challenging joint surfaces such as the hip (deep joint with difficult access) and wrist (small joint). The advantages of arthroscopic procedures include reducing recovery time and minimizing surgical insult. Triangulation is a difficult skill to master and can often pose a challenge for trainees.

The advent of MRI has reduced the need for direct diagnostic visualization, and as a consequence, the therapeutic possibilities have grown.

Equipment

- Arthroscope:
  - Typically rigid with fibreoptic illumination, lenses angled at 30° or 70° (choice depends on joint and surgery being performed).
  - Insert the cannula into the joint with a trocar.
  - Use saline to flush, and distend the joint prior to inserting the arthroscope.
  - Rotate the arthroscope to enable visualization of the joint.
  - Joint images are visualized on a display screen by the operator and assistants.
- Hand instruments:
  - Probe, punch, scissors, grabber, suture passer, etc.
- Power instruments:
  - Shaver—soft tissue or bone cutting, with suction to remove debris
  - Electrosurgery—for haemostasis and to cut or vaporize tissue.

Examples of joint-specific procedures

- *Knee:* meniscectomy or repair for a meniscal tear, removal of loose bodies (e.g. osteochondritis dissecans (OCD)), lateral retinacular release (for patellar maltracking), microfracture or fixation of an osteochondral defect (for further information, see ➲ Chapter 12, pp. 342–343).
- *Shoulder:* arthroscopic subacromial decompression (for impingement), rotator cuff repair (for further information, see ➲ Chapter 13, pp. 396–397).
- *Ankle:* cheilectomy (excision osteophyte) or 'footballer's ankle' (impingement from anterior osteophytic rim).
- *Elbow:* removal of loose body or osteophyte, synovectomy.
- *Wrist:* diagnostic mainly, but also for assistance of percutaneous scaphoid fracture fixation and debridement/repair of triangular fibrocartilage of the distal radioulnar joint.
- *Hip:* visualization and debridement of a labral tear.

Tendon repair

As a general rule, laceration of tendons are repaired if:
- *<25% of tendon torn:* any frayed or obvious flaps can be resected to ensure smooth, free-running tendon
- *<50% of tendon torn:* repair by using a running peripheral suture
- *>50% of tendon torn:* repair by using a core suture, in addition to a surrounding continuous peripheral suture.

Patients with restricted or difficult movement should be considered for a potential tendon injury—delay in diagnosis can lead to more challenging management.

Tendon structure
- Consists of predominantly type I collagen fibres and tenocytes arranged into fascicles surrounded by an endotenon:
  - Tenocytes include synovial cells and fibroblasts.
  - Blood vessels and nerves are present within the tendon unit.
- Fibrous epitenon covers the fascicles and is continuous with the mesotenon, which contains vinculae, the arterial supply to the tendon.
- Tendons are within a synovial-lined sheath at sites of excursion over joints (e.g. ankle and wrist/hand).
- Tendon shape and size depend on the site and functional requirements.
- Musculotendinous units are arranged in pairs around joints, so each has at least one antagonist muscle.
- Tendons are strong structures, capable of withstanding significant loads in tension.

Tendon repair
The strength of repair is proportional to the number of (equally tensioned) core strands and the calibre/characteristics of the suture used. Non-absorbable braided (strong and inelastic; size 3-0) suture is best for the core. For the running epitendinous suture, a smooth suture should be used such as a smooth monofilament like Prolene® (size 6-0), which stretches but also slides.

Core suture configurations and a circumferential running suture are recommended for round tendons. Flat tendons may be repaired with a simple, square, or mattress-type suture. Various core suture placement techniques have been described—all are designed to prevent direct pull-out through the striated structure (e.g. Bunnel, Kessler, Strickland) (Fig. 10.18).

Delayed repair can be very difficult, with retraction of the muscle/tendon and degeneration of tendon tissue. Augmented repair or use of a suitable graft, either harvested from another tendon or synthetic, may be required—otherwise consider an appropriate tendon transfer.

Healing
- *1 week:* inflammatory response and phagocytosis.
- *3 weeks:* fibroblastic proliferation and synthesis of new collagen, and angiogenesis.
- *8 weeks:* longitudinal, mature collagen fibrils present.
- *18 months:* tissue remodelling, replacement of type I collagen.

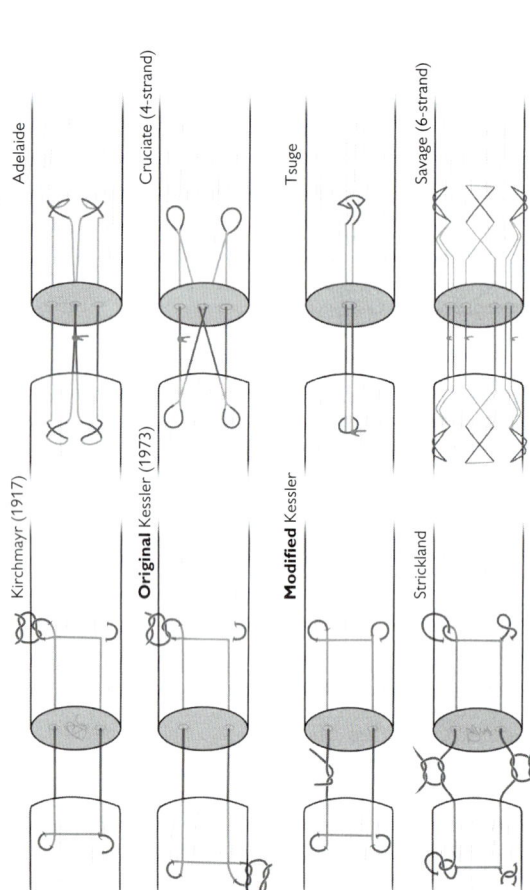

Fig. 10.18 Illustration of the original Kirchmayr flexor tendon core suture of 1917, and several more modern techniques.

Rehabilitation

Early controlled stressing of repaired tendons promotes healing/remodelling and maintains joint nutrition and cartilage viability, as well as prevents adhesion formation. Several specific regimes have been described (e.g. Belfast regime for hand flexor tendons). Extension block splints are useful after flexor repair, as they prevent eccentric contraction against extensor stretch but allow controlled tendon excursion. Early involvement and discussion with hand therapists are key to having the best outcomes following repair.

Soft tissue reconstruction and microvascular surgery

Principles of soft tissue management

To prevent further injury

Initially, establish adequate resuscitation, reduction of any deformities, and early skeletal stabilization. Any emergency management of vascular injury or compartment syndrome should be carried out expediently, and care should be taken to avoid any further contamination and desiccation (therefore, cover the wound).

Halsted's principles of tissue handling include:
- Gentle handling of tissue
- Meticulous haemostasis
- Preservation of blood supply
- Strict aseptic technique
- Minimum tension on tissues
- Accurate tissue apposition
- Obliteration of dead space.

'Debridement' or 'wound excision'

An open wound will be rapidly colonized by bacteria with variable capacity to multiply, spread along tissue planes, and create generalized sepsis. Necrotic tissue is a 'safe haven' for bacteria, which antibiotics cannot reach, and must be removed. Assess tissue and muscle viability by the four 'Cs': contractility, colour, consistency, and capacity to bleed. This can often require debridement of soft tissue and bone until a good bleeding bed for potential healing or coverage can occur, in severe cases leading to large areas of debridement. Bone additionally can be included in debridement and removed if loose—the 'tug test' is often used to identify viable bone.

Reconstruction

It is worth mentioning that this is predominantly the realm of the plastic surgery specialty, and joint involvement of orthopedics and plastic surgery is common practice. Reconstruction will depend on the extent of tissue deficit at the end of adequate wound debridement. In some cases, debridement may require a 'second look' in theatre, or on occasion a third or fourth to re-evaluate viability. Where primary closure is not possible, application of a suction sponge (vacuum) dressing is often used to maintain closed coverage, reduce local oedema, and remove residual bacteria. Caution should be taken in its use; application of 'vac' dressing after first debridement may lead to excessive blood loss, and use in very deep wounds can irritate local nerves.

Reconstructive ladder if primary closure not possible or safe

- *Healing by secondary intention:* allows the wound to heal by granulation from base and wound edge contraction; cosmesis by this method is generally poor. This may be augmented with use of negative-pressure dressings.
- *Delayed primary closure:* usually performed at subsequent surgery.
  - It is important to ensure the suture lines are tension-free.
- *Split skin grafting:* requires an appropriate bed of vascularized tissue and will not take on exposed bone, cartilage, or tendon unless the periosteum, perichondrium, or paratenon is intact.

- *Full-thickness or composite grafts:*
  - *Local flaps:* cutaneous, fasciocutaneous, myofascial section of tissue rotated on its vascular pedicle from a local site into the defect (e.g. gastrocnemius muscle flap to cover exposed bone in an open tibial fracture). This is then covered with a split skin graft.
  - *Free flaps:* whole section of tissue from a remote donor site. The vascular pedicle is divided and anastomosed to an appropriate vessel at the recipient site (e.g. gracilis and latissimus dorsi flaps).

Ideally it is best to replace tissue like for like. Defect coverage should be durable; it should protect underlying structures and have minimal donor site morbidity. If flap coverage is required following an open fracture, muscle is preferable, as it has an excellent blood supply which helps with sufficient distribution of nutrient factors, stem cells, and antibiotic delivery.

Microvascular surgical technique

Needed for surgical procedures involving structures so small that magnification is required (e.g. nerves, blood vessels). Microscopes provide 16–40 times magnification, or surgical loupes (worn like spectacles) up to five times. Use of these is essential for structures <2mm in diameter. Most microscopes are diploscopes or triploscopes, with additional ports for assistants and a television screen. Specialized microsurgical instruments are used, and fine nylon sutures range from size 8.0 to 12.0.

Replantation

Definition

Surgical reattachment of a traumatically amputated digit or limb. This involves shortening and stabilization of bone followed by an extensor and flexor tendon repair, arterial microvascular anastomosis, nerve repair, and finally vein anastomosis and closure.

Considerations

Expected comfort and function from replantation should significantly exceed that of management by amputation/prosthesis fitting.

Injury mechanism is important (clean and sharp amputations are better than crush injuries).

Important factors in decision-making

- Age.
- Severity of injury.
- Level of amputation.
- Warm ischaemic time (up to 6h, 12h if cooled).
- Multiple or bilateral amputations.
- Segmental injuries to amputated part.
- Comorbidity and rehabilitation potential.
- Economic factors.

Initial care of amputated part

Rinse gently with sterile saline, then either wrap in saline-soaked gauze and place in a plastic bag or immerse in saline in a bag, then place the bag on ice to cool, avoiding any direct contact with ice. (For Gustilo–Anderson classification, see ➲ Chapter 3, Open fractures, pp. 81–82.)

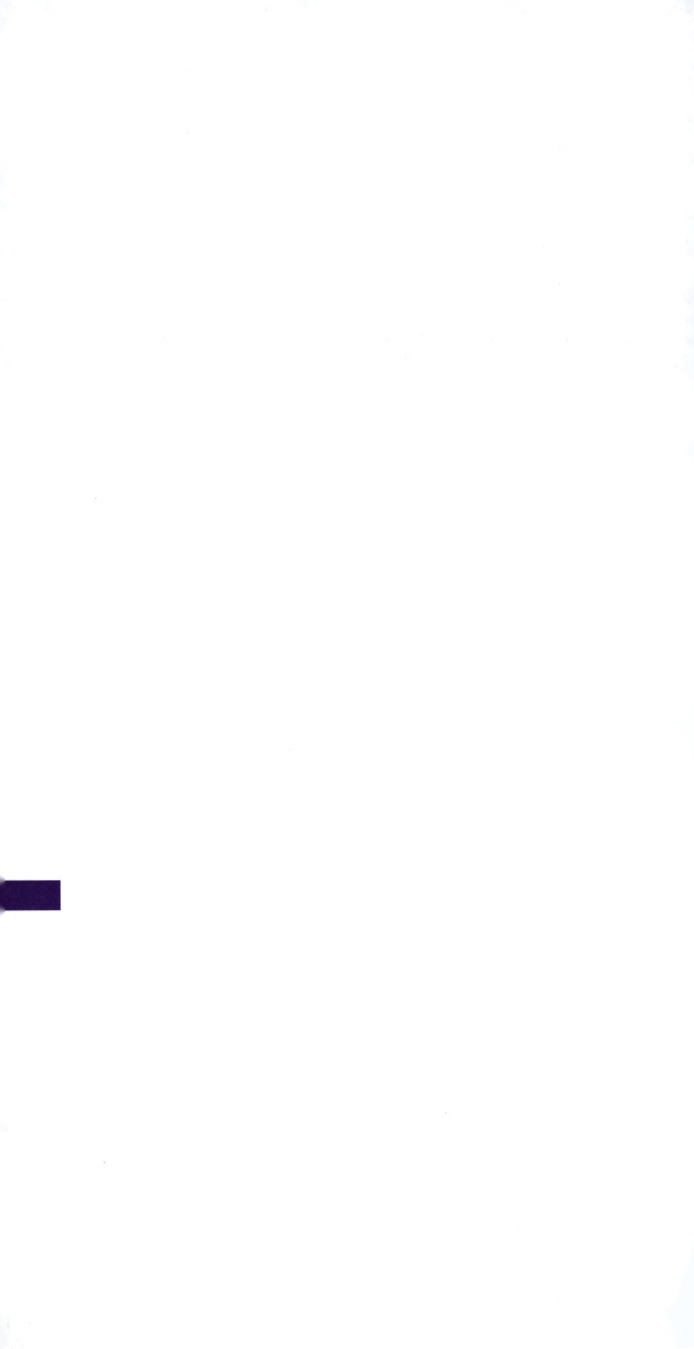

Adult orthopaedics: rheumatology

Osteoporosis

Osteoporosis is a metabolic bone disease characterized by low bone mass, with associated structural deterioration of bone tissue microarchitecture, leading to bone fragility and an ↑ risk of fracture (Fig. 11.1).

Risk factors

- *Include:* ♀ sex, older age, premature or post-menopause, oral steroids (especially longer-term use), smoking, alcohol excess, previous personal or family history of fragility fractures, underlying medical comorbidities (e.g. RA, inflammatory arthropathies).
- *Risk factors for secondary osteoporosis:* untreated hyperthyroidism, malnutrition, malabsorption disorders, hypogonadism, type 1 diabetes, chronic liver disease, low BMI (<18.5kg/m²).

Causes

- Primary:
  - *Type 1:* post-menopausal osteoporosis where there is a decline in oestrogen levels
  - *Type 2:* age-related osteoporosis where there is age-related ↓ in BMD.
- Secondary—related to medical conditions or medications that lead to acceleration in bone loss:
  - *Endocrine:* hyperparathyroidism, hyperthyroidism, hypogonadism, and diabetes mellitus
  - *GI disorders:* Crohn's disease, ulcerative colitis
  - *Liver disease:* biliary cirrhosis, chronic hepatitis
  - *Bone marrow disorders:* multiple myeloma, leukaemia, lymphoma
  - *Collagen vascular disease:* osteogenesis imperfecta, Ehlers–Danlos syndrome, Marfan syndrome
  - *Inflammatory disease:* RA
  - *Other:* Renal failure, osteomalacia, bone malignancy (metastasis).

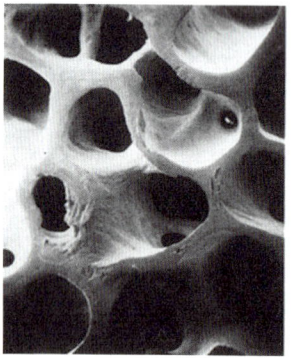 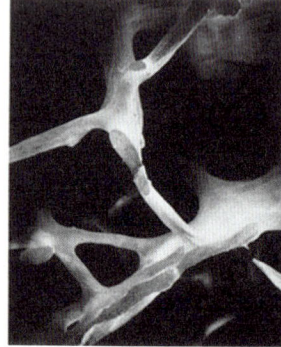

Fig. 11.1 Scanning electron microscopy appearance of normal and osteoporotic bone.

Reproduced from Bulstrode et al., Oxford Textbook of Orthopaedics and Trauma, with permission from Oxford University Press.

Clinical features

- For most of its course, osteoporosis is a silently progressive disease. End-stage osteoporosis culminates in a fragility fracture.
- Symptoms due to associated fractures. Spine example: back pain, loss of vertebral body height ≥4cm, de novo deformity in sagittal and/or coronal planes (kyphosis and scoliosis, respectively).
- Features of systemic diseases that cause secondary osteoporosis (e.g. Cushing's).

Diagnosis

- DEXA—remains the standard:
  - Calculate the FRAX® score (see below) prior to arranging a DEXA scan to measure the BMD or starting a bisphosphonate, except in the following groups who need DEXA:
    - Age >50 years with a history of fragility fractures
    - Age <40 years with a major risk factor for fragility fractures (consider referral to a specialist experienced in treatment of osteoporosis, depending on BMD T-score)
  - Following vertebral or hip fractures: starting treatment *without* DEXA should be considered if this is inappropriate or impractical.
  - WHO definitions:
    - *T-score*: comparison of a person's BMD with a healthy 30-year-old (peak bone mass) of the same sex and ethnicity
    - *Z-score*: comparison of a person's BMD with that of an average person of the same sex, ethnicity, and age
    - *Osteopenia*: T-score −1 to 2.5 SD below the mean
    - *Osteoporosis*: T-score more than −2.5 below the mean
- *Bloods*: FBC, U&Es, LFTs, erythrocyte sedimentation rate (ESR), vitamin D, calcium, protein electrophoresis, hormone profile (luteinizing hormone (LH), follicle-stimulating hormone (FSH), sex hormone-binding globulin (SHBG), testosterone), coeliac screen (tissue transglutaminase (TTG)), parathyroid hormone (PTH). Bone turnover markers can be useful for monitoring response and compliance to treatment but are not routinely checked in clinical practice.
- *Imaging*: to identify fractures and any underlying causes (e.g. malignancy—plain radiographs, MRI).
- FRAX® tool (Fig. 11.2):
  - Risk models developed from population-based cohorts in Europe, North America, Asia, and Australia
  - Algorithms give the 10-year probability of hip fracture and 10-year probability of a major osteoporotic fracture (clinical spine, forearm, hip, or shoulder fracture).

Fragility fracture prevention and management

- *Fracture liaison services (FLS)*: linked to trauma and orthopaedics fracture clinics and used to systematically identify patients with fragility fracture.
- Treatment aims to prevent osteoporosis:
  - Look for modifiable risk factors and causes of secondary osteoporosis.
  - Regular load-bearing exercise.
  - Proper nutrition, including calcium and vitamin D:

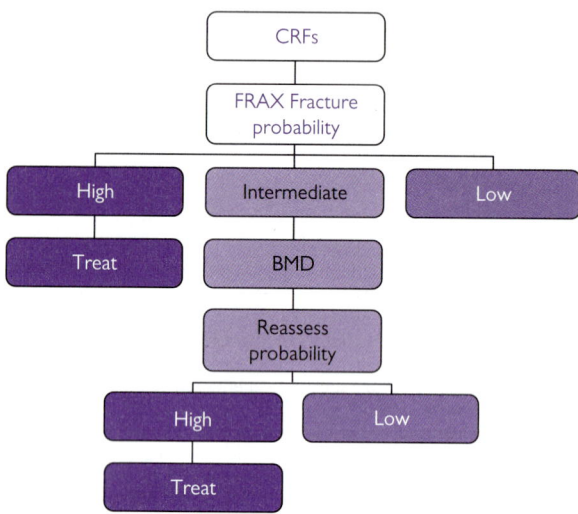

Fig. 11.2 FRAX® tool.

- ○ Daily calcium intake of 700–1200mg (ideally with diet ± supplements if necessary)
- ○ Post-menopausal women and men aged >50 years at ↑ risk of fracture: daily dose of 800IU colecalciferol. Calcium supplementation if dietary intake <700mg/day, and consider vitamin D supplementation in those at risk of, or with evidence of, vitamin D insufficiency. Ensure calcium and vitamin D are normal before starting bone-protective treatment with a bisphosphonate or any of the other agents listed further below.
- Avoidance of smoking and alcohol abuse.
- *Falls history:* in individuals at ↑ risk of fracture, and further assessment and appropriate measures undertaken in those at risk.
- *Pharmacological treatment:* offer bisphosphonates to patients with T-scores of ≤−2.5 if appropriate and no contraindications.
  - Post-menopausal women:
    - ○ Alendronic acid or risedronate are first line in most. Where oral bisphosphonates are not tolerated or are contraindicated, alternatives are IV zoledronic acid or denosumab; raloxifene and hormone replacement therapy are additional options. High cost of teriparatide, so restricted to those at very high risk (particularly of vertebral fractures).
    - ○ Romosozumab (sclerostin inhibitor) is a new class of osteoporosis treatment, that increases bone formation and reduces resorption, currently licensed for osteoporosis treatment for a 12 month period. It rapidly increases lumbar spine and hip BMD over 12 months, in both trabecular and cortical bone. Potential adverse effects include increased risk of cardiovascular disease,

hypocalcemia, osteonecrosis of the jaw and atypical femoral fractures. In females with higher risk of fractures, there is high certainty evidence that anabolic treatments (teriparatide or romosozumab) result in greater reduction in vertebral, non vertebral and hip fractures than bisphosphonates. However stopping anabolic treatments without subsequent anti resorptive therapy risks the loss of bone density gains.
- Bisphosphonates should be avoided in those who cannot follow dosing instructions (sitting upright for 30 minutes after taking the oral bisphosphonate), CKD with glomerular filtration rate (GFR) <30mL/min, Barrett's oesophagus, and following certain types of bariatric surgery.
- Treatment review after 3 years of zoledronic acid therapy and 5 years of oral bisphosphonate. Continuation of bisphosphonate treatment beyond 3–5 years generally recommended if age >75 years, history of hip/spine fracture, fracture on treatment, or on oral glucocorticoids. If treatment is discontinued, reassess fracture risk if new fracture occurs. If no new fracture occurs, reassess fracture risk after 18 months to 3 years. No evidence to guide treatment for >10 years (manage on case-by-case basis).
- Steroid (glucocorticoid-induced osteoporosis):
  - Women and men aged >65 years, with previous fragility fracture or on high doses of glucocorticoids (>7.5mg/day prednisolone), should be considered for bone-protective therapy.
  - In others, use FRAX®, with adjustment for glucocorticoid dose.
  - Treatment may be appropriate in some premenopausal women and younger men, particularly if previous fracture or on high steroid doses.
  - Alendronic acid and risedronate are first line. Where contraindicated or not tolerated, zoledronic acid and teriparatide are alternatives.
- Osteoporosis in men:
  - Alendronic acid and risedronate are first line. Where contraindicated or not tolerated, use zoledronic acid or denosumab, with teriparatide as a backup (treatment duration of teriparatide limited to 24 months).
  - DEXA T-scores should be based on National Health and Nutrition Examination Survey (NHANES) ♀ reference database. When using the online FRAX® tool, enter femoral neck BMD values (g/cm²) and the manufacturer of the densitometer.
- *Follow-up:* to manage adverse effects of bone-sparing treatment, treatment adherence, and the need to continue treatment after 3–5 years.
- *Surgical treatment:* fragility fracture sequelae (e.g. proximal (neck of) femur fracture—fixation/arthroplasty; persistent pain/instability after vertebral fracture—percutaneous vertebroplasty/balloon kyphoplasty with PMMA cement augmentation of body).

Further reading

FRAX. Available from: 🖰 www.sheffield.ac.uk/FRAX/

National Institute for Health and Care Excellence (2023). *Osteoporosis: prevention of fragility fractures.* Available from: 🖰 https://cks.nice.org.uk/topics/osteoporosis-prevention-of-fragility-fractures/

National Osteoporosis Guideline Group (NOGG). Available from: 🖰 www.sheffield.ac.uk/NOGG/

Rheumatoid arthritis

RA is a chronic, systemic inflammatory disease affecting the small synovial joints and extra-articular system.

Epidemiology

Affects 0.5–1% of the population. Commonest in young ♀ (30–50 years).

Aetiology

Complex interplay between genetic predisposition and environmental factors (e.g. smoking). T cell-mediated immune response. The inflammatory response is initially directed against the synovium, and later against cartilage and bone. Human leucocyte antigen (HLA)-DR4- and HLA-DW4 linked.

Clinical features

Often insidious onset of generalized joint aches and stiffness. Swollen, painful, and stiff hands and feet, usually worse in the morning, lasting >1h. Progressive symmetrical symptoms, often with fatigue, malaise, and anorexia.

Less common presentations include:
- Relapsing and remitting arthritis of different large joints (palindromic)
- Persistent monoarthritis (often of the knee)
- Systemic illness with minimal joint involvement
- Vague limb girdle discomfort
- Sudden-onset widespread arthritis
- Extra-articular manifestations such as interstitial lung disease (ILD) and necrotizing scleritis.

Articular examination
- Small joint swelling, especially MCPJ, PIPJ, and wrist.
- Later ulnar deviation and volar subluxation at MCPJs.
- Boutonnière and swan neck deformities of fingers and Z-thumbs.
- Wrist subluxation and prominence of the ulnar head (piano key).
- Extensor tendon rupture and muscle wasting.
- Similar changes in feet—claw toes and hallux valgus.
- Larger joint involvement rare.
- Atlanto-axial joint subluxation occurs and can threaten the spinal cord.

Extra-articular examination
- Rheumatoid nodules.
- Anaemia.
- Lymphadenopathy.
- Vasculitis.
- Multifocal neuropathies, carpal tunnel syndrome.
- Episcleritis, scleritis, keratoconjunctivitis, sicca syndrome.
- Pericarditis.
- Pulmonary fibrosis.
- Amyloidosis.
- Felty's syndrome—splenomegaly and neutropenia.
- Secondary Sjögren's syndrome—autoimmune exocrinopathy associated with RA.

Investigations

Radiograph findings (initially normal)
- Soft tissue thickening.
- Juxta-articular osteopenia.
- Loss of joint space.
- Periarticular erosions.
- Subluxed or dislocated joints.
- Protrusio acetabuli.

Blood tests
No test is specific for the disease:
- Rheumatoid factor (RhF)—positive in 80% (non-specific—may be positive in other diseases, including Sjögren's syndrome, sarcoid, and systemic lupus erythematosus (SLE)).
- Anti-cyclic citrullinated peptide (CCP) antibody (specificity 95–98%).
- ↑ in CRP and ESR.

Joint fluid assay
Confirms inflammatory arthritis with high polymorph counts, but it is non-specific.

Classification criteria (American College of Rheumatology (ACR)/European League Against Rheumatism (EULAR) 2010)

Need at least six out of 10 from four domains for a diagnosis; >1 joint with definite synovitis that is not explained by another disease (Table 11.1).

Management

Early multidisciplinary care can prevent complications. Refer to rheumatology early (guidance is within 3 working days of presentation). The concept of 'treat to target' is a guiding principle—choosing a target, measuring it, assessing progress towards a defined time point, and shared decision-making to change strategy if the target is not achieved.

Non-operative
- *Medical treatment:* NSAIDs, antimalarials, conventional disease-modifying agents (methotrexate, sulfasalazine, leflunomide), steroids. Biological drugs—tumour necrosis factor (TNF) inhibitors, anti-CD20 B cell depletor rituximab, interleukin (IL)-6 inhibitors, T cell co-stimulation inhibitor (CTLA4-Ig), JAK inhibitors. Most are immunosuppressive and confer a significant risk of infection; however, with more widespread use of biological agents, classic signs may not be present (e.g. patients on tocilizumab can have normal CRP despite infection).
- Exercise.
- Physiotherapy and occupational therapy.
- Orthoses.

Operative
Surgery to improve function and reduce pain/swelling. Options include synovectomy, soft tissue realignment, and arthroplasty. Synovectomy reduces pain but does not halt radiographic progression, delay the need for arthroplasty, or improve joint ROM. Soft tissue realignment has limited indication. All patients need a full clinical assessment of the cervical spine and

Table 11.1 American College of Rheumatology (ACR)/European League Against Rheumatism (EULAR) 2010 criteria

Criteria	Score
Joint distribution	
One large joint	0
Two large joints	1
1–3 small joints (large joints not counted)	2
4–10 small joints (large joints not counted)	3
>10 joints (at least one small joint)	5
Serology	
Negative RF AND negative ACPA	0
Low-positive RF OR low-positive ACPA	2
High-positive RF OR high-positive ACPA	3
Symptom duration	
<6 weeks	0
≥6 weeks	1
Acute phase reactants	
Normal CRP AND normal ESR	0
Abnormal CRP OR abnormal ESR	1

ACPA, anti-citrullinated peptide antibody; RF, rheumatoid factor.

cervical radiographs because of the risk of cervical instability (up to 90% of patients with RA) prior to anaesthesia.

Management goals
- To control destructive synovitis and pannus formation.
- To reduce pain.
- To maintain joint function.
- To prevent deformity.

Further reading

Aletaha D, Neogi T, Silman AJ, et al. 2010 rheumatoid arthritis classification criteria: an American College of Rheumatology/European League Against Rheumatism collaborative initiative. *Annals of the Rheumatic Diseases*. 2010;**69**(9):1580–8. Erratum in: *Ann Rheum Dis*. 2010;**69**(10):1892.

Kay J, Upchurch KS. ACR/EULAR 2010 rheumatoid arthritis classification criteria. *Rheumatology (Oxford)*. 2012;**51** Suppl 6:vi5–9.

Lundström E, Källberg H, Alfredsson L, et al. Gene–environment interaction between the DRB1 shared epitope and smoking in the risk of anti-citrullinated protein antibody-positive rheumatoid arthritis: all alleles are important. *Arthritis and Rheumatology*. 2009;**60**(6):1597–603.

National Institute for Health and Care Excellence (2018). *Rheumatoid arthritis in adults: management*. NICE guideline [NG100]. Available from: ℛ www.nice.org.uk/guidance/ng100

Silman AJ, Pearson JE. Epidemiology and genetics of rheumatoid arthritis. *Arthritis Research and Therapy*. 2002;**4**(3):1–8.

Whiting PF, Smidt N, Sterne JA, et al. Systematic review: accuracy of anti-citrullinated peptide antibodies for diagnosing rheumatoid arthritis. *Annals of Internal Medicine*. 2010;**152**(7):456–64; W155–66.

Systemic lupus erythematosus

SLE is a multisystemic autoimmune disease characterized by antinuclear autoantibodies (ANA). It can affect any part of the body, but major target organs are the skin, joints, bone marrow, kidneys, and brain.

Epidemiology

Affects mainly women of childbearing age, but increasingly common in those over 40 years of age among Europeans. Commoner in people of non-European descent. Prevalence was 1 in 1000 in 2012, and the age-standardized incidence is 8.3/100,000 per year for ♀ and 1.4/100,000 per year for ♂ in the UK.

Aetiology

Associated with HLA-DR2 and HLA-DR3. There is a higher concordance in monozygotic twins and first-degree relatives, but no single genetic cause has been identified. Environmental triggers are thought to initiate or exacerbate SLE and include medications (antibiotics, antidepressants), ultraviolet (UV) radiation, sex hormones, and stress.

Clinical features

- Patients commonly present with fatigue, malaise, joint pains, myalgias, and fever.
- *Musculoskeletal* (commonest, >80%): arthralgia, myalgia, myositis, and proximal myopathy. Arthritis affects mainly PIPJs and MCPJs, and the carpus and knees. Rheumatoid-like pattern, but is typically less destructive. There may be periarticular and tendon involvement. Progressively deforming, but non-erosive arthropathy (10–15%) is due to capsular laxity (Jaccoud's arthropathy). Aseptic bone necrosis, especially if treated with high-dose steroids.
- *Skin* (30%): photosensitivity, butterfly malar rash (over nasal bridge and spreading to cheeks and sparing the nasolabial folds), scarring alopecia, livedo reticularis (mottled lace-like purple discoloration), Raynaud's, purpura, oral and nasal ulceration, and urticaria. In 'discoid' lupus, there are three stages of the rash: stage 1, erythema; stage 2, pigmented hyperkeratotic oedematous papules; and stage 3, atrophic depressed lesions.
- *CNS:* broad range of symptoms—depression, psychosis, seizures, hemi- or paraplegia, cranial nerve lesions, cerebellar ataxia, chorea, myelitis, and meningitis occur in SLE. Headaches are common.
- *Renal:* painless haematuria or proteinuria. Lupus nephritis may lead to oedema, hypertension, and renal failure. Note renal and neurological manifestations are major causes of morbidity and mortality in SLE.
- *Pulmonary:* pleurisy, pneumonia, obliterative bronchiolitis, fibrosing alveolitis, shrinking lung syndrome, pleural effusion, pneumonitis, pulmonary hypertension or haemorrhage.
- *Cardiovascular:* pericarditis, endocarditis (Libman–Sacks: non-infective), myocarditis, and coronary artery disease.
- *Blood:* normochromic, normocytic anaemia, haemolysis (rare), leucopenia, lymphopenia, and thrombocytopenia. Splenomegaly. Lymphadenopathy is also common in SLE.

Diagnosis

Blood and urine tests

- Typically, positive for ANA and HLA-DR3 (minority are ANA-negative).
- High titre of anti-double-stranded (ds)DNA antibodies (Smith specific for SLE; ribonucleoprotein (RNP), Ro, and La also present in SLE and other connective tissue diseases (CTDs)). Also check for secondary antiphospholipid syndrome antibodies (anticardiolipin (ACL), lupus anticoagulant, and β2-glycoprotein).
- 40% RhF-positive.
- Low complement levels—indicate active disease.
- Raised CRP and ESR (former is a useful marker of infection, rather than of active SLE).
- Proteinuria and/or cellular casts (raised albumin:creatinine ratio (ACR) or protein:creatinine ratio (PCR)).

ACR/EULAR 2019 clinical diagnostic criteria

Positive ANA, at least one clinical feature out of below, and a score of ≥10:

- Serositis
- Mucocutaneous—oral/nasal ulcers, non-scarring alopecia, acute/subacute cutaneous or discoid lupus
- Musculoskeletal—arthritis
- Constitutional—fever
- Blood disorder
- Renal disorder (proteinuria >0.5g/24h, lupus nephritis on biopsy)
- Neurological disorder
- Immunology (see above).

Management

- *Non-operative:* the mainstay of management has been treatment with steroids, disease-modifying drugs (hydroxychloroquine, methotrexate, azathioprine, mycophenolate, cyclophosphamide, and rituximab). However, only steroid and hydroxychloroquine are licensed for SLE. More recently, belimumab, a monoclonal antibody that inhibits the soluble form of a B-cell survival factor (known as BLyS or BAFF), has been licensed to treat active SLE. Anifrolumab, a monoclonal antibody to type 1 interferon receptor has also been FDA appoved for treatment of moderate to severe SLE (but without lupus nephritis or neuropsychiatric lupus) in those who are already receiving standard therapies.
- *Operative:* splinting not usually successful. Fusion of small joints and arthroplasty for large joints can be successful.

Drug-induced lupus

Isoniazid, hydralazine, procainamide, chlorpromazine, anticonvulsants, and anti-TNF-α may induce lupus.

Antiphospholipid syndrome (secondary)

SLE features include arterial or venous thromboses, thrombocytopenia, and recurrent miscarriages. There are antiphospholipid antibodies (ACL antibodies or 'lupus anticoagulant') present in the blood.

Outcome

SLE has a relapsing, remitting course, with mortality related to infections and end-organ disease.

Further reading

Aringer M, Costenbader K, Daikh D, et al. 2019 European League Against Rheumatism/American College of Rheumatology classification criteria for systemic lupus erythematosus. Arthritis and Rheumatology. 2019;**71**(9):1400–12.

Deapen D, Escalante A, Weinrib L, et al. A revised estimate of twin concordance in systemic lupus erythematosus. Arthritis and Rheumatology. 1992;**35**(3):311–18.

Fanouriakis A, Kostopoulou M, Alunno A, et al. 2019 update of the EULAR recommendations for the management of systemic lupus erythematosus. Annals of the Rheumatic Diseases. 2019;**78**:736–45.

Gordon C, Amissah-Arthur MB, Gayed M, et al. The British Society for Rheumatology guideline for the management of systemic lupus erythematosus in adults. Rheumatology. 2018;**57**(1):e1–45.

Rees F, Doherty M, Grainge M, et al. The incidence and prevalence of systemic lupus erythematosus in the UK, 1999–2012. Annals of the Rheumatic Diseases. 2016;**75**(1):136–41.

Scleroderma (systemic sclerosis)

A condition in which there is progressive fibrosis and tightening of the skin. There is excessive collagen deposition and small-vessel obliteration, resulting in tissue ischaemia and atrophy.

This pathological process may extend beyond the skin to involve other organs. This is referred to as systemic sclerosis (SSc).

It affects ♀ more than ♂ and mainly in the fourth and fifth decades of life, with a prevalence of 38–341 per million persons per year.

ACR/EULAR 2013 classification criteria for scleroderma

(Please note these are not diagnostic criteria.) Skin thickening extending proximal to the MCPJs (sufficient criterion) or any of seven findings (with variable weighting associated with each):
- Digital ulcers
- Telangiectasia
- Dilated nail fold capillaries
- ILD
- Pulmonary hypertension
- Raynaud's syndrome
- Positive antibodies (SCL-70, centromere).

Other clinical features of systemic sclerosis

- Calcinosis—common at tips of fingers.
- GI tract hypomobility, pseudo-obstruction, malabsorption (secondary to bacterial overgrowth), and oesophageal involvement resulting in reflux and dysphagia.
- Renal involvement—causes severe hypertension and renal impairment or failure.
- Myocarditis and myositis.
- Joint stiffness and contractures.
- *CREST* syndrome (*C*alcinosis of subcutaneous tissues, *R*aynaud's phenomenon, disordered o*E*sophageal motility, *S*clerodactyly, and *T*elangiectasia) is a form of the disease with a more benign course.

Investigations

No single test. It is primarily a clinical diagnosis.
- Blood tests:
  - ↑ in ESR and immunoglobulins
  - ANA positive (>50%)
  - SCL-70 (anti-topoisomerase I) antibodies in progressive (diffuse cutaneous) SSc, higher risk of ILD
  - Anticentromere antibodies (limited cutaneous SSc) in CREST
  - Anti-polymerase III antibody in diffuse SSc associated with rapid skin involvement and scleroderma renal crisis
  - Raised creatine kinase (CK) in overlap myositis (OM).
- Urine proteinuria and/or cellular casts in renal scleroderma.
- Pulmonary function testing to look for restrictive ventilatory defect and reduced carbon monoxide diffusion.
- High-resolution CT (HRCT) is more sensitive than CXR in detecting ILD, even in those with normal pulmonary function tests.

- Echocardiography to assess for pulmonary hypertension (as well as for right heart catheterization, preferably via referral to a tertiary centre).
- GI investigations are guided by symptoms: upper GI endoscopy may show reflux oesophagitis, Barrett's oesophagus, infectious (*Candida*) oesophagitis, and oesophageal strictures. Oesophageal manometry may show a hypotensive lower oesophageal sphincter. Barium swallow may show air-filled oesophagus, aperistalsis, dilation of the oesophagus, and rapid transit of contrast.
- Radiology: subcutaneous calcinosis.

Management

- Early referral to a rheumatologist.
- Immunosuppression with disease-modifying drugs. Some cases may benefit from autologous stem cell transplantation, but the risk:benefit ratio needs careful consideration.
- Symptomatic treatment:
  - Raynaud's: heated gloves, calcium channel blockers, and angiotensin II receptor blockers
  - Critical ischaemia of digits: phosphodiesterase type 5 inhibitors, IV iloprost and antibiotics if infected, endothelin receptor antagonist. Digital sympathectomy in severe cases
  - Oesophageal disease: H_2 antagonists, PPIs, and motility stimulants
  - Malabsorption: intermittent broad-spectrum and rotational antibiotics, parenteral nutrition
  - Renal hypertension: ACEIs
  - Lung fibrosis: cyclophosphamide tocilizumab or rituximab
  - Pulmonary hypertension: refer to a tertiary specialist centre for treatment with licensed therapies (in agreement with clinical commissioning policies).
- Operative:
  - Proximal IPJ deformity with dorsal skin ulcer—arthrodesis
  - Calcific deposits—may need to be excised
  - Refractory fingertip ulcers—conservative tip amputation.

Prognosis

~75% survival at 5 years. Better prognosis with CREST variant.

Further reading

Denton CP, Hughes M, Gak N, *et al.* BSR and BHPR guideline for the treatment of systemic sclerosis. *Rheumatology*. 2016;**55**(10):1906–10.

Ingegnoli F, Ughi N, Mihai C. Update on the epidemiology, risk factors, and disease outcomes of systemic sclerosis. *Best Practice and Research: Clinical Rheumatology*. 2018;**32**(2):223–40.

Sobolewski P, Maślińska M, Wieczorek M, *et al.* (2019). Systemic sclerosis: multidisciplinary disease: clinical features and treatment. *Reumatologia*, **57**(4), 221–33.

Swales, C. Inflammatory connective tissue disease. In Bulstrode C, Wilson-MacDonald J, Eastwood D, et al., eds. Oxford Textbook of Trauma and Orthopaedics (2 edn). Oxford: Oxford University Press, 2011: pp. 810-13.

Van den Hoogen F, Khanna D, Fransen J, *et al.* 2013 classification criteria for systemic sclerosis: an American College of Rheumatology/European League against Rheumatism collaborative initiative. *Arthritis and Rheumatology*. 2013;**65**(11):2737–47.

Polymyositis and dermatomyositis

Idiopathic inflammatory myositis (IIM) can cause inflammation of muscles and systemic vasculopathy. Onset of symptoms is usually acute (several days) or subacute (several weeks to few months). Commonest in sixth decade; ♀ > ♂.

Dermatomyositis (DM) has a prevalence of 6 per 100,000 in the USA, and polymyositis (PM) 10 per 100,000.

PM can be seen in conjunction with other overlap conditions such as scleroderma, SLE, and Sjögren's syndrome.

Clinical features

- Musculoskeletal:
  - Proximal myopathy—progressive and symmetrical
  - Polyarthralgia.
  - Pain.
- Skin:
  - Skin involvement variable
  - Heliotropic rash (purplish rash of eyelids), with periorbital oedema
  - Scaly, erythematous rash on extensor surfaces of elbows, knees, and fingers (Gottron's papules)
  - Skin inflammation affecting the anterior upper chest (V sign) or posterior neck (shawl sign)
  - Raynaud's phenomenon
  - Mechanic's hands (thickened skin, periungal erythema, and cracked skin).
- GI: dysphagia.
- Respiratory: dysphonia, lung involvement, respiratory weakness.
- Cardiovascular: myocarditis or myocardial infarction (rare).

Be aware of amyopathic DM with only skin and lung involvement, but no muscle weakness or rise in CK.

Other

- Retinitis.
- Cancer risk: with ↑ age, there is a higher probability that myositis is associated with an underlying malignancy, usually adenocarcinoma of the breast or lung particularly with the TIF 1gamma and NXP2 antibodies. Malignant disease is usually apparent, and an extensive search for occult malignancy unjustified.
- Anti-synthetase syndrome: chronic autoimmune syndrome caused by autoantibodies to aminoacyl-transfer RNA (tRNA) synthetases associated with high risk of ILD.

Diagnosis

- ↑ in creatine phosphokinase (CPK) levels (10- to 50-fold in IIM), ↑ in ESR, EMG changes, muscle edema on MRI and abnormal muscle biopsy (pathognomonic inflammatory response).
- Autoantibodies: MDA-5 associated with ILD, Mi-2 with DM, TIF-1 with malignancy, and NXP-2 seen in children with calcinosis and tumours. Those individuals with anti-synthetase antibodies (anti-Jo-1, PL-7, PL-12, Ku, OJ, EJ) characteristically suffer from pulmonary fibrosis in association with myositis.

Management

Steroids (prednisolone) and immunosuppressive agents (azathioprine, mycophenolate, and methotrexate). Skin condition may respond to anti-malarials. In patients who are refractory to standard treatment, consider IV immunoglobulins (IVIG), rituximab, and cyclophosphamide.

Further reading

Ashton C, Paramalingam S, Stevenson B, *et al.* Idiopathic inflammatory myopathies: a review. *Internal Medicine Journal*. 2021;**51**(6):845–52.

Furst DE, Amato AA, Iorga SR, Gajria K, Fernandes AW. Epidemiology of adult idiopathic inflammatory myopathies in a U.S. managed care plan. *Muscle and Nerve*. 2012;**45**(5):676–83.

NHS England Specialised Services Clinical Reference Group for Specialised Rheumatology (2016). *Clinical Commissioning Policy: rituximab for the treatment of dermatomyositis and polymyositis (adults)*. Available from: www.england.nhs.uk/wp-content/uploads/2018/07/Rituximab-for-the-treatment-of-dermatomyositis-and-polymyositis-adults.pdf

Schmidt J. Current classification and management of inflammatory myopathies. *Journal of Neuromuscular Diseases*. 2018;**5**(2):109–29.

Swales, C. Inflammatory connective tissue disease. In Bulstrode C, Wilson-MacDonald J, Eastwood D, et al., eds. Oxford Textbook of Trauma and Orthopaedics (2 edn). Oxford: Oxford University Press, 2011: pp. 810-13.

Ankylosing spondylitis

AS is an inflammatory arthropathy of the spine with associated extraspinal features. Patients with AS can be classified as having radiographic (changes on X-ray) or non-radiographic AS (changes on MRI, combination of other findings, or both).

Epidemiology

Incidence is 0.1–0.3%. Prevalence in Europe is 23.8 per 10,000. In HLA-B27-positive patients, the incidence ↑ 100-fold but it is not a diagnostic test; <5% of those who are HLA-B27-negative have AS. The incidence ↑ 20-fold in first-degree relatives. Usually manifests in the third or fourth decade of life. Sex distribution is 3 ♂:1 ♀.

Pathophysiology

Inflammatory arthropathy affecting synovial and fibrous joints. The SIJs are affected in all patients. Inflammatory process leads to joint destruction and ankylosis.

Clinical features

Onset is insidious, and the course is characterized by flares and remissions. Inflammation is seen in ligaments, capsules, and subchondral bone. It is an axial arthritis, but girdle joints (hips and shoulders) are affected in 20%. Patients often have early morning stiffness, which improves during the day. There may be sacroiliac tenderness, ↓ spinal mobility, loss of lumbar lordosis, and flexion contraction of the hips. Extra-articular manifestations include: aortic insufficiency, conduction defects, ↓ chest expansion, uveitis (25%), Achilles tendonitis, plantar fasciitis, psoriasis, and inflammatory bowel disease (IBD). Complications include vertebral fragility fractures (commonest at the lower cervical spine). Of the three types of fractures (extension, flexion, and compression), the commonest is extension fracture.

Investigations

- *Blood tests:* HLA-B27, ESR, and CRP (raised in up to 70%, but normal results do not exclude AS).
- *Radiology:* radiographs show squaring of vertebral bodies in early stages; syndesmophytes, spinal fusion (bamboo spine), and osteopenia seen late. Joint space narrowing, sclerosis, erosion (begins on the iliac side where cartilage is thinner, compared to the sacral side), and ankylosis can be seen on X-ray of SIJs. Changes in SIJs are graded from 0 to 4, as per the Modified New York Criteria, and a diagnosis of AS needs at least bilateral grade 2 or unilateral grade 3. The grading is as follows:
  - Grade 0—normal; grade 1—suspicious, but no definite changes; grade 2—small, localized areas with erosions or sclerosis; grade 3—advanced sacroiliitis with sclerosis, erosions, partial ankylosis, and joint space widening or narrowing; and grade 4—total ankylosis of SIJs.
- Bone scan shows ↑ uptake in SIJs. MRI shows inflammation in the ligaments, capsule, and subchondral bone of SIJs.

Management

- *Non-operative:* exercise is the mainstay of treatment and is aimed at maintaining flexibility. Educate patient about the disease. Multidisciplinary care (GP, rheumatologist, ophthalmologist, physiotherapist, occupational therapist, orthopaedic surgeon) is needed. NSAIDs are the commonest type of drug used (at least two types for 4 weeks each, unless contraindications). Secondary drugs include corticosteroids and disease-modifying drugs for peripheral joint symptoms and anti-TNF inhibitors and IL-17 inhibitors JAK inhibitors and IL12/23 inhibitors for axial disease. Biological drugs are used for treating axial disease if failure to respond to standard treatment (NSAIDs) and high disease activity—assessed by Bath Ankylosing Spondylitis Disease Activity Index (BASDAI) score.
- *Operative:* surgery is reserved for complications—fixation of spinal fractures, correction of spinal deformity, and hip replacement (see ➔ Chapter 17).

Further reading

Dean LE, Jones GT, MacDonald AG, Downham C, Sturrock RD, Macfarlane GJ. Global prevalence of ankylosing spondylitis. *Rheumatology.* 2014;**53**(4):650–7.

Garcia-Montoya L, Gul H, Emery P. Recent advances in ankylosing spondylitis: understanding the disease and management. *F1000Research.* 2018;**7**:F1000 Faculty Rev-1512.

Linden SV, Valkenburg HA, Cats A. Evaluation of diagnostic criteria for ankylosing spondylitis. *Arthritis and Rheumatism.* 1984;**27**(4):361–8.

Westerveld L, Verlaan JJ, Oner FC. Spinal fractures in patients with ankylosing spinal disorders: a systematic review of the literature on treatment, neurological status and complications. *European Spine Journal.* 2009;**18**(2):145–56.

Psoriatic arthritis

Psoriatic arthritis is an inflammatory arthritis associated with psoriasis.

Epidemiology

Psoriasis is common, affecting 2% of the Caucasian population, and up to 25% may develop arthropathy. Sex distribution is equal (♂:♀). Usually seen at 30–50 years in patients with known psoriasis but may occur in childhood. Psoriatic arthritis may occur before the development of psoriasis (some patients will not have psoriasis).

Aetiology

Psoriasis, 50% association with HLA-B27, and there is often a strong family history of arthritis in a third of cases.

Clinical features

Presentations of psoriatic arthritis

- Asymmetrical oligoarthritis affecting finger joints—sausage finger and toes (dactylitis) (70%).
- Symmetrical polyarthritis similar to RA (15%).
- DIPJ arthritis with nail changes (5%).
- Arthritis mutilans with severe deformities secondary to osteolysis of affected joints (5%)—associated with sacroiliitis and widespread skin disease.
- Spondyloarthritis presenting as sacroiliitis and/or spondylitis (5%).

Clinical features in keeping with psoriasis, but nail changes (pitting, ridging, subungual keratosis, onycholysis) are commoner in those with psoriatic arthritis than those without (70% vs 30%, respectively).
  Periarticular manifestations include:

- Enthesitis—inflammation at the site of insertion of tendons, ligaments, and synovium into bone (Achilles tendinitis, plantar fasciitis)
- Tenosynovitis—inflammation of flexor tendons of the hands and ECU or tendons of the ankles
- Ocular—uveitis and conjunctivitis.

Investigations

- Radiology: radiographic changes include lysis of terminal phalanges, periostitis, new bone formation, pencil-in-cup deformity, erosions, and ankylosis of joints.
- MRI and USS detect soft tissue inflammatory changes and synovial effusions.
- Raised ESR and CRP (but may also be normal).

Management

Aimed at control of psoriasis and protection of joints.

- *Non-operative:* medications include NSAIDs, immunosuppressive drugs (methotrexate, sulfasalazine, leflunomide), and analgesics. Steroid injections may be helpful for localized disease. Avoid systemic steroid due to flare-up of skin psoriasis on steroid discontinuation. A range of biological drugs (anti-TNF inhibitors, IL-17 inhibitor, JAK inhibitors, IL-12/23 inhibitor, phosphodiesterase type 4 inhibitor) are available if treatment failure on standard disease-modifying antirheumatic drugs (DMARDs) (at least three swollen, tender joints despite two consecutive DMARDs). Splints are important in managing joint pain and deformities.

- *Operative:* reconstruction of joints helps to preserve function.

Complications

- Destruction of joints, ankylosis.

Further reading

Alinaghi F, Calov M, Kristensen LE, et al. Prevalence of psoriatic arthritis in patients with psoriasis: a systematic review and meta-analysis of observational and clinical studies. *Journal of the American Academy of Dermatology*. 2019;**80**(1):251–65.

Coates LC, Tillett W, Chandler D, et al. The 2012 BSR and BHPR guideline for the treatment of psoriatic arthritis with biologics. *Rheumatology*. 2013;**52**(10):1754–7.

Siannis F, Farewell VT, Cook RJ, Schentag CT, Gladman DD. Clinical and radiological damage in psoriatic arthritis. *Annals of the Rheumatic Diseases*. 2006;**65**(4):478–81.

Reactive arthritis

Reactive arthritis (a part of seronegative spondyloarthritis) is an aseptic inflammatory arthritis associated with urogenital, ocular, mucocutaneous, and musculoskeletal infections.

Epidemiology

Seen in young, sexually active adults, mostly men, but may be underdiagnosed in women due to subclinical *Chlamydia* infections. Affects Caucasian more than other racial groups; 70% associated with HLA-B27. Worldwide prevalence is 30–40 per 100,000, and incidence is 0.6–27 per 100,000.

Aetiology

Can be associated with urethritis, cervicitis, or diarrhoea. Triggering infective causes include *Chlamydia*, *Shigella*, *Salmonella*, *Campylobacter*, *Yersinia*, *Giardia lamblia*, and *Cryptosporidium*.

Clinical features

Asymmetrical, oligoarticular arthritis (90% have peripheral joint involvement) and dactylitis (tenosynovitis and soft tissue inflammation leading to sausage fingers). Skin lesions include psoriasiform lesions (keratoderma blenorrhagica), circinate balanitis, small oral ulcers, and opacity and thickening of nails.

Can also have spondyloarthritis similar to that in AS. May have urethritis, conjunctivitis, uveitis, erythema, photophobia, or diarrhoea. Systemic disease with fever and malaise. The triad of arthritis, urethritis, and conjunctivitis is present in under a third of patients initially. History, especially sexual, is very important in making the diagnosis.

Investigations

- Rule out septic arthritis by joint aspiration.
- Blood tests: may be unhelpful, but ESR and CRP are useful to monitor disease progression. Check RhF, anti-CCP, and HLA-B27 for prognostication.
- *Imaging:* sacroiliitis on MRI. Later joint destruction with recurrent disease. USS and MRI may also detect peripheral joint synovitis or tenosynovitis.

Management

- *Non-operative:* treatment is aimed at eradicating the triggering infection and relieving symptoms. NSAIDs and steroids, along with temporary splinting, are used to treat the acute phase. Joint injections with corticosteroids suppress synovitis and prevent irreversible joint damage. Disease-modifying drugs are used to treat chronic cases. Biological drugs may be used for failure to respond to standard DMARDs. Physiotherapy and exercise are necessary to preserve muscle strength and flexibility. Usually resolves in 3 months, but can become recurrent and up to 40% of patients have recurrent symptoms at 15 years. Antibiotic treatment of the sexual partner may prevent reinfection; long-term sequelae with recurrence.
- *Operative:* arthroplasty occasionally needed.

Complications

• Joint destruction, sterility.

Further reading

Schmitt SK. Reactive arthritis. *Infectious Disease Clinics*. 2017;**31**(2):265–77.
Townes JM. Reactive arthritis after enteric infections in the United States: the problem of definition. *Clinical Infectious Diseases*. 2010;**50**(2):247–54.

Enteropathic arthritis

Enteropathic arthritis is arthritis complicating IBD.

Epidemiology

It affects up to 46% of patients with IBD and is twice as common in patients with Crohn's disease as in those with ulcerative colitis.

Clinical features

Enteropathic arthritis may present as spondyloarthropathy or as peripheral arthritis. The spondyloarthritic form is unlikely to progress. The peripheral arthritis form may be more aggressive but does not usually destroy joints. Enthesitis and dactylitis may also occur.

Spondyloarthritis

Sacroiliitis is common with Crohn's disease and ulcerative colitis. There is a clear relationship between bowel disease flare-ups and arthropathy; 60% association with HLA-B27.

Peripheral arthritis

- *Type 1:* pauciarticular with acute, short-lived attacks often related to IBD activity. Associated with HLA-B27.
- *Type 2:* polyarticular with persistent symptoms less related to IBD attacks. Associated with HLA-B44.

Investigations

- *Radiology:* MRI useful for identifying isolated sacroiliitis.

Management

The spondyloarthritic form and type 1 peripheral form respond to control of IBD. Type 2 peripheral form is more likely to lead to joint deformity. Simple analgesics, intra-articular steroids, systemic steroids, and disease-modifying drugs, such as methotrexate and sulfasalazine, are used. NSAIDs may not be well tolerated with IBD. Anti-TNF therapy may successfully treat arthropathy and IBD. Those resistant to anti-TNF treatment may be offered IL-12/23 inhibitor (ustekinumab) as well as JAK inhibitors, which is used to treat Crohn's disease and psoriatic arthritis.

Further reading

Hatemi G, Akar S, Akpinar H, et al. 2019. FRI0392 evidence based recommendations for the management of enteropathic arthritis: a collaborative initiative. *Annals of the Rheumatic Diseases.* 2019;**78**(Suppl 2):881.1-881.

Olivieri I, Cantini F, Castiglione F, *et al.* Italian Expert Panel on the management of patients with coexisting spondyloarthritis and inflammatory bowel disease. *Autoimmunity Reviews.* 2014;**13**(8):822–30.

Poddubnyy D, Hermann KG, Callhoff J, Listing J, Sieper J. Ustekinumab for the treatment of patients with active ankylosing spondylitis: results of a 28-week, prospective, open-label, proof-of-concept study (TOPAS). *Annals of the Rheumatic Diseases.* 2014;**73**(5):817–23.

Behçet's disease

A rare immune-mediated, multisystem variable-vessel vasculitis.

Epidemiology

UK incidence estimated at 0.38 per 100,000. Pooled estimates of prevalence per 100,000 (1974–2015): Turkey, 119; Middle East, 31; Asia, 4.5; and Europe, 3. Onset usually between 20 and 40 years of age.

Aetiology

Exact cause unknown. Involves interplay between some well-characterized genetic factors and pathological pathways. HLA-B51 association.

Pathophysiology

Main histological finding is widespread vasculitis.

Clinical features

- Recurrent aphthous ulcers (often the first sign) are universal. Also large orogenital ulcers, skin lesions (erythema nodosum, acne, and pustulosis), eye disease (uveitis, retinal vasculitis), neurological (pyramidal and cerebellar signs, dementia, and psychiatric problems), recurrent thrombosis, and arterial aneurysms. Joint involvement is common with mono- or oligoarticular synovitis (may last several weeks).
- International Criteria for Behçet's Disease (ICBD) classification criteria mandates a score of 4 out of the following (variable weighting): ocular lesions, genital aphthous ulceration, oral aphthous ulceration, skin lesions, neurological manifestations, vascular manifestations, and positive pathergy test.

Investigations

- *Bloods:* FBC and inflammatory markers (ESR and CRP may be elevated).
- Test for, and exclude, other causes of oral and genital ulcerations (e.g. sexually transmitted infections, coeliac disease, IBD, nutritional deficiencies, CTDs).

Management

Steroids in the acute phase. Disease-modifying drugs, such as azathioprine, ciclosporin, tacrolimus, and mycophenolate, for eye disease. Methotrexate for inflammatory arthritis. Biologic drugs (usually anti TNF drugs and for refractory disease, can consider tocilizumab, interferon or rituximab. For refractory mucocutaneous disease, apremilast is an option) and/or cyclophosphamide for refractory ocular, neurological, GI, mucocutaneous, and vascular disease (see EULAR guidelines).

Further reading

Hatemi G, Christensen R, Bang D, *et al.* 2018 update of the EULAR recommendations for the management of Behçet's syndrome. *Annals of the Rheumatic Diseases.* 2018;**77**:808–18.

International Team for the Revision of the International Criteria for Behçet's Disease (ITR-ICBD). The International Criteria for Behçet's Disease (ICBD). *Journal of the European Academy of Dermatology and Venereology.* 2014;**28**(3):338–47.

Mahr A, Belarbi L, Wechsler B, *et al.* Population-based prevalence study of Behçet's disease: differences by ethnic origin and low variation by age at immigration. *Arthritis and Rheumatology.* 2008;**58**(12):3951–9.

Yazici H, Seyahi E, Hatemi G, Yazici Y. Behçet syndrome: a contemporary review. *Nature Reviews Rheumatology.* 2018;**14**(2):107–19.

Crystal arthropathies

Gout (monosodium urate deposition disease)

Gout is an inflammatory disease caused by deposition of monosodium urate (MSU) crystals in joints and other tissues. The formation of the crystals is the consequence of hyperuricaemia, a condition so called when serum uric acid (SUA) levels are >6.0mg/dL (360μmol/L). Gout is a disorder of purine metabolism. Uric acid is produced from xanthine by xanthine oxidase, and in gout, SUA levels are raised (hyperuricaemia). Hyperuricaemia is common and often asymptomatic.

Epidemiology

Gout is present in 1% of the population. Commoner in Afro-Caribbeans than in Caucasians. ♂ > ♀.

Clinical features

History

The natural history of gout is classically composed of three periods: asymptomatic hyperuricaemia, acute attacks with asymptomatic intervals (Inter-critical period), and chronic gout. The classic presentation of acute gout is characterized by a typical rapid development of severe pain and swelling, with overlying erythema and tenderness that reaches a maximum within 6–12h, often starting at night or in the early morning. Most often gout presents as acute monoarthritis and usually it involves a single joint in the lower extremity—in particular, the first MTPJ (podagra), which has been considered as a hallmark of the disease. Less often, the disease starts in other joints—tarsal and subtalar joints, ankle, knee, wrist, and MCPJs or IPJs of the hand can be affected. Inflammation at the Achilles tendon insertion, olecranon bursae, or patellar tendon is also common.

Comorbidities

Conditions associated with high cell turnover (e.g. some malignancies and psoriatic disease) may result in hyperuricaemia. This can be exacerbated when chemotherapy is given to treat such conditions. Patients should have prophylaxis against hyperuricaemia. In an important proportion of patients, hyperuricaemia is part of the metabolic syndrome and the presence of gout should alert the physician to this problem and its associated morbidities. These may require modification of dietary and lifestyle habits, and often medication.

Examination

Look for signs of gout inflammation: swelling, erythema, warmth, and tenderness. Clinical findings of acute gout may be indistinguishable from acute cellulitis. Tophi on extensor surfaces, such as elbows and ears, can be confused with rheumatoid nodules. The presence of tophi suggests long-standing hyperuricaemia.

Investigations

- *Bloods:* FBC, electrolytes, and SUA. Patients with gout may have normal SUA levels, especially during an acute episode.
- *Aspiration of joint effusion:* fluid is sent for microscopy and microbiological culture. Diagnosis confirmed with presence of negatively birefringent, needle-shaped crystals in the fluid examined with polarized light microscopy.

- *Radiographs:* may show erosions of bone slightly away from the articular surface (peri-articular) in gout.
- *USS:* MSU crystal deposits can be detected by sonography, which shows crystals deposited along the surface of the joint cartilage, and also in synovial tissue and tendons.
- *Dual-energy CT (DECT):* in cases where the diagnosis is uncertain and MSU crystal identification is not possible, this may be useful.

Differential diagnosis

Includes septic arthritis, pseudogout, seronegative peripheral spondyloarthritis, RA, and trauma.

Management

Non-operative

- *Acute episodes:* traditional medications are colchicine, NSAIDs, and steroids. Innovative/biological medications act as IL-1 inhibitors in patients with inadequate response or contraindication against/ intolerance of traditional medications.
- *Chronic gout:* three classes of medications are approved for urate-lowering treatment (ULT): xanthine oxidase inhibitors, uricosuric agents, and uricase agents.
  - Xanthine oxidase inhibitors block the synthesis of uric acid. Allopurinol has become the mainstay urate-lowering drug and so is used as the first-line ULT. NICE guidance recommends starting at a low dose of 50–100mg once a day (preferably taken with food), ↑ by 100mg increments approximately every 4 weeks, until the SUA level is below 300μmol/L.
  - Other medications available are febuxostat (non-purine-based xanthine oxidase inhibitor), probenecid, sulfinpyrazone, and benzbromarone (uricosuric drugs). However, each needs careful consideration after evaluating the risk:benefit ratio and some are on a named-patient basis only. Broadly speaking, these are contraindicated when eGFR<30 (except benzbromarone which has efficacy even when EGFR as low as 20) and in the presence of renal calculi.
- EULAR and ACR guidelines recommend that plasma or serum urate should be maintained at a concentration of <6mg/dL (360μmol/L).
- For all SUA-lowering drugs, it is an often-accepted rule that they should not be started until the gouty attack has fully resolved although data behind this concept does now show worsening of acute flare if ULT is started during an attack; furthermore, it must be kept in mind that initiation or ↑ in dosage of SUA-lowering therapy in patients with gout frequently results in a gouty attack if prophylactic colchicine is not co-administered (e.g. at 0.5–1mg/day).
- Duration of prophylaxis treatment with colchicine/NSAID/steroid varies from 2 weeks to 6 months, depending on the clinical picture.

Operative options

Joint washout can hasten the resolution of symptoms and aid in diagnosis. Joint reconstruction may become necessary if joint destruction worsens. Tophi can be excised if problematic, but healing may be prolonged and they often recur if SUA sub-optimally controlled.

Pseudogout (calcium pyrophosphate deposition disease)

Pseudogout is an inflammatory arthropathy caused by deposition of calcium pyrophosphate dehydrate crystals.

Epidemiology

Calcium pyrophosphate deposition disease (CPPD) is mainly a disease of the elderly. Prevalence of radiological CPPD in Caucasians is very low before 55–60 years of age but subsequently ↑: 15% in those aged between 65 and 74 years, 36% in those between 75 and 84 years, and 44% in those aged ≥85 years.

Clinical features

May present in a similar fashion to gout, although large joints are more commonly affected. Commonest joint affected is the knee and the wrist. Examination of the joint reveals OA with superimposed synovitis. CPPD can also be secondary to several metabolic diseases, including primary hyperparathyroidism, haemochromatosis, hypophosphatasia and hypomagnesaemia—some of which can also be familial.

Investigations

- *Radiographs:* may show chondrocalcinosis—mineralization within fibrocartilage structures such as the menisci of the knee. This finding may be present in several conditions and is neither diagnostic nor always symptomatic.
- *Joint aspiration fluid:* examined as for gout. Calcium pyrophosphate crystals are rhomboid in shape and weakly birefringent under polarized light.

Management

Treatment is essentially symptomatic with analgesics and NSAIDs. Low-dose colchicine (1mg/day) may be used as a preventative treatment in patients with frequently relapsing flares. Hydroxychloroquine was shown to be helpful in one placebo-controlled study. Methotrexate has been tested in a double-blind, placebo-controlled crossover study, but results have been disappointing, with no statistically significant reduction in the Disease Activity Score (DAS) 44 score, pain level, or secondary outcome. Painful joint effusions can be washed out arthroscopically.

Calcium hydroxyapatite deposition

Crystals of calcium hydroxyapatite are the major mineral content of bone. They can be deposited in other tissues such as tendons. If present in the synovial fluid, they can lead to an erosive arthritis that can be rapidly progressive and mistaken for collapse of osteonecrotic bone.

Differential diagnoses

A number of differential diagnoses must be considered when managing a joint affected by crystal arthropathy, including:

- RA—may start as a large joint monoarthropathy
- Seronegative arthritis
- Acute septic arthritis—fluid from joint aspiration should be sent for culture and sensitivity testing. Consider gonococcus in a sexually active younger patient.
- Reactive arthritis—joint swelling can occur in response to a systemic condition.

Further reading

Drug and Therapeutics Bulletin. Latest guidance on the management of gout. *BMJ*. 2018;**362**:k2893.

Finckh A, McCarthy GM, Madigan A, *et al.* Methotrexate in chronic-recurrent calcium pyrophosphate deposition disease: no significant effect in a randomized crossover trial. *Arthritis Research and Therapy*. 2014;**16**(5):458.

Hui M, Carr A, Cameron S, *et al.* The British Society for Rheumatology guideline for the management of gout. *Rheumatology*. 2017;**56**(7):e1–20.

Khanna D, Fitzgerald JD, Khanna PP, *et al.* 2012 American College of Rheumatology guidelines for management of gout. Part 1: systematic nonpharmacologic and pharmacologic therapeutic approaches to hyperuricemia. *Arthritis Care and Research*. 2012;**64**(10):1431–46.

Khanna D, Khanna PP, Fitzegarld JD, *et al.* 2012 American College of Rheumatology guidelines for management of gout. Part 2: Therapy and anti-inflammatory prohylaxis of acute gouty arthritis. *Arthritis Care and Research*. 2012;**64**(10):1447–61.

Ragab G, Elshahaly M, Bardin T. Gout: an old disease in new perspective—a review. *Journal of Advanced Research*. 2017;**8**(5):495–511.

Richette P, Doherty M, Pascual E, *et al.* 2018 updated European League Against Rheumatism evidence-based recommendations for the diagnosis of gout. *Annals of the Rheumatic Diseases*. 2020;**79**(1):31–8.

Roddy E, Choi HK. Epidemiology of gout. *Rheumatic Disease Clinics*. 2014;**40**(2):155–75.

Rothschild B, Yakubov LE. Prospective 6-month, double-blind trial of hydroxychloroquine treatment of CPDD. *Comprehensive Therapy*. 1997;**23**(5):327–31.

Adult orthopaedics: pathology

Musculoskeletal aspects of haemophilia

A bleeding disorder resulting from ↓ levels of clotting factor VIII (haemophilia A) or IX (haemophilia B/Christmas disease). X-linked recessive inheritance (one-third of cases caused by sporadic mutations). Incidence of 1:10,000 ♂ births.

Presentation

- Spontaneous bleeding/bruising or prolonged bleeding following minor injuries, surgery, or dental extractions. Family history in familial cases.
- Severity determined by clotting factor levels: mild (5–25% of normal), moderate (1–5%), and severe (<1%).

Musculoskeletal features

- Haemophilic arthropathy secondary to recurrent haemarthroses—triggers synovitis and cartilage damage.
- Subperiosteal/intraosseous bleeds causing local pressure effects ± pathological fracture.
- Intramuscular haematomas. Small risk of compartment syndrome and nerve compression.

Management

- Elective surgery by experienced staff in specialist centres (both orthopaedic and haematological).
- Haematological prophylaxis—factor VIII or XI therapy. ↑ levels perioperatively (soft tissue surgery, 40–50% of normal; skeletal surgery, 100%).
- Physiotherapy and splintage for acute bleeds.
- Intra-articular injections (early stages of arthropathy).
- Arthroscopic synovectomy (to reduce frequency of haemarthroses).
- Corrective osteotomy (to address abnormal limb axis and delay arthroplasty in young patients).
- Arthroplasty (severe arthropathy). Hip and knee replacements more predictable than ankle replacements. Knee arthroplasty most commonly performed due to high levels of synovial tissue.
- Revision arthroplasty (both aseptic and septic loosening relatively common in haemophilia).
- Arthrodesis (generally reserved as a salvage procedure).

Further reading

Kulkarni K, Dodd C, Pandit H. A bloody painful knee: delayed presentation of haemophilic arthropathy. *BMJ Case Reports*. 2014;**2014**:bcr2014205370.

Rizzo AR, Zago M, Carulli C, Innocenti M. Orthopaedic procedures in haemophilia. *Clinical Cases in Mineral and Bone Metabolism*. 2017;**14**(2):197–9.

Rodríguez-Merchán EC. The role of orthopaedic surgery in haemophilia: current rationale, indications and results. *EFORT Open Reviews*. 2019;**4**(5):165–73.

Tenosynovial giant cell tumour and pigmented villonodular synovitis

Tenosynovial giant cell tumours (TGCTs) are a group of benign neoplasms that arise from the synovium, bursae, or tendon sheaths. Classified by the WHO into two groups: localized and diffuse. These subtypes share a common aetiology but differ significantly in their clinical behaviour.

Presentation

- *Localized:* TGCTs form solitary nodular lesions. Typically presents as a painless, slow-growing mass or with mechanical symptoms. Can be intra- or extra-articular (intra-articular commonest in the knee).
- *Diffuse:* TGCTs (formerly known as pigmented villonodular synovitis (PVNS)). More aggressive than localized disease and, if left untreated, can cause severe joint destruction. Found throughout affected joint (classically knee, hip, and hindfoot/ankle). Usually presents with pain, stiffness, and swelling. Prone to recurrence after treatment.

Investigations

- *MRI:* essential for surgical planning and to define extent of disease.
- *Biopsy:* tissue diagnosis to rule out malignancy.
- *Synovial fluid analysis:* often brown or haemorrhagic in colour due to haemosiderin. Microscopy reveals multinucleated giant cells.
- *Radiographs:* soft tissue swelling and bony erosions in later stages.

Management

Localised

- Open marginal excision (arthroscopy runs the risk of seeding throughout the joint).

Diffuse

- Marginal excision with total synovectomy of affected joint as gold standard, although plagued with high recurrence rates (up to 50%).
- Arthroplasty with synovectomy at the knee (end-stage disease with severe, symptomatic joint arthropathy).
- Adjuvant external beam radiation (shown to reduce TGCT recurrence post-surgery—although risk of causing malignancy).
- Monoclonal antibodies (patients with extensive disease that is unlikely to be surgically resectable—pexidartinib undergoing trials).

Further reading

Bernthal NM, Ishmael CR, Burke ZD. Management of pigmented villonodular synovitis (PVNS): an orthopedic surgeon's perspective. *Current Oncology Reports.* 2020;**22**:1–6.

Lucas DR. Tenosynovial giant cell tumor: case report and review. *Archives of Pathology and Laboratory Medicine.* 2012;**136**(8):901–6.

Osteoarthritis

A degenerative disease of joints characterized by articular cartilage degeneration and bony remodelling. OA is common, with a symptomatic incidence in the hip and knee of 88 and 240 per 100,000, respectively. Although the prevalence ↑ with age, osteoarthritic collagen degrades differently to cartilage undergoing normal ageing (Table 12.1).

Table 12.1 Differences in structure of articular cartilage

Cartilage property	Age-related	Osteoarthritis
Collagen	Content relatively unchanged	Arrangement disordered Content ↓ Concentration ↑
Proteoglycan synthesis	Reduced	↑
Water content	↓	↑
Modulus of elasticity	↑	↓

Causes
- *Primary (idiopathic):* results from hereditary factors or general stresses on weight-bearing joints.
- *Secondary:*
  - Infection
  - Neuropathic (diabetes/syphilis)
  - Developmental (e.g. developmental dysplasia of the hip (DDH); Perthes' disease)
  - Biomechanical (malalignment/instability/incongruity)
  - Traumatic
  - Biochemical (haemochromatosis/gout/pseudogout).

Pathophysiology
Primary OA is a complex disorder influenced by multiple factors. Initially, molecular degradation results in cartilage softening (known as chondromalacia). Subsequent changes include synovitis, hypertrophic bone changes, and formation of osteophytes, before macroscopic cartilaginous disruption results in subchondral bone exposure.

Classification
- *Radiographic (Kellgren and Lawrence):* (1) minimal osteophytes; (2) osteophytes; (3) joint space narrowing; and (4) subchondral sclerosis.
- *Arthroscopic (Outerbridge):* (0) normal; (1) soft/swollen cartilage; (2) partial-thickness defects that do not reach subchondral bone or exceed 1.5cm in diameter; (3) fissuring to subchondral bone or diameter >1.5cm; and (4) full-thickness cartilage loss.

Presentation
- Pain (typically progressive worsens throughout day with activity).

- Swelling and stiffness (osteophytes, capsular thickening and/or effusion).
- Joint line tenderness and warmth.
- Muscle wasting and weakness.
- Crepitus
- Joint instability and deformity (severe cases).

Differential diagnosis

- *Monoarticular:* trauma, septic arthritis, gout, pseudogout.
- *Polyarticular:* reactive/inflammatory arthritis.

Management

Non-operative

- Weight loss/lifestyle modification to avoid load-bearing activities.
- Analgesia.
- Physiotherapy (to preserve range of motion/muscle strength).
- Cushioned footwear (to reduce impact of pain in lower limbs).
- Walking aids (to reduce lower limb joint reaction forces).
- Splints (to provide support/restrict ROM of involved joints).
- Corrective orthoses (to offload parts of joint causing pain).
- Intra-articular steroid/hyaluronic acid injections.
- PRP injections

Operative

- Arthroplasty (joint replacement)—successful for severe OA.
- Arthrodesis (joint fusion)—also effective in ankle, foot, wrist, and the majority of small joints of the hand (excluding MCPJs).
- Osteotomy—to correct malalignment and offload areas of joint affected the most.
- Discrete areas of cartilage loss in young patients may be treated with cartilage stimulation (microfracture), regeneration (autologous chondrocyte implantation), or transplant techniques (osteochondral autologous transfer system (OATS)). Some of these techniques are regarded as experimental.

Further reading

Iannone F, Lapadula G. The pathophysiology of osteoarthritis. *Aging Clinical and Experimental Research*. 2003;**15**(5):364–72.

National Institute for Health and Care Excellence (2019). *Platelet-rich plasma injections for knee osteoarthritis*. Interventional procedures guidance [IPG637]. Available from: ℜ www.nice.org.uk/guidance/ipg637

Aseptic bone necrosis (osteonecrosis)

Defined as death of bone due to ischaemia. Peri-articular lesions are termed avascular necrosis, whereas those in the dia-metaphysis are bone infarcts. Commonly involves the hip (femoral head), shoulder (humeral head), and talus. Also found in the lunate (Kienböck's disease), capitellum (Panner's disease), metatarsal head (Freiberg's disease), navicular bone (Kohler's disease), and scaphoid. Affected bone undergoes necrosis, resorption, and microfracture, and then subchondral collapse. Resulting joint incongruence leads to degenerative changes.

Causes
- Idiopathic.
- Trauma.
- Infection.
- Haematological diseases (leukaemia/lymphoma).
- Vascular microemboli (sickle-cell, haemoglobinopathies, polycythaemia, fat emboli, decompression nitrogen emboli).
- Drugs (corticosteroids, alcohol).
- Vasculitis (SLE).

Presentation
- Pain (charactersitically nocturnal). Adjacent joint irritability/effusion.

Investigations
- *Plain radiographs:* osteopenia, cystic or sclerotic changes, subchondral fracture, and collapse in peri-articular regions ('crescent sign').
- *MRI:* gold standard, diagnostic.
- *Isotope bone scan:* findings vary, based on stage. Superseded by MRI.

Management
- Depends on site and stage of disease.

Non-operative
- Remove/amend modifiable risk factors.
- Analgesia and intra-articular steroid injections.
- Physiotherapy (to maintain ROM/strength).

Operative
- Broadly divided into pre-collapse (decompression, revascularization, graft) vs post-collapse (osteotomy, fusion, arthroplasty):
  - Surgical decompression of peri-articular lesions (± revascularization)
  - Redirectional osteotomies—to offload peri-articular lesions
  - Arthroplasty/arthrodesis—salvage for degenerative joints.

Further reading
Petek D, Hannouche D, Suva D. Osteonecrosis of the femoral head: pathophysiology and current concepts of treatment. *EFORT Open Reviews.* 2019;**4**(3):85–97.

Osteochondroses

A diverse group of immature skeletal disorders involving the growth plates and their surrounding ossification centres. Exact aetiology poorly understood, although genetic, hormonal, traumatic, vascular, and mechanical factors have all been highlighted as potential causes. Involved bones undergo osteonecrosis followed by regeneration/recalcification. Radiographs show sclerosis followed by bony deformity and fragmentation, depending on disease stage.

Groups

Articular osteochondroses (joint space involvement)
- Panner's disease.
- Legg–Calve–Perthes' disease.
- Köhler's disease.
- Freiberg's disease.
- Kienbock's disease.

Monoarticular osteochondroses (apophysitis)
- Sinding–Larsen–Johansson disease.
- Osgood–Schlatter disease.
- Sever's disease.
- Epiphyseal osteochrondroses.
- Scheuermann's disease.
- Blount's disease (also affects the metaphysis).

Panner's disease (humeral capitellum)
- Common cause of lateral-sided elbow pain in children.
- May be associated with repetitive throwing.
- Commoner in dominant arm.
- Peak incidence in boys 5–12 years of age.
- Examination reveals elbow stiffness with capitellar tenderness.
- Early radiographs show an irregular capitellum followed by radiolucent areas—normal capitellum develops by 1–2 years.
- Treatment symptomatic (rest, analgesia, physiotherapy, surgery if unstable/loose fragment → arthroscopy, fixation, microfacture, OATS) (see ⊃ Chapter 15, Osteochondritis dissecans of the knee, pp. 487–488).

Köhler's disease (navicular)
- Presents with pain on dorsomedial foot (bilateral in 25% of cases).
- Peak incidence at 4–7 years.
- Examination reveals an antalgic gait and navicular tenderness.
- Treatment symptomatic (rest, analgesia, physiotherapy—if severe, may need period of immobilization).
- Usually resolves in 1–3 years.

Sever's disease (calcaneum)
- Causes heel pain exacerbated by exercise and ankle dorsiflexion (may be bilateral).
- Peak incidence in active children aged 10–15 years.
- Examination reveals calcaneal apophysis tenderness ± Achilles tightness.
- Self-limiting natural history.

- Treatment symptomatic—rest, ice, analgesia, protective heel cups, avoidance of repetitive exercises.

Scheuermann's disease (thoracolumbar spine)
(See ⮞ Chapter 22.)

Further reading

Dias JJ, Lunn P. Ten questions on Kienböck's disease of the lunate. *Journal of Hand Surgery (European Volume)*. 2010;**35**(7):538–43.

Disorders of osteoid

Osteogenesis imperfecta

A rare hereditary deficiency in type I collagen synthesis caused by *COL1A1/COL1A2* mutations. Characterized by ↑ bone fragility secondary to insufficient osteoid production by osteoblasts. Incidence of 1/15,000–1/20,000 live births (may be underestimated due to milder forms evading diagnosis). Histology shows ↑ Haversian canal and osteocyte lacunae diameter, but ↓ trabeculae and cortical thickness.

Musculoskeletal features

- Fragility fractures (heal normally but do not remodel).
- Ligamentous laxity.
- Short stature.
- Coxa vara.
- Long bone bowing.
- Scoliosis and codfish vertebrae (compression fractures).
- Basilar invagination (ataxia, myelopathy, apnoea, low GCS).
- Olecranon apophyseal fractures.
- Congenital radial head dislocations.

Non-orthopaedic manifestations

- Blue sclerae.
- Dysmorphic facies.
- Deafness.
- Dentinogenesis imperfecta.
- Cardiac pathology (mitral valve disease/aortic regurgitation).

Investigations

- *Radiographs:* generalized osteopenia, thin cortices, multiple fractures of different ages, bowing of long bones ('saber shins').
- *Genetic testing:* diagnostic.

Management

- MDT management (paediatrics, genetics, orthopaedics).
- Must rule out NAI.
- Bisphosphonates.
- Activity modification (protect from future fractures).
- Immobilize and treat acute fractures like for normal bone.
- Multiple long bone fractures may benefit from prophylactic intramedullary fixation.

Paget's disease

Metabolic disease characterized by abnormal bone remodelling. Primary abnormality is osteoclastic overactivity. This results in secondary osteoblastic overproduction of woven bone, which is prone to pathological fracture. Peak incidence in Caucasians in fifth decade.

Three phases (aide-memoire 'LAB': Lytic, Active, Burnt out) include:

- *Lytic* (intense osteoclastic resorption)
- *Mixed* (resorption and compensatory bone formation)—'*active*'
- *Sclerotic* or '*burnt-out*' phase (dense bone formation).

Clinical features

Asymptomatic in most people.
- Bone pain (during active phase of disease).
- Degenerative joint disease.
- Long bone bowing.
- Cranial nerve compression from enlarged skull bones.
- Small (1%) risk of sarcomatous change—beware of ↑ pain/rapid radiological progression.

Investigations
- *Radiographs*: bony expansion with coarse trabeculae. Lytic and/or sclerotic appearance, depending on phase.
- *Bone scan*: useful to determine disease phase and whether disease is monostotic or polyostotic. ↑ uptake unless burnt-out phase.
- *Bloods*: raised ALP levels characteristic, normal calcium levels.
- *Urine*: raised urine hydroxyproline.

Management
- *Analgesia*.
- *Physiotherapy* (maintain ROM/strength).
- *Bisphosphonates* (inhibit osteoclastic activity).
- *Arthroplasty*: for established degenerative disease. Perform during cold phase. Beware of ↑ risk of bleeding, fracture, malalignment, and high-output cardiac failure.

Osteoporosis

Age-related ↓ in bone density (i.e. quantitative reduction in bone mass). Histology shows thin trabeculae, ↓ osteon size, and enlarged marrow spaces. Associated with low-energy fragility fractures, classically affecting the distal radius, vertebrae, and hips.

Risk factors
- ♀ gender (♂:♀ ratio 1:4).
- Race (highest incidence among Caucasians).
- Low BMI.
- Poor mobility.
- Poor dietary intake of calcium and vitamin D.
- Endocrine disorders (hypothyroidism, steroid use, Cushing's syndrome).
- Smoking.
- Alcohol excess.

Investigations
- *DEXA scan*: used to calculate a patient's T- and Z-scores.
  - *T-score*: number of standard deviations of a patient's bone density away from the bone density of a sex- and race-matched 30-year old (peak bone mass)
  - *Z-score*: number of standard deviations of a patient's bone density from the bone density of an age-, sex-, and race-matched. A Z-score of <2.5 is diagnostic of osteoporosis.

Management
- Lifestyle and dietary advice for all.
- Calcium and vitamin D supplements.

- *Fracture risk assessment tool (FRAX®):* used to calculate 10-year risk of major osteoporosis-related fracture. Determines need for pharmacological agents in borderline cases.
- Bisphosphonates (alendronic acid, ibandronic acid, and risedronate sodium)—inhibit osteoclastic activity.
- Denosumab (second line).
- Raloxifene (selective oestrogen receptor modulator—secondary prevention).
- Teriparatide (recombinant human PTH—secondary prevention).

Further reading

National Osteoporosis Guideline Group (2017). Available from: ℘ www.sheffield.ac.uk/NOGG/

Sözen T, Özışık L, Başaran NÇ. An overview and management of osteoporosis. *European Journal of Rheumatology.* 2017;**4**(1):46.

Tu KN, Lie JD, Wan CK, et al. Osteoporosis: a review of treatment options. *Pharmacy and Therapeutics.* 2018;**43**(2):92.

Valenzuela EN, Pietschmann P. Epidemiology and pathology of Paget's disease of bone: a review. *Wiener Medizinische Wochenschrift.* 2017;**167**(1–2):2–8.

Van Dijk FS, Cobben JM, Kariminejad A, et al. Osteogenesis imperfecta: a review with clinical examples. *Molecular Syndromology.* 2011;**2**(1):1–20.

Disorders of cells

Hyperparathyroidism

↑ PTH that occurs in 0.1% of the population (commoner in women). PTH stimulates osteoclastic activity via osteoblastic release of RANK ligand. This leads to excessive bone resorption (cortical > cancellous) and resulting hypercalcaemia.

Clinical features

- Symptoms and signs related to hypercalcaemia:
  - Renal stones
  - Pancreatitis, peptic ulcer disease
  - Psychological disturbance
  - Proximal myopathy.

Investigations

- *Radiographs:* brown tumours (focal demineralization), osteopenia, deformity, fracture.
- *Bloods:* PTH, vitamin D, calcium, phosphate.

Classification and management

May be primary, secondary, or tertiary.

- Primary hyperparathyroidism:
  - Excessive PTH secretion from parathyroid adenoma/hyperplasia
  - *Management:* surgical parathyroidectomy.
- Secondary hyperparathyroidism:
  - Parathyroid hyperplasia due to sustained parathyroid gland stimulation from prolonged hypocalcaemia
  - PTH glands function appropriately, so serum calcium levels may be normal
  - *Management:* treat underlying cause of hypocalcaemia.
- Tertiary hyperparathyroidism:
  - Autonomous parathyroid adenoma develops following prolonged secondary hyperparathyroidism
  - PTH secreted regardless of serum calcium levels
  - *Management:* surgical parathyroidectomy.

Cushing's syndrome

A collection of signs and symptoms caused by excessive circulating glucocorticoid hormones.

Causes

- Iatrogenic steroid treatment (commonest).
- Pituitary adenoma producing excessive adrenocorticotrophic hormone (ACTH)—known as Cushing's disease.
- Adrenal adenoma (adrenal Cushing's).
- Ectopic ACTH production (paraneoplastic production of ACTH—most commonly lung cancer).

Clinical features

- Central obesity.
- Hyperglycaemia.
- Hypertension.

- Symptoms of diabetes (polydipsia, polyuria).
- Immunosuppression/recurrent infections.
- Psychological disturbance—euphoria/depression.
- Bone abnormalities—osteoporosis/AVN.
- Weakness/myopathy.
- Hirsutism.

Investigations
- *Bloods:* hyperglycaemia (cortisol is gluconeogenic), hypokalaemia (cortisol activates aldosterone receptors), high serum cortisol levels, serum ACTH (helps to localize causative pathology).
- *Urine cortisol:* 24h urine collection.
- *Low-dose dexamethasone suppression test:* use if ACTH high to differentiate pituitary from ectopic ACTH production.

Management
Treat primary cause:
- Stop/reduce exogenous steroid, if possible
- Surgical excision of adrenal, pituitary, or lung tumours
- Medical management: metyrapone and ketoconazole (cortisol synthesis inhibitors).

Acromegaly

A rare condition characterized by excessive growth hormone (GH) after growth plates have fused. Either found in isolation or in conjunction with other endocrine disorders (multiple endocrine neoplasia type 1, McCune–Albright syndrome). Most commonly caused by GH-producing pituitary adenomas (90% of cases). Results in overgrowth of organ systems, bones, joints, and soft tissues.

Clinical features
Large hands, feet, skull, jaw, nose, and tongue; headaches and bitemporal hemianopia (local tumour effects), diabetes mellitus, hypertension, OA, nerve compression syndromes (20–40%).

Investigations
- Oral glucose tolerance test.
- GH serum assay.
- MRI of the brain: assess for pituitary tumour.

Management
- Trans-sphenoidal resection of pituitary tumour.
- Somatostatin analogues (also known as GH-inhibiting hormones) or GH receptor antagonists for inoperable cases.

Mucopolysaccharidoses

A group of inherited lysosome storage disorders. Incomplete glycosaminoglycan breakdown products accumulate, causing dysfunction in multiple organs. Results in stunted growth caused by hydrolase enzyme deficiencies.
There are four main types, including:
- Hurler's syndrome
- Hunter's syndrome
- Sanfilippo's syndrome
- Morquio's syndrome.

Clinical features
- Proportionate dwarfism, carpal tunnel syndrome, C1/2 instability, hip dysplasia, abnormal epiphyses, genu valgum.

Investigations
- Urinary excretion of glycosaminoglycans.

Management
- No known cure. Medical treatment aimed at treating systemic complications and improving quality of life.

Disorders of mineralization

Bone mineralization is regulated by three hormones: vitamin D, PTH and calcitonin. These act primarily on three organs: bone (mineral reservoir), intestine (dietary mineral absorption), and kidney (mineral excretion). Disorders of any of these organs or of vitamin D, PTH, or calcitonin production can lead to abnormal bone mineralization.

Osteomalacia/rickets

Metabolic bone disorders resulting in defective osteoid mineralization. Termed 'qualitative' bone disorders (compared to osteoporosis, which is a 'quantitative' bone disorder). Osteomalacia and rickets are manifestations of the same pathological process. Rickets occurs in children with open physes, whereas osteomalacia occurs in adults with closed physes.

Causes
- Poor dietary intake of minerals.
- Inadequate gut absorption (malabsorption).
- Inadequate reabsorption or excessive mineral excretion from kidneys.
- Insufficient exposure to UV light (required for vitamin D activation).
- Drugs (phenytoin, steroids).
- Alcohol excess.
- Inherited forms (rickets):
  - Vitamin D-resistant rickets (known as familial hypophosphataemic rickets—impaired renal phosphate reabsorption)
  - Vitamin D-dependent rickets (inherited defects in vitamin D metabolic pathway)
  - Hypophosphatasia (see ➲ Chapter 12, [heading title], pp. 353–354).

Clinical features
- Weakness (proximal myopathy/waddling gait), generalized bone pain, fatigue, pathological fractures.
- Rickets: leg bowing, enlarged costochondral junctions (rachitic rosary), dental abnormalities, slowed growth, hypotonia.

Investigations
- *Bloods:* calcium, phosphate, ALP, and PTH.
- *Urine:* urinary calcium.
- *Radiographs:* osteopenia, Looser's zones (insufficiency fractures), widened and irregular growth plates (rickets), rugger jersey spine (osteosclerosis), metaphyseal flaring.

Management
- Predominantly non-operative. Revolves around vitamin D, calcium, and phosphorus supplements, and treatment of primary cause. Surgery reserved for severe deformities.

Hypophosphatasia

Autosomal recessive metabolic bone disease characterized by low ALP and inorganic phosphate levels. Results in failure of newly formed osteoid to mineralize in the growth plate's hypertrophic zone.

Clinical features
- Similar to rickets—bow legs, genu varum, slow growth, dental abnormalities.

Investigations
- *Bloods:* ↓ ALP.
- *Urine:* presence of phosphoethanolamine is diagnostic.
- *Radiographs:* physeal widening, deossification of bone adjacent to growth plate.

Management
- Analgesia.
- Enzyme replacement therapy (although no known cure).

Renal osteodystrophy

Impaired bone mineralization secondary to chronic renal disease. Renal disease results in insufficient metabolism of vitamin D into its active form. This leads to reduced intestinal calcium absorption, which stimulates secondary hyperparathyroidism and ↑ osteoclastic activity to release calcium from bone reservoirs. Hyperparathyroidism is also triggered by inadequate urinary phosphate excretion.

Clinical features
- Weakness, bone pain, pathological fractures, bony deformities, symptoms of hypocalcaemia (Trousseau's/Chvostek's signs).

Investigations
- *Bloods:* low calcium, high phosphate, high PTH.
- *Radiographs:* similar appearances to osteomalacia (see ➋ Chapter 12, [heading title], pp. 353–354).

Management
- Treatment of chronic renal failure.

Septic arthritis

- Septic arthritis (SA) is defined as joint inflammation secondary to an infectious aetiology. The causative organism is usually bacterial, although it may be fungal, viral, or mycobacterial. Surgical emergency due to irreversible chondrolytic effects of localized infection; early diagnosis and treatment are crucial. The synovium is highly vascularized and lacks a basement membrane, making it prone to infection via haematogenous seeding. SA may also follow a direct injury or contagious bacterial spread from adjacent osteomyelitis in bones with an intra-articular metaphysis (shoulder, elbow, hip, ankle).

Epidemiology

- Incidence 2–6/100,000.
- Commoner in children than adults. Peak incidence 2–3 years.
- ♂ > ♀.
- *Risk factors:* extremes of age (neonates/elderly), immunocompromised, prematurity, haemophilia, joint prostheses, recent joint surgery/injection, OA, RA.

Aetiology

Children

- Commonest organism *Staphylococcus aureus* (70% of paediatric/adult cases).
- Group B *Streptococcus*, *S. aureus*, *Neisseria gonorrhoeae*, and Gram-negative bacilli common in neonates.
- Consider *N. gonorrhoeae* in sexually active adolescents.
- *Salmonella* associated with sickle-cell disease.
- *Kingella kingae* commonest Gram-negative bacterial cause.
- Beware of fungal infections in immunosuppressed.
- Puncture wounds associated with *Pseudomonas aeruginosa*.
- The hip joint is most commonly affected in children.

Adults

- Commonest organism *S. aureus*.
- *Streptococcus pneumoniae* significant source of infection.
- Knee most commonly affected joint (followed by hip).

Presentation

- Classically acute-onset monoarticular joint pain (rarely polyarticular), fever (40–60% cases), swelling (effusion), warmth, reduced movement (severe pain with passive movement), sepsis, malaise.

Differential diagnosis

- Irritable hip (reactive arthritis).
- Overlying soft tissue pathology (bursitis, tendonitis, cellulitis).
- Crystal arthropathy (gout/pseudogout).
- Calcific tendonitis (shoulder).
- Inflammatory arthritis (RA, psoriatic, SLE).
- Perthes'/slipped upper femoral epiphyses (paediatric hip).
- Trauma.
- Bone/soft tissue tumour.
- Adjacent osteomyelitis.

Investigations

- *Bloods:* FBC, ESR, CRP, uric acid, blood cultures, clotting.
- *Radiographs:* widened joint space (effusion), chondrocalcinosis, periarticular erosions.
- *Joint aspiration:* gold standard. Send for urgent Gram staining and microscopy, as well as for culture and antibiotic sensitivities. Synovial fluid white cell count (WCC) >50,000; >90% neutrophils suggest bacterial pathogen.
- *MRI:* can identify adjacent osteomyelitis (should not delay treatment).
- *USS:* can identify effusions/intra-articular debris in deep joints.

Kocher criteria

Allows prediction of SA in children. Based on the presence of inability to weight-bear, ESR >40, fever >38.5°C, and WCC >12,000. Likelihood of SA of 3% if one of these is present, 40% if two are present, 93% if three are present, and 99% if all four are present. Elevated CRP (>20mg/L) was later added by Caird *et al.*, changing the likelihood of SA to 98% with all five present, 93% with four present, and 83% with three present.

Management

- Urgent drainage of involved joint. Paediatric cases managed surgically— mode of joint clearance in adults more controversial.
- Options include open or arthroscopic washout vs repeated needle aspiration. Repeated washouts may be required.
- Empirical IV antibiotics after joint cultures obtained (unless sepsis necessitating urgent treatment at presentation).
- Targeted antibiotics once cultures and sensitivities are available. Duration determined in conjunction with microbiology, based on clinical response (usually shorter than 2-week IV course followed by 2- to 4-week oral course).

Further reading

Caird MS, Flynn JM, Leung YL, Millman JE, Joann GD, Dormans JP. Factors distinguishing septic arthritis from transient synovitis of the hip in children: a prospective study. *Journal of Bone and Joint Surgery*. 2006;**88**(6):1251–7.

Colston J, Atkins B. Bone and joint infections. *Clinical Medicine (Lond)*. 2018;**18**(2):150–4.

Iliadis AD, Ramachandran M. Paediatric bone and joint infection. *EFORT Open Reviews*. 2017;**2**(1):7–12.

Kocher MS, Zurakowski D, Kasser JR. Differentiating between septic arthritis and transient synovitis of the hip in children: an evidence-based clinical prediction algorithm. *Journal of Bone and Joint Surgery (American Volume)*. 1999;**81**(12):1662–70.

Long B, Koyfman A, Gottlieb M. Evaluation and management of septic arthritis and its mimics in the emergency department. *Western Journal of Emergency Medicine*. 2019;**20**(2):331.

Osteomyelitis

Defined as inflammation of bone caused by an infectious agent. Histologically, localized infection and abscess formation classically lead to walled-off areas of infarcted bone (*sequestrum*) impervious to host immune system and antibiotics. Pus may result in periosteal elevation, leading to new bone formation (*involucrum*) or tracking through cortical defects (*cloaca*), and eventually forming a discharging *sinus*. Once a sinus develops, symptoms may improve transiently. However, unless any sequestrum are treated, the process will repeat, resulting in a cyclical pattern of worsening symptoms and resolution.

Classification

Waldvogel classification system
- Groups cases based on their mechanism of development and chronology.
- Mechanisms:
  - *Haematogenous:* bacteria transported to bone via circulation, generally single bacteria, 85% of patients aged <17 years
  - *Contiguous spread:* bacterial inoculation from adjacent focus, generally polymicrobial
  - *Direct inoculation:* usually secondary to trauma, 50% of adult cases; association with vascular insufficiency (particularly diabetic feet).
- Duration of infection:
  - *Acute:* initial episode of osteomyelitis
  - *Chronic:* recurrence of acute cases.

Cierny and Mader classification system
- Groups cases based on extent on bony involvement and patient (or host) status. Mainly developed for long bones (see ➲ Chapter 21, Osteomyelitis in Children, Fig. 21.18).
- Bony involvement:
  - *Medullary:* usually acute haematogenous spread
  - *Superficial:* infection restricted to cortical bone
  - *Localized:* cortex and medulla involved, but continuous segment of uninvolved bone remains; bone stability preserved
  - *Diffuse:* infection involving entire bone circumference.
- Host type:
  - Healthy
  - Local or systemic compromise (e.g. smoker, diabetes, extensive scarring, or poor vascularity)
  - Severe compromise or treatment worse than disease.

Presentation

- Pain (continuous, often nocturnal), fever, malaise, localized warmth/ erythema (acute > chronic), swelling, discharging sinus.

NB beware of Marjolin's ulcers (cutaneous squamous cell carcinoma at site of chronic inflammation).

Investigations

- *Bloods:* FBC, ESR, CRP, serum IL-6, blood cultures.
- *Radiographs:* often normal in first 2 weeks of acute cases. Later may show sequestrum, involucrum, cloaca, or a lamellar periosteal reaction. Metalwork may also show signs of loosening.
- *CT:* useful to identify bony anatomy (sequestra) for surgical planning.
- *MRI:* the most useful modality for osteomyelitis. High specificity and useful for delineating soft tissue and bony involvement.
- *USS:* may be of use in younger patients to avoid sedation/anaesthesia required for MRI. Can identify soft tissue oedema, periosteal thickening, and subperiosteal collections.
- *Image-guided/open bone biopsy:* send for microbiology and histology if diagnostic doubt. Key to guiding antibiotic therapy. Ideally, any antibiotics should be stopped >2 weeks before sampling, and >3 samples sent.

Management

Antibiotics

Empirical antibiotics should be started after tissue samples are collected for microbiology in non-septic patients. *S. aureus* should be covered by initial antibiotics. Regime will be altered as culture results return.

Haematogenous osteomyelitis

- Majority of cases successfully managed with appropriate antibiotics.
- Routine surgical exploration not recommended.
- Surgery reserved for cases not responding to medical treatment (abscess no longer an absolute indication).
- No clear guidelines on length or route of administration of antibiotics—should be based on clinical response/bloods.

Acute post-traumatic osteomyelitis

- Acute infections should be treated with extensive surgical debridement and appropriate antibiotics.
- The key factor for successful treatment is quality of debridement. Copious wash with saline is essential to reduce bacterial load (3–9L).
- Antibiotic therapy usually lasts 4–6 weeks but can be tailored to patient response.
- Repeated washouts and removal/revision of metalwork ± external fixation may be required in refractory cases.

Chronic osteomyelitis

- In cases of chronic osteomyelitis, a choice between palliative suppressive antibiotics and curative surgery must be made.
- Suppressive antibiotics may be used to control symptoms when surgical treatment is contraindicated or would result in too high morbidity (type IV disease in type B/C host).
- The principles of curative surgical treatment are:
  - *Debridement/excision:* all sinuses must be excised, and the diseased segment fully exposed. Dead tissue should be resected with an almost oncological approach.
  - *Irrigation:* copious amounts—volume of irrigation used proportional to bacterial load removed.

- *Stabilizing bone:* if significant amounts of bone removed, fixation may be required (usually external fixation/circular frame).
- *Dead space management:* dead spaces should be filled to avoid large haematomas, which act as a culture medium for bacteria. Antibiotic-loaded cement, muscle flaps, or bone transportation, or a combination, are all options.
- *Post-operative antibiotics:* tailored to pathogen and patient response.

Even with optimal treatment, infection can recur, sometimes many years after treatment.

Further reading

Cierny G, Mader J, Penninck J. A clinical staging system for adult osteomyelitis. *Contemporary Orthopaedics.* 1985;**10**:17–37.

Waldvogel FA, Medoff G, Swartz MN. Osteomyelitis: a review of clinical features, therapeutic considerations and unusual aspects. *New England Journal of Medicine.* 1970;**282**(4):198–206.

Primary malignant bone tumours—principles

Primary malignant bone tumours arrising from connective tissue cell lines are rare and should be managed in specialist centres by MDTs. Appropriate imaging and biopsy are essential to accurately diagnose and stage a bone sarcoma, *before* the optimal treatment can be determined.

The commonest malignant bone lesions are skeletal metastases from breast, prostate, lung and kidney primaries (in order of most common to least common). More uncommon primary sources can be thyroid, melanoma and myeloma.

Presentation
- Pain.
- Bony lump.
- Pathological fracture.
- Incidental finding.

Investigations
- *Bloods:* FBC, ESR, CRP, bone profile, calcium, phosphate, LFTs, clotting profile, thyroid function tests (TFTs), prostate-specific antigen (PSA), serum free light chains and protein electrophoresis (myeloma).
- *Urine:* Bence-Jones protein (myeloma).

Local imaging
- *Plain radiograph (whole bone):*
  - Patient age (key to differential diagnoses)
  - Site of lesion (which bone; epiphysis, metaphysis, or diaphysis; central or eccentric)
  - Lesion appearance (sclerotic, lytic, or mixed)
  - Number of lesions
  - Lesion matrix (contents)—osteoid, chondroid, or fibrous
  - Lesion margins (zone of transition)—wide (aggressive) or narrow (benign)
  - Periosteal reaction (benign or aggressive)
  - Soft tissue mass present.
- *MRI (whole bone):*
  - Determines intra- and extraosseous spread of lesion
  - Identifies skip lesions or soft tissue masses in aggressive lesions.
- *CT:*
  - Identifies bony anatomy in most detail
  - Diagnostic for certain tumours (osteoid osteoma).

Distant imaging (if malignancy suspected)
- *Radioisotope bone scan:* multiple bony lesions.
- *CXR/CT chest ± abdomen/pelvis:* visceral metastases.
- *Whole-body MRI:* metastases.

Tissue diagnosis
- Required when malignancy remains a differential diagnosis after appropriate imaging.
- Provides histological diagnosis and tumour grade for prognostication.
- Should be performed in a specialist centre with experience in management of malignant bone tumours.

Principles of biopsy

(See ⬎ Chapter 2.)

Management principles

Benign primary bone tumour
- Treatment dependent on lesion histology and characteristics.
- Some tumours' natural history one of resolution–observe if asymptomatic.
- Symptomatic tumours at risk of pathological fracture may need more invasive treatment. This may involve excision ± stabilization, curettage ± bone graft or radiofrequency ablation.

Malignant primary bone tumours
- Curative treatment revolves around en bloc resection of tumour with an adequate margin of uninvolved tissue. Depending on tumour type, this should be combined with neoadjuvant and/or adjuvant chemotherapy ± radiotherapy.
- Primary aim of treatment is patient survival, followed by limb salvage.
- If tumour resection with adequate margins is not possible due to tumour size or key neurovascular structure involvement, amputation should be considered.

Further reading

British Orthopaedic Oncology Society. Available from: ℘ https://boos.org.uk/services/educational-resources

Primary bone tumours (bone-forming)

Osteosarcoma

An aggressive, malignant tumour most commonly found in rapidly developing metaphyseal bone around the knee or proximal humerus. Follows a bimodal age distribution—peaks in skeletally immature (caused by rapid growth) and during sixth decade (secondary cases of osteosarcoma (OS)).

Classification

- Subcategorized based on clinical, radiographic, and histological features.

Primary osteosarcoma
- *De novo* disease process of bone.
- *Intramedullary subtypes* (95% of overall cases, usually high grade):
  - *Conventional OS:* commonest (80% of cases). Subcategorized based on extracellular matrix produced (osteoblastic/chondroblastic/fibroblastic). Radiographs show sclerotic, destructive lesion breaching the cortex, creating 'Codman's triangle'/'sunburst' periosteal reaction
  - *Telangiectatic OS:* radiographs show eccentric, osteolytic lesion expanding or disrupting the cortex. Similar radiological appearances to aneurysmal bone cyst
  - *Low-grade intramedullary OS:* patients usually in third or fourth decade. Radiographs show relatively benign lesion.
  - *Small cell:* radiographs similar to conventional OS.
- *Surface subtypes* (5% of cases, low grade):
  - *Parosteal OS:* found on surface of long bones. Usually slow-growing. Radiographs show ossified lesion, classically on posterior distal metaphysis of distal femur. Medullary canal spared
  - *Periosteal OS:* more aggressive than parosteal variant. Radiographic appearances similar to parosteal OS, although sunburst/Codman periosteal reaction may be seen
  - *High-grade surface OS:* radiographs show surface lesion with tumour extension into the surrounding soft tissues and cortical disruption often present.

Secondary osteosarcoma
- Paget's/radiation-associated sarcoma—poor prognosis.

Investigations

- *Bloods:* ALP and lactate dehydrogenase (LDH)—reflect osteoblastic and osteoclastic activity, respectively. Poor prognosis if elevated.
- *Radiographs (whole bone):* two orthogonal views.
- *MRI (whole bone):* soft tissue extent and marrow invasion/skip lesions.
- *CT chest:* pulmonary metastases.
- *Technetium bone scan:* bone metastases.
- *PET-CT/whole-body MRI:* evolving roles for disease extent.

Management principles
- Should be managed by MDT experienced in primary bone tumours.
- Curative treatment consists of neoadjuvant chemotherapy and surgical resection of tumour, followed by further adjuvant chemotherapy.
- Mifamurtide—synthetic analogue of mycobacterial cell wall; triggers patient immune cells to target cancer cells via TNF and IL release.

Osteoid osteoma

Benign bone tumour <1.5cm in size. Can occur in any bone, although most commonly found in long bones. Usually diagnosed in second decade of life, most commonly in men (♂:♀ ratio 3:1).

Presentation
- Pain, particularly at night. Classically relieved by NSAIDs.
- Antalgic gait (if lower limb involved).
- Scoliosis (if spine involved).

Investigations
- *Radiographs:* well-defined lytic lesion containing a dense sclerotic central nidus.
- *CT (fine-cut):* confirms diagnosis.

Management
- *Analgesia:* symptoms classically improved with NSAIDs/aspirin.
- *CT-guided radiofrequency ablation:* less invasive than surgery, but often no tissue subsequently available to confirm diagnosis.
- *Surgical excision:* for lesions adjacent to key neurovascular structures (contraindicating ablation).

Osteoblastoma

Rare, benign bone tumour. Similar histological and radiological appearances to osteoid osteoma, although larger, more locally aggressive, and commoner in the axial skeleton. Unlike osteoid osteoma, patients' pain is also not usually worse at night and is less likely to be helped by NSAIDs.

Management

Analgesia. Surgery involves intralesional curettage or en bloc resection. Allows histology to be confirmed, aims to reduce recurrence rates, and eliminates any ongoing structural destruction of bony architecture.

Primary bone tumours (cartilage-forming)

Chondrosarcoma

A diverse group of malignant cartilaginous tumours with variable degrees of malignancy. Peak incidence in patients aged 40–75 years where they present as pain, a mass, or a pathological fracture. Most commonly occur in the pelvis and proximal limbs.

Classification

Chondrosarcomas (CS) categorized as primary (develop *de novo* in bone) or secondary (arise from benign cartilaginous lesion).

Primary chondrosarcoma (90%)
Subclassified as central or peripheral:
- *Central CS* (four subtypes):
  - Conventional CS: commonest (85–90% cases); subclassified according to grade (low/high grade)
  - Dedifferentiated CS: highly aggressive, 5-year survival <10%
  - Clear cell CS (epiphyseal)
  - Mesenchymal CS.
- *Peripheral CS:*
  - Periosteal CS.

Secondary (10%)
- *Osteochondroma (OC)* (<1% risk of malignant transformation):
  - Hereditary multiple exostoses (HME) (1–10% risk of transformation).
- *Enchondromas* (1% risk of transformation)—higher risk of malignant transformation in Ollier disease and Maffucci syndrome.

Investigations

- *Radiographs (whole bone):* cartilaginous lytic or blastic lesion. Low-grade CS—similar appearances to enchondroma with cortical thickening and endosteal erosion. High-grade CS have a permeative or moth-eaten appearance, with cortical destruction ± soft tissue extension. Intralesional mineralization may be seen (characteristic 'popcorn' or 'rings and arcs' calcification).
- *MRI (whole bone):* soft tissue and marrow involvement/skip lesions.
- *CT (local):* bone/cortical involvement.
- *CT chest:* pulmonary metastases.
- *Technetium bone scan:* bone metastases.
- *Whole-body MRI:* increasingly used for bone staging.

Management

Should be managed by MDT experienced in primary bone tumours.
- *Intralesional curettage:* low-grade CS in limbs.
- *Wide surgical excision:* mainstay of surgical treatment.
- *Oncological therapies:* chemotherapy generally reserved for a small number of high-grade tumours. Radiotherapy used following certain incomplete resections or as a definitive treatment for unresectable cases.

Osteochondroma (exostosis)

The commonest bone tumour incidentally identified in 1–2% of patients. Contains cortical and medullary components with narrow (pedunculated) or broad-based (sessile) stalks. Generally grow away from the joint. Stop growing after skeletal maturity (in the absence of malignant transformation). Present as solitary (85% of cases) or multiple lesions:

- *Solitary OCs:* a developmental abnormality that occurs when a fragment of the growth plate herniates through the periosteum. This fragment continues to grow, resulting in a metaphyseal cartilage-capped lesion. Can occur spontaneously (primary OC) or following radiation exposure/trauma (secondary OC).
- *Multiple OCs:* found in a syndrome called hereditary multiple exostosis.

Presentation

Commonly noted as a hard lump. Occasionally an incidental radiological finding. Pain and fractures are possible. Can occur in any bone that develops by endochondral ossification. Most commonly found in long bones (50%) (particularly around the knee), or the scapula or pelvis. Patients with solitary OCs usually present before the age of 40. Those with multiple lesions usually present during childhood, due to accompanying bony deformities.

Complications

- Local soft tissue irritation/bursitis.
- Neurovascular compression.
- 'Pathological' fracture—usually through stalk of pedunculated OC.

Malignant transformation

- Solitary OCs 1%; HME 5%.
- Beware of OC growth after skeletal maturity—cartilage cap thickening may indicate transformation; if >2cm, should be further investigated.
- Usually differentiates to low-grade CS.

NB the cartilage cap may undergo thickening in the absence of malignancy in skeletally immature patients during growth.

Investigations

- *Radiographs:* often diagnostic.
- *MRI:* to assess cartilage cap size/identify neurovascular compression.
- *USS:* to assess cartilage cap in children.
- *CT:* useful to characterize flat bone OCs (e.g. scapula /pelvic).

Management

- *Observation:* asymptomatic OC without suspicious features.
- *Surgical excision:*
  - Large, symptomatic lesions
  - Lesions with suspicious radiological or clinical features (large cartilage cap/growth in skeletally mature patient)
  - 2% recurrence rate.

Hereditary multiple exostoses/familial osteochondromatosis (diaphyseal aclasis)

- Autosomal dominant condition resulting in multiple OCs.
- Characterized by loss-of-function mutations in tumour suppressor genes *EXT1* and *EXT2* (inherited in 70% of cases, spontaneous in 30%).
- Usually present earlier than solitary OCs due to association with multiple other bony deformities, including leg length discrepancy, bowing, coxa valgus, genu valgus, and short stature.
- Higher risk of malignant transformation than solitary OCs—around 5%.
- Surgical intervention much commoner in HME than in solitary OCs— patients undergo an average of >5 surgical procedures.

Further reading

Czajka CM, DiCaprio MR. What is the proportion of patients with multiple hereditary exostoses who undergo malignant degeneration? *Clinical Orthopaedics and Related Research.* 2015;**473**(7):2355–61.

Hakim DN, Myutan Kulendran TP, Caris JA. Benign tumours of the bone: a review. *Journal of Bone Oncology.* 2015;**4**(2):37–41.

Enchondroma

Commonest intraosseous chondroma. Develop in childhood from islands of proliferating chondrocytes and growth plate cartilage. Associated with somatic mutations in the isocitrate dehydrogenase genes *IDH1* and *IDH2*. Usually solitary, although multiple enchondromas (known as enchondromatosis) are seen in Ollier disease and Maffucci syndrome.

Presentation

Usually an incidental radiological finding. Pain and pathological fracture not uncommon. Usually found in the metaphysis/diaphysis of bones formed by endochondral ossification. Commonest in hands and feet. Solitary enchondromas usually present in the second decade of life. Enchondromatosis presents earlier, usually before the age of 10.

Investigations

- *Radiographs:* well-defined lytic defects, with varying amounts of intralesional calcification. Larger lesions can cause endosteal scalloping and cortical expansion/thinning.
- *MRI:* identifies any features of malignancy, including cortical disruption or soft tissue expansion.
- *CT:* assesses cortical bone involvement/identifies pathological fracture.

NB despite appropriate imaging and even biopsy, it is often difficult to distinguish a benign enchondroma from an atypical cartilaginous tumour (ACT) like a low-grade CS.

Complications

- Pathological fracture.
- Malignant transformation: 1% risk in solitary lesions, higher in enchondromatosis. Painful, large lesions or those with significant cortical thinning or an associated soft tissue mass warrant further investigation.

Management

- *Observation:* asymptomatic lesions, with no concerning radiographic features.
- *Operative:* symptomatic or suspicious lesions. Usually involves curettage with bone grafting or cementation to fill defects; 10-year recurrence rate of around 0.04%.

Enchondromatosis syndromes

Ollier disease

- A rare syndrome (1 in 100,000) characterized by enchondromatosis.
- Enchondromas may be accompanied by bone shortening, bowing, or metaphyseal widening.
- Whole-body MRI may be useful in determining the extent of lesions.
- ↑ risk of malignant transformation. Reported incidence highly variable in the literature (5–40%). ↑ risk of malignancy elsewhere, including gliomas and acute myeloid leukaemia.

Maffucci syndrome

- Multiple enchondromas associated with soft tissue haemangiomas, vascular malformations, and bony deformities.
- Radiographs show enchondromatosis and phleboliths (chronic calcified venous thrombus that develop in cavernous haemangioma).
- Highest risk of malignant transformation—associated with a high number of malignancies, including pancreatic and hepatic adenocarcinoma, ovarian tumour, glioma, astrocytoma, and various sarcomas.

Further reading

Hakim DN, Myutan Kulendran TP, Caris JA. Benign tumours of the bone: a review. *Journal of Bone Oncology*. 2015;**4**(2):37–41.

Verdegaal SHM, Bovee JVMG, Pansuriya TC, *et al*. Incidence, predictive factors, and prognosis of chondrosarcoma in patients with Ollier disease and Maffucci syndrome: an international multicenter study of 161 patients. *Oncologist*. 2011;**16**(12):1771–9.

Ewing sarcoma

A highly malignant tumour composed of small round cells of neurogenic origin. Metastases present in 34% of cases at presentation, most commonly to the lungs, bone marrow, and other bones. Associated with t(11:22) translocation (95% of cases), which leads to production of the chimeric protein EWS–FLI1. Differential diagnoses include other small round tumours, including neuroblastoma, leukaemia, eosinophilic granuloma, lymphoma, and myeloma.

Presentation

Pain and swelling over the site of the sarcoma are noted. Systemic features of pyrexia and weight loss are common. Pathological fracture can occur from either the primary tumour or metastases. Median age at diagnosis of 15 years. Found in the pelvis, ribs, distal femur, proximal tibia, femoral diaphysis, and proximal humerus.

Investigations

- *Radiographs (whole bone):* permeative, moth-eaten lesion. Aggressive 'onion skin' or 'sunburst' periosteal reaction.
- *MRI (whole bone):* soft tissue mass (common)/skip lesions.
- *CT (local):* bone/cortical involvement.
- *CT chest:* pulmonary metastases.
- *Technetium bone scan:* bone metastases/high uptake in primary lesion.
- *Bloods:* anaemia, leucocytosis, raised ALP and LDH (poor prognosis), raised ESR/CRP.
- *Bone marrow biopsy:* to rule out bone marrow metastases.
- *Biopsy molecular analysis:* immunohistochemical identification of surface glycoprotein CD99/confirmation of Ewing sarcoma-associated translocation.

Management

Must be managed by MDT experienced in primary bone tumours—National Ewing Sarcoma MDT in the UK.
- *Chemotherapy:* part of standard treatment for Ewing sarcoma. Usually includes neoadjuvant and post-operative adjuvant treatment.
- *Radiotherapy:* also central to Ewing sarcoma management. May be used as definitive management (in sites where morbidity of resection is excessive, e.g. pelvis) or in combination with surgery.
- *Operative:* should include wide excision of all anatomical structures involved in pre-chemotherapy tumour volume when feasible.

Further reading

Ozaki T. Diagnosis and treatment of Ewing sarcoma of the bone: a review article. *Journal of Orthopaedic Science.* 2015;**20**(2):250–63.

Giant cell tumour of bone

Giant cell tumours (GCTs) of bone are locally aggressive primary bone tumours. Although they are generally considered benign, they have a low risk of metastasis, particularly after local recurrence. Histologically, GCTs consist of giant multinucleated cells with osteoclast-like function.

Presentation

Pain and pathological fracture. Most commonly seen around the knee (50% of cases) or in the sacrum/vertebrae. Peak presentation at 20–40 years.

Investigations

• *Radiographs:* lytic lesion usually located in the epiphysis. Juxta-articular lesions may extend up to the subchondral region. Surrounding cortices may be expanded, thinned, or breached in large lesions.
• *MRI:* tumour extension and periosteal reaction.
• *CT:* to assess bone cortices in detail.

NB GCTs are one of the few non-infective bone lesions found in the epiphysis. Others include chondroblastoma, clear cell CS, and aneursmal bone cysts.

Management

Operative treatment

• Typically involves curettage plus cryotherapy/phenol ablation to reduce local recurrence rates. The resulting defect may be packed with bone graft or cement to provide structural support.
• Large, recurrent tumours may need wider excision and joint replacement.

Non-operative treatment

• *Denosumab:* a monoclonal antibody that inhibits the osteoclastic activity of GCTs.

Further reading

Hakim DN, Myutan Kulendran TP, Caris JA. Benign tumours of the bone: a review. *Journal of Bone Oncology.* 2015;**4**(2):37–41.

Multiple myeloma

Multiple myeloma (MM) is a lymphoproliferative disease characterized by proliferation of plasma cells. This proliferation leads to replacement of the patient's physiological marrow, resulting in anaemia, leucocytosis, and thrombocytopenia. Eventually, lytic bone lesions develop weakening bone.

Presentation

- Pain (commonest).
- Pathological fracture (>50% of cases).
- Spinal cord or nerve root compression.
- Hypercalcaemia.
- Renal failure.
- Symptoms of bone marrow insufficiency (*anaemia*: fatigue; *leucocytosis*: infection; *thrombocytopenia*: bleeding).
- Median age at diagnosis 69 years.
- Bone lesions may involve flat (skull, spine, pelvis, ribs, and sternum) or long (proximal humerus and femur) bones.

Investigations

- *Radiographs:* 'punched-out' lytic lesions with classical 'moth-eaten' appearance.
- *CT:* more sensitive than radiographs at identifying bony lesions.
- *MRI:* to assess marrow infiltration, vertebral lesions, and neural elements.
- *Bloods:* low Hb/WCC/platelets, raised calcium/ESR/CRP. Serum free light chains.
- *Serum electrophoresis:* raised immunoglobulin protein (M protein).
- *Urine:* Bence-Jones protein (monoclonal light chain).

Management

Non-operative

- 'Non-intensive' or 'intensive' approach. 'Intensive' treatment involves higher drug doses and stem cell transplant.
- Drugs, including chemotherapy, steroids, and thalidomide or bortezomib.
- Radiotherapy may also be used to control local disease.

Operative

- *General indications:* impending/existing pathological fracture, spinal instability, spinal cord/nerve root compression, or intractable pain.
- *Aims:* to alleviate pain, restore mobility, and improve quality of life.

Further reading

The Surgeon's Committee of the Chinese Myeloma Working Group of the International Myeloma Foundation. Consensus on surgical management of myeloma bone disease. *Orthopedic Surgery.* 2016;**8**(3):263–9.

Metastatic bone disease

Metastases are the commonest malignant bone lesions identified in the adult population. Metastatic bone disease (MBD) may develop in two-thirds of cancer patients and is ↑ in incidence. Skeletal metastases most commonly arise from the breast, lung, prostate, kidney, and thyroid primaries. Malignant cells trigger osteoclastic activity, resulting in bone resorption and marrow replacement by fibrous tissue and cancer cells. This weakens the bone, causing pain and an ↑ risk of fracture.

Presentation

- Pain (constant, worse with weight-bearing).
- Pathological fracture.
- Hypercalcaemia.
- Spinal cord compression/back pain (vertebral MBD).

Investigations

- *Bloods:* FBC, U&Es, LFTs, bone profile, ESR/PV, CRP, and tumour markers (if primary unknown). Serum free light chains (to rule out myeloma).
- *Radiographs (whole bone):* often the first modality used but can miss small lesions. Metastases may be sclerotic, lytic, or mixed.
- *Local CT/MRI:* CT to define bone loss; MRI to identify marrow involvement and tumour extension.
- *Technetium bone scan:* ↑ uptake due to ↑ osteoblastic activity. Myeloma is the exception (cold on bone scans).
- *CT chest, abdomen, and pelvis:* to identify primary.
- *Angiography:* preoperative embolization (renal primaries).

Management

The aim of MBD surgery is to relieve pain, and maintain or restore function. The general principles include the following:

- A primary bone tumour must be excluded. A biopsy may be required for solitary lesions.
- Surgical constructs should allow immediate weight-bearing.
- It should be assumed that pathological fractures will not heal.
- Surgical fixations should last the patient's lifetime.
- All lesions in the affected bone should ideally be stabilized.
- Prophylactic fixation of long bone metastases is preferential to fixation of a pathological fracture.
- Radiotherapy should be used in all cases except en bloc resection to reduce recurrence.
- Samples should be sent for histological analysis during surgery.
- *Appendicular skeleton surgery*—general options are to:
  - Either support the affected bone with intramedullary nail or plate and screws augmented with cement; or
  - Resect metastases and reconstruct by using arthroplasty, endoprosthetic surgery, or rarely amputation
  - Endoprosthetic replacement for extensive bone destruction (usually renal primary) or tumours with good prognosis (long latency from primary).

Table 12.2 Mirel's scoring system

Variable/score	1	2	3
Site	Upper limb	Lower limb	Peritrochanteric
Pain	Mild	Moderate	Severe
Lesion	Blastic	Mixed	Lytic
Size*	<1/3	1/3–2/3	>2/3

* As seen on plain radiographs, maximum destruction of the cortex involved in any view.

Total score: 7 = 5% fracture risk; 8 = 15% fracture risk; 9 = 33% fracture risk.

- *Pelvic/acetabular surgery*—general principles are to:
  - Debulk as much tumour as possible
  - Fill or structurally bypass defects to create a durable hip joint for weight-bearing.
- *Spinal surgery*—objectives include:
  - Decompression of neural elements (preventing further neurological deficit)
  - Restoration of spinal stability
  - Decompression and stabilization, both of which are generally required.

Mirels scoring system

Mirels' system was devised to predict pathological fractures in long bone metastases (Table 12.2). It helps to guide when prophylactic fixation should be considered. A lesion's maximum possible score is 12. Prophylactic fixation should be considered if a lesion scores 9 or more.

Management

Includes bisphosphonates, denosumab, chemotherapy, hormone therapies, molecular agents, radiotherapy, radiofrequency ablation, and cementoplasty.

Follow-up

The prognosis of MBD patients continues to improve and survival of >5 years is not uncommon. Patients should be followed up for disease progression and fixation failure while they remain symptomatic.

Further reading

British Orthopaedic Oncology Society and British Orthopaedic Association (2015). *Metastatic bone disease: a guide to good practice*. Available from: ℘ https://www.boa.ac.uk/resource/boast-management-of-metastatic-bone-disease.html

D'Oronzo S, Coleman R, Brown J, Silvestris F. Metastatic bone disease: pathogenesis and therapeutic options: update on bone metastasis management. *Journal of Bone Oncology*. 2018;**15**:004–4.

Mirels H. Metastatic disease in long bones. A proposed scoring system for diagnosing impending pathologic fractures. *Clinical Orthopaedics and Related Research*. 1989;249:256–64.

Soft tissue tumours—principles

Benign soft tissue tumours are common and can generally be managed conservatively. In contrast, primary malignant soft tissue tumours (soft tissue sarcomas (STS)) are rare and need aggressive treatment. This should be done in a specialist centre by an MDT. Caution is needed to avoid mistaking an STS for a benign lesion and managing it inappropriately. An inadvertent STS resection in such a scenario (a 'whoops' procedure) will directly worsen the prognosis.

Presentation
- Lump (± pain/tenderness).
- Distal neurovascular deficit (rare in benign tumours).
- Overlying skin changes (ulceration /erythema/warmth/punctum).

Clinical red flags warranting further investigations
- Size >4cm.
- Pain.
- ↑ size.
- Location deep to deep fascia.
- Recurrence following previous tumour resection.

Investigations
- *Bloods:* FBC, ESR, CRP, clotting profile.

Local imaging
- *USS:*
  - The most commonly used modality (ready available, cheap, can accurately identify lipomata)
  - Can record tumour size, homogeneity, vascularity, and depth.
- *MRI:*
  - Provides most accurate description of tumour size, location, margins, and infiltration into adjacent tissues (including neurovascular structures).

NB appropriate imaging modalities ± biopsy in any equivocal cases is essential to make an accurate diagnosis, stage any malignant tumours, and guide appropriate treatment.

Distant imaging (if malignancy suspected)
- *CT chest ± abdomen/pelvis:* visceral metastases (most commonly in the lung in STS).
- *Whole-body MRI:* soft tissue metastases in certain STS subtypes.
- *PET-CT:* to characterize indeterminate pulmonary lesions during staging.

Tissue diagnosis
- Image-guided (usually USS) biopsy required when diagnosis unclear after appropriate imaging.
- Should be undertaken after discussion with an MDT experienced in management of STS.
- Principles of biopsy should be adhered to (see ⊃ Chapter 2).
- Excision biopsy may be suitable for small, superficial, indeterminate lesions after discussion with appropriate MDT.

Management principles

Benign primary soft tissue tumours
- The majority of asymptomatic benign soft tissue tumours can be treated conservatively. This includes lipomata—the commonest soft tissue tumour.
- Pain, enlarging lesions, or neurovascular symptoms due to local compression may necessitate surgery.

Malignant primary soft tissue tumours
- The keystone of curative treatment for STS is planned resection with (neo)adjuvant radiotherapy (see ➜ Soft tissue sarcomas, pp. 376–377 for more detail).
- STS are generally resistant to chemotherapy, with the exception of a few subtypes (synovial sarcoma, rhabdomyosarcoma)—therefore, chemotherapy generally reserved for metastatic disease.
- Isolated metastases or oligometastatic disease may be suitable for excision or radiofrequency ablation.
- Isolated limb perfusion may be used in cases of locally advanced extremity STS.

Soft tissue sarcomas

STS are rare primary malignant soft tissue tumours that are derived from mesenchymal stem cells. Although there are over 50 different histological STS subtypes, they still only make up <1% of all new cancer diagnoses. They can occur at almost any anatomical site and affect patients of any age, and are much rarer than benign soft tissue tumours (ratio 1:100). This makes a high index of suspicion key to avoid the misdiagnosis of an STS and its inappropriate treatment. STS most commonly metastasize to the lungs, with a few exceptions (e.g. myxoid liposarcoma—soft tissue/abdominal metastases; alveolar soft part or clear cell sarcoma—brain).

Presentation

- Enlarging lump.
- Pain/tenderness (not always).
- Overlying skin changes (ulceration).
- Neurovascular deficit (signifying local tumour invasion or nerve tumours).
- Abdominal pain/bowel obstruction/weight loss (retroperitoneal tumours).
- Systemic features: weight loss, anorexia, lethargy.

Investigations

- *Bloods:* FBC, ESR, CRP, clotting profile.
- USS.
- MRI.
- Image-guided tissue biopsy.
- *CXR/CT chest, abdomen, and pelvis:* to detect metastases.
- *Whole-body MRI:* to identify soft tissue metastases in certain subtypes.
- *PET-CT:* to characterize indeterminate pulmonary nodules.

Tumour grading and staging

Every STS must be graded and staged prior to treatment.

- *Grading:* STS are generally graded by using the *Fédération Nationale des Centres de Lutte Contre le Cancer (FNCLCC) grading system*. This categorizes tumours as grade 1, 2, or 3, based on their cellular differentiation, mitotic cells, and necrosis.
- *Staging:* STS are subsequently staged by using the *American Joint Committee on Cancer (AJCC)/International Union Against Cancer staging system*. This stages a tumour based on its grade, location, and size, and the presence or absence of any distant disease, allowing prognosis to be predicted and appropriate treatment instigated.

Management

- STS should only be managed by an MDT in specialist centres.
- Early referral is key to ensuring appropriate treatment.

Surgical margin classification

STS surgical margins are classically described by using the Enneking classification. This system judges the adequacy of a resection and the need for any adjuvant treatment.

Depending on their plane, surgical resections are categorized as:
- *Intralesional*—a resection that enters the STS
- *Marginal*—removes all of the STS but travels through its pseudocapsule (or reactive zone)
- *Wide*—removes the STS and its pseudocapsule
- *Radical*—removes the entire anatomical compartment containing the STS.

Curative treatment
- Wide or planned marginal surgical resection with (neo)adjuvant radiotherapy.
- Small, superficial, widely resected tumour may not require radiotherapy.
- Chemotherapy in selected STS subtypes (minority of cases)—usually adjuvant, but in some cases neoadjuvant.

Palliative treatment
- Chemotherapy.
- Radiotherapy.
- Palliative surgical resections—reserved for rapidly enlarging tumours to prevent fungation/aid nursing (may involve amputation).

Outcome

Long-term outcome heavily dependent on disease stage; 5-year survival rates of 10%, 52%, 72%, and 86% reported for stage 4, 3, 2, and 1 tumours, respectively. Pulmonary metastatic recurrence carries an extremely poor prognosis, with a 5-year survival rate of only 15%.

Further reading

BMJ Best Practice (2023). *Soft-tissue sarcoma*. Available from: ℘ https://bestpractice.bmj.com/topics/en-us/271; https://www.nature.com/articles/s41416-024-02674-y

Edge S, Byrd DR, Compton CC, *et al. AJCC Cancer Staging Manual*, 7th edn. New York, NY: Springer, 2010; pp. 347–76.

Benign soft tissue tumours

Lipoma

Lipomas (lipomata) are benign adipose tumours mostly found in subcutaneous tissues. Lipomata are the commonest soft tissue tumours (incidence 1 in 1000). May be single or multiple (lipomatosis).

Presentation

Obvious palpable lump. Soft and usually non-tender. Common over back and chest wall. Can present at any age, although commonest in fifth decade. If diagnostic doubt, investigate with USS ± MRI. If concerning features (large, pain, rapid growth, deep, nodularity, neurovascular symptoms), then further imaging warranted.

Variants

- *Familial multiple lipomatosis:* autosomal dominant condition characterized by lipomatosis.
- *Gardner's syndrome:* autosomal dominant condition involving lipomatosis, intestinal polyposis, cysts, and osteomas.
- *Dercum's disease:* a rare condtion characterized by painful lipomata, asthenia, and psychiatric disturbances.

Management

- *Observation:* small, asymptomatic lesions.
- *Marginal excision:* large (>5cm), painful, or rapidly growing lesions.

Vascular malformations

A heterogeneous group of benign vascular tumours. Comprise abnormal vascular anatomy and fibrous tissue. Assessed with Doppler USS, MRI, or angiography. Categorized based on flow, and further subgrouped according to the pathophysiology and structures involved:

- *Low-flow:*
  - *Capillary malformation:* referred to as 'port-wine stain'—a macular pink or purple discoloration
  - *Venous malformation:* dependent lesions—predisposition to thrombosis and pathognomonic phleboliths
  - *Lymphatic malformation:* vascular channel or pouches filled with lymphatic fluid.
- *High-flow:*
  - *AV malformations:* develop from an abnormal shunt linking the arterial and venous systems.

Presentation

- Incidental phlebolith on radiographs.
- Lump (may be painful).
- Bleeding if lesion is superficial.

Management

- *Observation:* asymptomatic lesions.
- *Interventional radiology:* sclerotherapy or embolization.
- *Surgical resection:* consider preoperative embolization in large lesions.

Peripheral nerve sheath tumours—schwannoma and neurofibroma

Schwannoma

A benign encapsulated nerve sheath tumour consisting of Schwann cells. Characterized by their slow, non-infiltrating growth, which displaces (rather than destroys) nerve fascicles. Symptoms result from nerve fascicle compression. Malignant transformation extremely rare, although reported. MRI is the imaging modality of choice.

Presentation

- Lump (may be painful/Tinel's test positive).
- Distal neurovascular symptoms/radicular pain.
- Incidental finding.
- Peak incidence 20–50 years.

Management

- *Microsurgical resection:* can usually be excised, with little or no damage to nerve fascicles, due to eccentric, non-infiltrating growth pattern.

Neurofibroma

The commonest benign nerve tumour. Most cases occur sporadically, although 10% are associated with neurofibromatosis type 1 (NF1). Based on their growth pattern, neurofibromas are classified as localized, diffuse, or plexiform. Plexiform neurofibromas are strongly associated with NF1 and malignant transformation. Can also be classified as 'stump neurofibromas' (with no distal nerve fascicles) or 'neurofibromas in continuity' (found midway along a nerve).

Presentation
- Painful lump (Tinel's test positive).
- Neurological symptoms—dysaesthesia, hyperaesthesia, paraesthesiae, cold intolerance.
- Peak incidence 20–30 years.

Management
- Observation.
- Surgical excision.

NB excision of a neuroma in continuity may result in significant deficit—must be discussed with the patient. Selective neuroma excision or nerve stump reconstruction may help to maximize residual function.

Desmoid fibromatosis

Defined by the WHO as an intermediate soft tissue tumour characterized by fibroblastic proliferation. Desmoid fibromatosis (DF) has a uniquely complex natural history, with some cases undergoing spontaneous regression when observed, and others progressing rapidly. A significant proportion of DF cases occurs in women who are pregnant or have recently given birth.

Cases of DF are broadly categorized into two groups containing sporadic or familial adenomatous polyposis (FAP)-associated cases:

- *Sporadic DF:* ~85% of cases. Driven by somatic β-catenin activating mutations in *CTNNB1*
- *FAP-associated DF:* the incidence of DF in FAP patients is 10–20%—a relative risk of 852, compared with the general population. FAP-associated DF is driven by mutations in *APC* and is usually found in the abdomen.

Management

Should be managed by an MDT experienced in benign and malignant soft tissue tumours.

- *Active surveillance:* has become increasingly popular in recent years. Spontaneous regression may allow more invasive treatments to be avoided.
- *Surgical resection:* historically primary treatment for DF—now generally avoided due to high recurrence rates and significant iatrogenic morbidity.
- *Radiotherapy:* can be used in isolation or as an adjunct to surgery.
- *Hormone therapy (tamoxifen):* tumour response explained by oestrogen receptors in DF tissue.
- *NSAIDs:* most effective when used alongside hormonal therapy.
- Chemotherapy.
- Tyrosine kinase inhibitors.

Bone tumour-like conditions

Unicameral (simple) bone cysts

- Benign, fluid-filled lesion found near the physis.
- Over 90% of cases found in proximal humerus.
- Peak incidence at age <20 years.
- May grow during skeletal growth before healing spontaneously.
- Often asymptomatic, but may present with pathological fracture.
- *Radiographs:* concentric, lytic, well-demarcated metaphyseal lesion. May result in cortical thinning.
- *Management:* treat conservatively unless symptomatic. If intervention required, consider cyst decompression, steroid injection, or curettage/ bone grafting ± internal fixation.

Aneurysmal bone cyst

- Benign, locally aggressive lesion containing multiple blood-filled cavities.
- May extend into surrounding soft tissues.
- Commonest in long bones (metaphyseal) and spine (posterior elements).
- Peak incidence at age <20 years.
- Presents with pain and swelling ± pathological fracture.
- *Radiographs:* expansile, eccentric lytic lesion.
- *MRI:* multiple cavities with fluid lines.
- *Management:* excision or curettage with bone grafting if symptomatic.

Bone island (enostosis)

- A piece of cortical bone found in an area of the skeleton that is usually cancellous.
- Aetiology unknown.
- Usually asymptomatic—may need to exclude malignancy in large, painful lesions.
- *Radiographs:* rounded foci of cortical bone within medullary space.
- *Management:* nil required.

Fibrous cortical defect

- Benign lesion characterized by proliferation of fibrous tissue and histiocytes.
- Large fibrous cortical defects called non-ossifying fibromas (same histology).
- Commonest in long bone metaphysis (80% in leg).
- Peak incidence in skeletally immature.
- Most spontaneously resolve/reossify by third decade.
- Usually asymptomatic. Often incidental finding after minor trauma. Rarely present as pathological fracture.
- *Radiographs:* eccentric, lytic lesion surrounded by a sclerotic rim. Narrow zone of transition. Cortex may be thinned. Lesions become more sclerotic as they resolve.
- *Management:* observation as mainstay of treatment. Curettage with bone grafting for large, symptomatic lesions at risk of fracture.

Fibrous dysplasia

- Developmental bony abnormality characterized by abnormal lamellar bone development.
- May present as a solitary lesion (80%, monostotic) or at multiple sites (20%, polyostotic).
- Associated with mutations in the *GNAS* gene.
- Common in long bones (particularly proximal femur) and ribs.
- Peak incidence at age <30 years.
- There is 1% risk of malignant transformation.
- Usually asymptomatic/incidental finding.
- May be associated with certain syndromes:
  - *McCune–Albright syndrome:* polyostotic fibrous dysplasia (FD), café-au-lait spots, endocrine abnormalities
  - *Mazabraud syndrome:* polyostotic FD, intramuscular myxomas.
- *Radiography:* concentric, lytic lesion with characteristic 'ground-glass' appearance. May be accompanied by other bony deformities (bowing/'shepherd's crook' deformity of proximal femur).
- *Management:* observation for asymptomatic patients. Bisphosphonates may be used for symptomatic polyostotic FD. Surgical stabilization for symptomatic lesions at risk of fracture.

NB autologous bone graft contraindicated (turns into fibrous dysplastic bone on incorporation).

Soft tissue tumour-like conditions

Nodular fasciitis

- Benign subcutaneous tumour consisting of fibroblasts and myofibroblasts.
- Can occur anywhere, although 50% of cases in the upper limb.
- Peak incidence at age <40 years.
- Presents as growing lump (may be painful).

Management
- Marginal excision.

Myositis ossificans

- A reactive process that leads to abnormal formation of bone in soft tissues.
- Occurs following trauma and the formation of intramuscular haematoma.
- Most commonly found in the quadriceps, brachialis, and gluteal muscles.
- Peak incidence in young ♂ (♂:♀ ratio 2:1).
- Presents as a persistent, painful lump, with associated stiffness, following an injury.
- Natural history self-limiting—classically, lesions begin to shrink 1 year after injury.
- *Radiographs:* peripheral calcification with central lucency. Calcification first evident 2–6 weeks of injury.
- *Management:* treat symptomatically. Reserve surgery for mature symptomatic lesions (required in minority of cases).

Further reading

British Orthopaedic Oncology Society and British Orthopaedic Association (2015). *Metastatic bone disease: a guide to good practice*. Available from: ℘ https://baso.org.uk/media/61543/boos_m bd_2016_boa.pdf

Cox JA, Bartlett E, Lee EI. Vascular malformations: a review. *Seminars in Plastic Surgery*. 2014;**28**(2):58–63.

Dangoor A, Seddon B, Gerrand C, *et al.*; British Sarcoma Group. UK guidelines for the management of soft tissue sarcomas. *Clinical Sarcoma Research*. 2016;**6**:20.

Eastley N, McCulloch T, Esler C, *et al.* Extra-abdominal desmoid fibromatosis: a review of management, current guidance and unanswered questions. *European Journal of Surgical Oncology*. 2016;**42**(7):1071–83.

Eberlin KR, Ducic I. Surgical algorithm for neuroma management: a changing treatment paradigm. *Plastic and Reconstructive Surgery Global Open*. 2018;**6**(10):e1952.

Gerrand C, Athanasou N, Brennan B, *et al.*; British Sarcoma Group. UK guidelines for the management of bone sarcomas. *Clinical Sarcoma Research*. 2016;**6**:7.

Gosk J, Gutkowska O, Urban M, *et al.* Results of surgical treatment of schwannomas arising from extremities. *BioMed Research International*. 2015;**2015**:547926.

Hakim DN, Myutan Kulendran TP, Caris JA. Benign tumours of the bone: a review. *Journal of Bone Oncology*. 2015;**4**(2):37–41.

Adult orthopaedics: shoulder and elbow

Shoulder and elbow osteoarthritis

Primary OA of the upper limb is not as common as that of the lower limb.
Secondary OA of the upper limb may be due to a precipitating cause such as trauma or inflammatory arthropathy.

Epidemiology

- Incidence ↑ with age (more likely >60 years).
- Commoner in women.

Shoulder girdle

- *Sites:* OA may affect the GHJ or, more commonly, the ACJ. ACJ arthritis may cause irritation of the underlying rotator cuff muscles and present with impingement or rotator cuff tears (Fig. 13.1). GHJ OA may follow large rotator cuff tears where superior migration of the humeral head and narrowing of the acromiohumeral interval occur. This is termed 'cuff arthropathy'.

Acromioclavicular joint

Clinical

Patients with joint arthritis have pain and tenderness localized to the ACJ. Pain aggravated by overhead activity, pressing motion, and shoulder adduction. Often develops after repetitive microtrauma. Clinically, patients demonstrate tenderness over the ACJ and are positive for the scarf/cross arm adduction test.

Investigations

- *Radiographs:* Zanca view is best; however, often evident on plain radiographs without clinical signs or symptoms.
- *Local anaesthesia:* injection of lidocaine into the joint can be used to confirm the diagnosis if it alleviates symptoms.

Management

- *Non-operative:* most patients with ACJ arthritis respond to non-operative treatment—modification of activities, NSAIDs, and corticosteroid injections.
- *Operative:* resection of 5–10mm of distal clavicle, either as an open procedure or arthroscopically.

Glenohumeral joint

Clinical

Glenohumeral OA pain is felt deep within the shoulder and lateral aspect of the arm. The pain is often worse with movement of the shoulder and resolves with rest. Osteophytes may act as blocks to the range of motion. Characteristics on examination include ↓ ROM (particularly external rotation), sensation of crepitus with movements, and pain throughout the ROM.

Investigations

Diagnostic injections of local anaesthetic into suspected sites. Radiographs show typical features of OA and may show a high-riding humeral head, suggesting dysfunction of rotator cuff muscles.

(A)   (B)

(C)   (D)

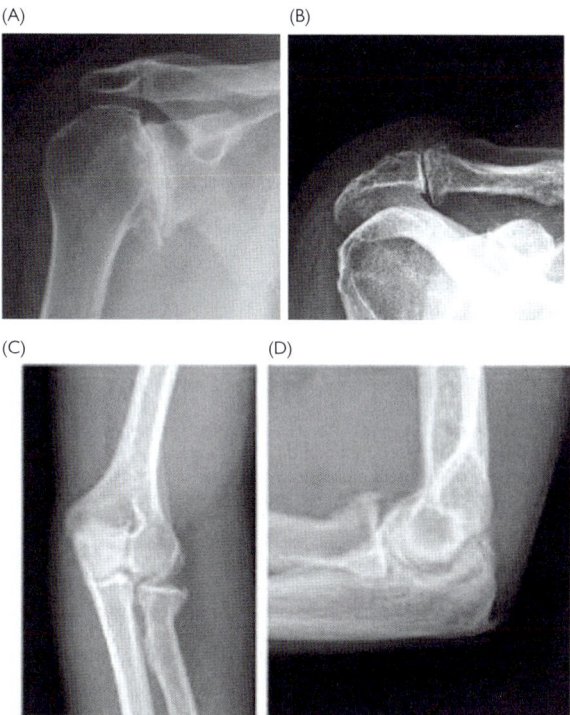

Fig. 13.1 Osteoarthritis of the glenohumeral (A), acromioclavicular (B), and elbow (radio-capitellar and ulno-humeral) joints (C, D).

Management
- *Non-operative:* includes analgesia ± anti-inflammatories. Physiotherapy and intra-articular injections of corticosteroids can be beneficial in retaining the ROM and strength.
- *Operative:* arthroplasty has good results (10-year survival rate of 90–95%). Arthroplasty options are dependent on the status of the rotator cuff. Intact rotator cuff/deltoid function allows anatomical stemmed replacement or resurfacing arthroplasty. Rotator cuff arthropathy requires reverse-geometry shoulder arthroplasty. Complications include glenoid/humeral component loosening, infection, scapular notching, and fracture.

Elbow

Clinical

Present with pain around the elbow, typically at end range of motion, not mid-range, and loss of terminal extension. Symptoms of ulnar neuropathy at the elbow present in 50% of patients. Loose bodies may cause intermittent locking of the joint. Extension may be blocked by osteophytes in the olecranon fossa and anterior capsule contractions. Further passive extension causes pain due to impingement. Flexion can also be blocked by anterior osteophytes at the tip of the coranoid process or fossa. Pronation and supination may be affected by radiocapitellar involvement.

Investigations

- *Plain radiographs:* usually sufficient to demonstrate arthritis and any bony loose bodies.
- Occasionally, *high-definition CT* may be helpful.

Management

- *Non-operative:* similar to those used for the shoulder joint.
- *Operative:*
  - Ulnar neuropathy in the presence of a flexion deformity may benefit from anterior transposition of the ulnar nerve.
  - Symptomatic loose bodies can be excised by an open procedure or arthroscopically. In the olecranon fossa, this can be performed directly from the back. Anterior loose bodies can be removed arthroscopically or through a window made in the base of the olecranon fossa from posteriorly (OK procedure).
  - Joint replacement—may be indicated in older patients (>65 years) with severe arthritis and lower demand, for relief of pain. Long-term results are not excellent, and longevity is reduced in all but low-activity individuals. Results are not as good as when performed for inflammatory arthropathy.

Further reading

Hay S, Kulkarni R, Watts A, *et al*. The provision of primary and revision elbow replacement surgery in the NHS. *Shoulder and Elbow*. 2018;**10**(2 Suppl):S5–12.

Thomas M, Bidwai A, Rangan A, *et al*. Glenohumeral osteoarthritis. *Shoulder and Elbow*. 2016;**8**(3):203–14.

Rheumatoid arthritis of the upper limb

The most visible effects of RA can be seen in the upper limb, especially in the hands. Arthritis of the lower limbs may ↑ demands on the upper limbs during mobilization, and this should be taken into consideration when deciding on management.

Upper limb functions

Include ADLs (feeding, washing, dressing), communication, mobility (sticks and wheelchairs), and sensory organs (through touch). RA can significantly impact the ability to manage these activities.

Clinical features

Patients with RA involving the upper limbs present with pain, loss of function, and deformity. In addition to the disease, patients can present with problems related to treatment (e.g. steroid use resulting in osteonecrosis). Careful assessment of the cervical spine must be performed to rule out instability or compression of neural structures. As patients with RA have numerous problems, it is important to take a history focused on the currently most disabling issue. However, it is important to consider joint involvement in the context of local and systemic problems, alongside overall goals. To achieve this, each patient should have an MDT looking after them that includes a rheumatologist, an orthopaedic surgeon, a physiotherapist, and an occupational hand therapist.

Presenting symptoms include:
- *Pain:* multiple possible sources, including cervical spine, joints, nerve entrapment, and soft tissue problems
- *Deformity:* sudden onset may indicate tendon rupture. Swelling may be due to synovitis, rheumatoid nodule, or joint subluxation
- *Loss of function:* the summation of deformities, pain, stiffness, and neurological impairments result in progressive disability

Investigations

- *Haematological and biochemical tests:* to monitor disease.
- *Radiology:* includes plain radiographs, CT, MRI, and USS. Imaging modality use depends upon diagnostic/treatment question being asked.

Management

- *Non-operative:* may include NSAIDs, immunosuppressive agents, disease-modifying agents, and corticosteroids. Physiotherapy and occupational therapy to maintain movements. Splintage can be helpful.
- Modification of home and use of modified utensils.
- *Operative:* surgical options can be classified as preventative (synovectomy), corrective (tendon transfers, soft tissue reconstruction, synovectomy, nerve decompression), and salvage (arthroplasty and arthrodesis).

Rheumatoid arthritis of the upper limb: clinical problems

Shoulder

Clinical

Patients are younger and tend to be ♀. They typically have multiple joint involvement, synovitis, joint erosion, and rotator cuff dysfunction. Marked muscle atrophy may be present. High incidence of rotator cuff abnormalities.

Management

- *Non-operative:* may include NSAIDs, immunosuppressive agents, remittive agents, and corticosteroids. Physiotherapy and occupational therapy to maintain movements. Splintage can be helpful.
- *Operative:* rotator cuff tears can be repaired if systemic disease is under control. Symptomatic joint degeneration would be an indication to consider arthroplasty. The aim is to provide pain-free movement.

Elbow

Clinical

Some patients develop stiff elbows (↓ ROM), whereas others become very mobile (unstable). Function may be very good despite dramatic appearances on radiographs; hence, history is essential. Examination must include assessment of soft tissues around the joint and radial and ulnar nerves.

Management

- *Non-operative:* may include NSAIDs, immunosuppressive agents, remittive agents, and corticosteroids. Physiotherapy and occupational therapy to maintain movements. Splintage can be helpful.
- *Operative:* surgery indicated for intractable pain and progressive deformity. Surgical options include synovectomy (contraindicated in severe instability and stiffness), capsular release, radial head excision, and arthroplasty (interposition or replacement—reliable procedure for RA).

(See ➲ Chapters 11 and 14 for further details.)

Rotator cuff tear

The rotator cuff is a confluence of tendons that insert onto the proximal humerus. Muscles that help to form this tendon are the supraspinatus, infraspinatus, subscapularis, and teres minor.

Tears of the rotator cuff can be acute or chronic. As we age, our rotator cuff tendons degrade and weaken. This degenerative process can cause pain but is often asymptomatic. The cuff tendons may rupture (rotator cuff tear), including with minor trauma and/or no recalled injury. The supraspinatus is most commonly torn, although large tears may involve several tendons. Tears can be partial or full thickness (Fig. 13.2); both can be painful, although full-thickness tears usually cause more weakness.

History

Age usually >50 years; prevalence ↑ with age. Features include:
- Pain, weakness, loss of function following a low-energy traumatic event
- A history of shoulder problems suggestive of impingement
- Difficulty with activities where the arm is held above shoulder height
- In younger patients, the cuff may be torn due to high-energy trauma.

Examination

- Findings will depend on which tendon is torn and the extent of the tear (Table 13.1).
- Inspection may reveal muscle wasting or asymmetry.
- Tenderness over the greater tuberosity, which may be minimal.
- Active abduction may be limited to 30° and associated with a 'shrug' as the whole scapula is raised. Compensatory movements of the whole body are common and may mask the severity of active motion loss.
- Passive movements may be nearly normal (can be sustained by the deltoid).
- Rupture of the long head of the biceps tendon may also be evident.

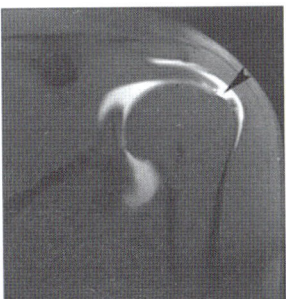 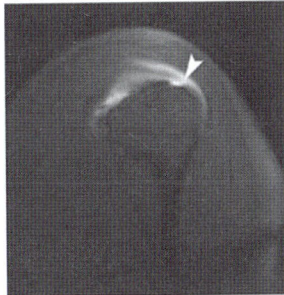

Fig. 13.2 Full-thickness infraspinatus tendon tear on magnetic resonance arthrography.

Table 13.1 Physical examination in rotator cuff tear

Cuff muscle	Impaired movement	Special tests
Supraspinatus	Weakness to resisted elevation in Jobe position	Jobe test (pain) Drop arm test
Infraspinatus	ER weakness at 0° abduction	ER lag sign
Teres minor	ER weakness at 90° abduction and 90° ER	Hornblower's sign
Subscapularis	IR weakness at 0° abduction	Excessive passive ER Belly press test Lift-off test IR lag sign

ER, external rotation; IR, internal rotation.

Investigations

- *Plain radiographs:* the humeral head may be noted to migrate superiorly due to unopposed pull of the deltoid. In long-standing tears, there may be secondary arthritic changes ('cuff arthropathy').
- *USS:* allows for dynamic examination. In experienced hands, partial- or full-thickness tears can be detected. The size of the tear can be assessed.
- *MRI:* diagnostic standard for rotator cuff pathology. The size, shape, and degree of retraction can be evaluated. Significant muscle fatty infiltration indicates a long-standing tear and makes it less likely that the patient will do well with a repair. *NB in asymptomatic patients, ~28% of those aged >60 years and ~65% of those aged >70 years have tears on imaging.*

Classification of full-thickness tears

Tears are classified by partial or full thickness, and by the size of the tear (amount of retraction of the tendon):
- Small: <1cm
- Medium: 1–3cm
- Large: 3–5cm
- Massive: >5cm.

Management

Rotator cuff tears may be asymptomatic, and initial conservative management is indicated for most. Partial-thickness tears are commonly more painful but will usually respond to analgesia and anti-inflammatory medication. Physiotherapy with rotator cuff and scapula stabilizer strengthening over 3–6 months is often beneficial.

Surgery is indicated in active individuals who fail to respond to non-operative measures. The aims of treatment are pain relief, removal of the cause for the tear, and restoration of function. In planning treatment, it must be remembered that the cuff tendons are degenerate. Surgical options include:

- Arthroscopic debridement—in select patients with low-grade, painful partial-thickness tears and minimal weakness
- Mini-open or arthroscopic reattachment of the cuff followed by a structured rehabilitation programme—in patients with small to large full-thickness tears who fail non-surgical treatment. Acute traumatic tears should be surgically repaired early
- Tendon transfers—in young patients with massive cuff tears that are not amenable to reattachment, especially if the muscle is contracted
- Superior capsular reconstruction—graft (cadaveric, fascia lata) attached to the glenoid and humeral head, preventing superior migration; potential option in younger patients without severe arthritis. Must have repairable or intact subscapularis and some infraspinatus present
- Graft jacket—allograft acellular dermal matrix used to augment larger and otherwise primarily irreparable tears
- Balloon interposition arthroplasty—biodegradable spacer that acts to depress the humeral head and enable deltoid activation; trials ongoing in older patients with irreparable tears and progressive arthropathy
- Reverse shoulder arthroplasty—may be indicated in patients with cuff arthropathy. In the presence of a degenerative GHJ, cuff repair alone is not indicated.

Further reading

Karjalainen TV, Jain NB, Heikkinen J, Johnston RV, Page CM, Buchbinder R. Surgery for rotator cuff tears. *Cochrane Database of Systematic Reviews*. 2019;**12**:CD013502.

Schemitsch C, Chahal J, Vicente M, et al. Surgical repair versus conservative treatment and subacromial decompression for the treatment of rotator cuff tears: a meta-analysis of randomized trials. *Bone and Joint Journal*. 2019;**101-B**:1100.

Wong I, Burns J, Snyder S. Arthroscopic graft jacket repair of rotator cuff tears. *Journal of Shoulder and Elbow Surgery*. 2010;**19**(2 Suppl):104–9.

Subacromial shoulder pain

Often referred to as subacromial impingement (SAI) or subacromial impingement syndrome (SIS), this refers to a combination of shoulder symptoms and clinical examination findings that can be explained by the compression of structures with shoulder elevation. Such compression causes persistent pain and dysfunction. This is the commonest cause of shoulder pain, accounting for 30–35% of shoulder disorders.

Pathophysiology

Consists of a spectrum of clinical findings rather than of injury to a specific structure. The underlying mechanism of injury occurs when the rotator cuff, subacromial bursa, and other tissues (e.g. long head of the biceps) are compressed between the humeral head and the undersurface of the acromion, ACJ, or coracoacromial arch. Several mechanical and anatomical factors play a role, including:

- ↑ proximal translation of the humeral head
- Shape of the acromion predisposes to impingement
- Reduced distance between the humeral head and the underside of the acromion
- Osteophytic changes of the ACJ.

Neer (1983) identified three stages, as shown in Table 13.2.

Presentation

Often aged 40–60 years. Common in athletes/workers with repetitive activity above the shoulder. Insidious onset of presenting symptoms:

- *Pain:* typically as the shoulder is abducted/flexed, felt over the lateral aspect of the arm. May be 'painful arc' or pain with overhead activities
- *Sleep disturbance:* pain worse when lying on the affected shoulder.

Examination

- Examination of the neck, both upper limbs, and neurology is essential.
- Local wasting, swelling, instability, and tenderness are important signs. Measure both active and passive ROM of both shoulders.
- Pain may be experienced through the painful arc, although further passive movement may be possible and sustainable once achieved.

Table 13.2 Neer stages of subacromial impingement syndrome

Stage	Age (years)	Pathology	Course	Treatment
I	<25	Oedema and haemorrhage	Reversible	Conservative
II	25–40	Fibrosis and tendonitis (rotator cuff tendinopathy)	Activity-related pain	Conservative and/or acromioplasty
III	>40	Spur formation and cuff tear	Progressive disability	Acromioplasty and/or repair

- At the point of impingement pain, external rotation may relieve the pain and internal rotation worsens the pain (*Hawkins test*).
- Injection of local anaesthetic into the subacromial space may relieve pain within minutes, allowing ↑ passive forward flexion (*Neer's test*).
- Although painful, the cuff muscle power should be intact.

Differential diagnoses

- Calcific tendonitis.
- Rotator cuff tear.
- Referred pain from the neck or cervical radiculopathy.

Investigations

- *Plain radiographs:* three views at 90°. Typical signs include acromion undersurface sclerosis ('sourcil' sign), greater tuberosity cyst formation, osteophytes of the ACJ, and narrowing of the subacromial space (with cuff tear). Lateral view may show 'hooked' acromion or os acromiale.
- *USS:* can identify site of impingement and tendons involved.
- *MRI:* evaluate degree of rotator cuff pathology and evidence of bursitis.

Management

Most rotator cuff disease can be managed *non-operatively* with:
- Changes in activity and analgesics, including NSAIDs
- Injection—subacromial local anaesthetic and steroid injection
- Physiotherapy and exercise programme—aimed at improving rotator cuff muscle strength and ensuring the humeral head is centred in the glenoid.

Surgical management is reserved for failed conservative treatment (~30%):
- Arthroscopic/open subacromial decompression (acromioplasty).

Further reading

Khan M, Alolabi B, Horner N, *et al*. Surgery for shoulder impingement: a systematic review and meta-analysis of controlled clinical trials. *CMAJ Open*. 2019;**7**:E149.

Steuri R, Sattelmayer M, Elsig S, *et al*. Effectiveness of conservative interventions including exercise, manual therapy and medical management in adults with shoulder impingement: a systematic review and meta-analysis of RCTs. *British Journal of Sports Medicine*. 2017;**51**:1340.

Adhesive capsulitis (frozen shoulder)

Idiopathic condition associated with initial pain followed by ↓ ROM, with a gradual, often incomplete, recovery over months to years. The criterion for diagnosing adhesive capsulitis is a painful shoulder, with restricted active and passive glenohumeral and scapulothoracic motion, with no clear underlying cause.

Can be *primary* (idiopathic) frozen shoulder, or more often is *secondary* to other conditions, after shoulder trauma (such as proximal humerus fractures) or surgery, or even after other upper limb injuries (such as distal radius fractures). Systemic disorders (diabetes mellitus, hypothyroidism, hyperthyroidism, hypoadrenalism) are associations. In particular, diabetic patients have a lifetime prevalence of 10–20%.

Pathology

- Aetiology unclear, but autoimmune responses, biochemical changes, neurological dysfunction, trauma, and psychological problems implicated.
- Histological changes in the capsule are consistent with chronic inflammation and resemble changes seen in Dupuytren's disease.
- Capsule is avascular, tense, and adherent to humeral head, resulting in reduced joint volume. Coracohumeral ligament often tightly contracted.

History and examination

- Three defined stages have been established: 'freezing'—gradual onset of diffuse pain and worsening loss of ROM (6 weeks to 9 months); 'frozen'—pain improves, but fixed reduced ROM affecting ADLs (4–9 months +); and 'thawing'—gradual return of ROM (5–26 months).
- Symptoms are often worse at night. Typically, global reduction in active and passive movements. Loss (and return) of passive external rotation is a good clinical marker to serially monitor, alongside overall range of motion.
- There may be a preceding, sometimes minor, traumatic event. Examine both shoulders, the cervical spine, and the trunk to exclude other pathology.

Investigations

- *Radiographs:* usually normal. Important in excluding other causes of stiff shoulder (glenohumeral OA, cuff arthropathy, locked chronic dislocations).
- *MRI:* not usually necessary but can exclude other pathology. Loss of axillary recess can indicate capsule contracture. Arthrography is difficult—contrast cannot be injected easily into constricted joint space.

Differential diagnoses

- Rotator cuff disorders.
- Dislocation—may be missed, especially in confused patients/ polytrauma.
- Arthritis—osteophytes or articular damage may result in painful stiffness.
- Any painful condition of the shoulder—tumour, SAI, brachial neuritis, and infection are vital to exclude.

Management

Freezing stage
During the early painful stage, analgesia and physiotherapy (gentle, active assisted exercises) can help. Corticosteroid injections aid in pain control.

Frozen stage
Pain is less of a problem, but limited ROM can limit function. Physiotherapy is essential to maintain and improve ROM. Intra-articular corticosteroid injections appear to help, leading to improved ROM and pain reduction. There is evidence that up to three injections can be beneficial (limited evidence for up to six). Furthermore, the combination of structured physiotherapy alongside corticosteroid injections is more effective than either therapy alone. If not progressing with natural recovery, several further options are available, including:

- *MUA:* with the patient under general anaesthesia, the capsular adhesions are torn by manual force in a sequenced manipulation with short lever arms (one hand stabilizing the scapula, the other holding the humerus close to the shoulder). The humerus is gently forced into abduction, flexion, external rotation, and internal rotation until the adhesions are released. Repeating each movement once there has been some release with other movements is beneficial. The GHJ is then injected with corticosteroid and local anaesthetic to limit the inflammatory response and provide early analgesia. Post-operatively, the patient should start physiotherapy early. Risks include fracture of the humerus or dislocation.
- *Hydrodistension (dilatation):* saline and anaesthetic are infused into the glenohumeral capsule to expand the joint space under US guidance. May be an effective short-term treatment.
- *Arthroscopic interval release:* aims to divide the contracted tissues in the rotator interval. Reserved for patients with osteopenia, rotator cuff thinning, or failed manipulation/non-operative measures. The benefit of these procedures, compared with simple manipulation, is unclear.

The UK FROST RCT showed no significant clinical superiority of MUA, arthroscopic capsular release (highest risk), or early structured physiotherapy (most cost-effective).

Further reading

Favejee MM, Huisstede BM, Koes BW. Frozen shoulder: the effectiveness of conservative and surgical interventions: systematic review. *British Journal of Sports Medicine*. 2011;**45**:49.

Maund E, Craig D, Suekarran S, *et al*. Management of frozen shoulder: a systematic review and cost-effectiveness analysis. *Health Technology Assessment*. 2012;**16**:1.

Rangan A, Brealey SD, Keding A, *et al*. Management of adults with primary frozen shoulder in secondary care (UK FROST): a multicentre, pragmatic, three-arm, superiority randomised clinical trial. *The Lancet*. 2020;**396**(10256):977–89.

Shah N, Lewis M. Shoulder adhesive capsulitis: systematic review of randomised trials using multiple corticosteroid injections. *British Journal of General Practice*. 2007;**57**:662.

Acute shoulder dislocations

The shoulder has the greatest ROM of all joints in the body. Instability may develop. Shoulder dislocations comprise 50% of all joint dislocations. Shoulder dislocations can be described by:
- *Direction:* majority are anterior (95–97%); some are posterior (2–4%) and, more rarely, inferior (0.5%)
- *Timing:* acute (<3 weeks) or chronic (>3 weeks)
- *Aetiology:* traumatic or atraumatic
- *Patient factors:* recurrent, habitual (able to perform voluntarily), or obligatory (occurs with the limb in a particular position).

Acute anterior dislocation

Clinical
- Usually follows a traumatic event (e.g. contact sport, fall from height). Usually occurs with the arm abducted and externally rotated.
- Presents with pain and inability to move the arm. Deformity may be present due to the humeral head bulging anteriorly; may be absent in large individuals.
- Important to assess neurological and vascular function of upper limb (including axillary nerve sensation over lateral arm—'regimental badge area' and deltoid function) prior to any intervention.

Investigations
- *Plain radiographs:* AP, scapular Y, and axial/axillary views to confirm diagnosis and exclude a fracture dislocation (Fig. 13.3). Clinically important fractures occur in ~25% of shoulder dislocations. A posterior humeral head impaction fracture (Hill–Sachs lesion) to the posterior aspect of the humeral head can be seen if large.
- *MRI:* can show damage to the anterior labrum (Bankart lesion).

Management
- Prompt reduction of dislocation. This should not require excessive force and can often be done without sedation (Entonox®/oral analgesia, intra-articular local anaesthetic injection). Reduction should not be

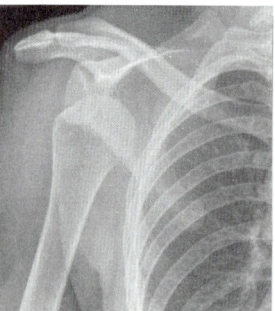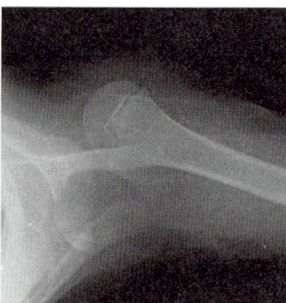

Fig. 13.3 Anterior shoulder dislocation (anteroposterior and axial views).

attempted without radiographs. Isolated fractures of the greater tuberosity should not preclude a cautious closed reduction attempt, but beware of difficult-to-spot surgical neck fractures. Some cases may require general anaesthesia with muscle relaxant.

- Awake sedation with analgesia is an option but should only be conducted by experienced clinicians. Monitoring and resuscitation facilities are needed. Infiltration of the joint with local anaesthetic is equally successful, albeit with fewer adverse effects than sedation.

- *Technique of closed reduction:* no clear evidence exists supporting the superiority of any one of the many methods used to reduce anterior shoulder dislocations. Techniques that are quick, simple, and require neither significant force nor IV medication are ideal. Start with scapular manipulation, and if unsuccessful, attempt the external rotation technique (± Milch technique). If this fails, then traction–countertraction or an alternative technique may be used. Blocks to reduction include muscular contraction or long head of the biceps/fracture fragment interposition. Confirm reduction and exclude iatrogenic fracture with check radiographs. Re-document neurovascular function.

- *Post-reduction management:* prolonged immobilization does not reduce the risk of recurrence. Aim for early, active mobilization, as comfort allows, and strengthening exercises to improve rotator cuff function. Immobilization in external rotation may reduce the risk of recurrence but is generally impractical. Early orthopaedic referral.

- *Recurrence* is directly proportional to age and sex; younger ♂ patients have the highest risk of redislocation (e.g. in men: 78% in an 18-year old; 56% in a 25-year old; 29% in a 35-year old).

Acute posterior dislocation

Clinical

Occurs after either high-energy trauma to the anterior shoulder or strong muscular contraction (seizures, electric shock). The profile of the shoulder girdle may be deceptively normal, especially if bilateral. Arm may be held adducted and internally rotated, with limited external rotation (hence mistaken for frozen shoulder, particularly if chronic).

Investigations

- *Radiographs:* AP view may show the humeral head in an oblique profile ('light bulb' sign) (Fig. 13.4), but may appear almost normal. Other views (axial/axillary preferably) are mandatory to exclude dislocation.

- *CT:* impaction fracture of the posterior glenoid lip or anterior humeral head (reverse Hill–Sachs lesion) may be present. Always perform CT for chronic/subacute (>24h) cases to identify any bony block to reduction.

Management

Closed reduction by using longitudinal traction. The humeral head can be disimpacted with internal rotation of the humerus. If open reduction is required, an anterior approach is the preferred option. Some authors advocate external rotation bracing post-reduction.

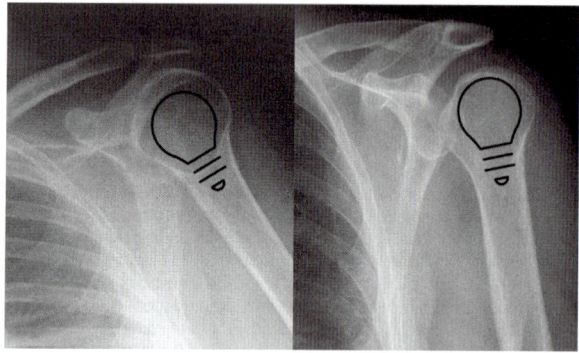

Fig. 13.4 Posterior dislocation, demonstrating the 'light bulb' sign.

Acute inferior dislocation
- *Clinical:* rare; presents with inability to adduct arm (luxatio erecta).
- *Management:* closed reduction with longitudinal traction is indicated.

Inferior subluxation
- *Clinical:* following shoulder trauma or surgery, a joint effusion/ haemarthrosis combined with inhibition of the rotator cuff muscles allows the humeral head to drift inferiorly with the effect of gravity on the upper limb. Should not be confused with true dislocation.
- *Management:* no specific treatment required.

Missed dislocation
Old (>3 weeks) missed dislocations usually require planned, rather than emergent, open reduction and reconstruction. CT first. Occasionally, in elderly, low-demand patients, function is maintained despite the dislocation and the risks of open reduction outweigh the benefits. These patients are more suitably managed with a physiotherapy rehabilitation programme if pain is not a major problem.

Further reading
British Elbow and Shoulder Society. *Patient care pathways and guidelines*. Available from: ℘ https:// bess.ac.uk/patient-care-pathways-and-guidelines/

Itoi E, Sashi R, Minagawa H, Shimizu T, Wakabayashi I, Sato K. Position of immobilization after dislocation of the glenohumeral joint: a study with use of magnetic resonance imaging. *Journal of Bone and Joint Surgery*. 2001;**83**(5):661–7.

Shoulder instability

Recurrent shoulder instability

Description

Subluxation or dislocation may occur recurrently when any of the stabilizing structures are deficient. The pathology varies, depending on whether the initial dislocation was traumatic (with associated injuries) or relatively atraumatic.

- *Traumatic:* instability is most commonly anterior.
  - Bankart lesion—avulsion of the glenoid labrum from the glenoid
  - Glenohumeral ligament avulsion or tear from the glenoid or humerus (humeral avulsion of the inferior glenohumeral ligament (HAGL)).
  - Hill–Sachs lesion—impaction fracture of the posterior humeral head in anterior dislocations (reverse Hill–Sachs in posterior dislocations), which reduces the contact area of the humeral head with the glenoid.
- *Atraumatic:* instability is more likely to be multidirectional.
  - Generalized ligamentous laxity—may be familial or inherited as part of a recognized syndrome (e.g. Ehlers–Danlos syndrome). Other joint laxity may be evident (e.g. knees, elbows, hands). Patients are usually young.
  - Rarely, the glenoid may be hypoplastic or abnormally orientated.

Clinical

Important things to note include:

- Age: <25 years—high risk (up to 90%) of recurrence following traumatic dislocation; >40 years—lower risk of recurrent dislocation, but need to assess for acute rotator cuff tears that may warrant early surgery.
- Wilful dislocation and relocation: if this is the patient's 'party trick' or method of gaining attention, it is less likely to respond to surgical intervention. This is termed habitual dislocation. Surgery should be avoided.
- Symptoms may be non-specific in young patients who compensate well with dynamic stabilizers. Pain, arm paraesthesiae, and apprehension may be present. If these follow a traumatic episode, suspect subtle instability.

Examination

On examination, look for the following:

- *Signs of laxity:*
  - Generalized ligamentous laxity (Beighton score; see ⊃ Chapter 1, History and examination, p. 7)
  - Sulcus sign—pulling arms inferiorly produces ↑ subacromial space, evident as a visible and palpable skin sulcus
  - Load shift sign—by holding the scapular neck firmly with one hand and the humeral head with the other, the humerus can be displaced in an anterior or posterior direction more on the affected side
- *Signs of instability:*
  - Apprehension/relocation—for anterior instability. The abducted arm is externally rotated, and the patient resists the movement (apprehension +ve). When repeated, with anterior pressure over the humeral head, the patient is more comfortable (relocation +ve)
  - Posterior apprehension—posterior force on a flexed arm reproduces patient symptoms.

Investigations
- *Radiology:*
  - Plain radiographs—looking for fractures or Hill–Sachs lesions
  - CT arthrography—can show disruption to the labrum or capsular structures, and delineate bony trauma.
  - MRI or magnetic resonance arthrography—excellent soft tissue definition; however, sensitivity is poor and clinical examination is key.
- *Examination under anaesthesia (EUA):* negates the effects of dynamic muscular stabilizers.
- *Arthroscopy:* may be required in less obvious cases to decide on the exact pathology.

Management
Fig. 13.5 shows UK British Elbow and Shoulder Society algorithm on the management of first-time shoulder dislocations.

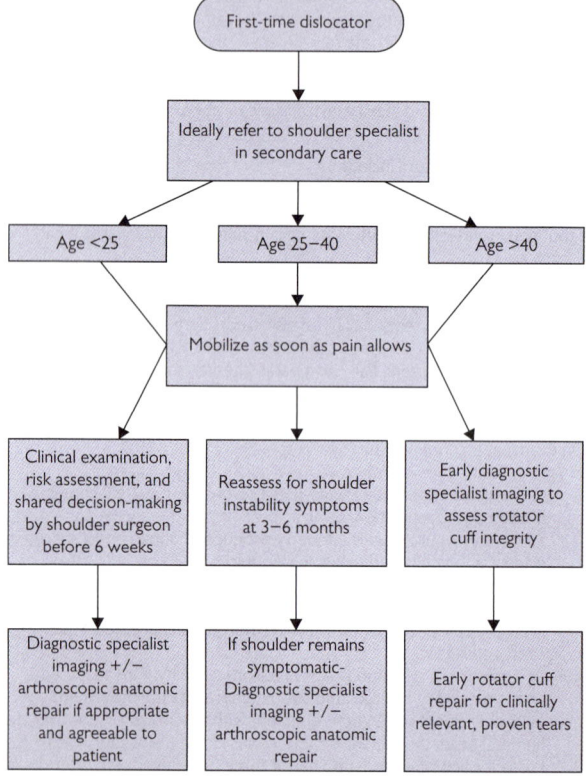

Fig. 13.5 UK British- Elbow and Shoulder Society algorithm on the management of first-time shoulder dislocations.
Taken from ✆ https://bess.ac.uk/patient-care-pathways-and-guidelines/

Anterior instability—in patients aged <25 years

Recurrence is so common in this group that early intervention aimed at correcting the pathology is often indicated. Sporting and ligamentously lax individuals are more at risk of recurrence. Surgical options include repair of the labrum to the glenoid and tightening of the inferior glenohumeral ligament, subscapularis advancement, and operations to address glenoid bone loss such as transfer of the tip of the coracoid to the anterior aspect of the glenoid (Latarjet procedure). Specific risks of such interventions include recurrence, axillary nerve damage, loss of external rotation, and late arthritic changes.

Anterior instability—older patients

With ↑ age, the risk of recurrence ↓, as the risk of stiffness ↑. Need to assess rotator cuff integrity. An early structured physiotherapy programme following 1 or 2 weeks of immobilization is appropriate. Less commonly, stabilization procedures are required. Acute rotator cuff tears should be repaired. Physiotherapy is aimed at cuff muscle strengthening exercises and maintaining range of motion.

Multidirectional instability

First-line treatment is physiotherapy (3- to 6-month programme), aiming to strengthen the dynamic stabilizers. Surgical intervention is possible with capsular shift procedures. However, there is a high failure rate, and it is vital to ensure all conservative options have been exhausted and any psychological problems are addressed. Many younger patients presenting like this will stabilize as they grow older. The Stanmore classification can be used to better categorise patients (Fig. 13.6).

Management summary (after Matsen)

- *TUBS:* Traumatic aetiology, Unidirectional instability, Bankart lesion present, and Surgical management.
- *AMBRI:* Atraumatic, Multidirectional instability, Bilateral involvement, Rehabilitation vital, and Inferior capsular shift is a surgical option.

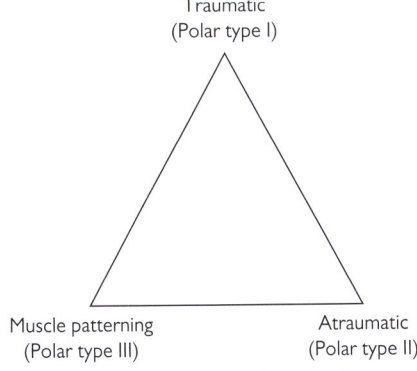

Fig. 13.6 Stanmore classification of glenohumeral joint instability.

SLAP tears

The superior labrum is the upper portion of the cartilage rim that attaches to the edge of the glenoid. This upper part of the glenoid and labrum is also the attachment for the long head of the biceps tendon. Occasionally, a SLAP tear extends into the biceps tendon itself (Fig. 13.7). The term SLAP means 'Superior Labrum Anterior and Posterior' to biceps.

Pathophysiology

Can occur either in isolation or as part of a more widespread shoulder instability picture. SLAP tears in younger patients are likely traumatic or sports-related; in patients aged >40 years, they are normally degenerate.
  Mechanisms of injury include:
- Repetitive overhead activities (e.g. crossfit or throwing athletes)
- Fall on outstretched arm with tensed biceps
- Traction on the arm.

History and examination

- Often vague. May recall a precipitating traumatic event, 'hearing a pop', but delay in onset to symptoms. Vague deep shoulder pain. May have symptoms of popping, clicking, or fatiguability.
- No one specific test. O'Brien's test and Crank test can be useful.

Imaging

- MRI ± arthrography: sensitivity ~50%, specificity ~90%. Associated paralabral ganglion cyst highly specific for labral tear.

Management

- Rest, activity modification, analgesia, and physiotherapy are first line.
- Surgery: arthroscopic SLAP repair ± biceps tenotomy or tenodesis; 85% have a good outcome by 6 months.

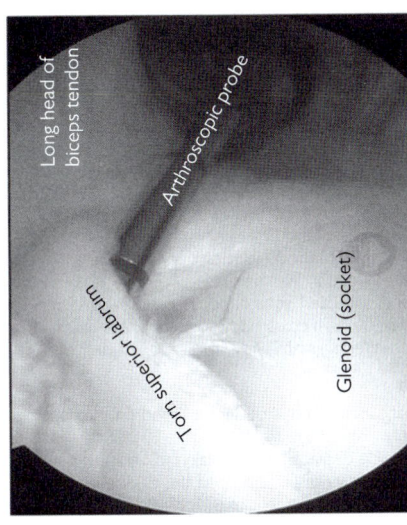

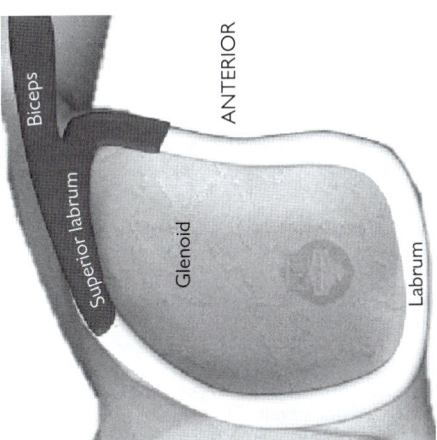

Fig. 13.7 *Face-on view of the shoulder socket (glenoid)—labral cartilage rim with the superior labrum and long head of biceps tendon in red.* Arthroscopic photograph of an unstable SLAP tear. The long head of the biceps tendon is sometimes destabilized by this injury. This patient's injury was repaired.

Acromioclavicular joint disruption

The ACJ is usually disrupted by a direct blow to the top/point of the shoulder. Initially, the capsule and ligaments of the ACJ are damaged, but with ↑ energy, the supporting coracoclavicular (CC) and acromioclavicular (AC) ligaments, along with the adjacent supporting muscles, may be disrupted. CC ligaments are the trapezoid and conoid (3cm and 4.5cm from the lateral end of the clavicle, respectively).

History and examination

There is a history of trauma resulting in pain and swelling over the ACJ. The injury usually occurs in young athletes playing contact sports. Open dislocations are rare. Localized tenderness may be the only sign in ACJ sprains. With ligament disruption, the lateral end of the clavicle becomes more prominent. In late presentations, examine the contralateral side to compare ACJ mobility. In high-energy injuries, cervical spine and neurovascular injuries must be excluded.

Stability of the shoulder should be assessed—horizontal (anterior–posterior) stability, through cross-body adduction, evaluates AC ligaments; vertical (superior–inferior) stability evaluates CC ligaments.

Classification

Rockwood classification of displacement is based on the depth of the ACJ on AP radiographs (Fig. 13.8):
- Type I—no clavicle displacement on plain radiographs; a sprain
- Type II—slight superior displacement of the clavicle (<25%)
- Type III—25–100% displacement of the clavicle (Fig 13.9)
- Type IV—posteriorly displaced; clavicle buttonholes through the trapezius
- Type V—>100% displacement of the clavicle
- Type VI—clavicle displaced inferiorly under the coracoid process.

Investigations

- *Plain radiographs*: bilateral AP views of the ACJs should be obtained. AP view of the clavicle is important; can be improved with 10° cephalic tilt (Zanca view). Axillary lateral view to diagnose posterior displacement (type IV).
- Stress views—rarely used; can help to differentiate between types II and III.

Management

In general, types I–III should be managed non-operatively, and types IV–VI should be reduced and stabilized.
- *Types I and II:* 1 week of rest in broad arm sling, followed by active full range of motion.
- *Type III:* non-surgical treatment as for types I and II usually sufficient despite prominence of the clavicle. Typical return to normal function is 6–12 weeks. In some patients, especially manual labourers and elite athletes, open reduction and ligamentous reconstruction with temporary CC fixation may be advisable.
- *Types IV–VI:* a good outcome is unlikely unless treated by open reduction and reconstruction of the ligaments.

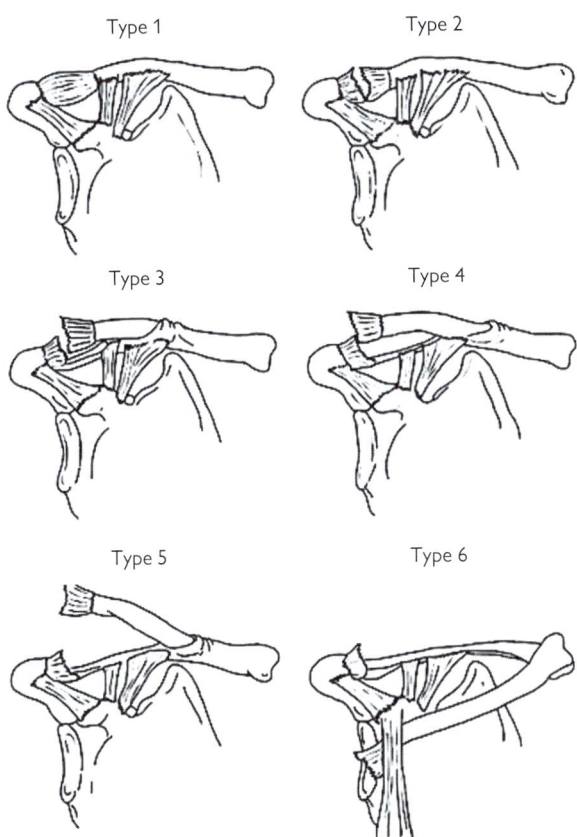

Fig. 13.8 Rockwood classification of acromioclavicular joint dislocations.

- Surgical techniques for CC interval restoration include fixation or ligament reconstruction. Ligament reconstruction with soft tissue graft can be through modified Weaver–Dunn, autograft, allograft, or synthetic ligaments. This can be performed open or arthroscopically. Open fixation includes use of hook plates, CC screws, cortical flip buttons (such as Dog Bone), and sutures. Rehabilitation usually includes 6 weeks of sling immobilization before building up with active-assisted ROM.

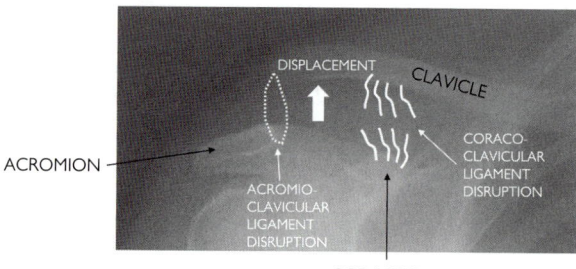

Fig. 13.9 Radiographic appearances of type III acromioclavicular joint dislocation.

Further reading

Rockwood CA Jr, Williams GR, Young DC. Injuries to the acromioclavicular joint. In: Rockwood CA, Green DP, Bucholz RW, *et al.*, eds. *Fractures in Adults*, vol. 2, 4th edn. Philadelphia, PA: Lippincott-Raven, 1996; p. 1341.

Tamaoki MJS, Lenza M, Matsunaga FT, Belloti JC, Matsumoto MH, Faloppa F. Surgical versus conservative interventions for treating acromioclavicular dislocation of the shoulder in adults. *Cochrane Database of Systematic Reviews*. 2019;**10**:CD007429.

Weaver JK, Dunn HK. Treatment of acromioclavicular injuries, especially complete acromioclavicular separation. *Journal of Bone and Joint Surgery (American volume)*. 1972;**54**:1187.

Calcific tendinopathy

Calcific tendinopathy of the shoulder is characterized by the presence of macroscopic deposits of hydroxyapatite (crystalline calcium phosphate) in any tendon of the rotator cuff, usually the supraspinatus. Tendon inflammation located around the deposits and ↑ intratendinous pressure are thought to contribute to pain.

Aetiology
- Remains controversial.
- Early hypothesis—↑ in calcium deposits is due to degenerative calcification. However, patients have a relatively young age at peak incidence. There is spontaneous resolution in many cases (in contrast to degenerative tendinopathy).
- Four distinct phases: formative—tendon undergoes fibrocartilaginous transformation, and calcification occurs; resting—calcific deposits stable; resorptive—inflammatory reaction may occur, and macrophages and giant cells absorb deposit; post-calcific—fibroblasts reconstitute the collagen pattern of tendon.

History and examination
- Pain is the cardinal symptom, and onset is gradual and not associated with trauma. May report ↑ pain at night and inability to lie on the affected shoulder. Activities with overhead motions often painful.
- Chronic course, with symptoms over 1 year in a third of patients, with intermittent periods of pain.
- During resorptive phase, may have acute ↑ in pain from leakage of calcium crystals into overlying bursa.
- Pain commonly radiates from the point of the shoulder to the deltoid insertion and is aggravated by elevation of the arm above shoulder level or by lying on the shoulder. Stiffness, catching, or weakness of the shoulder are other symptoms. Often marked overlap with impingement signs.

Investigations
The calcific deposit can be characterized by its location (i.e. which tendon is affected) and its size. The appearance may change rapidly over days.
- *Plain radiographs:* show an area of calcification; in supraspinatus tendonitis, this is just proximal to the greater tuberosity. This should not be mistaken for an avulsion fracture. Radiological appearance of calcific deposits can occur after the start of pain.
- *USS:* highly sensitive for detecting calcifications. Pain caused by compression from the transducer, while the deposit is visualized, suggests the deposit is contributing to symptoms.

Differential diagnoses
- Neuralgic amyotrophy or brachial neuralgia—a post-viral condition associated with intense shoulder girdle pain.
- Rotator cuff syndrome—chronic calcific depositions may be present on imaging but are not the source of pain. Impingement pain is the principal finding.

Management

- Acute phase (conservative):
  - Rest
  - NSAIDs
  - Physiotherapy
  - Subacromial injection with steroid preparation and local anaesthetic.
- Persistent symptoms:
  - Extracorporeal shock wave therapy
  - Ultrasound guided barbotage can be performed using a needle to break up the calcium deposits and help them to dissolve.
  - Surgical decompression can be performed as an open procedure or arthroscopically. Either technique can be combined with subacromial decompression.

Natural history

This condition is self-limiting in all cases. Intervention should only be considered where pain relief is not achieved with simple measures within 3–6 months.

Biceps rupture—proximal and distal

Proximal biceps

The biceps muscle has two distinct tendons at its proximal end (short head and long head). The short head is outside the shoulder joint and rarely causes problems. The long head passes through the shoulder joint and attaches to the top of the glenoid—it frequently contributes to pain in the shoulder and occasionally ruptures (Fig. 13.10).

Presentation

Rare in patients aged <40 years. May be associated with traumatic SLAP lesion in this group. Degenerative tendon ruptures commonest in those aged >60 years. Often present with sudden tearing pain, bruising tracking down the arm, and cramping and fatigue of the biceps. The muscle can retract down the arm, causing a 'Popeye sign'. Imaging not usually required (clinical diagnosis unless tendinopathy suspected (MRI)).

Management

Symptoms usually resolve within 3–4 weeks with non-operative management. Active patients may complain of cramping in the arm with repetitive tasks. Surgery (biceps tenodesis) indicated for patients who want to restore muscle contour and reduce (but not eliminate) cramping. Patients suffering from symptoms of biceps tendinopathy (as opposed to rupture) may benefit from biceps tenotomy procedure.

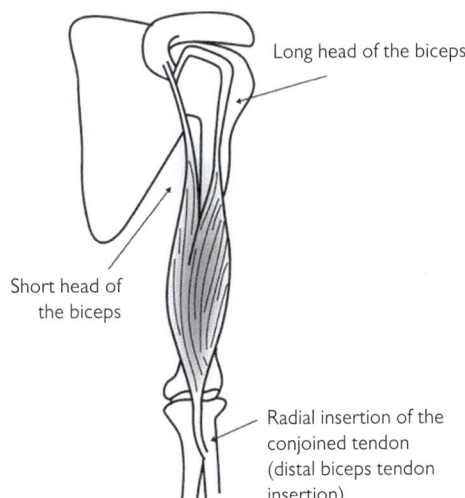

Long head of the biceps

Short head of the biceps

Radial insertion of the conjoined tendon (distal biceps tendon insertion)

Fig. 13.10 Sites of biceps tendon rupture.

Distal biceps

Epidemiology

Vast majority in men, 86% in dominant elbow. Most commonly occurs when lowering heavy weights (eccentric tension) or in sports such as rugby when attempting to tackle. Risk factors include anabolic steroid use, smoking (7.5 times greater risk), and hypovascularity.

Presentation

May be a painful 'pop', weakness, and pain (primarily on supination). On examination, may see proximal retraction of the muscle belly ('reverse Popeye sign') and bruising, and palpate a defect (absence of tendon on 'Hook' test; NB an intact lacertus fibrosus can give a false positive). Loss of supination power greater than loss of flexion.

Investigations

- *Plain radiographs:* may show small avulsion of bone from the radial tuberosity.
- *USS:* aid in diagnosis and identifying retraction.
- *MRI:* useful for surgical planning; helps to distinguish between:
  - Complete and partial tear
  - Tear in tendon and muscle substance
  - Degree of retraction.

Management

- *Non-operative:* for older/low-demand patients or partial tears. Outcomes for full tears:
  - 50% loss of sustained supination power
  - 45% loss of supination strength
  - 30% loss of flexion strength
  - 15% loss of grip strength.
- *Operative:* should occur within a few weeks of injury to avoid retraction and scarring of the distal biceps tendon. Tendon secured to the tuberosity by anchors, buttons, or sutures; 95% of patients have full restoration of flexion and supination. Caution to avoid damage to PIN (1–2%) and lateral antebrachial cutaneous nerve (LABCN; 9%).

Sternoclavicular joint dislocation

SCJ dislocation is much rarer than ACJ disruption, but important to recognize. It can be traumatic or atraumatic (subluxation). There can be anterior (commonest) or posterior dislocation. Posterior SCJ dislocation can be associated with major vascular injuries and airway compromise. The injury is often caused by RTAs or direct trauma. In the case of atraumatic subluxation, this is typically associated with hypermobility/ligamentous laxity conditions in younger patients.

History and examination

Usually due to high-energy injury. Anterior dislocation will present with a visible deformity that may ↑ with arm abduction and elevation. Posterior dislocation patients will not have a palpable deformity but may have dyspnoea, dysphagia, and stridor, which is made worse on lying supine. Important to note whether there is: (1) history of trauma; and (2) generalized laxity.

Investigations

- *Plain radiographs:* AP and serendipity views (beam at 40° cephalic tilt).
- *CT:* modality of choice as allows visualization of mediastinal structures and can distinguish from medial physeal fractures (pseudodislocation; clavicle physis to fuse, at around 20–25 years).

Management

- For acute anterior SCJ dislocations, non-operative treatment is generally indicated. Closed reduction is debatable in this highly unstable injury because a high proportion redislocate and reduction techniques are not without risk. A sling may be worn for comfort.
- Conversely, posterior dislocations with compressive symptoms need to be reduced promptly to prevent life-threatening complications. This can be performed closed or open, but should be with thoracic surgical support. Persistent pain and instability can be managed surgically through a variety of means—no technique has been shown to outperform another.
- Chronic instability may be addressed by physiotherapy ± stabilization by using a tendon graft (e.g. sternocleidomastoid, palmaris longus), with surgery demonstrating good outcomes if traumatic in aetiology.

Further reading

Athanatos L, Singh HP, Armstrong AL. The management of sternoclavicular instability. *Journal of Arthroscopy and Joint Surgery.* 2018;**5**(2):126–32.

Scapular winging

Imbalance and abnormal motion of the scapula secondary to dysfunction of stabilizing muscles. Can have medial or lateral winging, defined by movement of the inferior border of the scapula. Patients are often young and athletic, or have a history of recent surgery to the neck.

Winging can occur because of nerve injury (>50% traction for medial; lateral largely iatrogenic), bony abnormality, muscle contracture, intra-articular disease, and brachial neuritis (Parsonage–Turner syndrome). Nerve injuries include:

- *Medial winging:* long thoracic nerve injury (serratus anterior palsy)
- *Lateral winging:* spinal accessory nerve (trapezius palsy), dorsal scapular nerve (rhomboid palsy).

Presentation

Vague, non-specific shoulder girdle pain for both varieties. Discomfort sitting against chair. May also have subjective sensation of shoulder instability, weakness with overhead activity, and symptoms of brachial plexus neuropathy.

Examination

(Fig. 13.11)

- *Medial*: inferior medial scapula elevates and protrudes posteriorly and medially (exaggerated by forward arm flexion).
- *Lateral*: superior medial scapula drops downward and protrudes posteriorly and laterally (exaggerated by arm abduction and resisted external rotation).

Management

Scapular stabilization tends to improve pain for both types.

Medial

- *Non-operative:* physiotherapy (minimum of 6 months) focus on serratus anterior strengthening, bracing.
- *Operative:* pectoralis major split transfer ± autologous hamstring graft.

Lateral

- *Non-operative:* controversial as usually iatrogenic. Physiotherapy focuses on trapezius strengthening.
- *Operative:* neurolysis, Eden–Lange transfer (levator and rhomboids transferred laterally), scapula–thoracic fusion.

MEDIAL WINGING   LATERAL WINGING

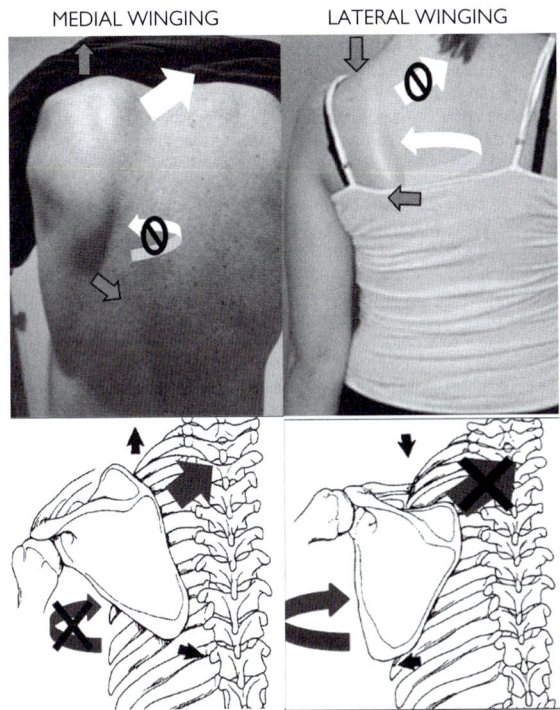

Fig. 13.11 Scapular winging—medial and lateral.

Thoracic outlet syndrome

Thoracic outlet syndrome (TOS) is a condition that causes chronic neck, shoulder, and arm pain. Distinct terms are used to describe the predominantly affected structure: neurogenic (nTOS) from brachial plexus compression; venous (vTOS) from subclavian vein compression; and arterial (aTOS) from subclavian artery compression. nTOS is commonest (~95%).

Aetiology

- The brachial plexus runs between the scalenus anterior and the scalenus medius, along with the subclavian artery. The subclavian vein runs in front of the scalenus anterior.
- Any abnormality in this region may cause compression of neurovascular structures in certain arm positions. The commonest compressive forces arise from a cervical rib (an extra rib; occurs in 1 in 200 people); 10% who have a cervical rib develop TOS.
- Other causes include fibromuscular bands or muscle hypertrophy.
- Less common causes include an aneurysm of the subclavian artery and repeated trauma.

Differential diagnoses

TOS must be differentiated from cervical spine disease, in particular cervical radiculopathy. Other differentials include:
- Musculoskeletal pain
- Subclavian vascular steal syndrome
- Peripheral nerve entrapment
- Raynaud's disease.

History

- Patients with nTOS often have a prior history of repetitive occupational physical stress or neck trauma. Compression of the brachial plexus leads to upper extremity numbness, weakness, and altered sensation, which may not have a specific nerve distribution.
- vTOS is highly associated with repetitive movements, particularly overhead arm movements. Venous compression may cause DVT and extremity swelling.
- Arterial compression can lead to arm pain with claudication, distal thromboembolism, or acute arterial thrombosis.

Examination

- A full peripheral neurological and vascular examination is required in any atypical arm pain presentation.
- Examine the cervical spine for evidence of nerve root compression.
- nTOS presents with often unilateral progressive weakness, numbness, and altered sensation. Tenderness over the scalene muscles is often present.
- vTOS often leads to upper venous thrombosis with swelling and cyanosis.
- aTOS typically presents as thromboembolism to the hand or arm with features of ischaemia, including pain, paraesthesiae, pallor, and coolness.

- Special tests aim to reproduce the provocative position. Arm abduction and neck rotation are typical positions used to provoke symptoms. However, Adson test is of little clinical value and should not be relied upon to make a diagnosis of any of the three types of TOS.

Investigations
- These will be indicated by history and examination.
- Plain radiographs of the cervical spine. Look for cervical rib or elongated C7 transverse process.
- MRI of the cervical spine and posterior triangle of the neck.
- Arterial or venous duplex USS is the initial diagnostic test for aTOS or vTOS, followed by angiography.
- Electrophysiological studies can exclude a more peripheral cause of symptoms or cervical root problem.
- Infiltration of the anterior or middle scalene muscle with local anaesthetic can be used as a confirmatory test.

Management
- Operations that may be required include:
  - Cervical rib excision
  - Repair of subclavian aneurysm
  - Fibrous band/muscle release
  - Transaxillary approach for first rib resection—80–90% of patients report a satisfactory result. Despite surgical intervention, symptoms recur in 15–20% of patients and usually in those with involvement of the upper cervical nerve roots.
- nTOS: non-operative measures such as postural and muscle strengthening exercises may control or alleviate symptoms. If related to muscle hypertrophy (e.g. body builders), resting the muscles involved may ease symptoms.
- vTOS: thrombolysis and early thoracic outlet decompression relieve extrinsic vein compression. Excellent long-term outcomes in certain patients.
- aTOS: patients with thromboembolism undergo decompression with embolectomy, thrombolysis, or anticoagulation. Without surgery, the rate of recurrent embolism is high. Repair of aneurysm is occasionally needed.

Elbow epicondylitis

Tendinopathies around the elbow comprise two main conditions: lateral ('tennis elbow') and medial epicondylitis ('golfer's elbow').

Epidemiology

Not exclusive to athletes, these conditions affect 1–3% of the population. Risk factors include smoking, obesity, age 40–50 years, repetitive movements for ≥2h daily, and working with loads >20kg.

Anatomy and pathology

- *Tennis elbow:* overuse injury of common extensor origin, predominantly ECRB (felt at the tip of lateral epicondyle) and occasionally EDC (just posterior and distal to the tip of lateral epicondyle).
- *Golfer's elbow:* overuse injury of common flexor origin, pronator teres, and FCR (originate at medial epicondyle).
- *Pathology:* represents chronic tendinosis rather than an acute inflammatory process as the name suggests (misnomer). Degenerative angiofibroblastic hyperplasia within the tendon origin has been described.

Clinical evaluation

- Activity-related pain around the medial or lateral epicondyle.
- Local tenderness at the epicondyle.
- Pain on resisted wrist or finger extension (tennis elbow) or wrist flexion (golfer's elbow).

Investigations

- *Radiographs:* often normal (may see calcification in lateral epicondylitis).
- *USS or MRI:* may be useful if diagnostic doubt.

Management

- *Non-operative:* rest, activity modification, counterforce brace, physiotherapy (and eccentric exercises), NSAIDs. Steroid injections (into the tendon, not the epicondyle) show evidence of improved short-term symptoms but do not prevent recurrence. Evidence for PRP/autologous blood product injections and extracorporeal shock wave therapy is mixed; 90% will resolve with non-operative management in 2 years.
- *Operative:* surgical release of common extensor or flexor origin. *Tennis elbow approach*: Kocher's incision and approach between ECRL and anconeus; release common extensor origin and remove any abnormal ECRB tendon. *Golfer's elbow*: direct medial incision over medial epicondyle; excise degenerative tissue; protect (± release) the ulnar nerve.

Further reading

Smidt N, Van Der Windt DA, Assendelft WJ, Devillé WL, Korthals-de Bos IB, Bouter LM. Corticosteroid injections, physiotherapy, or a wait-and-see policy for lateral epicondylitis: a randomised controlled trial. *The Lancet.* 2002;**359**(9307):657–62.

Elbow instability

Instability of the elbow may be acute, chronic, or recurrent. An acute traumatic dislocation is common and may lead to chronic instability. (Also see ➲ Chapter 18, Adult elbow injuries, pp. 595–596.)

Anatomy and pathology

The elbow is a complex hinge joint, consisting of three articulations within a common joint capsule:

- Ulno-humeral joint
- Radio-capitellar joint
- Proximal radioulnar joint.

Stability is provided by the bones, the joint capsule, muscular action, and the ligamentous restraints. Important ligaments are the MCL (especially its anterior band) and lateral ligament (which consists of the lateral ulnar collateral ligament (LUCL), annular ligament, and radial collateral ligament, with the LUCL being the most important), which form the primary static stabilizers with the ulno-humeral articulation. Muscles that cross the elbow joint (anconeus, brachialis, triceps) act as dynamic stabilizers by applying a compressive force to the joint.

A dislocation is named according to the direction in which the radius and ulna move relative to the humerus—most commonly posterior or posterolateral (80%) after a fall onto the outstretched hand. Occasionally, the ulna and radius are separated by the injury (divergent dislocation).

Acute dislocation

Types of injury

- Open or closed.
- Simple—no associated fracture (50–60% of all dislocations).
- Complex—associated with fracture, commonly coronoid, radial head or neck, and capitellum or epicondyles.
- Terrible triad—dislocation with LUCL tear, and radial head and coronoid fractures. This has a bad reputation, with a predisposition to recurrent instability and poor prognosis.

Clinical evaluation

- History: mechanism of injury.
- Neurovascular status.
- Radiographs: AP and lateral views.
- MRI: assessment of soft tissue injuries.
- CT: assessment of bony injuries.

Management

- Closed reduction: by traction on forearm/countertraction on arm.
- Assess post-reduction stability.
- Repeat radiographs to ensure concentric reduction.
- If soft tissue dislocation, with no fractures, then no immobilization is required and early ROM is advised.
- Splint elbow in 30–90° flexion in unstable injuries, for 5–10 days, followed by early therapy for simple soft tissue injuries.

Post-reduction management
- Simple: if stable after reduction, mobilize early (7–10 days in splint). Can then start active assist ROM with stable arc. Immobilization for >3 weeks results in poor ROM outcomes.
- Complex: fractures may require internal fixation; radial head/neck fractures require replacement if not reconstructable. Coronoid fractures of <10% in size do not require repair. If instability persists after ORIF, then address the need for ligament repair/reconstruction or hinged external fixation.

Chronic instability

This is an uncommon condition that can be secondary to:
- Repetitive trauma in the throwing athlete—usually to the MCL complex, producing valgus instability
- Previous elbow dislocation
- Inflammatory arthropathy.

Posterolateral rotatory instability
Usually a consequence of insufficiency of the LUCL. Symptoms may be elbow pain, clicking, or clunking. Examination may reveal no abnormality, but the lateral pivot-shift test (or difficulty with pushing off an armchair) may reveal the instability.

Treatment of chronic instability
- Activity modification.
- Bracing for provocative activities.
- Ligament reconstruction or repair.

Further reading

O'Driscoll SW, Jupiter JB, King GJ, Hotchkiss RN, Morrey BF. The unstable elbow. *Journal of Bone and Joint Surgery.* 2000;**82**(5):724.

O'Driscoll SW, Jupiter JB, King GJ, *et al.* The unstable elbow. *Instructional Course Lectures.* 2001;**50**:91.

Savvidou OD, Koutsouradis P, Kaspiris A, *et al.* Displaced olecranon fractures in the elderly: outcomes after non-operative treatment: a narrative review. *EFORT Open Reviews.* 2020;**5**:391–7.

Watts AC, Singh J, Elvey M, Hamoodi Z. Current concepts in elbow fracture dislocation. *Shoulder and Elbow.* 2021;**13**(4):451–8.

Radioulnar synostosis

Bony union of the radius and ulna limiting forearm rotation is a rare condition seen most commonly after high-energy comminuted forearm fractures. May also occur as a congenital abnormality.

Congenital radioulnar synostosis

Due to *in utero* failure of longitudinal segmentation of the radius and ulna (4–7 weeks). Usually affects proximal forearm (lack of forearm rotation); may not present until late childhood or adolescence; 60% bilateral. Usually sporadic. One-third of cases associated with other skeletal abnormalities.

Anatomy and pathology

Range of synostosis from proximal fibrous union to total synostosis of the radius and ulna. Limits forearm rotation; commonest clinical presentation is a fixed pronation deformity.

Investigations

- *Radiographs:* AP and lateral.
- *CT:* if uncertain whether fibrous or bony union.

Management

Often no treatment needed as patients compensate well with shoulder movement. Surgery is considered in severe cases, usually when fixed in marked pronation. Surgical excision of synostosis with soft tissue interposition often fails due to re-fusion. Rotational osteotomy to a more functional position (20–30° supination) may yield better results.

Post-traumatic radioulnar synostosis

Occurs with 3–9% of forearm fractures. Seen mostly in association with the following factors:

- High-energy injury/polytrauma/open fractures
- Head injury
- Both bone fractures being at same level/ORIF of both through single incision
- Delayed fixation.

Management

Surgical resection indicated for mature (4–6 months old) post-traumatic synostosis that impairs function. Can supplement with interposition of inert material (synthetic material, fat graft), irradiation, or indomethacin to prevent recurrence. Outcomes poor, except in mid-shaft disease.

Further reading

Cleary JE, Omer Jr GE. Congenital proximal radio-ulnar synostosis. Natural history and functional assessment. *Journal of Bone and Joint Surgery.* 1985;**67**(4):539–45.

Dohn P, Khiami F, Rolland E, Goubier J-N. Adult post-traumatic radioulnar synostosis. *Orthopaedics and Traumatology: Surgery and Research.* 2012;**98**(6):709–14.

Chapter 14

Adult orthopaedics: wrist and hand

Osteoarthritis of the wrist and hand

Wrist

Clinical

OA of the wrist usually follows trauma (e.g. post-fractured scaphoid non-union advanced collapse (SNAC) or osteonecrosis, scapholunate ligament disruption—scapholunate advanced collapse (SLAC)) or other instability patterns (e.g. as a sequela of Kienböck's disease of the lunate). Pain and stiffness are usual complaints, resulting in reduced function, affecting both employment and hobbies. Grip strength is reduced. Pronation and supination may be maintained if the distal radioulnar joint (DRUJ) is preserved, but other movements are reduced.

Investigations

Radiographs show arthritic changes that may initially be localized to one articulation.

Management

- *Non-operative:* depends on site of degenerative change and patient's requirements. Includes analgesia/NSAIDs and intra-articular corticosteroids. Splintage is often therapeutic and also simulates wrist fusion if this is being considered (can serve as a trial to aid in decision-making).
- *Operative:*
  - Wrist denervation (AIN/PIN neurectomy)
  - Radial styloidectomy
  - Proximal row carpectomy
  - Fusion—can be partial or complete. Partial fusions (e.g. 4-corner) retain some movement, but complete transcarpal (wrist) fusion has a more predictable outcome. The position is chosen after a careful assessment of the patient's needs
  - Wrist arthroplasty—classically reserved for low-demand patients with inflammatory arthropathy, although indications are growing as implant technology evolves.

Hand

Clinical

Most commonly affected hand joints are finger DIPJs and thumb CMCJ. IPJ OA can present with pain, stiffness, deformity (DIPJ osteophytes—Heberden's nodes, PIPJ—Bouchard's nodes), or mucous cysts (a ganglion-like cyst arising from a degenerate joint).

Investigations

- Radiographs of the hand—PA and oblique views of the hand, lateral views of digits, Robert's view of the thumb.

Management

- *Non-operative treatment:* analgesia, thumb spica splintage, corticosteroid injections, and hand therapy may be beneficial.
- *Operative options:* surgical treatment options for IPJ OA include debridement, arthroplasty, and arthrodesis. For OA involving the thumb CMCJ, trapeziectomy ± ligament reconstruction or CMCJ arthroplasty may be indicated for advanced disease. CMCJ fusion is an option for young patients (<50 years) with high demands, as this may

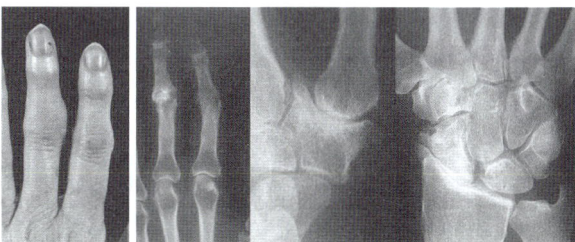

Fig. 14.1 Osteoarthritis of the fingers, thumb base, and wrist.

preserve some pinch strength, but outcomes are variable. No single technique has proven statistically superior for all patients; trapeziectomy is commonest and most established, while CMCJ arthroplasty is increasingly popular, with more rapid post-operative recovery and improving outcomes.

Further reading

Berber O, Garagnani L, Gidwani S. Systematic review of total wrist arthroplasty and arthrodesis in wrist arthritis. *Journal of Wrist Surgery*. 2018;**7**(5):424–40.

Davis TR, Brady O, Dias JJ. Excision of the trapezium for osteoarthritis of the trapeziometacarpal joint: a study of the benefit of ligament reconstruction or tendon interposition. *Journal of Hand Surgery*. 2004;**29**(6):1069–77.

Herren DB, Marks M, Neumeister S, Schindele S. Low complication rate and high implant survival at 2 years after Touch® trapeziometacarpal joint arthroplasty. J Hand Surg Eur Vol. 2023 Oct;48(9):877-883. doi: 10.1177/17531934231179581. Epub 2023 Jun 13. PMID: 37310049.

Wajon A, Vinycomb T, Carr E, *et al.* Surgery for thumb (trapeziometacarpal joint) osteoarthritis. *Cochrane Database of Systematic Reviews*. 2015;2:CD004631.

Watson HK, Ballet FL. The SLAC wrist: scapholunate advanced collapse pattern of degenerative arthritis. *Journal of Hand Surgery*. 1984;**9**(3):358–65.

Rheumatoid arthritis of the wrist and hand: clinical problems

(Also see ➲ Chapters 11 and 13.)

Wrist

Clinical

The effects of the disease on the joint and volar ligaments result in dissociation of the DRUJ and dorsal subluxation of the ulnar head. Reduction of this may be painful ('piano key' sign). The radiocarpal joint becomes eroded and subluxes volarly and ulnarward, and rotates into radial deviation. Must distinguish from extensor lag caused by PIN compression neuropathy (seen in RA due to elbow synovitis).

Management

- *Non-operative:* may include NSAIDs, immunosuppressive agents, remittive agents, and corticosteroids. Physiotherapy and occupational therapy to maintain movements. Splintage can be helpful.
- *Operative:* distal radioulnar resection at the distal ulna (Darrach procedure), hemiresection interposition technique, or fusion of the DRUJ and creation of pseudarthrosis in the distal ulna (Sauvé–Kapandji procedure). Radiocarpal reconstruction: tendon transfers, partial or total wrist arthrodesis, or wrist arthroplasty.

Hand

Clinical

Clinical problems that develop include (see Fig 14.2):

- MCPJ subluxation due to synovitis destroying the capsule and abnormal pull of tendons
- Swan neck deformities (hyperextension of the PIPJ and flexion of the DIPJ) due to laxity of volar structures at the PIPJ (volar plate, FDS) or dorsal structures at the DIPJ (mallet finger)
- Boutonnière deformity (flexion of PIPJ, with hyperextension of DIPJ) because of damage to the central slip over the PIPJ, allowing subluxation of the lateral bands of the extensor mechanism which hyperextend the DIPJ
- The thumb that can develop either swan neck or boutonnière deformity, or become unstable at the CMCJ or MCPJ.

Management

- *Non-operative:* may include NSAIDs, immunosuppressive agents, DMARDs, and corticosteroids. Physiotherapy and occupational therapy to maintain movements. Splintage can be helpful.
- *Operative:* soft tissue reconstruction, provided some cartilage is preserved and the deformity is flexible (synovectomy, tendon transfers, tendon relocation, capsular reefing). Arthroplasty or arthrodesis used in more advanced disease.

Patients with RA who require joint reconstruction or salvage procedures should be treated in a specialized hand unit.

Tendons

Clinical

Tendon ruptures occur due to attrition over bony prominences or is-chaemia in a fibro-osseous tunnel exacerbated by synovitis.

- *Vaughan–Jackson syndrome:* rupture of the digital extensor tendons over the DRUJ. Often begins with little digit tendon and tendons sequentially rupture from ulnar to radial.
- *Mannerfelt lesion:* rupture of the FPL tendon at the distal radius or scaphoid tubercle due to a bony spur.

Management

- Treated with tendon transfer or fusion (for advanced disease).

Nerves

Peripheral compressive neuropathies are common (e.g. carpal tunnel).

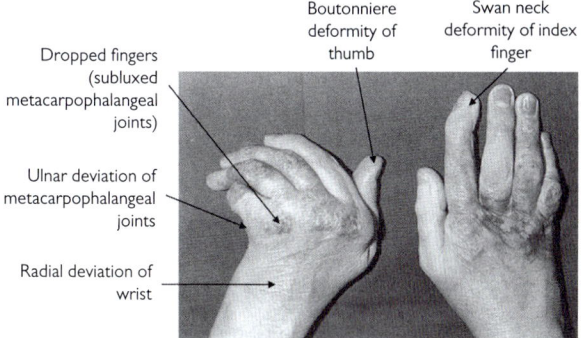

Dropped fingers (subluxed metacarpophalangeal joints)

Ulnar deviation of metacarpophalangeal joints

Radial deviation of wrist

Boutonniere deformity of thumb

Swan neck deformity of index finger

Fig. 14.2 Rheumatoid hand and wrist deformities.

Further reading

Hindley CJ, Stanley JK. The rheumatoid wrist: patterns of disease progression: a review of 50 wrists. *Journal of Hand Surgery.* 1991;**16**(3):275–9.
Trieb K. Treatment of the wrist in rheumatoid arthritis. *Journal of Hand Surgery.* 2008;**33**(1):113–23.

Avascular necrosis of the carpal bones

Most sporadic cases of AVN are of the lunate and scaphoid; others are rare.

Avascular necrosis of the lunate (Kienböck's disease)

Kienböck's disease (pronounced 'keen-bock'), or lunatomalacia, is an uncommon, but important, differential diagnosis of wrist pain. Management remains controversial as the natural history of the condition is unknown.

Anatomy and pathology
The lunate is the keystone of the carpus, transmitting 50% of compressive load across the wrist (80% load transmission via the radius, 20% via the ulna). Mostly covered by articular (hyaline) cartilage. Blood supply is usually by vessels entering the dorsal and volar poles, with a rich anastomotic (intraosseous) network within the bone; compromise causes AVN. Aetiological theories include (single/repetitive micro-) trauma and association with a relatively short ulna (negative ulnar variance).

Clinical evaluation
• Insidious onset of wrist pain, stiffness, and weakness often in the young adult. Localized dorsal lunate tenderness.

Investigations
• PA and lateral plain radiographs. MRI (low-signal change on T1).
• Arthroscopy can be helpful in determining the status and number of affected articular surfaces.

Management
Dependent on symptoms and radiographic/arthroscopic stage (Box 14.1; Fig. 14.3). See Bain and Begg classification reference in 'Further reading'.

Box 14.1 Imaging Classification of radiographic stages (Lichtman) and potential management options

• Stage I: no plain radiographic changes visible, changes seen on MRI only. Non-operative treatment → lunate unloading, steroid injections (pain relief).
• Stage II: sclerosis of the lunate, ↑ density. Radioscaphoid angle <60°. Consider radial forage, radial shortening (lunate unloading), revascularization.
• Stage III: sclerosis and fragmentation of the lunate—(1) radioscaphoid angle <60°; (2) radioscaphoid angle >60° (carpal collapse, prox migration of the capitate). Radial shortening (if no scaphoid rotation) or scaphoid-trapezium-trapezoid (STT)/scapho-capitate fusion, proximal row carpectomy (PRC).
• Stage IV: degenerative arthritis in adjacent joints. PRC, total wrist fusion

---

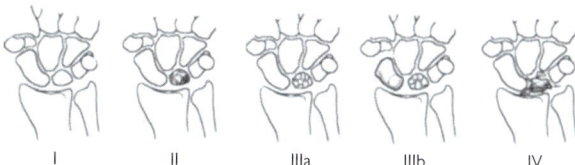

Fig. 14.3 Classification of radiographic stages (Lichtman).

Avascular necrosis of the scaphoid (Preiser's disease)

Preiser's disease (pronounced 'prizers') is a rare condition of idiopathic AVN. Scaphoid AVN is most commonly seen post-fracture (see ➲ Chapter 18, Adult Wrist Injuries - Scaphoid Fracture, p. 586). Average age of onset 40 years. May respond to immobilization. End-stage arthritis may require salvage procedures.

Further reading

Bain GI, Begg M. Arthroscopic assessment and classification of Kienbock's disease. Tech Hand Up Extrem Surg. 2006 Mar;10(1):8-13. doi: 10.1097/00130911-200603000-00003. PMID: 16628114.
Dias JJ, Lunn P. Ten questions on Kienböck's disease of the lunate. *Journal of Hand Surgery (European Volume)*. 2010;**35**(7):538–43.

Carpal instability

Carpal instability is a dysfunction of the carpus, and should be considered after any wrist trauma and in any case of chronic wrist pain.

Anatomy

The carpus comprises a proximal row (scaphoid, lunate, triquetrum) and a distal row (trapezium, trapezoid, capitate, hamate). The pisiform lies separately in the tendon of the FCU. The proximal row acts as an intercalated segment between the tightly bound distal row and the radiocarpal joint.

Intrinsic ligaments bind bones within the same carpal row. The important proximal row ligaments are the scapholunate and lunotriquetral ligaments. Extrinsic ligaments span >2 bones or the radiocarpal joint.

Kinematics

Flexion/extension can occur at both the radiocarpal and mid-carpal joints. During radial deviation, the scaphoid flexes and the triquetrum extends.

Classification of carpal instability

May be categorized by chronicity, severity (static or dynamic), aetiology, location (e.g. radiocarpal, mid-carpal, intercarpal), direction, or pattern.

Direction of instability
(Fig. 14.4)
- *Dorsal intercalated segment instability (DISI):* the lunate is angled dorsally (extends with an intact lunotriquetral ligament), scapholunate angle >70°. Causes: scapholunate dissociation, scaphoid fracture.
- *Volar intercalated segment instability (VISI):* the lunate is angled volarward (flexes with an intact scapholunate ligament), scapholunate angle <30°. Causes: lunotriquetral ligament disruption.

Patterns of instability
- *Carpal instability dissociative (CID):* within a row.
- *Carpal instability non-dissociative (CIND):* between rows.
- *Carpal instability combined (CIC):* both within and between rows.
- *Carpal instability adaptive (CIA):* secondary to pathology outside the carpus (e.g. malunion of a distal radius fracture).

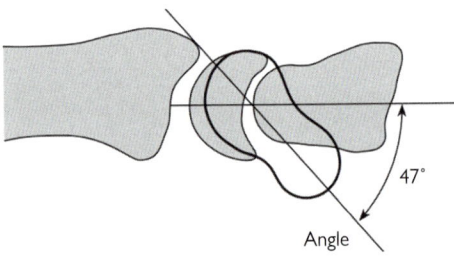

Fig. 14.4 Lateral scapholunate is measured by the angle subtended by the axes of the scaphoid and the lunate. The normal value is 47°, with a range of 30–60°.

Reproduced from Bulstrode *et al.*, *Oxford Textbook of Orthopaedics and Trauma*, with permission from Oxford University Press.

MAYFIELD CLASSIFICATION

Stage I   Scapholunate dissociation

Stage II   Stage II: + lunocapitate disruption

Stage III   Stage II: + lunotriquetral disruption, "perilunate"

Stage IV   Lunate dislocated from lunate fossa (usually volar), associated with median nerve compression

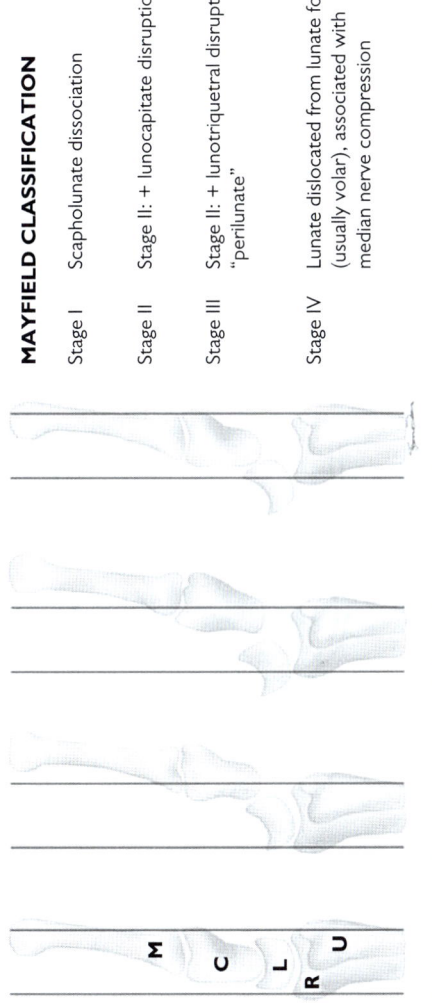

Normal   Perilunate dislocation   Mid-carpal dissociation   Lunate dislocation

Fig. 14.5 Spectrum of lunate/perilunate injuries and the Mayfield classification.

Mayfield classification

A classification of progressive perilunate instability (a CIC type). Ranges from stage 1 (scapholunate ligament tear) to 4 (lunate dislocation) (Fig. 14.5). Injuries do not always follow this pattern.

Clinical assessment

- History of an acute trauma, or failure of a 'wrist sprain' to resolve.
- Examination requires detailed palpation of wrist landmarks and assessment of neurovascular status.
- Be alert to median nerve compression in acute injuries.
- Special tests—for example, Watson's test for scapholunate instability (see ➲ Chapter 1, Hand and wrist examination, p. 15), Reagan's shuck test (shears the lunotriquetral joint).
- PA and lateral wrist plain radiographs: normal features—scapholunate angle = 30–60°. Smooth arc of carpal rows and Gilula's lines (Fig. 14.6). Scapholunate interval ≤3mm (widening (diastasis) of this interval = Terry Thomas sign).
- Magnetic resonance arthrogram (with contrast)/wrist arthroscopy may help in occult diagnosis.

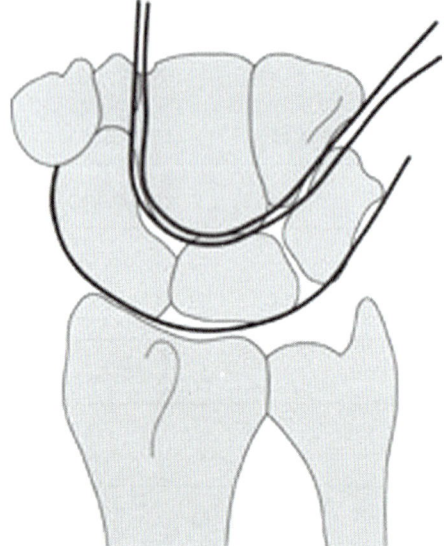

Fig. 14.6 Gilula's lines.

Reproduced from Bulstrode et al., *Oxford Textbook of Orthopaedics and Trauma*, with permission from Oxford University Press.

Management

- *Acute lunate/perilunate dislocation:* reduction, stabilization ± ligament reconstruction. Median nerve decompression as clinically indicated.
- *Acute ligament ruptures:* open repair and/or stabilization.
- *Chronic ligament disruptions:* options include ligament reconstruction, capsulodesis, and fusion procedures for irreducible deformity and/or degenerative change.

Complications

- Degenerative changes may occur in the intercarpal and radiocarpal joints (e.g. SLAC in chronic scapholunate dissociation).

Further reading

Larsen CF, Amadio PC, Gilula LA, Hodge JC. Analysis of carpal instability: 1. Description of the scheme. *Journal of Hand Surgery (American Volume)*. 1995;**20**:757–64.

Mayfield JK. Mechanism of carpal injuries. *Clinical Orthopaedics and Related Research*. 1980;**149**:45–54.

Schmitt R, Froehner S, Coblenz G, Christopoulos G. Carpal instability. *European Radiology*. 2006;**16**(10):2161–78.

Dupuytren's disease

Proliferative thickening and subsequent contracture of the palmar fascia of the hand. It is highly prevalent in the Scandinavian population (30% of men in Norway aged >60 years; 'Viking disease') and is also common in the UK (15% of men in England aged >60 years). Pre-contracture can present with palmar nodules and pitting. Most commonly affects the ring and little fingers.

Risk factors/aetiology

Genetics (family history, ♂ sex), age. Associations with smoking, alcohol, diabetes mellitus, AEDs, and climbing.

Anatomy and pathology

Dupuytren's disease affects the palmar and digital fascia of the hand. *Bands* of fascia are referred to as *cords* when affected.
- Pre-tendinous cords run longitudinally from the proximal palm to the base of the digit.
- The spiral cords are made up of the diseased pre-tendinous band, spiral band, lateral band, and Grayson's ligament. They pull the neurovascular bundle towards the midline, proximally, and superficially (Fig 14.7).
- Histology: the normal fascia is replaced by a proliferating fibroblast and myofibroblast population, producing cords of thicker—and, in the case of contracture, shorter—bands of fascia, with a higher type III-to-type I collagen ratio than normal.
- *Dupuytren's diathesis* is an aggressive form of the disease affecting younger individuals, (onset <50 years), radial sided disease, and ecoptic disease, including fibromatosis in the plantar fascia (Lederhosen's disease), penis (Peyronie's disease), and Garrod's (knuckle) pads.

Clinical evaluation

- Ask about risk/diathesis factors.
- Look and feel for cords, skin nodules, and pits in both hands.
- Assess symptoms, cosmesis, and function (face washing, ability to put hand in pocket or glove). Pain is usually absent.
- Measure MCPJ and PIPJ contracture. Screen for significant contracture by the ability to put the hand flat on the table (Hueston's tabletop test).
- Digital Allen's test to assess arterial supply to the fingers.

Management

- *Non-operative:* splintage has no proven benefit. Steroid injection may help with pain but does not affect contracture. Collagenase *Clostridium histolyticum* (CCH) are no longer readily available in the UK.
- *Surgery:* many options and factors to consider, including incisions, skin, fascia, and joints that all need to be dealt with. Aim is to improve function by straightening the digits, not to 'treat' as does not address the underlying cause (Figs 14.8 and 14.9):
  - *Incision:* Brunner zigzag or straight
  - *Fascia:* either needle (percutaneous) aponeurotomy or a small, curved palmar incision (segmental fasciectomy) for isolated pre-tendinous cord with predominantly MCPJ contracture. Alternative is limited fasciectomy (removal of fascia), which separates and protects

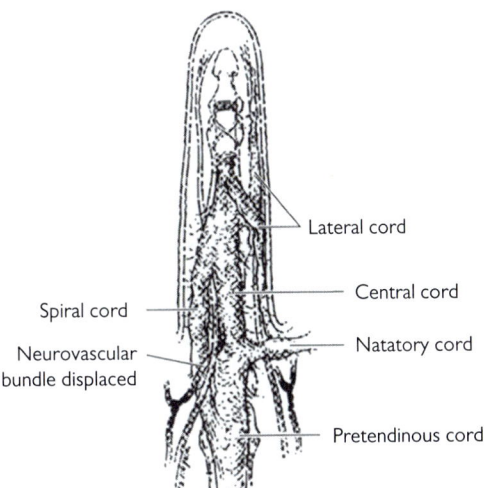

Fig. 14.7 Common patterns of fascia involvement.

Lateral cord

Central cord

Spiral cord

Natatory cord

Neurovascular
bundle displaced

Pretendinous cord

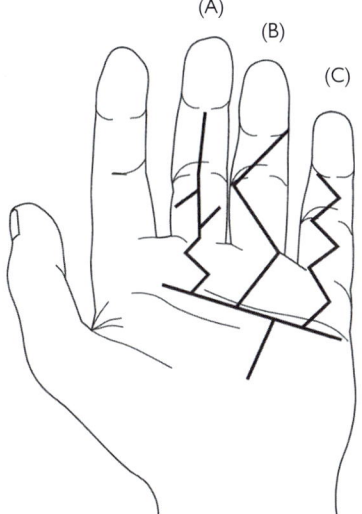

(A)

(B)

(C)

Fig. 14.8 Incisions for Dupuytren's fasciectomy. (A) Midline longitudinal incision converted to Z-plasty in the proximal segment of the finger. (B) Brunner zigzag incision. (C) Modified Brunner's incision.

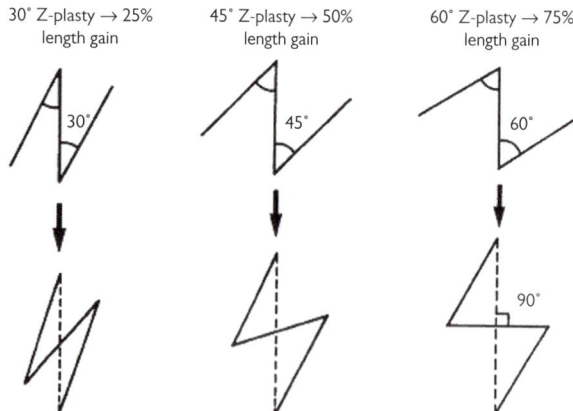

Fig. 14.9 Z-plasties to gain length after contracture release.

the neurovascular bundle removing diseased Dupuytren's tissue causing contracture
- *Skin:* small wounds, particularly in the palm can be left open (McCash open palm technique), if necessary, to heal by secondary intention. In the fingers, extra length can be gained by VY or Z-plasties. Skin grafts are sometimes required for coverage. A more radial technique, dermofasciectomy, aims to remove both skin and fascia, utilising a full thickness skin graft (FTSG) to act as a 'firebreak', to act as a 'firebreak' to try and prevent recurrence—especially with diathesis or recurrence. Post-op 3-months night splinting is common.
- *Joints:* almost any degree of MCPJ contracture is correctable. PIPJ contracture is more difficult to deal with. It may correct with passive manipulation; otherwise sequential releases (e.g. flexor sheath, palmar plate, accessory collateral ligaments) may be required.

Indications for surgery

Symptomatic significant or progressive contracture. Recurrence is common (>50% at 10 years) but may not require further surgery. Salvage procedures—PIPJ fusion, amputation.

Complications of surgery
- Delayed wound healing.
- Digital nerve or artery injury; chronic regional pain syndrome.
- Recurrence.
- Persistent or incomplete PIPJ correction.
- Loss of flexion (i.e. stiff, straight finger which may be more disabling than the original contracture).
- Infection.

Further reading

Dias, J., Tharmanathan, P., Arundel, C., Welch, C., Wu, Q., Leighton, P., Armaou, M., Johnson, N., James, S., Cooke, J. and Bainbridge, L., 2024. Collagenase Injection versus Limited Fasciectomy for Dupuytren's Contracture. The New England journal of medicine, 391(16), p.1499.

Dias JJ, Aziz S. Fasciectomy for Dupuytren contracture. *Hand Clinics*. 2018;**34**(3):351–66.

Dias JJ, Braybrooke J. Dupuytren's contracture: an audit of the outcomes of surgery. J Hand Surg Br. 2006 Oct;31(5):514-21. doi: 10.1016/j.jhsb.2006.05.005. Epub 2006 Jul 11. PMID: 16837113.

McGrouther DA. The microanatomy of Dupuytren's contracture. Hand. 1982 Oct;14(3):215-36. doi: 10.1016/s0072-968x(82)80055-7. PMID: 7152372.

Smith P. Dupuytren's disease. In: *Lister's The Hand*, 4th edn. London: Churchill Livingstone, Harcourt Publishers, 2002.

Ullah AS, Dias JJ, Bhowal B. Does a 'firebreak' full-thickness skin graft prevent recurrence after surgery for Dupuytren's contracture?: a prospective, randomised trial. J Bone Joint Surg Br. 2009 Mar;91(3):374-8. doi: 10.1302/0301-620X.91B3.21054. PMID: 19258615.

Upper limb nerve compression neuropathies

A peripheral nerve consists of the axons of sensory, motor, and autonomic nerves supported by Schwann cells producing myelin sheaths and connective tissue with a rich vascular supply. Various substances travel along the axons from the cell body in the dorsal root ganglion (sensory) or anterior horns of the spinal cord (motor). Anything disrupting this transport or the vascular supply of the nerve results in dysfunction.

Entrapment syndromes occur when compression of the nerve is present in one of the fibrous, muscular, or osseous tunnels through which the nerve passes. The nerve may be surrounded by fibrosis.

Specific nerve entrapments can occur at almost any point along the course of a nerve, so it is vital to know the normal anatomy and common variants of the peripheral nervous system.

Although most upper limb nerve entrapments are idiopathic, there are several conditions which can predispose to developing neuropathy or cause swelling in the tissues surrounding the nerve.

- Predisposing conditions to exclude: diabetes mellitus, alcoholism, B12 deficiency, and medications.
- Triggers of nerve compression: synovitis due to rheumatoid disease or other causes, pregnancy, myxoedema (hypothyroidism), space-occupying lesions (SOLs), fibrous bands.

Treatment of these conditions usually relieves the compression, and symptoms associated with pregnancy usually resolve with childbirth.

The differential diagnosis includes viral neuritis and radiation neuritis.

Clinical

Presenting features of nerve root entrapment include:
- Pain—often poorly localized to the area of compression or the course of the nerve
- Paraesthesiae—the exact site of 'pins and needles' can be crucial in the diagnosis, as the distribution reflects the sensory innervation distal to the site of compression
- Numbness—↓ or loss of sensation in the innervated region. Can be quantified with threshold testing by using filaments of various thickness (Semmes–Weinstein monofilaments)
- Weakness of innervated motor units—a late sign or symptom as other motor units hypertrophy to compensate
- Others—swelling, soft tissue wasting (pulp of digits), altered temperature or hydration, stiffness, loss of dexterity.

Provocative tests—these are positive if they reproduce the symptoms with which the patient presents. Percussion over the nerve produces an electric shock-like pain in the distribution of that nerve, suggesting an underlying degenerative lesion (Tinel's sign). Compression of the nerve with digital pressure or a joint position which reduces the size of the fibro-osseous canal may also reproduce the symptoms.

Investigations

- Plain radiographs—with abnormal presentations may reveal bony protuberances which may compress the nerve.
- USS/MRI—may reveal fibrous bands or a SOL causing compression.
- Neurophysiology—may show slowing of conduction across the region of compression (normal in upper limb is >50m/s), suggesting demyelination. Reduced amplitude implies loss of the total number of axons available (see ➜ Chapter 2, Investigations, p. 55). EMG may reveal denervation fibrillation potentials. Normal tests do not exclude compression, and vice versa. EMG testing may suggest cervical radiculopathy (nerve root compression) and a 'double crush' of the peripheral nerve.

Management

- *Non-operative:* once the site of compression has been identified, the entrapment can be addressed.
  - Physiotherapy—aimed at stretching tight muscles or bands. Nerve gliding exercises are tailored to individual nerves and may promote improved perfusion of the nerve.
  - Splintage—especially night splintage. Prevents patient from adopting provocative postures such as wrist flexion compressing the median nerve or elbow flexion compressing the ulnar nerve. Splints may be off-the-shelf or custom-moulded for the patient.
  - Steroid injection—around the nerve. Can reduce inflammation. Useful if there is evidence of synovitis.
- *Operative:*
  - Surgical decompression or transposition. Common syndromes usually respond well to decompression at the site of compression; the same is not true for less common syndromes.
  - Surgery usually results in rapid relief of paraesthetic symptoms. Sensory and motor losses take longer to recover and may do so only incompletely. It is important to warn patients of this.
  - Long-standing motor deficits may not recover, and nerve/tendon transfers may be required to restore function.

Specific nerve entrapment: median nerve

Proximal compression

- May involve the whole nerve or just the AIN which has no cutaneous sensory distribution.

Anterior interosseous syndrome

- Testing the AIN involves getting the patient to form an 'O' with their index finger and thumb (the 'OK' sign) and to pinch hard. Hyperextension of the IPJ of the thumb and DIPJ of the index finger occurs due to weakness of the FPL and FDP to the index finger. The PQ is also supplied by the AIN, and its strength can be assessed with resistance to pronation of the forearm, with the elbow in flexion.
- Treat non-operatively: symptoms resolve by 18 months, so patient counselling is important. There is no indication for exploration.

Pronator syndrome

Compression of the median nerve occurs where it passes between the two heads of the pronator muscle. Forearm pain is usually caused or worsened by resisted flexion of the elbow, with the forearm pronated. The syndrome requires surgery if muscle weakness persists despite non-operative care. Rarely may need to explore the area between the heads of the pronator muscle, lacertus fibrosus, and arch of the FDS.

Other sites of compression
- Supracondylar spur, ligament of Struthers, proximal edge of the FDS.
- Carpal tunnel (see ⮌ Chapter 14, Carpal tunnel syndrome, pp. 444–446).

Specific nerve entrapment: ulnar nerve

Proximal compression: cubital tunnel syndrome
The ulnar nerve can be compressed by the following: in the arcade of Struthers, between Osborne's ligament and the MCL, and between the two heads of the FCU muscle.
- *Clinical:* the patient complains of pain or paraesthesiae in the ulnar one-and-a-half digits on the palmar aspect of the hand, but also more proximally, including the dorsal ulnar border of the hand supplied by the dorsal branch of the ulnar nerve. Symptoms worsen with elbow flexion such as holding a phone or magazine. Patients may be woken from sleep with symptoms. Wasting of the intrinsic muscles of the hand (excluding those supplied by the median nerve) can be seen in the space between the metacarpals ('guttering'), especially in the first webspace. Froment's test examines this specifically and is positive if thumb adduction is replaced by flexion at the IPJ by the FPL. Claw hand leads to hyperextension of the MCPJs and flexion of the PIPJs of the ulnar two digits due to unopposed action of the FDS and FDP tendons.
- *Management:* prolonged elbow flexion should be avoided. If splintage and physiotherapy fail to relieve symptoms, surgical options are decompression with or without transposition (subcutaneous or submuscular) and with or without medial epicondylectomy. Occasionally, the ulnar nerve subluxes over the epicondyle, with elbow flexion causing symptoms. This must be excluded before operations are performed around the elbow.

Distal compression: Guyon's canal—ulnar entrapment syndrome
- *Clinical:* entrapment at this site may produce motor signs, sensory signs, or both due to branching of the nerve in the canal—altered sensation, pain, or weakness. Hyperaesthesia in the ulnar two digits, muscle atrophy, and reduced filling of the ulnar artery may occur.
- *Management:* rest and immobilization, and avoidance of repetitive trauma. Surgical decompression if symptoms persist.
- Ulnar paradox—distal entrapment of the ulnar nerve produces a greater claw hand deformity, as the FDP is unaffected and so its action is unopposed.

Specific nerve entrapment: radial nerve

The radial nerve and its main branches—the PIN (a motor nerve) and superficial radial nerve (SRN) (a sensory nerve)—are less commonly involved in entrapment syndromes. *Aide-memoire:* 'FREAS'—*F*ibrous bands at the elbow, *R*adial recurrent vessels (leash of Henry), *E*xtensor carpi radialis brevis (fibrous border of the ECRB), *A*rcade of Frohse (the fibrous proximal border of the superficial portion of the supinator), Supinator (distal border).

Radial nerve: posterior interosseous nerve

- *Clinical:* compression of the PIN at the proximal edge of the supinator (arcade of Frohse) may produce a motor syndrome (PIN syndrome) with weakness of the ED or ECRB, or a sensory syndrome (radial nerve syndrome) with pain in the forearm (the PIN has sensory fibres from the wrist joint), but no sensory loss. The sensory syndrome must be differentiated from tennis elbow (see ➲ Chapter 13, Elbow epicondylitis, p. 420). The so-called 'Saturday night' palsy may develop from prolonged pressure on the radial nerve in the spiral groove.
- *Management:* most resolve spontaneously. Surgical decompression (rarely) if symptoms persist.

Specific nerve entrapment: suprascapular nerve

Entrapment of the suprascapular nerve occurs either as it passes under the transverse scapular ligament at the suprascapular notch or via mass effect (e.g. spinoglenoid ganglion cyst or labral tear) at the spinoglenoid notch. Investigate with MRI/NCS if unclear diagnosis.

- *Clinical:* rare condition. There may be a history of (repetitive) trauma (e.g. overhead activities). Patients present with deep, diffuse pain in the paravertebral area of the shoulder and wasting/weakness of: (1) either both the supraspinatus and infraspinatus muscles (suprascapular notch entrapment); or (2) only the infraspinatus (spinoglenoid notch entrapment).
- *Management:* can initially manage non-operatively with physiotherapy; surgical decompression if failure of non-operative management ± clear structural lesion on MRI.

Carpal tunnel syndrome

Carpal tunnel syndrome is a collection of clinical features due to compression of the median nerve as it passes beneath the transverse carpal ligament in the wrist.

Anatomy

The carpal tunnel is made up of a floor with carpal bones and a roof with the transverse carpal ligament running from the pisiform and hook of the hamate medially to the scaphoid tubercle and trapezium laterally. It transmits the median nerve, four tendons of the FDP, four tendons of the FDS, and one tendon of the FPL (Fig. 14.10).

Incidence

- 1 in 1000 per year; middle age; the commonest peripheral nerve entrapment.

History

- Typically, nocturnal dysaesthesia that wakes the patient and is relieved by shaking the hand or hanging it over the side of the bed.
- Pain or paraesthesiae when gripping (e.g. holding a steering wheel, telephone, or book).
- The paraesthesiae should be in the distribution of the median nerve: thumb, index, and middle fingers. There may be wrist pain ± proximal radiation, and patients have difficulty with performing fine tasks due to numbness (e.g. picking up a needle or doing up buttons).

Examination

- Blunting of sensation in the median nerve distribution (thenar eminence sensation should be intact—supplied by the palmar cutaneous branch of the median nerve, which originates proximal to the carpal tunnel).
- Weakness, even wasting, in the 'LOAF' muscles supplied by the median nerve distal to the carpal tunnel (lateral two lumbricals, opponens pollicis, abductor pollicis brevis—most reliably, flexor pollicis brevis).

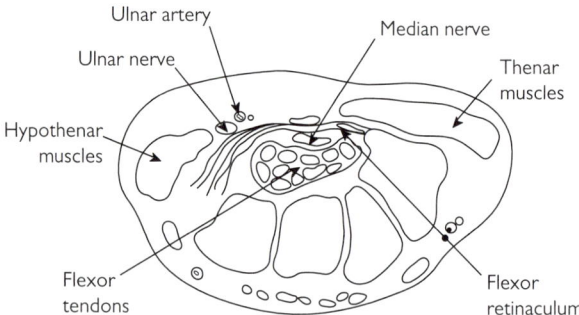

Fig. 14.10 Cross-section of the carpal tunnel.

- *Tinel's test:* tapping over the median nerve in, or just proximal to, the carpal tunnel produces tingling in the median nerve distribution or reproduces the patient's symptoms in a positive test.
- *Phalen's test:* hold both wrists fully flexed for 1min; a positive test provokes paraesthesiae in the median nerve distribution. Applying direct pressure over the median nerve with the wrist in the flexed position may reinforce this test (*Durkan's test*).
- Exclude other causes of wrist pain (e.g. De Quervain's, basal thumb OA) and other causes of neurological symptoms (e.g. thoracic outlet compression syndrome, cervical root impingement).

Investigations

- *Neurophysiology:* nerve conduction velocity is reduced across the carpal tunnel, with ↑ latency and reduced amplitude. Often not required in clinically clear cases of primary carpal tunnel syndrome, but use varies across centres; most helpful in investigating recurrence or if unclear clinical picture (including 'double crush' phenomenon—compression of nerve at neck and carpal tunnel or combined carpal/cubital tunnel compression).
- *Steroid injection:* both diagnostic and therapeutic (see ➲ Management below). Unclear mechanism of action, as this is not an inflammatory condition.

Causes of carpal tunnel syndrome

Idiopathic (majority) 'sick' nerve; wrist ratio (more 'square' wrists, i.e. an individual's anatomy), ♀ sex, and obesity are predisposing factors. Associations with trauma (distal radius fracture, lunate/perilunate dislocation), endocrine/inflammatory/autoimmune pathology (Cushing's disease, RA, myxoedema—hypothyroidism, acromegaly, amyloidosis, diabetes, sarcoid, SLE), compressive mass lesions (tumours, ganglia), and pregnancy.

Management

- *Non-operative:*
  - Nocturnal neutral position wrist splints may help with night symptoms and may be worn for daytime provocative activities.
  - Steroid injections into the tunnel (not into the nerve) may provide relief in the early stages (<6 months from onset).
- *Operative:*
  - Open decompression—longitudinal release of the transverse carpal ligament in line with the radial border of the ring finger. Soft tissue dissection superficial to the ligament should be performed with care to avoid damage to the palmar cutaneous branch of the median nerve. Release from distal fat pad to 2-3cm proximal to wrist crease.
  - Arthroscopic (endoscopic) or USS-guided decompression—not universally performed (learning curve), but evidence suggests possible quicker return to function and good patient satisfaction.
  - Complications: infection, pillar pain, wound problems, weakness, nerve damage, CRPS, recurrence (<10%).

Prognosis

Aim of surgery is primarily to relieve paraesthesiae, and secondarily to prevent further sequelae of prolonged nerve compression. Duration of symptoms may not influence the final functional outcome after surgery. Preoperative severity does seem to indicate a worse final outcome, but surgery is still beneficial; most patients are satisfied, despite surgery not necessarily resolving all symptoms. Weakness and numbness may not always recover, as these are usually secondary to more significant or chronic nerve compression/damage. In refractory peripheral nerve compression cases, consider clinical genetics referral for Hereditary Neuropathy with Liability to Pressure Palsies (HNPP) testing (alteration on chromosome 17 affecting the PMP22 gene).

Further reading

Agee JM, McCarroll Jr HR, Tortosa RD, Berry DA, Szabo RM, Peimer CA. Endoscopic release of the carpal tunnel: a randomized prospective multicenter study. *Journal of Hand Surgery*. 1992;**17**(6):987–95.

Burke FD, Wilgis EF, Dubin NH, *et al*. Relationship between the duration and severity of symptoms and the outcome of carpal tunnel surgery. *Journal of Hand Surgery (American Volume)*. 2006;**31**:1478–82.

Moghtaderi A, Izadi S, Sharafadinzadeh N. An evaluation of gender, body mass index, wrist circumference and wrist ratio as independent risk factors for carpal tunnel syndrome. *Acta Neurologica Scandinavica*. 2005;**112**(6):375–9.

Padua, L., Coraci, D., Erra, C., Pazzaglia, C., Paolasso, I., Loreti, C., Caliandro, P. and Hobson-Webb, L.D., 2016. Carpal tunnel syndrome: clinical features, diagnosis, and management. *The Lancet Neurology*, 15(12), pp.1273-1284.

De Quervain's syndrome

This is a painful disorder of the first extensor compartment. The cause is unknown; overactivity is not causal but often aggravates symptoms. Commoner in ♀ (may arise during/after pregnancy).

Anatomy and pathology

Affects APL and EPB (first dorsal compartment of the wrist) (Fig. 14.11). May be fibrillation or delamination of the tendon surface with collagen fibril thickening and fibrocartilage metaplasia. Not an inflammatory condition (cf. often referred to as 'tenosynovitis', a misnomer).

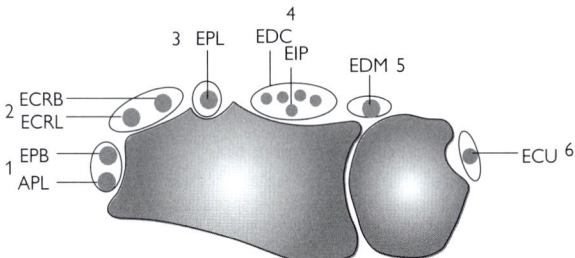

Fig. 14.11 The six extensor compartments of the wrist.

Clinical evaluation

- Pain, swelling, tenderness over first dorsal compartment; worse during thumb use (especially resisted extension).
- Special provocative tests: Eichhoff's (patient actively places thumb within the hand and clenches tightly with the other fingers; hand is then passively abducted ulnarward by the examiner) and Finkelstein's (place patient's wrist on the table edge, examiner asks the patient to actively ulnarly deviate the wrist before grasping the patient's thumb and passively flexing it into the palm); latter is less uncomfortable and more specific.
- Exclude other causes of dorso-radial wrist and thumb base pain (basal thumb arthritis, scaphoid injury, radio-carpal osteoarthritis).

Management

- *Non-operative:*
  - Rest, analgesia, ice
  - Splintage with thumb immobilization (thumb spica or gauntlet splint)
  - Steroid injection (avoid subcutaneous injection—leads to skin atrophy and depigmentation), beware multiple sub-sheaths and tendon slips, especially of APL, which may limit efficacy.
- *Operative (surgical release of first extensor compartment):*
  - Skin incision over compartment (transverse or longitudinal) under LA, avoid superficial branches of the radial nerve (damage may result in neuroma), longitudinal dorsal release of the compartment and any subsheaths/compartments.

Further reading

Finkelstein H. Stenosing tendovaginitis at the radial styloid process. *Journal of Bone and Joint Surgery (American Volume)*. 1930;12:509–40.

Wu F, Rajpura A, Sandher D. Finkelstein's Test Is Superior to Eichhoff's Test in the Investigation of de Quervain's Disease. J Hand Microsurg. 2018 Aug;10(2):116-118. doi: 10.1055/s-0038-1626690.

Triangular fibrocartilage complex

The TFCC is a collection of structures at the ulnar side of the wrist. Its role is to bridge/support the DRUJ and ulno-carpal joint, particularly during movements (e.g. gripping, rotation).

Composition

Akin to the knee meniscus, the peripheral third is well vascularized, with the central portion being largely avascular. Components include:
- Dorsal and volar radioulnar ligaments (the TFCC starts whether these originate at the sigmoid notch of the radius and terminates where they converge and insert at the base of the ulnar styloid)
- Ulnar collateral ligament
- Ulnolunate and ulnotriquetral ligament origins
- Central articular disc
- Meniscus homologue
- ECU (extensor carpi ulnaris) tendon subsheath.

Triangular fibrocartilage complex tears

Ulnar wrist pain (e.g. turning a key), weakness, clicking. History of trauma may be present. Note tenderness in soft spot (between ulnar styloid and FCU tendon, volar aspect of ulnar head and pisiform); pain on wrist ulnar deviation (TFCC compression), or radial deviation (TFCC tension). Exclude differentials: ulnocarpal abutment/impaction, ulnar styloid fracture, ulnar nerve entrapment (Guyon's canal) hook of hamate fracture, pisotriquetral arthritis, ECU tendon subluxation.

Classification

Contrast MRI and/or arthroscopy help classification (table 14.1) and management.

Table 14.1 Palmer classification of TFCC injuries.

Type 1—traumatic	
1A	Central perforation or tear
1B	Ulnar avulsion (without ulnar styloid fracture)
1C	Distal avulsion (origin of UL and UT ligaments)
1D	Radial avulsion
Type 2—degenerative	
2A	TFCC wear and thinning
2B	Lunate and/or ulnar chondromalacia + 2A
2C	TFCC perforation + 2B
2D	Ligament disruption + 2C
2E	Ulnocarpal and DRUJ arthritis + 2D

DRUJ, distal radioulnar joint; TFCC, triangular fibrocartilage complex; UL, ulnolunate; UT, ulnotriquetral.

Management

- *Non-operative:* all acute type 1, all type 2—widget/Futuro splint, analgesia (NSAIDs), steroid injection, physiotherapy (ECU/pronator quadratus strengthening).
- *Operative:* type 1A—arthroscopic debridement. Type 1B/C/D—open/arthroscopic repair (most regain movement and strength if injury <3 months). Type 2 (and ulnar positive variance)—ulnar shortening osteotomy; (no variance)—Wafer procedure. Type 2D—limited ulnar head resection. NB always evaluate and address bony problems first (e.g. malunion), and assess (e.g. arthroscopy) for degenerative change before considering TFCC repair procedures for instability.

The paralytic hand

Paralysis of any of the muscles of the hand leads to compromise of this vital functional unit. Assessment and treatment should occur within a specialist unit.

Anatomy and pathology

Causes of paralysis of the hand muscles are related to pathology of the CNS (e.g. cerebral palsy (CP)), brachial plexus, peripheral nerves, or muscles/tendons. The commonest aetiology is traumatic.

Clinical evaluation

A careful history and examination must be performed to identify the cause and muscles affected by the paralysis. Most importantly, the functional difficulties that the patient experiences in their ADLs and employment must be carefully evaluated.

Management

- Treatment must be directed towards clearly identified goals:
  - To prevent contractures
  - To preserve existing ROM and power
  - To maximize use of functioning units.
- *Non-operative:* occupational, hand and physiotherapy. Splints may often facilitate certain functions (e.g. splinting a wrist drop in extension aids in grip strength).
- *Operative* (for CP, see ➲ Chapter 14, Cerebral palsy: hand problems, p. 453):
  - Consider nerve transfers, tendon transfers (Table 14.2), or arthrodesis. Aim is to replace/restore the function of a paralysed muscle unit and/or return balance to a paralysed hand.
  - Suitable donor nerves need to be available for nerve transfers; tissue equilibrium must be achieved before consideration of tendon transfer; arthrodesis (e.g. of the wrist) provides a good platform for more distal function.

Table 14.2 Common tendon transfers

Pathology	Functional loss	Tendon transfer
Ruptured EPL (e.g. distal radius)	Thumb extension	EIP transfer
EDM, EDC rupture (e.g. rheumatoid synovitis)	Finger extension	EIP transfer
Radial nerve palsy	Wrist extension	Pronator teres to ECRB
	Finger extension	FCU/FCR to EDC
	Thumb extension	Palmaris longus to EPL

EPL, extensor pollicis longus; EIP, extensor indicis proprius; EDM, extensor digiti minimi; EDC, extensor digitorum communis; ECRB, extensor carpi radialis brevis; FCU/FCR, flexor carpi ulnaris/radialis.

- *Key questions to ask are:*
  - What function is missing?
  - What is available for transfer?
  - How are these best combined?
  - Is the patient compliant with post-operative therapy?
- *Criteria for a transferable tendon:* synergism, supple overlying scar-free skin, expendable, with adequate amplitude strength, length, excursion, glide, and correct line of pull on a mobile joint.

Volkmann's contracture

Contracture and paralysis of the upper limb originally described in 1881 by Richard von Volkmann. It is due to muscle necrosis and fibrosis secondary to an untreated ischaemic insult.

Anatomy and pathology

Venous stasis and/or disruption to arterial flow lead to tissue ischaemia. Subsequent tissue oedema and swelling further compromise tissue blood supply, leading to further ischaemic muscle damage. The muscles most severely affected are the FDP and FPL, followed by the FDS and pronator teres.

Ischaemic nerve damage occurs, leading to irreversible sensory changes and motor paralysis.

Causes

- Vascular injury.
- Direct trauma.
- Compartment syndrome.

Management

The key to management of this condition is prevention. Volkmann's contracture is most frequently seen as the sequela to compartment syndrome. High vigilance and prompt intervention are vital in patients at risk of compartment syndrome, to avoid the irreversible changes of Volkmann's ischaemic contracture.

Injury phase

In the early stages of ischaemia, emergency steps should be taken to restore vascularity to the upper limb and, if necessary, perform fasciotomies to alleviate compartment syndrome.

Established contracture

Careful functional evaluation must be performed of this difficult condition by a specialist with an interest in this field. In most cases, non-operative management is indicated.

Cerebral palsy: hand problems

CP is an evolving disorder of movement, posture, and motor function due to a non-progressive abnormality in the immature brain. Upper limb involvement is present in all types of CP patients, and the hand is affected to a varying degree.

General evaluation

A MDT is required to manage CP patients—carers, occupational therapists and physiotherapists, social workers, paediatricians, and surgeons should all be involved in their assessment. This will be an ongoing process, over several visits, and over a significant period.

Hand function is affected by the condition of the rest of the upper limb and by the general neurological state. Surgery is therefore individualized and should be designed to meet very specific goals. Only a small proportion of patients with hand involvement can be helped by surgery.

Evaluation of the hand

Important elements of the examination include:
- Sensation—stereognosis, sensory thresholds (by using Semmes–Weinstein monofilaments), proprioception, temperature perception. A hand that is ignored may be insensate, and surgery is unlikely to restore function
- Muscle examination—strength, degree of spasticity, coordination for each major muscle. Also assess proximal control of the upper limb (i.e. shoulder and elbow function—for hand placement)
- Joints—determine if deformities are static (fixed joint contracture) or dynamic (correctable by overcoming spasticity or changing the position of adjacent joints)
- Note resting position of the hand and ability to grip and release.

Non-operative management

Daytime splinting usually impedes function, and spasticity is abolished in sleep. Splints and therapy are therefore most used post-operatively.

Goals of surgery

- To improve hand function—to allow grasp and release.
- To correct deformities that hinder hygiene, dressing, or mobilization.
- Cosmetic improvement.

Principles of surgery

- Spastic deformities respond best to soft tissue surgery. Surgery is less helpful in other forms of CP, unless arthrodesis is required for joint stability.
- Abnormal joints should be restored to a functional position.
- The muscular forces on that joint should be rebalanced to prevent recurrent deformities.

Operative options

- Lengthenings or releases—of tendon, musculotendinous junction, fractional lengthening of the muscle or release from its origin.
- Tendon transfer.

- Tenodesis.
- Joint procedures—joint excision, arthrodesis, or capsular release.

Common situations

- Wrist flexion deformity—dynamic deformities can be treated by flexor releases/lengthening and a tendon transfer. There are many motors that can be transferred to the ECRB (e.g. FCU, FCR, ECU). Release of the flexor–pronator origin has been used for more severe deformities. Wrist fusion reserved for severe contractures.
- Thumb-in-palm deformity—in the commonest type, release of the adductor pollicis ± Z-plasty of the webspace is required. With flexion deformities of the thumb, release of the FPB ± FPL is needed. Stabilization of the MCPJ may be necessary if it is in hyperextension. Thumb abduction may require augmentation by tendon transfer.
- Finger flexion deformities—require lengthening of the flexors and augmentation of finger extension (by the FDS, FCR, or FCU). If using the FDS, this can also power the wrist.
- Swan neck deformity of fingers (Fig. 14.12)—treated by central slip tenotomy or FDS tenodesis.

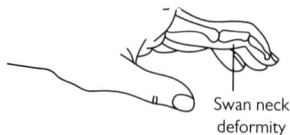

Swan neck deformity

Fig. 14.12 Swan neck deformity.

Reproduced from Davies, R, and Everitt, H, *Musculoskeletal Problems*, 2006, ISBN 978-0-19-857058-5, with permission from Oxford University Press.

Further reading

Saeed WR. Cerebral palsy of the upper extremity: the surgical perspective. *Current Orthopaedics.* 2003;**17**:105–16.

Trigger finger

Trigger finger, or stenosing tenosynovitis, is a common cause of pain and disability in the hand.

Anatomy and pathology

Trigger finger in the adult is due to nodular thickening on the flexor tendon, accompanied by stenosis of the first annular pulley (A1) at the level of the MCPJ. It is commonest in middle-aged ♀ and usually affects the ring finger, middle finger, and thumb. It is mostly idiopathic but is seen more commonly in rheumatoid, diabetic, and renal dialysis patients (amyloid deposition). Note that paediatric (often termed 'congenital') trigger thumb is a distinct entity in which children present with a flexion deformity of the thumb IPJ; if this does not resolve by the age of 4-6 years (increasingly being left until later), then A1 pulley release is indicated (note the proximity of the radial digital nerve).

Clinical evaluation

Patients present with painful nodule (grade 1), actively or passively releaseable, clicking (grade 2-3), or fixed locking (grade 4) of the finger in flexion/extension. Often the finger is found locked in the palm on waking and needs to be straightened by the opposite hand (often very painful). Although the patient often points to the IPJ as the problem, tenderness and palpable clicking are felt over the site of pathology at the A1 pulley.

Management

- *Non-operative:*
  - May resolve spontaneously (up to 50% by 1-2 years)
  - Night splintage in extension
  - Steroid injection of tendon sheath (60–70% success of first injection).
- *Operative:*
  - Indicated after failure of conservative management
  - Surgical release of the A1 pulley under local anaesthesia
  - Transverse or longitudinal skin incision over A1 pulley at MCPJ
  - Protect neurovascular bundle, then perform longitudinal release of A1 pulley
  - Consider regional anaesthesia in rheumatoid patients to allow for synovectomy.

Trigger thumb

Trigger thumb is commoner in young children and often presents with a painless flexion deformity of the IPJ. Initial treatment is with observation and/or night splintage; failure of resolution post-toddler years can be treated with surgery.

Further reading

Baek GH, Kim JH, Chung MS, Kang SB, Lee YH, Gong HS. The natural history of pediatric trigger thumb. J Bone Joint Surg Am. 2008 May;90(5):980-5. doi: 10.2106/JBJS.G.00296. PMID: 18451388.

Ganglia

Fluid-filled cysts which originate from a joint and usually present as sub-cutaneous lumps, which may fluctuate in size. They are most commonly found in the hand and account for 50% of all hand swellings. May not be the cause of the pain to which they are attributed (rather this may be due to underlying pathology such as microtrauma to the joint capsule from where they originate).

Presentation

• Dorsal wrist ganglia are the commonest and originate from the dorsal wrist capsule at the scapholunate interval. Usually only a cosmetic nuisance, but may cause discomfort with wrist extension.
• Palmar wrist ganglia are usually found on the radial side of the wrist and originate from the scapholunate or scaphotrapezial joint.
• Flexor tendon sheath ganglia are usually small, hard, tender lumps found over the proximal digital crease. May cause pain on gripping.
• Digital mucous cysts are a form of ganglia originating from an arthritic DIPJ. Present as swellings to the side of the midline at the base of the nail. Growth of the nail may be affected (ridging).
• Intraosseous ganglia are rare.

Examination

Transilluminate when sufficiently large. Usually non-tender and may be fluctuant/mobile, especially if attached to the joint by a long pedicle.

Investigations

• Usually none required.
• Radiographs may be useful in dorsal digital ganglia to show arthritic change in joints or to rule out other causes of pain.
• USS or MRI for occult ganglia.

Management

• Reassurance—most are best left alone and will resolve spontaneously (may take a few years).
• Historically, rupture was performed by a blow from the family Bible!
• Aspiration of the ganglion cyst contents can be reassuring for patients, but recurrence is common. Aspiration, then steroid injection probably does not reduce the incidence of recurrence (rates of up to 50%).
• For flexor sheath ganglia, aspiration is usually not advisable.
• For the recurrent symptomatic wrist ganglion, surgical excision of the sac, with excision of the pedicle back to the joint of origin, has a lower incidence of recurrence (recurrence rates may be around 30%).
• Digital mucous cysts can be excised, and the skin defect may need a local skin flap for coverage (do not treat the underlying cause which is DIPJ degenerative change; fusion if the joint is stiff and painful will prevent recurrence).

Further reading

Dias JJ, Dhukaram V, Kumar P. The natural history of untreated dorsal wrist ganglia and patient reported outcome 6 years after intervention. *Journal of Hand Surgery (European Volume)*. 2007;**32**(5):502–8.

Infection in the hand

Paronychia

Infection (usually *Staphylococcus aureus*) of the eponychial fold. Treatment involves release of pus under pressure by probing the nail fold or by formal incision and drainage under digital nerve block. Symptoms usually settle quickly. Oral antibiotics may hasten resolution.

Felon

Pulp space infection. Often exquisitely painful due to ↑ compartment pressure between unyielding fibrous septae of the pulp. Treat with incision and drainage through a mid-lateral incision, releasing septae from bone (approach from the ulnar side of the digit, except the thumb and little finger).

Bite injuries

- *Human bites*: often follow a punch injury over the knuckle ('fight bite'). MCPJ frequently violated, mandates formal exploration and irrigation. Plain radiograph to exclude fracture or tooth fragment in metacarpal head. Organisms include α-haemolytic *Streptococcus*, *S. aureus*, and *Eikenella corrodens*. All puncture wounds should receive antibiotics (e.g. co-amoxiclav (amoxicillin/clavulanic acid)), even if the joint/tendon sheath is not apparently involved.
- *Animal bites*: organisms include α-haemolytic *Streptococcus*, *Pasteurella multocida*, *S. aureus*, and anaerobes. Treatment similar to that for human bites; special care with cat bites, as sharp canines often puncture joint or tendon sheath, mandating surgical drainage.

Tendon sheath infection

- *Kanavel's cardinal signs:*
  - Fusiform (sausage) swelling
  - Flexed posture
  - Tenderness along tendon sheath
  - Pain on passive extension.

Early diagnosis and prompt treatment with elevation/IV antibiotics are essential. Open drainage and washout are required in most cases of tendon sheath infection. Delayed treatment can lead to fibrosis, joint contracture, or extension of infection to deep palmar spaces: index finger and thumb to the thenar space; middle, ring, and little fingers to the mid-palmar space.

Deep space infections

- *Webspace abscess:* form on either side of the transverse metacarpal ligament, leading to swelling on the palm and dorsum of the hand and abduction of the adjacent fingers. Drain through dorsal and volar incisions to avoid scars in the webspace, which heal with contracture. On the dorsum, infections may spread to the dorsal subaponeurotic space (fig 14.3).
- *Deep palmar infections:* thenar, mid-palmar, and hypothenar spaces; remember that the thumb and little finger bursae communicate proximal to the wrist (space of Parona), causing a 'horseshoe abscess'.

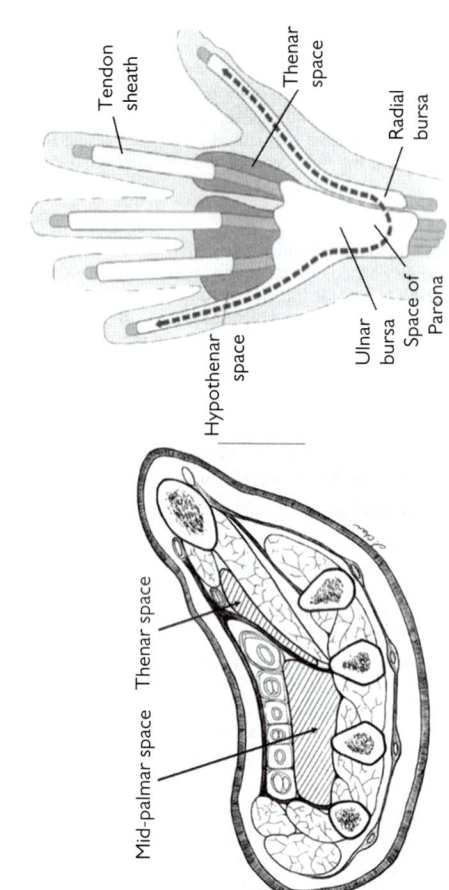

Fig. 14.13 Deep spaces of the hand.

Present as tender, boggy volar swellings, with pain on movement of tendons passing through the space. Treatment involves open drainage (palmar approach) followed by elevation and IV antibiotics. Splintage should be in the Edinburgh position (MCPJ flexed, IPJ extended) to avoid contracture of collateral ligaments and permanent stiffness.

Tumours of the hand

Hand tumours are common, but the vast majority are benign.

History

- *Age:* primary bone tumours occur in younger age groups. Metastatic tumours in older age groups.
- *Pain:*
  - Night pain—associated with neoplasia
  - Throbbing—associated with infection.
- *Trauma:* possible fracture callus or malunion.
- *Constitutional symptoms:* night sweats, malaise, fatigue, weight loss.
- *Family history:* multiple exostoses (HME), NF.
- *Past medical history:* malignancy, gout, RA.

Examination

Examine for site, size, shape, etc., as you would for any lump. Of particular relevance to the hand:

- Large ganglia may transilluminate.
- Check for mobility/tethering to adjacent structures.
- Always examine regional lymph nodes.

Investigations

- Blood tests: Ca^{2+}, ALP, uric acid, inflammatory markers.
- Blood cultures if patient pyrexial.
- Imaging:
  - Plain radiograph: to look for any bony involvement
  - MRI: gives excellent definition to the tumour—the gold standard
  - USS: to ascertain whether the tumour is cystic.
- Biopsy: often excisional, which may be the only treatment required.

Tumour classification

Non-neoplastic lesions

- Ganglion cyst—the commonest hand swelling (palmar or dorsal wrist ganglia, digital mucous cyst, ganglion of tendon sheath).
- Others (e.g. dermoid cyst).

Tumours of bone

- Benign: exostosis (may be multiple, think of HME), osteoid osteoma (occasionally occurs in phalanges/metacarpals).
- Malignant: osteosarcoma, Ewing's sarcoma—extremely rare.

Tumours of cartilage

- Benign: enchondroma (quite common, may be an incidental finding, if multiple—Ollier disease/Maffucci syndrome).
- Malignant: chondrosarcoma.

Tumours of vascular apparatus

- Benign:
  - Glomus tumour—usually under nail bed, exquisitely tender, gives bluish tinge (Love's and **Hildreth's tests**).
  - AV malformations—capillary haemangiomas (strawberry naevi/port-wine stain) or more substantial arterial/venous abnormalities.
- Malignant: haemangiosarcoma.

Tumours of nerves
- Benign: schwannoma/neurilemmoma.
- Malignant.

Tumours from other cell origin
- Benign: giant cell tumour of the tendon sheath (common, localized form of pigmented villo-nodular synovitis—treatment is excision).
- Malignant: synovial sarcoma, epithelioid sarcoma.

Tumours of skin cells
- Basal cell carcinoma.
- Squamous cell carcinoma.
- Melanoma.

Metastases
- Rarely present in the hand.

Further reading

Hsu CS, Hentz VR, Yao J. Tumours of the hand. *The Lancet Oncology*. 2007;**8**(2):157–66.

Adult orthopaedics: hip and knee

Osteoarthritis of the hip

A progressive, benign degenerative condition of the hip joint characterized by loss of articular cartilage and associated bone remodelling. This leads to progressive stiffness of the joint.

Incidence

One to 2% in those aged <55 years, with a slight ♂ preponderance. Over this age group, the literature suggests 8–10% of the population will have symptomatic hip OA, with the ratio skewed more towards ♀. The prevalence is much lower in black and Asian minority ethnicities (1–2%), compared with Caucasians, suggesting a genetic component. The lifetime risk of symptomatic hip OA is 18.5% for men and 28.6% for women.

Causes

- *Primary*: idiopathic, age-related change which may be associated with a strong family history, and genetic predisposition.
- *Secondary*: previous trauma, AVN, infection, prior paediatric conditions (Perthes' disease, DDH, SCFE).

History

- Persistent groin, thigh, or buttock pain frequently in the classic 'C' shape distribution. May be referred to anterior thigh or knee.
- Pain is exacerbated by activity, upon excessive weight-bearing, and at night when there is significant deterioration of the joint.
- Stiff movements, with loss of flexion and internal rotation first (e.g. limitation in putting on shoes and socks, or cutting toenails).
- Reduced walking distance due to pain, development of a stiff or limping gait.

Clinical features

- Antalgic or Trendelenburg gait, stiff circumduction in ankylosed hip.
- FFD, as revealed by Thomas' test.
- Reduced ROM, commonly loss of internal rotation.
- Trendelenburg sign (pelvic tilt on single leg stance—'lifted leg lags').
- Leg length measurements may show some discrepancy (especially if, for example, prior DDH or shortening after fracture).
- FABER test (*F*lexion to 90°, *AB*ducted hip, and *E*xternally *R*otated) can help to differentiate if SIJ pain is the main component.
- FADIR test (*F*lexion to 90°, *AD*duction, and *I*nternal *R*otation) is useful in assessing for anterior labral pathology and femoroacetabular impingement.

Investigations

- *Radiographs*: AP pelvis and lateral hip views. Mainstay of diagnosis, along with history and examination. Cardinal features include narrowing of joint space, subchondral sclerosis, subchondral cysts, and osteophyte formation. Shenton's line is a reliable method to assess subluxation of the joint. In cases of congenital or acquired anatomical difference, a reduced centre-edge angle (of Wiberg) is observed, along with a crossover sign, to suggest an altered acetabular version.

- *CT and 3D reconstruction:* may be useful in preoperative planning, especially if significant bone loss or abnormal anatomy.
- *MR arthrography:* may be useful in young patients if labral pathology or AVN is suspected, and hip preservation may be considered.
- *Bloods:* FBC, ESR, and CRP to rule out inflammation and infection.

Management

- *Non-operative:* activity modification, weight loss, walking aid in contralateral hand, physiotherapy (ROM, abductor strengthening exercises, and non-impact exercise programmes have good results in early OA), oral analgesics (stepwise escalation from non-opioid analgesics and NSAIDs to opioids). Image-guided steroid injections to temporarily relieve inflammation and pain or to differentiate hip vs back pain.
- *Operative:*
  - *Hip preservation:* femoral or acetabular osteotomy and realignment in the young where cartilage is still preserved. An underlying structural abnormality needs to be identified and targeted (e.g residual dysplasia leading to acetabular retroversion).
  - *Joint replacement:* total hip arthroplasty (THA) is the gold standard treatment for failed non-operative management, with good results. Hip resurfacing arthroplasty is still offered in select individuals, with close surveillance with regular imaging and serum metal ion levels. Ongoing debate on cemented vs uncemented techniques, implants (manufacturers), and choice of head/acetabulum bearings (e.g. metal/ceramic on polyethylene).
  - *Excision arthroplasty:* Girdlestone's procedure—removing the native joint, leaving behind a pseudarthrosis—poor mobility and function, infrequently used, mainly in immobile/unfit patients.
  - *Arthrodesis:* mainly historic, utilized in young patients or TB infection. Significant impact on function, hence not routinely used.

Complications of total hip replacement

Infection (1%), thrombosis (1–2%), dislocation of joint (1%), leg length discrepancy, periprosthetic fracture (dependent on implant type), nerve and vessel injuries (<1%; sciatic nerve most at risk), heterotopic ossification, future revision surgery. Primary THA early complication rate is low, with a very high satisfaction rate (>90%). Survivorship of modern implants at 10 years of ≥90% (see ℘ www.njrcentre.org.uk/).

Rheumatoid arthritis of the hip

The hip is a common joint to be affected by RA. The pathology starts as synovitis and soft tissue inflammation, leading to pannus formation and joint destruction. One per cent of all THAs in the UK in the over 50s are for RA. In the young, the rate is higher at 8%. Patients with RA tend to have a higher risk of fractures around the hip, in part due to medicinal side effects (e.g. steroid use) and associated osteopenia. Diagnosis is mainly clinical, with the American College of Rheumatology/European League Against Rheumatism (ACR/EULAR) criteria.

History

- Polyarthralgia, often with bilateral hip involvement.
- Patients may be younger in age.
- Morning stiffness.
- Severe restriction in movement.
- May have associated malaise and extra-articular signs.
- Current medication/DMARD use is important for surgical planning (biological agents are usually stopped preoperatively).

Clinical features

- May have generalized tenderness/pain around the hip, which is non-specific due to synovitis.
- Contracture of soft tissue may be present, leading to a fixed flexion deformity.
- Range of motion can be limited due to arthrosis or pain. Typically, internal rotation and adduction of the hip bear the worst pain.
- Assess for extra-articular features and association with medical treatment (e.g. osteopenia, fragile skin, respiratory symptoms, generalized muscle wasting, peripheral joint involvement).

Investigations

- *Bloods:* FBC, ESR, CRP.
- *RhF:* positivity is found in 80% of patients but may be absent in early disease. Anti-CCP is more specific for RA.
- *Radiographs:* classic signs are uniform joint space loss, periarticular osteopenia, and marginal erosions. Protrusio acetabuli is common in patients with hip RA and makes surgical management challenging. General survey of peripheral joints with radiographs to confirm diagnosis. C-spine examination/radiographs pre-anaesthesia to screen for atlanto-axial instability (risk of cord damage and neurology during positioning/airway manoeuvres for general anaesthesia).

Management

- *Non-operative:* patients may have radiographical deterioration with minimal symptoms if RA is under control. Close liaison with rheumatologists is important in optimizing control and providing pain relief and cartilage preservation. Modern biological therapies (and other DMARDs) have reduced the need for earlier surgical intervention. Physiotherapy to maintain joint movement and muscle strength.

Adjuvant support with occupational therapy and walking aids. Intra-articular steroid injections for temporary pain relief.
* *Surgical:* hip preservation surgery has not shown good results in RA. THR has a good clinical outcome, but the complication rate can be higher than THR in the context of OA, particularly with periprosthetic joint infection (PJI) (3–4%) and fracture. In protrusio, more complex reconstruction is required. Mid-term survivorship is equivalent to that of OA cases, but there is a higher rate of acetabular revision at 10 years, regardless of prosthesis type in RA, according to several studies.

Further reading

Mäkelä KT, Eskelinen A, Pulkkinen P, Virolainen P, Paavolainen P, Remes V. Cemented versus cementless total hip replacements in patients fifty-five years of age or older with rheumatoid arthritis. *Journal of Bone and Joint Surgery.* 2011;**93**(2):178–86.

Ranawat CS, Dorr LD, Inglis AE. Total hip arthroplasty in protrusio acetabuli of rheumatoid arthritis. *Journal of Bone and Joint Surgery (American Volume).* 1980;**62**(7):1059–65.

Osteonecrosis of the hip

Loss of blood supply to the femoral head, leading to pain, deterioration, and eventual collapse of the femoral head. Often referred to 'avascular necrosis', but the term 'osteonecrosis' is preferred as this does not allude to a particular underlying (ischaemic) pathophysiology. Progression can lead to secondary degenerative changes and significant loss of function. May be idiopathic or secondary to various risk factors. Regardless of aetiology, the histological picture is the presence of empty lacunae in the trabecular bone.

Epidemiology

Commoner in men. Typically presents in the late 30s to early 40s.

Risk factors

- Idiopathic (30%).
- Trauma.
- Corticosteroids—either low dose and long term or high dose and short term.
- Excessive alcohol intake.
- Coagulopathies and haemoglobinopathies (e.g. sickle-cell disease).
- Caisson's disease (decompression sickness).
- Gaucher's disease (lysosomal storage disorder).
- Viral illnesses (cytomegalovirus (CMV), hepatitis, HIV).
- Hyperlipidaemia.

Symptoms and signs

- Insidious groin pain, exacerbated by ambulation and activity.
- Pain may be severe for a few weeks and then subside.
- Pain usually present before radiographic changes.
- Stiffness.
- Early disease may be asymptomatic and incidentally noted on imaging.

Differential diagnosis

- Hip OA (but can get secondary osteonecrosis due to OA).
- Septic arthritis of the hip joint.

Classification

Various systems have been proposed, including Ficat and Arlet, Steinberg, and ARCO. The modified Ficat and Arlet systems aim to correlate symptoms with imaging and pathology.

- *Stage 0 (preclinical):* no symptoms, normal plain radiograph, no MRI changes.
- *Stage 1 (pre-radiological):* no or mild symptoms, normal plain radiograph; MRI may show bony oedema and early signs of ischaemia. Histology shows abundant dead marrow cells, osteoblasts, and osteogenic cells.
- *Stage 2 (pre-collapse):* mild symptoms, density changes in femoral head on plain radiograph, ↑ uptake on bone scan; MRI changes are classical signs. Sphericity remains of the femoral head. Classically pre-collapse stage.
- *Stage 3 (collapse):* loss of sphericity and collapse of femoral head, ↑ uptake on bone scan, subchondral fracture ('crescent sign'), collapse, compaction and fragmentation of necrotic segment, dead bone trabeculae and marrow cells on both sides of fracture line.

- *Stage 4 (degenerative):* moderate to severe symptoms, joint space narrowing with acetabular changes, ↑ uptake on bone scan, osteoarthritic changes with degeneration of acetabular cartilage.

Investigations
- *Plain radiographs*: changes seen later than MRI/bone scan (Fig. 15.1A).
- *MRI*: ↓ signal from ischaemic marrow on T1 images; double line sign on T2 images—100% sensitivity, 98% specificity (Fig. 15.1B).
- *Bone scan*: 75–80% sensitivity for stages 1 and 2. ↑ uptake on both sides of joint may suggest OA.
- *Single-photon emission CT (SPECT)*: 3D isotope scanning. Useful in mapping of osteonecrosis and treatment follow-up.

Management
Broadly divided into: (1) joint preservation if the patient is identified pre-collapse; and (2) reconstruction post-collapse.
- *Non-operative:*
  - Protective weight-bearing
  - Reversal of risk factors such as steroid use
  - Bisphosphonate use to delay collapse of femoral head.
- *Operative treatment* (Table 15.1):
  - Core decompression—with or without vascularized graft or implant (e.g. tantalum rod); main option if symptomatic pre-collapse

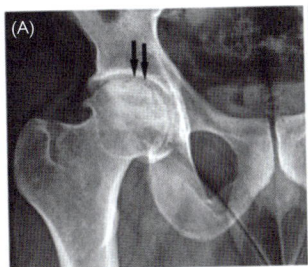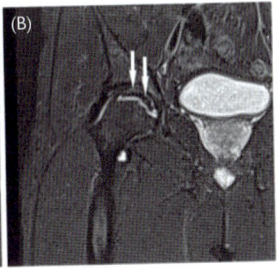

Fig. 15.1 Avascular necrosis of the hip. (A) Radiograph of the right hip (anteroposterior projection) showing a curvilinear radiolucent area just below the articular surface of the head of the femur, called the 'crescent' sign (arrows). (B) STIR sequence of MRI of the right hip (coronal section), showing hypointensity.

Table 15.1 Operative options for osteonecrosis of the hip

Treatment	Stage of disease
Decompression	Pre-collapse
Bone grafting	Pre-collapse
Osteotomy	Pre-collapse
Total hip replacement	Collapse/collapse with OA

- Bone grafting—vascularized or not, undertaken for pre-collapse
- Osteotomy—to offload AVN portion of femoral head in pre-collapse
- THR—post-collapse with associated degenerative changes. Patients should be counselled regarding a higher risk of revision the younger their age at time of surgery.

Further reading

Agarwala S, Jain D, Joshi VR, Sule A. Efficacy of alendronate, a bisphosphonate, in the treatment of AVN of the hip. A prospective open-label study. *Rheumatology*. 2005;**44**(3):352–9.

Ficat RP. Idiopathic bone necrosis of the femoral head. Early diagnosis and treatment. *Journal of Bone and Joint Surgery. (British volume)*. 1985;**67**(1):3–9.

Femoroacetabular impingement

Abnormal contact between the femoroacetabular joint surfaces, usually presenting with pain that is worse on hip flexion, secondary to a combination of asphericity/incongruency at the joint and resultant chondral/labral injury.

Epidemiology

Common in the general population and often asymptomatic. There may be a history of prior hip pathology (e.g. SCFE).

Pathophysiology

Two main types (can be combined) (Fig. 15.2):
- *Cam*: aspherical femoral head; broad head/neck bone, reduced head:neck ratio, reduced offset, retroversion. Asphericity causes chondrolabral junction shearing, resulting in labral detachment and delamination of the cartilage.
- *Pincer*: overhang of (anterosuperior) acetabulum; broad acetabular bone/labrum with overhang/overcoverage; acetabular retroversion or protrusio; coxa profunda. The femoral neck impinges onto the labrum, resulting in tears and associated cartilaginous injury.

Clinical features

- *Symptoms*: groin pain, worse on hip flexion (e.g. sports, sitting); clicking/grinding; altered gait (and associated pain at neighbouring joints).
- *Examination findings*: restricted ROM (flexion/internal rotation); FADIR pain (flexion, adduction, internal rotation).

Imaging

- *Radiographs*:
  - AP and true lateral views. Other views can be performed (e.g. Dunn lateral)
  - 'Pistol grip' deformity (cam); 'crossover sign' (acetabular retroversion with pincer); 'posterior wall sign'
  - Alpha angle (on frog-leg lateral radiograph): <42° normal (>50–55° suggests cam)
  - Head–neck offset ratio: >0.17 normal (<0.17 suggests cam)
  - Centre-edge angle of Wiberg: <40° normal (Fig. 15.3)
  - Acetabular index (Tonnis roof angle): >0° normal (Fig. 15.3).
- *CT*: aids in operative planning.
- *MRI/MR arthrography*: to evaluate cartilage lesions/labral tears.

Management

- *Non-operative*: analgesia (NSAIDs), activity modification, physiotherapy.
- *Operative*: hip arthroscopy (osteoplasty). Open surgical hip dislocation and osteoplasty (rarer now). Peri-acetabular osteotomy for acetabulum retroversion/dysplasia. Arthroplasty (THA) in the presence of symptomatic degenerative changes.

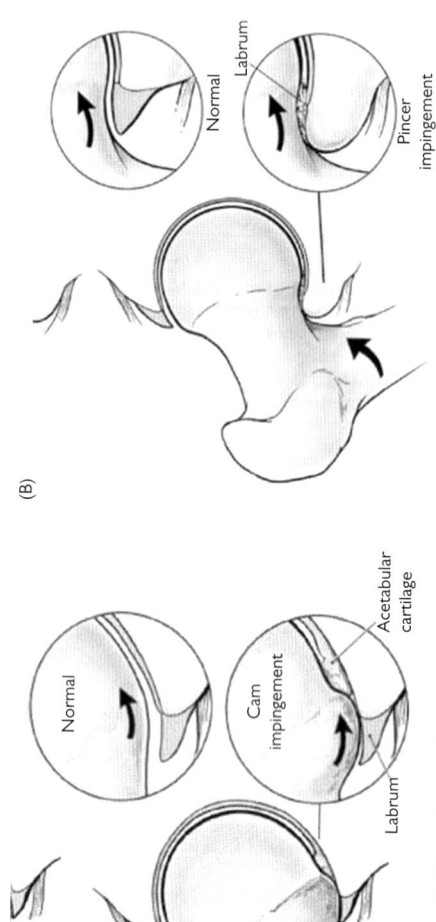

Fig. 15.2 Cam (A) and pincer (B) deformities causing femoroacetabular impingement.

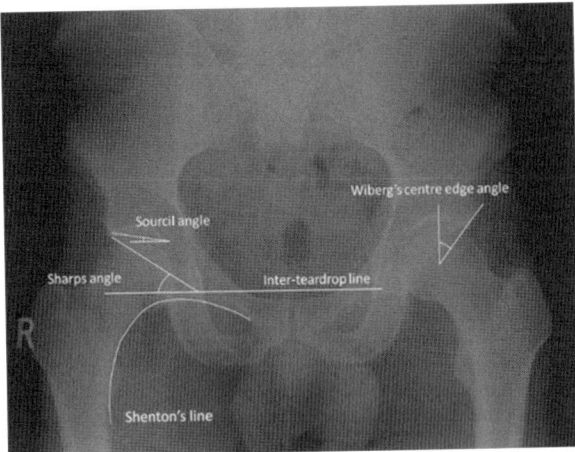

Fig. 15.3 Common radiographic angles. Acetabular angle (of Tonnis) or sourcil angle, normal value of 0–10°. Vertical centre-edge angle (of Wiberg), normal value of ≥25°. Note small cam lesion in the left hip.

Further reading

Griffin DR, Dickenson EJ, O'Donnell J, et al. The Warwick Agreement on femoroacetabular impingement syndrome (FAI syndrome): an international consensus statement. *British Journal of Sports Medicine*. 2016;**50**(19):1169–76.

Total hip replacement

Surgical approaches

- *Posterior:* most commonly used. Patient positioned laterally, with operative side facing up (see ➲ Chapter 9 for details).
- *Anterolateral:* more 'traditional' approach. Patient positioned laterally, with operative side up. Abductor tendons need to be elevated from the femur, hence making post-operative limp commoner.
- *Direct anterior:* most modern, but less commonly used approach. Patient supine. Negates abductor weakness and risk to sciatic nerve. Intermuscular and internervous planes. Presumed more rapid recovery.
- Decision of approach is usually dictated by surgeon experience/ preference, but other factors include previous incisions, dislocation risk, deformity, and occasionally implants used.

Prosthesis designs

Femoral components

- *Uncemented:* implants are initially fixed via a press-fit mechanism, but subsequent biological fixation occurs due to the coating upon the implant. Implants can be proximally, distally, or fully coated. Coating is usually hydroxyapatite. Higher risk of intraoperative and post-operative periprosthetic fracture.
- *Cemented:* widely used. Bone cement acts as a grout to create a buffer between the stiff implant and the relatively less stiff bone. Results in initial and long-term fixation. Taper slip implants have shown >30 years' survival in some series.

Acetabular components

- *Uncemented:* utilize biological coating or trabecular metal to provide initial press-fit fixation with long-term biological fixation. Screws can occasionally be used to reinforce initial fixation. Relatively more bone preserving than cemented implants.
- *Cemented:* more flexible to compensate for bony deficits in the acetabulum and not reliant on bone quality of the patient.

Combinations

- *Fully cemented:* both femoral and acetabular components cemented.
- *Full uncemented:* both components uncemented.
- *Hybrid:* femoral cemented, acetabular uncemented.
- *Reverse hybrid:* femoral uncemented, acetabular cemented.

Bearing surfaces

- The bearing surfaces make up the articulation between the femoral and acetabular components. These are modular, and combinations are available to accommodate differing patient anatomy.
- *Metal-on-polyethylene:* the femoral head is metal and the acetabular bearing is polyethylene. Widely used with long-term data.
- *Ceramic-on-polyethylene:* the femoral head is made from ceramic in this case. Lowest revision rates on the UK NJR.
- *Ceramic-on-ceramic:* this hard-on-hard combination has excellent wear characteristics in laboratory settings. Specific complications include a squeak and ceramic fracture.

- *Metal-on-metal:* another hard-on-hard combination with excellent wear characteristics. Less forgiving to malposition of components. Specific complications include the release of metal ions which can have devastating consequences to local tissues and bone (adverse reaction to metal debris, ARMD).

Complications

- *Infection:* 0.5% risk. Can occur at time of surgery (direct) or via haematogenous spread. If acute (<3–6 weeks), then the implant might be saved via surgical washout, debridement, antibiotics, and change of modular components, but retention of implants ('DAIR'). If chronic (>3–6 weeks), then the implant is likely coated with biofilm-containing organisms and will need to be revised. Diagnosed via use of serum inflammatory markers, joint aspiration, and biopsies.
- *Leg length discrepancy:* small leg length discrepancy is common. Rarely a cause for reoperation. Usually managed with shoe raise on opposite side.
- *Dislocation:* 1–3%; 75% of these occur in first few months following surgery. General hip precautions provided to all patients for prevention. Usually reduced closed. If recurrent, then can be a cause for revision surgery to reposition implants or provide a more constraint implant design to prevent dislocation.
- *Periprosthetic fracture:* can be intraoperative or post-operative. Immediate check radiographs should be scrutinized for fractures.
- *Heterotropic ossification:* frequently seen, rarely a clinical issue. Diagnosed on radiographs. Can be surgically excised, but patient will be on prophylactic radiotherapy and NSAIDs to prevent reformation.
- *Iliopsoas impingement:* under-recognized cause of ongoing groin pain and weakness following THR. Diagnosed with image-guided injection. Treatment can be surgical release, which is performed endoscopically.
- *Aseptic loosening:* macrophage-induced inflammatory response, which leads to osteolysis and loosening of implants. Start-up pain is classic symptom. Need to rule out infection prior to revision surgery.
- *Nerve injury:* rare.

Outcomes

Satisfaction rate 90–95%; 90% of patients with moderate or severe pain preoperatively report their pain to be mild or non-existent at 5 years following THR. Revision is performed in 0.5–1.0% per year.

Knee osteoarthritis

Causes
- *Primary:* no known cause, progressive degenerative changes.
- *Secondary:* secondary to an underlying cause, often following trauma/AVN/infection, chronic instability, meniscal defunctioning.

Risk factors
- Obesity.
- Instability (e.g. ACL insufficiency).
- Angular malalignment of limb.
- Trauma.
- Previous meniscectomy.

History
- Pain around knee—activity-related, generalized vs specific to involved compartments (e.g. medial pain for medial compartment OA, anterior knee pain for patellofemoral involvement).
- (Anterior) pain/grinding/crepitus aggravated by stair climbing and squatting suggests patellofemoral OA.
- Pain at rest and night suggests more severe OA.
- Impact on function—mobility, level of activity, ADLs, change to higher-impact activities (sports).
- Previous history of trauma or infection.
- Past interventions—activity modification, weight control, physiotherapy, injectables.
- Patient expectations and demands.

Examination
- Alignment—coronal plane (front on) alignment may be varus (bow legs), valgus (knock knees), or neutral. Sagittal plane (side on) alignment may show a FFD.
- Effusion (sweep test, patellar tap).
- Range of motion.
- Stability of the knee (collaterals, cruciates)—has an impact on surgical planning and the degree of constraint required from arthroplasty.

Investigations
- *Weight-bearing (standing) AP and lateral view radiographs:* show alignment of limb under physiological load and confirm diagnosis with four cardinal features of OA.
- *Weight-bearing flexion view of knee (Rosenberg):* can detect early OA with greater sensitivity than standard radiographic views.
- *Skyline view of patella (Merchant):* better evaluation of patellofemoral joint.
- *Maquet views:* long leg radiographs to assess weight-bearing coronal alignment.
- *MRI:* to identify isolated cartilage loss and other causes for knee pain (e.g. acute meniscal tear, ligamentous injury). Used to assess chondral surfaces when considering unicompartmental knee replacement.
- *Pelvic radiograph:* if clinical picture unclear, exclude hip OA with radiation of pain.

Management

- *Non-operative:* weight loss and lifestyle/activity modifications; physiotherapy to strengthen quadriceps mechanism; analgesics/short-term NSAIDs.
- *Intra-articular corticosteroid:* for temporary pain relief only. There is some evidence that repeated use can ↑ rate of cartilage loss.
- *Osteotomy:* joint preservation surgery to offload a degenerative compartment. Usually coronal plane correction only. Varus knees with medial compartment OA need high tibial osteotomy. Valgus knees with lateral compartment OA need undergo distal femoral osteotomy. Severe deformities may warrant double osteotomy.
- *Unicompartmental arthroplasty:* patient selection is key. If isolated compartment arthritis with no significant stiffness or loss of alignment, unicompartmental knee replacements are increasingly used, with good results and quicker recovery, compared with total knee arthroplasty. However, revision rates are higher compared with TKR.
- *Total knee arthroplasty:* remains the most reliable option for pain relief in advanced OA with failed conservative management. Level of constraint used depends on ligamentous stability of the knee. 'Constraint ladder'—unconstrained cruciate retaining, unconstrained posterior stabilized, unlinked constrained (high tibial post), linked constrained (hinge).
- *Arthrodesis:* rarely used, usually an option for failed PJI treatment. Only indicated primarily if there is no functioning extensor mechanism to allow arthroplasty.

Complications of total knee replacement

- <5%: wound healing problems, pain, bleeding, thrombosis (without prophylaxis), stiffness, wear/loosening.
- <1%: infection, periprosthetic fracture, nerve and vessel injuries. Other: future revision surgery, death.
- Satisfaction rates generally 85% (lower than THA).
- Survivorship of modern implants at 10 years of ≥90% (see ℰ www. njrcentre.org.uk/).

Meniscal injuries

The menisci play an important role in the functioning of a knee (see ➲ Chapter 6). Meniscal tears are more frequent in the medial side. Blood supply to the meniscus is poor; hence, tears have a high rate of non-healing without surgery. Degenerate tears are common in the over 40s, with many being asymptomatic and picked up incidentally on MRI.

Classification of tears (descriptive based on shape)

- Longitudinal.
- Radial.
- Horizontal cleavage.
- Bucket handle.
- Flap and inverted flap tears.
- Complex tears (tears occurring in two or more planes).

Blood supply of meniscus and location of tear

- Relative avascular structure, blood supply sourced laterally from branches of genicular vessels coming in from capsular tissue:
  - *Red zone*—peripheral third of meniscus, best blood supply, and highest chance of healing if repaired
  - *Red-white zone*—middle third of meniscus, has some capillary diffusion, equivocal chances of healing a tear in this region
  - *White zone*—inner third of meniscus, avascular section, does not heal if repaired.

History and examination

- Mechanism is often a twisting injury under axial load.
- May have associated swelling; a large immediate effusion suggestive of a root avulsion tear in the red zone (or ligamentous injury, i.e. ACL rupture).
- Tenderness along the joint line of the compartment involved.
- Positive McMurray's test: clicking or pain along the joint line on forced knee flexion and rotation—often very uncomfortable for the patient and not always used in practice.
- Deep squats and duck-walking are painful.
- In large acute tears (e.g. bucket handle), a true (mechanical) 'locked' knee may be present (i.e. the knee will not fully extend passively).
- Symptoms of pseudo-locking (catching) of the knee with giving way and sharp pain may occur due to the torn fragment catching in the joint.
- Tears often occur in conjunction with ligament injuries such as ACL rupture.

Imaging

- MRI is the gold standard in diagnosing meniscal injuries, with good sensitivity in detecting tears. It can also help to rule out differentials and concomitant injuries (e.g. ACL injuries with lateral meniscal tears).

Management and prognosis

- *Non-operative:* activity modification, reducing pivoting actions. First choice in stable, degenerative tears.

- *EUA for acutely locked knee:* if confirmed to be locked, then proceeding to arthroscopic surgery is advised. Partial meniscectomy or meniscal repair can be performed to unlock the knee.
- *Arthroscopic partial meniscectomy:* indicated for unstable tears with ongoing mechanical symptoms that are not amenable to repair (location of tear or its complexity). Care is taken to only excise the unstable portion and to preserve the remnant meniscus to reduce the rate of future degenerative change to the articular cartilage. Less commonly performed in modern practice.
- *Meniscal repair:* successful repair is dependent on age of patient and pattern/location of tear. Repair is more likely to fail in unstable knees (e.g. if ACL is not reconstructed in the same sitting). Usually repaired arthroscopically now by using various techniques.
- *Meniscal transplant:* occasionally, meniscal deficiency can result in significant compartment pain and early degeneration. Meniscal allograft transplant can be used to improve symptoms and prevent rapid joint degeneration. Currently reserved for young patients with preserved alignment, a stable knee, and minimal degenerative change. Performed in limited specialist centres. Avoid if high BMI.

Knee ligamentous disorders

Ligaments about the knee are important in maintaining stability and function. Injuries can occur with associated damage to other structures (e.g. meniscus, chondral surfaces). Chronic ligamentous injuries can also cause secondary damage to the menisci and chondral surfaces. Often, associated injuries will not resolve without restoring stability of the knee. MRI is the gold standard investigation to confirm these injuries, along with physical examination findings.

Classification of sprains

- *Grade I*: stretching of the ligament with no detectable instability.
- *Grade II*: further stretching of the ligament with detectable instability, but with some fibres in continuity.
- *Grade III*: complete disruption of the ligament.

Anterior cruciate ligament

- ACL injuries account for half of all sporting injuries to the knee.
- The mechanism is often a pivoting injury, with a planted foot, the knee in a flexed position, and application of a valgus force.
- Common in ♀, thought to be due to neuromuscular modulation and biomechanics.
- *Incidence:* peaks in third decade, although ♀ tend to be younger. In children, injury may be an ACL avulsion fracture (tibial origin).
- *Clinical presentation:* acute injuries are associated with pain, immediate swelling (haemarthrosis), and instability, with a mechanism as above. Clinically, a positive Lachman or anterior drawer test (either ↑ translation or soft end point, compared with the other leg) will be present (Table 15.3). A positive pivot-shift test suggests rotatory instability (but often difficult to do acutely unless patient is anaesthetized). Those with chronic injuries often describe frequent instability.
- *Management:* should be individualized. Non-operative management indicated in isolated injuries, with minimal symptoms of instability. Strengthening of secondary stabilizers with physiotherapy is the mainstay, especially in low-demand patients. Early reconstruction indicated for young patients, high-demand (pivoting sport) patients, or those with significant associated injuries.
  - Direct repair—usually in acute injuries in the paediatric or adolescent population. Not recommended in high-demand adults.
  - Reconstruction with an autograft is the gold standard. Different techniques described, including bone–patellar tendon–bone, quadriceps tendon or hamstring (semitendinosus ± gracilis) tendon(s) grafted in a single or double band. This is performed arthroscopically.
  - Addition of lateral extra-articular tenodesis (part of ITB wrapped around LCL) can reduce the risk of re-rupture in high-risk young patients.
  - Associated injuries (e.g. meniscal tears, chondral injuries) should be addressed at the same time.
  - Allografts or synthetic material—reserved for revision procedures. Both have higher failure rates and complications.

- Risks of surgery include arthrofibrosis (scarring, stiffness). Pre- ('pre-hab') and post-operative rehabilitation with physiotherapy crucial to achieving successful outcomes.
- In chronic cases, consider the role of high tibial osteotomy (older patients, varus malalignment, medial degeneration + ACL deficient) and posterolateral corner (PLC) laxity (which may warrant reconstruction).

Posterior cruciate ligament

- Primary restraint to posterior translation of the tibia. Twice as strong as the ACL.
- Injuries to the PCL are much less common than those of the ACL. The menisci are rarely damaged. Combined injuries of the other ligaments can occur, especially following knee dislocation.
- *Clinical presentation:* usually after a fall on a flexed knee, or a sudden hyperextension or 'dashboard' injury. Symptoms may be subtle, particularly if in conjunction with other ligamentous injury; rule out dislocation and vascular injuries (popliteal artery). Posterior drawer test positive and resting posteriorly subluxed position, which is best judged with the knees flexed to 90° (compare tibial tubercle position with the other side) (Table 15.3).
- *Management:* the majority can be managed non-operatively with a brace to reduce posterior translation while the PCL heals. In bony avulsion injuries with instability, acute repair may be offered. If patients are symptomatic of instability after physiotherapy, then consider reconstruction. PCL surgery is technically more challenging, with less predictable outcomes, compared with ACL reconstruction.

Medial collateral ligament

- Commonest knee ligament injury.
- Two layers: the superficial layer is the main restraint against valgus stress at 30° knee flexion; the deep layer is attached to the medial meniscus and adds further stability to valgus stress, particularly in full extension.
- *Clinical presentation:* medial pain following forced valgus stress to the knee. There may be localized swelling and instability. Valgus stress test in 30° flexion identifies the injury due to pain for laxity, compared with the contralateral knee (Table 15.3). Cruciate ligament injuries may coexist, so they must be checked for carefully.
- *Management:* isolated MCL injuries are usually treated conservatively, as this broad ligament tends to heal well. Grade 1 injuries need no bracing, and weight-bearing as pain allows. Grade 2 injuries benefit from 2–4 weeks of hinged knee bracing and weight-bearing as pain allows. Grade 3 injuries should be placed in a hinged knee brace for 6 weeks with limited deep flexion to 90° and partial weight-bearing. A hinged knee brace can be used to protect the ligament while it heals, avoiding valgus stress. If non-operative treatment fails and the patient is left with grade 3 laxity, then reconstruction can be an option. This can be performed by using autograft, allograft, or synthetic material.

Lateral collateral ligament

- LCL injuries are less common than MCL injuries. They are usually more extensive, involving the cruciates and/or the PLC structures of the knee. These injuries may represent a spontaneously reduced knee dislocation, and careful neurovascular assessment is necessary.
- *Clinical presentation:* lateral joint pain with some swelling. Varus stress causes pain and opening of the joint when the knee is flexed at 30° and in full extension. Presence of any excess external rotation needs to be checked in comparison with the contralateral side with the dial test— patient prone, knees together and flexed at either 30° (isolated PLC injury) or 90° (PLC + PCL injury) (Table 15.2). Check peroneal nerve function.
- *Management:* dependent on extent of associated injuries. If PLC or cruciate involvement, surgery is necessary to avoid long-term instability. Reconstruction may involve the use of tendon autograft or allograft or synthetic material. With PLC involvement, stiffness and ongoing instability can remain in the long term.

Table 15.2 Clinical assessment of specific knee ligamentous injuries

Ligament	Clinical test
MCL	Valgus stress at 30° knee flexion (reduces posterior capsule involvement)
LCL	Varus stress at 30° knee flexion (reduces posterior capsule involvement). Dial test at 30° and 90° to confirm posterolateral corner injury
ACL	Anterior drawer test and Lachman test positive Positive pivot-shift or glide to suggest rotatory instability
PCL	Posterior drawer test Posterior tibial sag Quadriceps active test at 90° Dial test at 90°

MCL, medial collateral ligament; LCL, lateral collateral ligament; ACL, anterior cruciate ligament; PCL, posterior cruciate ligament.

Instability of the knee

The ability to maintain alignment under physiological load is important to allow stable functioning of the knee joint and mobility. This is determined by:

- *Bony anatomy:* congruency of the shape of the femoral condyles with the tibial plateau
- *Ligamentous stability:* ACL and PCL for AP translation and rotation, MCL and LCL for varus–valgus stability.
- *Joint capsule:* posterior capsule can act as a secondary restraint (hence, testing collaterals is undertaken with the capsule relaxed at 30° flexion).
- *Muscles:* secondary support structures that help in dynamic stability, namely the quadriceps and hamstrings.

Posterolateral corner instability

Rotatory instability where the lateral tibial plateau translates posteriorly with rotation, leading to abnormal opening of the knee joint.

Clinical examination
- Important to differentiate between isolated LCL or PCL injuries and a complete PLC injury, as their function and management is different. This can be done with the following tests:
- Varus stress test
- External rotation of the tibia (patient prone, dial test at 30° and 90°)
- External rotation recurvatum test
- Reverse pivot-shift test
- Remember to check peroneal nerve function in such injuries.

Imaging
- *Plain radiographs:* an avulsion fracture fragment laterally (now known to be of the anterolateral ligament) is strongly associated with an ACL injury ('Segond' fracture). Varus stress view can show instability.
- *MRI:* to assess the PLC, ACL, PCL, and site of any other injuries or occult fractures.

Management
Invariably, surgery is necessary. Structures that may need to be addressed are the LCL, popliteus attachments, biceps tendon, ITB, arcuate ligament, and capsule. In a multi-ligament injury, the timing/order of ligament reconstruction remains controversial.

Patellofemoral instability

Patellofemoral joint instability may present as recurrent anterior knee pain, episodes of subluxation, or dislocation of the patella.

Risk factors
- *Bony anatomy:*
  - Femoral trochlear dysplasia (shallow femoral groove)
  - Patella alta (high-riding)
  - Patella shape
- *Mechanical axis malalignment:*
  - ↑ genu valgum
  - ↑ femoral anteversion
  - External tibial torsion.

NB these all lead to an ↑ Q angle, predisposing to dislocation and maltracking.

- Soft tissue:
  - Ligamentous laxity—either secondary to an underlying hyperlaxity condition (e.g. Ehlers–Danlos syndrome) or post-traumatic (acute medial patellofemoral ligament (MPFL) rupture)
  - Strength and tone of vastus medialis oblique (VMO) muscle— maintains medial tracking of patella in trochlea.

Clinical examination

A focused history is required to determine whether: (1) there has been a preceding traumatic event; or (2) the dislocation is spontaneous (atraumatic). If unilateral symptoms, it is crucial to examine the contralateral knee and patella.

- Inspect for muscle bulk.
- Q angle evaluation (normal between 12° and 18°) and coronal plane alignment—the presence of valgus is significant (Fig. 15.4).
- J sign—lateral translation of the patella on the trochlea with active knee extension.
- Palpation of patellar facets—for pain, suggests osteochondral injury may be present.
- Medial patella tenderness—can be a sign of MPFL injury.
- Apprehension test—often unable to do immediately following injury, usually assessed after a few weeks.
- Assess how much the patella glides laterally and medially to quantify (in quarters) the degree of laxity.
- Beighton score to assess the degree of ligamentous laxity (see ➲ Chapter 1, General principles of history and examination, pp. 4–7).

Imaging

- *Lateral knee radiograph* (in 30° of flexion) (Fig. 15.5):
  - The superior pole of the patella should be beneath a line extended from the central part of the distal femoral growth plate = Blumensaat's line
  - Numerous measures of patellar position, including Insall–Salvati ratio (length of patella-to-length of patella tendon, normally 1; >1.2 and <0.8 are abnormal) and Blackburne–Peel index (length of patella articular surface relative to distance of its inferior margin from the tibial plateau; normally 0.8–1.1).
- *Skyline view radiograph:*
  - Trochlear signs—look for dysplastic condyles and trochlear depth (normally <8mm)
  - Sulcus angle (normally 126–150°)
  - Congruence angle: angle between a line bisecting the sulcus angle and a line through the lowest point of the patella articular ridge. Positive on the lateral side, negative on the medial side (normal +16°).
- *CT:* helps to delineate rotational abnormalities such as tibial tuberosity to trochlear groove distance (TT–TG: abnormal if >20mm). Can also be used to dynamically assess patella tracking by having scans with the quadriceps relaxed and then contracted.
- *MRI:* to look at associated injuries and signs of trauma such as chondromalacia and acute MPFL rupture.

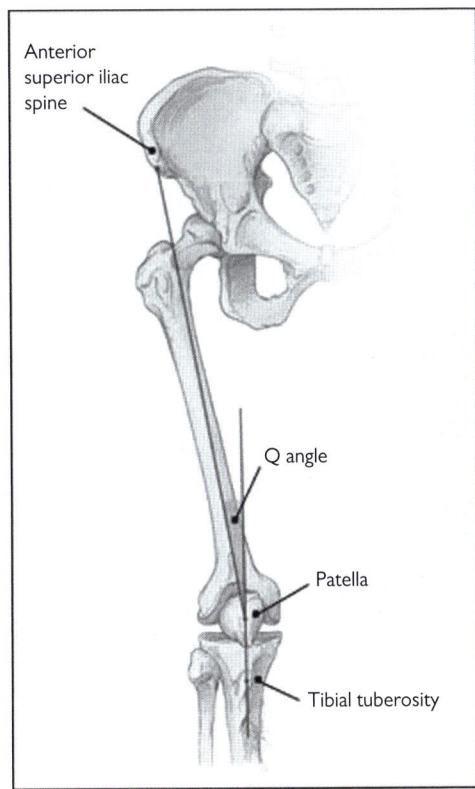

Anterior
superior iliac
spine

Q angle

Patella

Tibial tuberosity

Fig. 15.4 Q angle—usually 10° for men and 15° for women.

Management
Tailored to the individual, according to radiological and clinical findings. Avoid surgery in habitual dislocators with ligamentous laxity, as it does not achieve desirable outcomes. Surgery should be aimed at correcting morphological abnormalities.
- *Physiotherapy:* muscle balance and tracking exercises.
- *Orthotics:* braces and taping of patella. Useful for dynamic instability during certain activities.
- *Patella alta:* corrected with tibial tubercle osteotomy and distalization.
- *Tibial tubercle external rotation:* corrected with tibial tubercle osteotomy and medialization.
- *Femoral anteversion:* femoral derotational osteotomy.

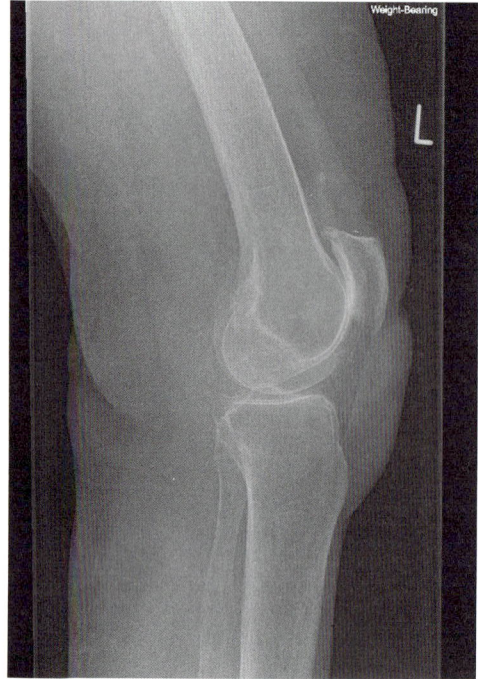

Fig. 15.5 Lateral radiograph of the knee demonstrating osteoarthritis of the patellofemoral joint.

- *Genu valgum:* distal femoral coronal plane osteotomy.
- *Trochlear dysplasia:* trochleoplasty.
- *MPFL reconstruction:* this should be considered as an adjunct to any procedure in patients with instability.

Osteochondritis dissecans of the knee

OCD is a benign lesion that affects the subchondral bone in a joint (commonly the knee) and can result in separation or instability of the overlying articular cartilage.

Aetiology and epidemiology

- Commonest in adolescents (10–16 years) but does have an adult form.
- Commonest in the medial femoral condyle (around 70–80%).
- Can be secondary to trauma or vascular injury, leading to subchondral damage.

Clinical examination

- Symptoms may be vague and poorly localized.
- Joint pain and swelling, intermittent in nature at first.
- Locking may occur if a loose body is present due to displacement of OCD. This is the commonest presentation in adults.
- Progressive degenerative arthritis due to irregular articular surface.
- May find effusions, quadriceps weakness, and loss of full extension.
- Wilson's test: flex knee to 90° while internally rotating the tibia—positive if pain is elicited at 30° and relieved with external rotation.

Imaging

- *Radiographs:* AP, lateral, Merchant, and tunnel views—can detect irregularity of subchondral bone or the presence of loose bodies or osteochondral defect.
- *MRI:* can detect early OCD by detecting oedema in subchondral bone; can size the lesion and identify any isolated loose bodies.

Classification

Lesions are classified according to the integrity of articular cartilage and the stability of the underlying subchondral bone. The final classification is done on inspection at the time of surgical investigation, based on the International Cartilage Regeneration and Joint Preservation Society:

- *Grade I:* intact articular surfaces, but softening due to underlying oedema
- *Grade II:* articular cartilage breach, but stable attachment on probing
- *Grade III:* fully detached lesion but remains *in situ*
- *Grade IV:* empty defect with loose body.

Natural history

The natural history is directly dependent on age at presentation. The *adult* type (closed physis) has a poorer prognosis because of limited healing potential. In general, the prognosis of OCD is better in younger patients, but also depends on the location, size, grade, and depth of the lesion.

Management

A locked knee warrants urgent surgical intervention. Alternatively, non-operative treatment can involve physiotherapy, weight loss, activity modification, and analgesia. In adults, these lesions are unlikely to heal.

Surgical treatment is based on the grade and extent of the lesion:
- Removal of loose bodies arthroscopically
- Arthroscopic or open fixation of unstable fragments by using headless metal screws, bioabsorbable darts, or OATS surgery
- Osteochondral autograft or allograft if fragment is not salvageable
- Microfracture to encourage fibrocartilage cover of an osteochondral defect (used in adults rather than in children)—note that normal hyaline cartilage cover cannot occur, rather 'scarring' fibrocartilage
- Autologous chondrocyte implantation (ACI)—when defects are larger than 4cm².

Subchondral insufficiency fracture of the knee

Formerly known as spontaneous osteonecrosis of the knee (SONK) or Ahlbäck disease, this condition may have devastating consequences and result in degenerative changes in the knee. Classified into *spontaneous* type with no obvious preceding cause, or *secondary* to an insult.

Epidemiology

Commoner in the over 50s, with a preponderance for women. Usually occurs as a single focal lesion, commonly in the medial femoral condyle. Secondary lesions usually occur in younger patients as a result of an underlying factor and may be multifocal.

Pathophysiology

Various theories have been proposed.

- *Vascular theory:* initially thought to be the primary cause of the event, although novel research suggests this is a secondary event (hence a change in the nomenclature from SONK).
- *Trauma theory:* microfracture in the subchondral bone. This allows fluid to enter through the articular cartilage into the subchondral bone and marrow space, creating ↑ interosseous pressure and pain. This ↑ pressure in a closed space interferes with the blood supply and triggers the cycle of compromised circulation and results in osseous ischaemia. However, only 10% of patients give a history of trauma.
- *Meniscal root tear theory:* ↑ compartment pressure may result from an unnoticed meniscal root tear. The meniscus then becomes non-functional, leading to strain on chondral surfaces.
- *Insufficiency theory:* insufficiency stress fracture in osteopenic bone, leading to interosseous ischaemia.
- *Secondary causes:* steroids, alcohol, renal transplantation, coagulopathies, sickle-cell disease, myeloproliferative disorders, haemoglobinopathies.
- *Post-arthroscopy:* rare variant observed after arthroscopic surgery, especially associated with a full meniscectomy.

Clinical examination

- Acute onset of knee pain, often with no preceding/minor trauma.
- Night pain.
- Specific joint line tenderness of the involved portion (usually the medial femoral condyle).
- Joint effusion.
- ROM limited by pain.
- In cases of collapse—may have malalignment.

Imaging

- *Plain radiographs:*
  - Stage 1—normal
  - Stage 2—slight flattening of the condyle
  - Stage 3—area of radiolucency surrounded by subchondral sclerosis. Collapse of subchondral bone plate

- Stage 4—radiolucency is surrounded by a definite sclerotic halo of variable thickness and density
- Stage 5—secondary arthritic changes.
- *MRI:*
  - Most sensitive diagnostic tool
  - Can detect early disease and allows evaluation of the extent of bone involvement
  - T1—discrete low-intensity signal in the femoral condyle
  - T2—corresponding low-intensity signal area in the central lesion, with a high-intensity signal around the margin (surrounding oedema).

Differential diagnosis

- OCD.
- Primary OA.
- Radiologically—transient osteoporosis of the knee, bone marrow oedema.

Prognosis

- Related to the size, site, and number of lesions.
- Lesions may progress to degenerative joint disease.
- Larger lesions (>50% of the width of the femoral condyle, or >5cm²) have a poorer prognosis in terms of joint preservation.

Management

- *Non-operative:* if detected early and smaller lesions. Protected weight-bearing, reduce secondary risk factors, bisphosphonates (may reduce the rate of collapse), appropriate analgesia.
- *Pre-collapse surgery:* depends on size of lesion. Strategies include core decompression (with or without bone grafting), offloading tibial/femoral osteotomy (if single compartment).
- *Post-collapse surgery:* consider osteochondral autograft/allograft in the young, but if not salvageable, then will need reconstruction with either partial or total knee arthroplasty.

Jumper's knee and adolescent apophysitis

Painful conditions of the adult and adolescent knee extensor mechanism due to repeated mechanical overload. Caused by repetitive jumping/landing on a semi-flexed knee, loading the extensor mechanism. Pain arises from the patellar tendon itself or its insertion to the inferior patella or tibia. Quadriceps insertion into the superior pole is less commonly affected. In adolescents, similar activities cause traction apophysitis of the inferior patellar pole (Sinding–Larsen–Johansson (SLJ) disease) or tibial tuberosity (Osgood–Schlatter (OS) disease).

Risk factors

- Frequent sports with rapid acceleration/deceleration/direction change, particularly jumping sports.
- Poor quadriceps flexibility overloading tendons (eccentric exercises).

Clinical examination

- Insidious onset of anterior knee pain following activity.
- Swelling with pain on kneeling with SLJ and OS disease.
- Local tenderness at site of pain, but knee itself is normal.
- Tightness and wasting of quadriceps muscle.

Investigations

- *Plain radiographs:* ossicle formation in tendon near bony attachments through avulsions in OS/SLJ disease; may persist into adult life.
- *USS:* inflammatory changes, tendon thickening, structural heterogeneity.
- *MRI:* useful in surgical planning and checking to ensure no rupture or retraction of tendon. Key finding is tendon thickening.

Management

Adolescent apophysitis

- Maintain athletic activities as much as possible; treat symptoms.
- Periods of rest as required—occasionally splint/plaster immobilization for 6 weeks to rest the tendon.
- Can excise persistently symptomatic ossicles in OS disease at skeletal maturity (10% of cases).

Adult tendonosis

- Physiotherapy (quadriceps/hamstring stretches; local ice; eccentric strengthening exercises).
- Occasionally rest ± immobilization.
- Platelet-rich plasma (PRP) injection: controversial, mixed evidence.
- Debridement of degenerate tendon, with excision of any ossicles.
- Repair or reconstruction of ruptured tendons, then rehabilitation.

Failure of hip and knee arthroplasty

Although joint replacement surgery numbers are rising, with THR and TKR both having very high satisfaction rates, the implants will inevitably fail over time. A number of factors can contribute to this and may account for earlier-than-expected failure. Many countries now track and analyse national survival rates with arthroplasty registries (e.g. the UK's NJR). This allows long-term implant survivorship to be monitored and helps to determine common causes of failure. Most established THR and TKR implants now provide 10-year survival rates of over 90%, and this is the benchmark expected for this type of surgery (for Orthopaedic Data Evaluation Panel ratings, p. 212).

Clinical history and examination

There remains a rate of patient dissatisfaction and unexplained pain (TKR > THR), but this is a diagnosis made after a detailed evaluation and exclusion of other causes of a problematic replacement, particularly infection:

- History of the implant and original surgery. Any earlier complications, prior function, and change in function
- Start-up pain is a common symptom of loose components (groin—acetabular component; thigh—femoral). Night pain may be present
- Acute systemic illnesses can seed infection of the joint
- Examine the scar for signs of sinus and integrity
- Examine passive movements of the joint
- Serial interval radiographs can show an implant failing over time.

Aseptic loosening

- Commonest indication for revision THR/TKR surgery.
- Infection must be excluded prior to surgery.
- Can reconstruct in one setting.

Periprosthetic joint infection

- Critical to diagnose, as difficult to eradicate. Various consensus statements exist on how to define a PJI (Table 15.3).
- Timing of infection changes treatment options (Table 15.4).
- For implant preservation with a DAIR procedure there are novel decision making tools available (Table 15.5)
- Stability of the implant fixation requires assessment prior to planning definitive management.
- MDT-led management recommended in planning complex treatment, in conjunction with microbiology support.
- Chronic infection is associated with biofilm formation around implants, reducing the ability of antibiotic penetration into the bacterial colonies.
- Long-term suppression may be an option in failed surgical candidates or patients unsuitable for major surgery.
- Surgery is best performed in specialist, high-volume regional centres.

Instability

Instability is uncommon with TKR and is more of a problem with THR components, with a ~1% lifetime risk. Factors that can lead to recurrent dislocation of a THR that need to be assessed before deciding on definitive management include:

- *Implant:* relates to the design of the implant used primarily, such as the head:neck ratio, with a smaller diameter of the femoral head potentially increasing the risk of instability
- *Surgical:* intraoperative malpositioning of components beyond Lewinnick's safe zones can ↑ the risk of recurrent dislocation. Variations in the natural anatomy of the patient must be considered
- *Patient:* poor compliance with post-operative instructions, poor abductor state, spino pelvic tilt, and neuromuscular conditions all ↑ the risk of instability.

Due to the nature of revision surgery and major reconstruction, the risk of dislocation and other complications is generally higher.

Mechanical failure

- Mode of failure depends on which joint is involved (THR/TKR) and the type of implant. Cemented and uncemented components fail differently.
- Often, wear particles (third body wear) cause a secondary inflammatory response by the body, leading to an osteolysis cascade around components, and subsequent loosening and migration of components.
- Metal-on-metal hip resurfacings are at risk of a phenomenon termed 'adverse reaction to metal debris' (ARMD), resulting in a higher rate of early failure and formation of pseudo-tumours. The UK MHRA guidance advises close observation of resurfacings, including monitoring of serum metal ion levels (cobalt, chromium) and MARS MRI if concerns.
- Initial stability of implants, including cemented (quality of the implant–cement–bone interface) and uncemented (implant–cement interface), can help to determine if an implant is likely to fail early.

Periprosthetic fracture

- Increasing burden of disease in trauma, mainly fragility fracture in an ageing population.
- Often requires complex reconstruction or revision, depending on location of fracture and stability of implant.
- High complication and 1-year mortality rates.
- Aim of treatment is to control pain and allow stability to enable the patient to start mobilizing again and fully weight-bearing.

Investigation of a painful arthroplasty

- Key points from history of surgery and perioperative period.
- Location of pain—is it from another source referred to the joint (e.g. spine)?
- Surrounding impingement of soft tissue/muscle.
- Plain radiographs for component geometry and gross radiographic signs of loosening and/or infection, often easier to evaluate if compared with previous radiographs.
- WCC/inflammatory markers for infection.
- ^{99m}technetium bone scan: ↑ uptake suggestive of loosening and/or infection (not recommended if implant has been in for <12 months as post-operative inflammation).
- Labelled white cell scan to identify low-grade infection.
- Joint aspiration for microscopy, culture, and sensitivities is key to rule out PJI.
- Immediate bedside testing of aspirate with either alpha-defensin or leucocyte esterase to confirm the presence of PJI (e.g. Synovasure™).

Table 15.3 New scoring-based definition for periprosthetic joint infection

Major criteria (at least one of the following)	Decision
Two positive cultures of the same organism	Infected
Sinus tract with evidence of communication to the joint or visualization of the prosthesis	

Minor criteria	Score	Decision
Preoperative diagnosis		
Serum		≥6 infected
Elevated CRP or D-dimer	2	2–5 possibly infected[a]
Elevated ESR	1	0–1 not infected
Synovial		
Elevated synovial WBS count or LE	3	
Positive alpha-defensin	3	
Elevated synovial PMN (%)	2	
Elevated synovial CRP	1	
Inconclusive preop score or dry tap[a]	**Score**	**Decision**
Intraoperative diagnosis		
Preoperative score	–	≥6 infected
Positive histology	3	4–5 inconclusive[b]
Positive purulence	3	≤3 not infected
Single positive culture	2	

NB proceed with caution in the presence of adverse local tissue reaction, crystal deposition disease, and slow-growing organisms.

[a] For patients with inconclusive minor.

[b] Consider further molecular diagnostics such as next-generation sequencing.

CRP, C-reactive protein; ESR, erythrocyte sedimentation rate; LE, leukocyte esterase; PMN, polymorphonuclear; WBC, white blood cell.

Table 15.4 Timing classification of periprosthetic joint infection

Infection	Management options
Acute (<4 weeks post-operatively)	Debridement with implant retention (DAIR)
	Chronic suppression
Chronic (>4 weeks post-operatively)	One-stage revision (if criteria met)
	Two-stage revision
	Chronic suppression
Acute haematogenic (<4 weeks' symptoms in well-functioning joint and preceding systemic illness)	DAIR
	One- or two-stage revision
	Chronic suppression

Table 15.5 Indications, risk factors to consider in the decision-making process, and contraindications for a DAIR (debridement, antimicrobial therapy, and implant retention) procedure in periprosthetic hip and knee

Indications	Risk factors*	Not recommended°
• Well-fixed prosthesis	• Early acute: 4-12 weeks after index arthroplasty	• Loose prosthesis
• Acute PJI:	• Multiple previous revision surgeries	• >12 weeks after index arthroplasty
• Early acute: ≤4 weeks after index arthroplasty	• Host and clinical factors:	• >3 weeks of symptoms
• Late acute: <3 weeks of symptoms after an uneventfil postoperative period	• Rheumatoid arthritis	• Presence of a sinus tract
	• COPD	• Compromised soft tissue
	• Immunosuppressive therapy	
• Good conditions of the surrounding soft tissue without a sinus tract	• *S.aureus* infection (late acute PJI)	
	• Difficult to treat microorganism – no biofilm active antimicrobial therapy available – and fungal infections	
	• Bacteraemia	

*These host and clinical factors can be associated with a higher risk of failure of DAIR

° If cure is intended, in patients fulfilling these factors, a full revision of the whole implant should be considered.

Reference:

Sigmund, I. K., Wouthuyzen-Bakker, M., Ferry, T., Metsemakers, W.-J., Clauss, M., Soriano, A., Trebse, R., and Sousa, R.: Debridement, antimicrobial therapy, and implant retention (DAIR) as curative surgical strategy for acute periprosthetic hip and knee infections: a summary of the position paper from the European Bone & Joint Infection Society (EBJIS), J. Bone Joint Infect., 10, 139–142, https://doi.org/10.5194/jbji-10-139-2025, 2025.

Further reading

McNally M, Sousa R, Wouthuyzen-Bakker M, *et al*. The EBJIS definition of periprosthetic joint infection. *Bone and Joint Journal*. 2021;**103-B**(1):18–25. [EBJIS consensus statement on PJI]
National Joint Registry (NJR). Available from: ℘ www.njrcentre.org.uk
Orthopaedic Data Evaluation Panel (ODEP). Available from: ℘ www.odep.org.uk/
Parvizi J, Tan TL, Goswami K, *et al*. The 2018 definition of periprosthetic hip and knee infection: an evidence-based and validated criteria. *Journal of Arthroplasty*. 2018;**33**(5):1309–14. [MSIS criteria of PJI]

Chapter 16

Adult orthopaedics: foot and ankle

Osteoarthritis of the ankle

Epidemiology

Primary OA (7%) is uncommon, compared with OA in other joints (knee, 98%; hip, 90%). Most cases present in middle age and are related to a post-traumatic incident (~80%).

Aetiology

- Primary.
- Secondary to trauma (related to angular deformity after fracture or due to minor repeated trauma).
- Chronic ankle instability.
- As part of systemic inflammatory arthropathy (12%).
- Osteochondral defects.
- Osteonecrosis.
- Infection.
- As a complication of bleeding disorder.

History

Pain, loss of function, and past history of injury.

- *Ankle OA:* pain over anterior ankle joint, associated with walking uphill, with loss of dorsiflexion, pain at night, dull in nature, generalized stiffness with start-up pain.
- *Subtalar OA:* pain from lateral heel to foot dorsum.

Examination

- Examine the patient seated and standing.
- Examine the patient's shoes for uneven wear pattern.
- Observe gait: heel strike (inability suggests limited ankle dorsiflexion), time in standing phase (short in antalgic gait).
- Assess for:
  - Swollen joints and scars
  - Deformity (usually visualized from posterior)
  - Joint line tenderness (anterior for ankle, laterally for subtalar joint)
  - Palpable osteophytes (usually felt dorsally over distal tibia)
  - ↓ or painful ROM
  - Ligament integrity (particularly lateral ligament complex)
  - Neurological and vascular status.

Investigations

- *Radiology:* obtain a full set of ankle radiographs—AP, lateral, and mortice views—ideally standing (weight-bearing) for a true view. Look for:
  - Loss of joint space, sclerosis, cyst formation, and osteophyte formation
  - Loose bodies
  - Talar dome flattening
  - Deformity in coronal images
  - Soft tissue shadow may show swelling.
- *MRI scan:* may show evidence of early arthritis and other hindfoot joint involvement.

Management

- *Non-operative:* analgesics and NSAIDs, corticosteroid injections, weight loss activity, and shoe wear modification. Orthoses—ankle brace, rocker-bottom sole shoe, heel insoles for subtalar OA.
- *Operative:* indicated if non-operative treatment fails after 3–6 months. Surgery includes:
  - Arthroscopy and debridement (can improve symptoms for 3–5 years), dependent on the degree of arthritis, not indicated in severe OA
  - Osteotomy: for mild to moderate arthritis affecting one-half of the joint
  - Arthrodesis: 'gold standard', with good long-term results, but ↑ loads on other joints, leading to adjacent degenerative changes (e.g. subtalar), and has a non-union rate of 5–10%; this ↑ in the diabetic population. Can be performed arthroscopically or open. May be better for younger patients with more physical jobs
  - Arthroplasty: growing popularity; total ankle replacement has been shown to have survivorship of 86% at 10 years in the ankle. May be better for lower-demand patients.

Further reading

Hassouna H, Kumar S, Bendall S. Arthroscopic ankle debridement: 5-year survival analysis. *Acta Orthopaedica Belgica.* 2007;**73**(6):737.

Park JH, Kim HJ, Suh DH, *et al.* Arthroscopic versus open ankle arthrodesis: a systematic review. *Arthroscopy: The Journal of Arthroscopic and Related Surgery.* 2018;**34**(3):988–97.

Tanaka Y. Current concepts in the treatment of osteoarthritis of the ankle. In: Canata G, d'Hooghe P, Hunt K, Kerkhoffs G, Longo U, eds. *Sports Injuries of the Foot and Ankle.* Berlin, Heidelberg: Springer, 2019.

Valderrabano V, Horisberger M, Russell I, Dougall H, Hintermann B. Etiology of ankle osteoarthritis. *Clinical Orthopaedics and Related Research.* 2009;**467**(7):1800.

Rheumatoid arthritis of the ankle and foot

Incidence

RA affects 90% of foot and ankle joints, which is almost always bilateral. In 17% of RA patients, the joints of the feet are the first to be affected. The forefoot is most commonly involved, but the subtalar and ankle joints are involved in one-third of patients.

Natural history

RA of the foot and ankle progresses through three stages:
- Chronic synovitis destroying the supporting structures, leading to subluxation and eventual dislocation
- Joint erosions, tendon dysfunction, and instability
- Progressive deformities (dorsal subluxation and eventual dislocation of the MTPJs), loss of intrinsic–extrinsic muscle balance, and claw toe deformity.

Clinical findings

Careful history taking and medication regime. Important to ascertain whether the disease is currently in an active or a quiescent stage. Evaluation of vascular status of leg and condition of skin (as well as history of skin healing potential).
- Hindfoot—valgus of ankle joint and hindfoot (resulting in tight Achilles tendon); posterior tibial tendon dysfunction is also very common, as the tendon overcompensates for a weakened ligamentous medial arch.
- Midfoot—flattening of the longitudinal arch, flattening and pronation of the foot. Talonavicular and naviculocuneiform articulations usually affected.
- Forefoot—painful plantar callosities (secondary to subluxed metatarsals), present or past ulcerations, hallux valgus, swelling of MTPJs with dorsal subluxation or dislocation (due to synovitis) and large plantar bursae, interdigital neuromas, severe hammer toe and claw toe deformities, tendon ruptures, tarsal tunnel syndrome.
- Also look for associated features—PVD/vasculitis, neurology.
- Diagnostic local anaesthetic injections help to localize the source of pain.

Investigations

- *Radiology:* AP, lateral, and weight-bearing views. Bilateral involvement is usually asymmetrical.

Management

- *Non-operative:* optimal rheumatological therapy, managed via an MDT approach. Analgesia, NSAIDs, physiotherapy to stretch the Achilles tendon and maintain range of motion of the hindfoot and MTPJs, taping, foot orthosis, walking aids and crutches, local injections of steroids to joints or tendon sheaths (tendon rupture is a potential risk).
- *Operative:* pre-surgical skin condition and blood supply review, discuss immunotherapy/DMARD 'holiday' with the rheumatologist to reduce

complication rates. Consider alignment of whole lower limb. Main goal is to alleviate pain and achieve stability. If severe hip and knee deformity exists, it must be corrected before that of the ankle and foot.

Ankle
- Initial synovitis can be treated with synovectomy (open or arthroscopic).
- If there is joint destruction but no deformity, ankle arthroplasty or arthrodesis may be considered.
- If the joint is significantly deformed, then primary arthrodesis is the operation of choice.

Hindfoot
- RA in the hindfoot can cause either a loose mobile joint in planovalgus, which responds poorly to surgery, or a stiff joint which can be fused (e.g. talonavicular or triple fusion in subtalar joint subluxation). Patients should remain non-weight-bearing in a short leg cast for 6 weeks post-operatively.

Midfoot
- The tarsometatarsal and intertarsal joints are less frequently involved in RA. Custom-moulded soft orthosis may be used. In severe cases, arthrodesis is indicated.

Forefoot
- This is the commonest part of the foot affected by RA.
- Arthrodesis of the first MTPJ. The lesser MTPJs can be corrected by releasing the extensor tendons and resection arthroplasty (excising the heads of the metatarsals and reducing the displaced fat pad).
- Claw toes can be corrected by an open procedure and Kirschner wire stabilization for 4 weeks.

Further reading
Wilson O, Hewlett S, Woodburn J, Pollock J, Kirwan J. Prevalence, impact and care of foot problems in people with rheumatoid arthritis: results from a United Kingdom based cross-sectional survey. *Journal of Foot and Ankle Research*. 2017;**10**(1):46.

Ankle instability

There are two categories of instability:
- *Functional:* pain that causes the ankle to give way
- *Mechanical:* weakened static ankle restraints that lead to excessive lateral ankle movement and resultant pain. Ligamentous laxity syndromes and neuromuscular conditions may present with this type of instability.

Incidence

Ankle sprains are the commonest sports injuries, but only 20% of patients will have residual symptoms.

Classification

Three grades exist for lateral collateral ankle ligament injuries:
- Grade I—confined to the ATFL, with little ligamentous laxity on examination
- Grade II—injury to the ATFL and calcaneofibular ligament (CFL), with mild laxity
- Grade III—as grade II, with significant laxity and no palpable end point.

Clinical findings

- Tenderness over the ATFL and/or CFL.
- Positive anterior drawer test.
- Positive inversion test (talar tilt).
- Pain on squeezing the tibia and fibula together (suggests concurrent syndesmosis injury).
- Painful external rotation of the foot.
- Subtalar instability is difficult to diagnose. Clinical examination alone fails to distinguish between tibiotalar and subtalar instability (requires X-ray). Abnormal tibiotalar tilt is defined as between 3° and 15° relative to the contralateral side and talar translation on the tibia of >3mm.

Imaging

- AP, mortise, and lateral views of the ankle and foot. AP and lateral standing views.
- EUA and stress X-rays (operator-dependent).
- USS of the ankle ligamentous structures.
- MRI (when osteochondral injuries or inconclusive USS).
- CT (when fractures are suspected).

Management

- *Non-operative:*
  - Ankle and hindfoot sprains are initially treated with RICE (rest, ice, compression bandage, elevation), with a walking boot for support.
  - Most patients with ankle instability will improve with early weight-bearing and rehabilitation (this includes a gradual programme of strengthening the peronei and dorsiflexors, stretching of the tendoachilles, isometric exercises with Therabands, and proprioceptive training).
  - In severe strains, protect the ankle with a pneumatic brace or taping for sports for 3–6 months.

- Warn the patient that pre-injury status can take up to 12 months for full function.
- *Operative:* the primary aim of anatomical reconstruction is functional stability. Surgical options include:
  - Arthroscopy: note that 25% of patients having arthroscopy for instability symptoms have another intra-articular pathology.
  - If the residual lateral ligamentous tissues are amenable to repair, then imbrication of the ATFL and/or CFL with augmentation of the inferior extensor retinaculum is carried out (e.g. modified Broström–Gould repair).
  - Alternatively, the peroneus brevis, semitendinosus, or gracilis tendons can be used as augmentation grafts (e.g. Chrisman–Snook procedure).
  - Bioabsorbable or metallic suture anchors have been used to achieve primary fixation.
  - If hindfoot varus coexists with lateral ankle instability, then valgus calcaneal osteotomy may be indicated.

Tibialis posterior tendon dysfunction

The tibialis posterior tendon is a key dynamic stabilizer of the medial arch. A spectrum of pathology may compromise its function; progressive inflammation, degeneration, and/or rupture of the tendon with associated ligamentous degeneration ultimately lead to secondary changes in the foot and ankle shape, with resultant functional deficits.

Risk factors

Obesity, hypertension, middle age, ♀ sex, diabetes, collagen disorders, previous ankle fracture, injury or surgery (medial), local steroid injection, seronegative arthropathy.

Symptoms and signs

Initially pain ± swelling posteromedially at the ankle and into the foot. Usually no clear history of trauma. As the valgus deformity progresses, impingement of the fibula on the calcaneus causes lateral pain.

Look for characteristic medial heel wear of shoes. Observe gait. View from behind to assess for valgus deformity of the hindfoot and for the 'too many toes' sign (>2 toes visible laterally) (Fig. 16.1) due to forefoot abduction. Also assess the medial longitudinal arch; loss leads to classic pes planus deformity. Examine all deformities to see if they are *flexible* or *rigid*.

Assess strength of heel inversion while palpating the tendon. Ask the patient to perform single leg heel rise—usually impossible in stage 2 or 3 disease (i.e. inability to support body weight and maintain stability when standing on tiptoes of one foot).

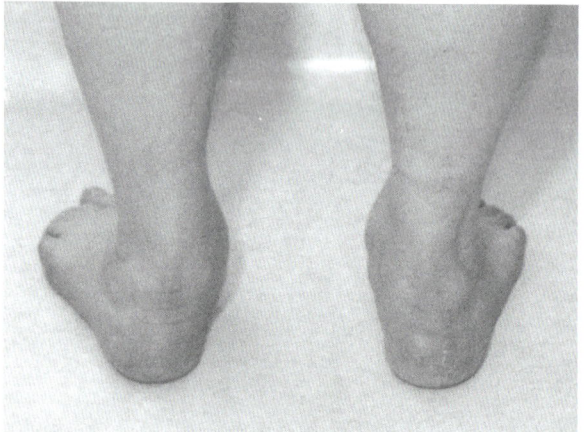

Fig. 16.1 'Too many toes' sign.
Reproduced Luqmani, Raashid et al. (ed.), *Rheumatoid Arthritis* (2010) with permission from Oxford University Press.

Staging of disease: Johnson and Strom

- Stage 1: tenosynovitis with intact tendon.
- Stage 2a: ruptured tendon with flexible deformities (flexible flat foot).
- Stage 2b: flexible flat foot, flexible hindfoot, forefoot abduction (too many toes).
- Stage 3: ruptured tendon with rigid deformities, rigid abduction, and rigid hindfoot valgus.
- Stage 4: as stage 3, with valgus angulation, arthritis of the talus in the ankle mortice, deltoid compromise.

Differential diagnosis

- Of acquired pes planus (flat foot): neuropathic (Charcot) foot, midfoot OA, rupture of spring ligament.
- Of medial ankle/foot pain: tarsal tunnel syndrome, deltoid ligament strain, AVN of the head of the talus or navicular.

Investigations

- *Plain radiographs:* abnormal in only 50% of cases. May show uncovering of talar head, abnormal talometatarsal angles, or arthritic changes at ankle, subtalar, and talonavicular joints.
- *MRI:* can image the tendon directly.

Management

- *Non-operative:* rest, NSAIDs, well-fitted footwear, orthoses (corrective for flexible deformity, accommodative if rigid), cast immobilization (stage 1 disease).
- *Operative:* these are complex and dependent on disease stage, synovectomy, debridement and repair of the tendon, flexor tendon transfers (e.g. flexor digitorum longus (FDL)), calcaneal medial shift osteotomy, lateral column lengthening (for earlier stages); triple arthrodesis for painful degenerative changes (for later stages, i.e. stage 3 or 4 disease).

Further reading

Johnson KA, Strom DE. Tibialis posterior tendon dysfunction. *Clinical Orthopaedics and Related Research.* 1989;**1**(239):196–206.

Kohls-Gatzoulis J, Angel JC, Singh D, Haddad F, Livingstone J, Berry G. Tibialis posterior dysfunction: a common and treatable cause of adult acquired flatfoot. *BMJ.* 2004;**329**(7478):1328–33.

Myerson MS. Adult acquired flatfoot deformity. Treatment of dysfunction of the posterior tibial tendon. *Journal of Bone and Joint Surgery (American Volume).* 1996;**78**:780–92.

Tarsal tunnel syndrome

This is an entrapment neuropathy of the tibial nerve, or its branches (medial and lateral plantar nerves, calcaneal branch), as it passes through the tarsal tunnel (by the flexor retinaculum as it courses around the medial malleolus).

Incidence

An uncommon cause of heel/plantar foot, and medial distal calf pain. Often vague in nature. May have paraesthesiae and numbness. Isolated pain may be confused with plantar fasciitis.

Anatomy

The tibial nerve has three branches: medial, lateral plantar, and medial calcaneal nerves.

Causes

- SOLs within the tarsal canal, including ganglion cysts, varicosities, bony prominences, lipomas, tenosynovitis, and schwannoma.
- Anatomical deformity: heel valgus.
- Systemic disorders (e.g. RA, diabetes, PVD).
- Trauma.

History

Pain and numbness in the heel and sole of the foot exacerbated by activity, although not always completely settled with rest. Careful past medical history for medical causes of peripheral neuropathy.

Examination

- Reduced sensation—distribution of medial and lateral plantar nerves and calcaneal branches.
- Atrophy of the intrinsic foot muscles may be noted in long-term cases.
- Foot eversion and dorsiflexion may exacerbate symptoms.
- Tinel's sign (radiation of pain and paraesthesiae along the course of the nerve) may be induced by percussion over the course of the nerve.

Differential diagnosis

- Plantar fasciitis.
- Calcaneal/talar process fracture.
- Lumbar radiculopathy.
- Peripheral neuropathies.

Investigations

- Plain radiographs may show osteophytes, deformity, and neuroarthropathy (i.e. Charcot disease) in long-standing neuropathies.
- Electrophysiology studies—but negative findings do not rule out the diagnosis.
- MRI/USS if suspected mass lesion in tarsal tunnel—a ganglion being common.

Management

- *Non-operative:* should be tried for 6–12 weeks.
  - NSAIDs
  - Immobilization of the ankle
  - Orthotics altering hindfoot alignment
  - Low-dose neurotropic medications (e.g. amitriptyline).
- *Operative:*
  - Reserved for those in whom diagnosis is secure and who have not responded to conservative management.
  - Decompression (tarsal tunnel release)—incise along course of the tibial nerve from deep investing fascia of the lower leg to origin of abductor hallucis. Open flexor retinaculum and fascia of abductor hallucis origin fully. Non-weight-bearing for 4 weeks, then mobilize.
  - Complications—iatrogenic injury to the nerve or posterior tibial artery could have significant deleterious effects on foot function. Failure to adequately release the retinaculum along the entire course may lead to treatment failure and secondary insult from post-operative scar contraction.
  - Prognosis—surgical decompression relieves pain in 50–75% of cases. Redo procedures are less successful.

Achilles tendinopathy

Insertional tendinopathy

Inflammatory and degenerative tendon changes at insertion of the Achilles tendon to the calcaneum. Pathology can include bursitis adjacent to the Achilles tendon—the retrocalcaneal bursa, anterior (deep) to the tendon or posterior (superficial) to the tendon or inflammation of the paratenon (peritendonitis). Tendon changes are seen on imaging and a Haglund's deformity is common.

Incidence
Common, especially in physically active individuals. Also seen in association with inflammatory disorders. Commonly in middle age.

History
Chronic posterior heel pain. Usually worse with activity or post-activity. Unilateral or bilateral. Lump noticed (a 'pump bump'). Ask regarding recent change in activity level or footwear, and for evidence of an underlying inflammatory disorder.

Examination
- Local tenderness and warmth, superficial or deep to the tendon around its insertion.
- Possible palpable bony mass at the affected site.
- Ensure the tendon is intact (calf squeeze test).

Differential diagnosis
- Non-insertional Achilles tendonitis.
- Achilles tendon rupture.
- Calcaneal injury/fracture.
- Arthritis of ankle joint.

Investigations
- Plain radiographs (Haglund's deformity).
- Blood markers—ESR, CRP—if suspicion of generalized inflammatory disorder.
- USS to assess for tendinosis or tendon degeneration.
- MRI to review for intrasubstance tears.

Management
- *Non-operative:*
  - Rest or activity modification
  - Walker boot usage to enable tendon rest
  - Ice treatment
  - NSAIDs
  - Change of footwear to some, with absent or cushioned back
  - Physiotherapy—mainstay of treatment; strengthening of the muscle–tendon complex and stretching will improve symptoms in most
  - Steroid injection generally not recommended because of risk of tendon rupture.
- *Operative:*
  - Removal of Haglund's deformity
  - Excision of implicated bursa

- Debridement of Achilles tendon to remove degenerative thickened tendon
- Repair of partial tears
- Local marrow stimulation techniques to initiate healing cascade.

Prevention
- Well-fitting shoes, careful stretching prior to exercise, maintenance strengthening.

Complications
- Chronic pain. Rupture of Achilles tendon.

Non-insertional tendinopathy

Inflammatory change in the paratenon (peritendonitis)—the soft tissue sheath that surrounds the Achilles tendon. May coexist with tendinosis (degenerative change of the tendon itself).

Risk factors
Physical exertion in context of poor running technique/footwear causing irritative rubbing over a bony protuberance, biomechanical abnormalities (e.g. overpronated foot); ↑ age; inflammatory conditions (e.g. RA, diabetes, steroid use).

Incidence
- Reported to be as high as 10% in runners.

History
May be a precipitating change in activity level or training regime. Gradual onset of posterior ankle pain and stiffness, particularly when mobilizing. May reduce with exercising or applying heat, but recurs. More acute onset suggests a rupture.

Examination
Fusiform swelling, thickening and tenderness of the tendon, with palpable crepitus. Usually 2–6cm from insertion. Presence of calf atrophy indicates chronicity. Nodules within the tendon imply an underlying tendinosis.

Investigations
- Primarily a clinical diagnosis.
- *Plain radiographs:* may show soft tissue swelling, calcifications, calcaneal avulsion fractures, or Haglund's deformity.
- *USS:* useful if rupture suspected; will show inflammation in paratenon.
- *MRI:* can show any degenerate change in the tendon (tendinosis).
- If other suggestive features, consider investigation for underlying medical condition (e.g. diabetes, RA).

Management
- *Non-operative:*
  - Rest, often for several weeks, or activity modification
  - Ice treatment
  - NSAIDs
  - Physiotherapy—mainstay of treatment; strengthening of the muscle–tendon complex and stretching will improve symptoms in most
  - Appropriate shoes ± customized orthoses to control foot position if biomechanics not optimized

- Weight loss if obese
- Corticosteroid injection generally contraindicated.
- *Operative:*
  - Treatment of the underlying cause is imperative for symptom improvement.
  - Release ± excision of paratenon—release is performed on the dorsal, medial, and lateral aspects of the tendon. Avoid the anterior sheath as may compromise blood supply. Running may begin 6–10 weeks after surgery.

Prognosis

'Excellent' results reported in 75% of cases with non-operative treatment, with mean recovery time of 5 weeks. Operative outcomes variable.

Prevention

- Good stretching, footwear, and training programme.

Further reading

Alfredson H, Cook J. A treatment algorithm for managing Achilles tendinopathy: new treatment options. *British Journal of Sports Medicine*. 2007;**41**(4):211–16.
Lopez RG, Jung HG. Achilles tendinosis: treatment options. *Clinics in Orthopedic Surgery*. 2015;**7**(1):1–7.

Achilles tendon rupture

Complete or partial discontinuity of the Achilles tendon. Commonly occurs 5cm proximal to its insertion into the calcaneum at the point of the 'vascular watershed' (the hypovascular region), although it can happen at any point in its length.

Epidemiology

- Peak age 30–50 years; ♂:♀ 4:1. Incidence: 31:100,000.

Risk factors

- Acute physical exertion, often unaccustomed.
- Previous rupture.
- Underlying tendinosis.
- Recent epitendinous steroid injection.
- Systemic medication—steroids and quinolone antibiotics have been implicated.

History

Sudden sensation of, or even audible, snap in back of the heel while undertaking physical activity. Usually painful but can have minimal pain. Patient may believe they have been hit or kicked. Difficulty walking/climbing stairs/standing on tiptoes. Previous rupture or non-specific heel pain (suggestive of underlying tendinopathy).

Examination

- Local soft tissue swelling/bruising.
- Palpable gap at the site of rupture.
- Degree of active plantar flexion does not exclude the diagnosis (intact deep flexor tendons), but power would be subnormal.
- Calf squeeze test: with the patient prone, calf muscles are squeezed—induced plantar flexion should be comparable with normal side; reduced if rupture.

Differential diagnosis

- Non-insertional Achilles tendonitis.
- Ankle or calcaneal avulsion fracture.
- Musculo-tendinous junction tear.
- Gastrocnemius/soleus muscle tear.

Investigations

- *Plain radiograph:* to exclude avulsion fracture.
- *USS:* to confirm clinical diagnosis (complete or partial tear) and estimate gap between tendon ends (if <5mm, may indicate low re-rupture rate with non-operative treatment).
- *MRI:* for neglected/long-standing cases; may provide useful information.

Management

There remains controversy as to the best treatment option with regard to non-operative or operative intervention. Recent evidence suggests that re-rupture rates are close to equivalent for functional rehabilitation regimes vs operative intervention.

- *Non-operative:* regimes vary—below is a guideline.
  - Initial immobilization in gravity equinus plaster cast—this is generally applied in the ED.
  - At next clinic visit, the plaster is exchanged for an adjustable removable boot for 4 weeks, 30° locked plantigrade, fully weight-bearing.
  - Progressively ↓ the amount of plantar flexion over weeks 4–6, dynamized weight-bearing 15–30°.
  - Weeks 6–8, dynamized 0–30°.
  - Total time in boot 8 weeks.
  - Refer to physiotherapy for progressive mobilization and strengthening.
- *Operative:*
  - May be performed as an open or percutaneous technique.
  - End-to-end repair may be augmented with plantaris or peroneal tendons or gastrocnemius fascia (but usually reserved for re-rupture or late-presenting cases).
  - Surgery reduces re-rupture rate—the risk difference is 1.6%, but at the cost of a significantly higher number of complications (wound dehiscence, infection, sural nerve damage).

Further reading

Aujla RS, Patel S, Jones A, Bhatia M. Non-operative functional treatment for acute Achilles tendon ruptures: the Leicester Achilles Management Protocol (LAMP). *Injury.* 2019;**50**(4):995–9.

Aujla R, Sapare S, Bhatia M. Acute Achilles tendon rupture treatment: where are we now? *Journal of Arthroscopy and Joint Surgery.* 2018;**5**(3):139–44.

Ochen Y, Reinier BB, van Heijl M, et al. Operative treatment versus nonoperative treatment of Achilles tendon ruptures: systematic review and meta-analysis. *BMJ.* 2019;**364**:k5120.

Plantar fasciitis

Definition
Degenerative change of the plantar fascia (sole of the foot).

Epidemiology
Common in adults, usually in third to fifth decades. Commonest cause of heel pain.

Pathogenesis
Develops with repetitive tensile overload of soft tissue attachments to the plantar aspect of the heel.

Pathology
Chronic degeneration at the origin of the plantar fascia. It is a degenerative, not an inflammatory, condition. The central part of the deep fascia is attached to the medial plantar tubercle of the calcaneum.

Aetiology
Idiopathic, obesity, inflammatory conditions, prolonged standing, trauma, unaccustomed exercise, footwear.

Symptoms
Gradual onset of pain at the origin of the plantar aponeurosis that is worse in the morning or after rest, and ↑ with weight-bearing. A relative heel cord contracture ↑ the symptoms, and pain is more distal than in other causes.

Examination
Assess the ankle and foot profile. Establish if the point of maximal tenderness is related to the medial calcaneal tuberosity. ↑ pain with dorsiflexion of toes, which tensions the plantar fascia. Tenderness over the medial longitudinal arch may occur.

Differential diagnosis
Heel pain triad—plantar fasciitis, posterior tibial tendon dysfunction, and tarsal tunnel syndrome. Other causes of heel pain are calcaneal apophysitis, gout, pseudogout, Paget's disease, inflammatory arthritides or enthesopathies, heel fat pad atrophy, and tumours.

Investigations
- *Radiology*: standing AP and lateral radiographs. 'Saddle sign' is present in 60% of cases of heel pain—radiolucency proximal to plantar calcaneal spur, indicating fatigue of the calcaneal tuberosity. Heel spurs are not in the plantar fascia, as is commonly thought, but are found at the origin of the short flexors. A 45° medial oblique view is useful to diagnose a stress fracture. An axial view may detect an occult bone tumour.
- *MRI*: demonstrates partial tears and inflammation.
- *Bone scan*: in plantar fasciitis, there is a focal ↑ in uptake at the origin of the fascia.
- *Other*: chronic cases may require screening to exclude metastatic and inflammatory conditions, including HLA-B27 if spondyloarthropathy is suspected.

Natural history

- Usually a self-limiting condition.

Management

- *Non-operative:* heel cord and plantar fascia stretching—physiotherapy, ice stretching, orthotics (gel heel insert), night splints, analgesics and NSAIDs, and extracorporeal shock wave therapy. A medial arch support that tilts the heel into varus may be helpful in treatment of plantar fasciitis in patients with pes planus. Steroid injection—this is controversial as the injection itself can lead to fat pad atrophy and its effects are transient.
- *Operative:* after failure of non-operative treatment (<5%). Commonest procedure is plantar fascia release. Excision of the plantar spur (located at the origin of the flexor digitorum brevis (FDB) and not at that of the plantar fascia) is sometimes recommended. Gastrocnemius lengthening is also an option.

Further reading

Guijosa A. Plantar fasciitis: evidence-based treatment review. *Reumatologia Clinica*. 2007;**3**(4):159–65.
League AC. Current concepts review: plantar fasciitis. *Foot and Ankle International*. 2008;**29**:358–66.
Orchard J. Plantar fasciitis. *BMJ*. 2012;**345**:e6603.

Hallux valgus

Definition

Lateral deviation of the great toe at the MTPJ, with medial deviation of the first metatarsal.

Aetiology

Positive family history in up to 65% of patients. Common in patients with hyperlaxity syndrome or acquired laxity due to RA, gout, or injury. Metatarsus primus varus (medial deviation of the first metatarsal) or acquired hallux valgus from narrow shoewear and splayed foot (weak intrinsics with ↑ age) are less common.

Anatomical factors

Distal metatarsal articular angle (DMAA), intermetatarsal angle (IMTA), hallux valgus angle (HVA), congruency of the MTPJ, and interphalangeal angle (IPA) (Fig. 16.2).

Prevalence

• Occurs in up to 30% of individuals. ♀ affected more than ♂.

Normal angles

• Normal—IMTA <10°, HVA <15°, no incongruency, DMAA <10°.

Classification

• *Mild:* IMTA <13°, HVA <20°, no incongruency.
• *Moderate:* IMTA 13–15°, HVA 20–40°, incongruency.
• *Severe:* IMTA >16°, HVA >41°, incongruency.

History

Family history, age of onset, progression, shoewear, main complaint (pain vs appearance), site of pain, activity level, and expectations of surgery. Usually presents with pain over medial aspect of MTPJ. May have discomfort due to impingement of second toe.

Examination

Gait—look for normal push-off. Foot inspection—presence of a large bunion, great toe deformity at MTPJ and IPJ, lesser toe deformities, overriding and underriding of lesser toes, pronation of the foot, site of pain. Ankle and subtalar movements, plantar callosities, metatarsal–cuneiform movement (if proximal procedures required). MTPJ, evidence of pain on movement. MTPJ (hallux rigidus). Neurovascular assessment.

Differential diagnosis

• Gout, fracture malunion, congenital deformity.

Imaging

Weight-bearing AP and lateral radiographs to measure angles. HVA, IMTA, DMAA, MTPJ congruency, evidence of degenerative changes of first MTPJ and IPJ, plantar opening of the first metatarsal cuneiform joint, relative lengths of the first and second metatarsals. Assess position of the sesamoids.

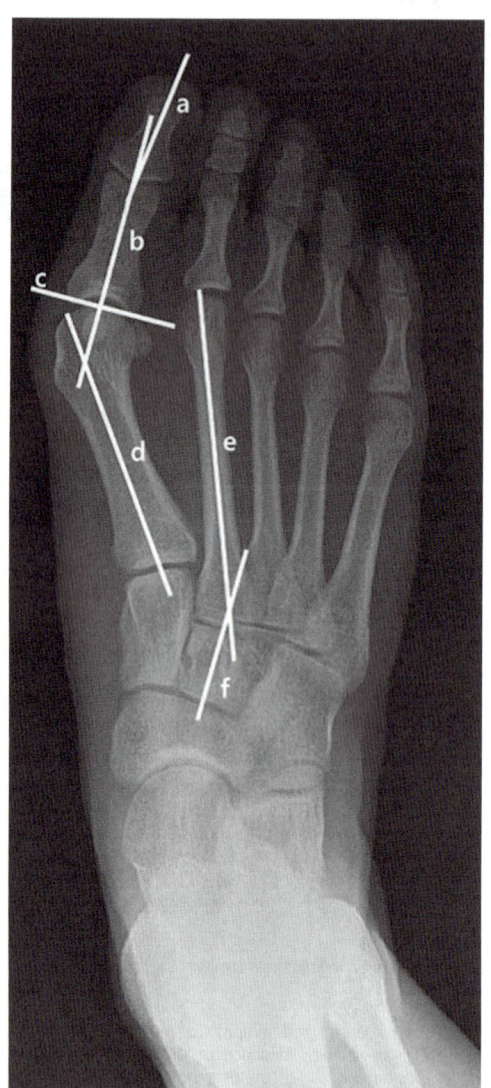

Fig. 16.2 An AP radiograph of the right foot. Distal metatarsal articular angle (angle between c and d); hallux valgus angle (angle between b and d); and interphalangeal angle (angle between a and b).

Reproduced from Kyoung Lee, Soyeon Ahn, Chin Chung, et al. Reliability and Relationship of Radiographic Measurements in Hallux Valgus, *Clinical Orthopaedics and Related Research* **470**:9, 2012, with permission from Wolters Kluwer.

Management

- *Non-operative:* always consider first. Wider shoes supplemented with a wide toe-box to prevent rubbing of the bunion, metatarsal head pads, toe spacers for lesser toes, prescription shoes.
- *Operative options:* surgery aims to establish a congruent first MTPJ with sesamoid realignment, and to correct IMTA and HVA. Resect medial eminence (bunion), and retain the first MTPJ motion and foot biomechanics.
- *Indications:* failure of non-operative treatment, progressing deformity and pain, restricted function; cosmesis is not an indication for surgery.
- *Groups:* (1) congruent MTPJ; (2) incongruent or subluxed MTPJ; and (3) hallux valgus with arthritis of MTPJ.

The wide array of operative procedures indicates that there is disagreement on the best operative procedure (i.e. which osteotomy to use).

Soft tissue and bony procedures

- *Congruent MTPJ:* Chevron and Mitchell's, with or without distal soft tissue procedures.
- *Incongruent joint:* treatment depends on the severity:
  - Mild—Chevron osteotomy, Mitchell's osteotomy, distal soft tissue procedure
  - Moderate—Mitchell's osteotomy, distal soft tissue and proximal osteotomy
  - Severe—scarf osteotomy, first MTPJ arthrodesis, Lapidus procedure.

Osteotomies

- *Chevron:* 'V'-type osteotomy at level of metatarsal neck, with the centre of the metatarsal head used as the apex. The plantar cut is at 60° to the metatarsal base and should avoid damage to plantar vascularization. The dorsal cut is 45° to the cortex. Allows displacement to 50% of the width of the metatarsal head. Used to treat mild to moderate hallux valgus. The osteotomy is stable and may correct DMAA. Maximum displacement (30%). AVN occurs in up to 20% of cases.
- *Scarf:* consists of a horizontal cut and two transverse cuts, allowing for a wide range of angular corrections. The procedure allows for medial and lateral translations, IMTA or DMAA correction, lowering/elevation of the metatarsal head, and shortening/elevation of the first metatarsal. Technically difficult and has a learning curve. Internal fixation is required. However, it is a popular option for all severities.
- *Akin's:* medial closing wedge osteotomy at the level of the proximal phalanx base. Used to correct hallux interphalangeus. Often performed with a definitive hallux valgus procedure. Requires internal fixation, usually with staples.
- *Lapidus osteotomy:* for moderate to severe deformities, hypermobility of proximal metatarsal leads to severe valgus deformity. May be combined with other hallux valgus procedures. There is no shortening of the first metatarsal. Less commonly performed, compared with other distal osteotomies.

Complications

- Recurrence, failure to correct the deformity, hallux varus and transfer metatarsalgia, AVN of metatarsal head. Non-union of osteotomy.
- Adolescents: up to 30% rate of recurrence post-correction. This may be due to inadequate soft tissue release and failure to correct alignment.

Further reading

Fraissler L, Konrads C, Hoberg M, Rudert M, Walcher M. Treatment of hallux valgus deformity. *EFORT Open Reviews.* 2016;**1**(8):295–302.

Malagelada F, Sahirad C, Dalmau-Pastor M, *et al.* Minimally invasive surgery for hallux valgus: a systematic review of current surgical techniques. *International Orthopaedics.* 2019;**43**(3):625–37.

Hallux rigidus

Definition
Degenerative changes at the first MTPJ.

Epidemiology
- Joint most commonly affected by OA in the foot. Occurs in 1 in 40 people >50 years. Twice as common in women. Rare in children.
- Adolescents—localized lesions. Adults—generalized arthrosis.
- Typically dorsal cartilage loss, and hence dorsal osteophyte common.

Causes
Antecedent trauma, RA/inflammatory arthritis, gout, osteochondral defect in first metatarsal head, congenital elevation of the first metatarsal.

History
Insidious onset of pain and stiffness of the great toe, ↑ on walking, running, and wearing high-heeled shoes. Burning and paraesthesiae can occur. Leading to continuous pain.

Examination
- Initial swelling and tender first MTPJ. Reduced dorsiflexion. Later, dorsomedial osteophyte (loss of motion, skin irritation) and elevated (and long) first metatarsal.
- Pseudohallux rigidus—nodular swelling of the proximal FHL limiting hallux dorsiflexion. FHL becomes constricted within its fibro-osseous tunnel; motion is restored on ankle plantar flexion.

Radiology
Joint space narrowing, widening and flattening of first metatarsal head and base of proximal phalanx, subchondral sclerosis and cysts, formation of dorsal osteophytes at the metatarsal head and proximal phalanx.

Management
- *Non-operative:* aimed at reducing MTPJ movement and relieving dorsal pressure. Stiff shoe or rocker-bottom shoe, NSAIDs, MUA, intra-articular steroid injection (evidence does not support hyaluronic acid), and cushioned shoe wear.
- *Operative:* indication is failure of non-operative treatment.
  - *Adolescents:* osteotomy of base of proximal phalanx—requires preoperative 30° plantar flexion
  - *Adults:*
    - Cheilectomy—will relieve only dorsal impingement (dorsal spur and one-third of metatarsal head)
    - Arthrodesis—following failed cheilectomy or where advanced degenerative changes are present
    - Interpositional arthroplasty—shows promising short- to mid-term results, but arthrodesis remains the gold standard.

Further reading

Anderson MR, Ho BS, Baumhauer JF. Current concepts review: hallux rigidus. *Foot and Ankle Orthopaedics*. 2018;**3**(2). Available from: ⚲ https://doi.org/10.1177/2473011418764461

Chan O. Hallux rigidus: a review. *Orthopaedics and Trauma*. 2020;**34**:23–9.

Daniels TR, Younger ASE, Penner MJ, *et al*. Midterm outcomes of polyvinyl alcohol hydrogel hemiarthroplasty of the first metatarsophalangeal joint in advanced hallux rigidus. *Foot and Ankle International*. 2017;**38**(3):243–7.

Morton's neuroma

Aetiology
- Due to compression of a common digital nerve between the metatarsal heads as it passes deep to the intermetatarsal ligament to enter the webspace.
- Third webspace is most commonly affected, followed by the second webspace.
- Patients are commonly middle-aged and ♀.

Pathology
- Histologically, the nerve shows fibrous tissue formation around the nerve and nerve degeneration.

History
- Symptoms range from a dull ache, including a 'pebble in shoe' sensation, or a burning paraesthetic pain on the medial and lateral borders of the affected toes.

Examination
- A positive Mulder's click test (squeezing the metatarsal heads together while applying AP compression with the other examining hand) helps to clinically diagnose the condition.
- Review for paraesthesiae of the digital nerve of the affected toe.

Investigations
- *Plain radiograph*: will indicate any osteologic (deformity) which can be affecting the nerve.
- *USS*: operator-dependent, so may not always yield a diagnosis in inexperienced hands.
- *MRI*: gold standard investigation if there is doubt regarding the diagnosis or multiple neuroma is expected.

Management
- Corticosteroids remain the gold standard of treatment.

Further reading
Thomson L, Aujla RS, Divall P, Bhatia M. Non-surgical treatments for Morton's neuroma: a systematic review. *Foot and Ankle Surgery*. 2020;**26**(7):736–43.

Hammer toe deformity

Definition
Abnormal fixed flexion posture of the PIPJ of the lesser toe, with associated hyperextension of the MTPJ (Fig. 16.3). Associated with a contracture of the FDL tendon.

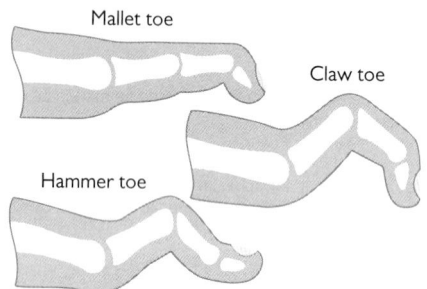

Fig. 16.3 Various lesser toe deformities.

Associated conditions
Often a mechanical cause; long second metatarsal, high heels and narrow shoes. RA, diabetes mellitus, crossover deformity. May be iatrogenic, post-plantar release.

Epidemiology
Commonest is the second toe. May accompany hallux valgus.

Differential diagnosis
Interdigital neuroma, claw toe, and MTPJ synovitis.

History
Pain on plantar aspect of the metatarsal head, dorsum of the proximal phalanx and apex of the toe (can be with associated thick skin), deformity worse on walking (hammer toes are accentuated on weight-bearing when the intrinsics are relaxed).

Examination
Callus formation over the dorsum of PIPJ ± volar tip of the toe. Distinguish between a supple and a fixed hammer toe (DIPJ remains supple). When there is contracture of the FDL tendon, then plantar flexion of the ankle will straighten the toe, with dorsiflexion worsening the deformity (± evaluate for subluxation of the stability of MTPJ hyperextension).

Management
- *Non-operative:* pads over corns and daily stretching of PIPJ. Hammer toe-straightening orthotics + taping of toe to prevent further deformity.

- *Operative*: surgery is indicated for disabling pain. Flexibility (i.e. fixed or flexible deformity) determines the techniques used to correct hallux valgus first:
  - Flexible and mild deformity of PIPJ alone—isolated tenotomy of FDL tendon, flexor-to-extensor transfer
  - Moderate deformity and fixed contracture at PIPJ—arthroplasty, arthrodesis
  - Severe deformity—partial proximal phalangectomy (poor cosmesis).

Claw toe deformity

Definition
Hyperextension at the MTPJ and flexion at the PIPJ and DIPJ.

Pathogenesis
Imbalance between the extrinsic extensor tendons (which indirectly extend the MTPJ) and the intrinsics (which flex the MTPJ). The deformity results from simultaneous contraction of extensors and flexors and leads to the metatarsal fat pad being pulled distally through its attachment to the proximal phalanx.

Associated
Pes cavus, Charcot–Marie–Tooth disease and its neurological associations. Always consider whole-spine MRI and EMG to exclude an underlying cause.

Differential diagnosis
Hammer toes (±MTPJ hyperextension).

Precipitating conditions
Age, RA, diabetes mellitus, post-traumatic compartment syndrome, polio, hereditary sensory motor neuropathy (HSMN), CVA.

History
Pain under metatarsal heads, deformity, callosities, catching of the toes on walking, and neurological symptoms.

Examination
- Neurological examination of upper and lower limbs, and look for a cavus foot.
- Is the deformity correctable? Assess flexibility of the toes with the ankle in plantar flexion and dorsiflexion; if the claw toe deformity disappears with plantar flexion, then it is considered flexible. Determine the degree of MTPJ hyperextension and PIPJ flexion.
- Look for trophic changes of the foot.
- Assessment during gait: does the clawing become more pronounced during the stance/swing phase?
- Swing phase weakness: may indicate weak ankle dorsiflexors and overcompensation of toe extensors.
- Stance phase weakness: may indicate weak triceps surae and overcompensation of the long toe flexor.

Management
- *Non-operative:* corn pads, metatarsal pads, and wide toe-box in shoe wear.
- *Operative:* surgical correction depends on the size of the deformity and flexibility of the joints.
  - Flexible claw toe implies that there is no contraction of the MTPJ or PIPJ—FDL flexor to extensor tendon transfer with capsulodesis of the MTPJ.
  - Fixed claw toe:

- ○ MTPJ subluxation: MTPJ soft tissue release—extensor Z lengthening and EDB tenotomy, release of collateral ligaments ± shortening at the base of the proximal phalanx to aid reduction of the MTPJ
- ○ MTPJ dislocation: Stainsby procedure/DuVries metatarsal head arthroplasty with release of EDL, dorsal capsule, and MCL
- ○ PIP deformity: PIPJ fusion or resection arthroplasty (removing distal third of proximal phalanx)
- ○ Arthrodesis MTPJ: for severe or recurrent deformity, or when associated with neurological disturbance of forefoot.

Stainsby procedure: dorsal incision over the MTPJ (single) or webspace (multiple). Extensor tenotomy, remove three-quarters of proximal phalanx. Suture distal extensor tendon end to the flexor tendon. Stabilize with a k-wire.

Lesser toe deformities

Common problems often leading to pain, deformity, and footwear problems. May be associated hallux valgus to correct first.

Aetiology

Constrictive footwear which restricts normal movement of the lesser toe joints, impeding intrinsic muscle function.

Examination

Is the deformity correctable? Presence of callosities, neurovascular abnormality, subluxation of the MTPJ, hallux valgus, or tight FDL? Do deformities become more pronounced on gait?

Deformities

- *Hammer toe:* flexion at the PIPJ ± hyperextension of the MTPJ. Usually acquired. Often flexible early, and fixed contracture late (for treatment, see ➲ Hammer toe deformity, p. 522).
- *Mallet toe:* flexion contracture of the DIPJ. Patients complain of toe stubbing, which may lead to toe-tip pain.
  - *Management—operative options:* flexible FDL tenotomy at the DIPJ; fixed—DIPJ fusion and FDL tenotomy.
- *Claw toe:* hyperextension at the MTPJs and flexion at the PIPJ and DIPJ. Usually involves several toes and may be associated with a neurological deformity.
  - *Management:* non-operative treatment should be attempted—a deep and wide toe-box shoe, corn padding, and soft metatarsal pads. For operative treatment, see ➲ Claw toe deformity, p. 522.
- *Curly toes:* flexion at both the PIPJ and distal DIPJ, malrotation of one or more toes. A common disorder in childhood. May be related to contracture of FDL and FDB tendons.
  - *Management:* reassurance of parents and initially non-operative. Operative options for pain, progression of deformity, and problems with footwear or walking. FDL/FDB tenotomy (age 3–4 years).
- *Overlapping fifth toe:* a dorsal adduction deformity of the fifth toe. There may be malrotation with EDL contracture. The deformity is often familial and bilateral. Often asymptomatic, but can cause difficulty with footwear, dorsal toe pain, callus, or a bunionette.
  - *Management:* most treated *non-operatively* with strapping. *Operative options* include DuVries correction and Butler's or Lapidus procedure.
- *Bunionette deformity:* soft corn over the dorsal aspect of the fifth toe.
  - *Classification:* (1) enlargement of the metatarsal head; (2) lateral bowing of fifth metatarsal; (3) wide fourth to fifth IMTA. A symptomatic plantar callus is secondary to plantar flexion of the fifth metatarsal.
  - *Management: non-operative* initially (wide footwear, metatarsal pads, and chiropodist treatment). Soft tissue surgery unlikely to be successful. *Operative options* for type 1: Chevron osteotomy; for types 2 and 3: mid-shaft medial displacement oblique osteotomy.

Ingrown toenails

Also known as onychocryptosis.

Epidemiology

Common, occur in adolescents and young adults, with ♂ affected more frequently. Usually affects the hallux, but other nails may be involved. Bilateral on occasion.

Pathology

Nail plate penetration of the lateral nail fold. A sharp spike of nail presses against the soft tissues and lateral nail fold. Excessive inflammatory response, with granulation tissue that grows over the nail.

Aetiology

Tight-fitting shoes, poor foot care, inappropriate nail cutting (longitudinal).

History

Pain (especially on wearing shoes), bacterial/fungal infections (which are often recurrent), soft tissue oedema in distal phalanx.

Management

- *Non-operative:* regular salt soaking and foot washing, well-fitting shoes, education on nail cutting (transversely), and chiropodist referral.
- *Operative:* failure of non-operative treatment, recurrent infection, pain. The nail can be removed by avulsion of the whole nail or wedge resection of the involved side of the nail and mechanical (Zadek's procedure)/chemical (phenolization) nail plate ablation. This has a 95% success rate.

Complications include recurrence and persistent infection. Two-stage procedure: in the presence of infection, the first stage involves removal of the nail to allow resolution of infection and the second stage involves the Zadek's procedure.

Further reading

Park DH, Singh D. The management of ingrowing toenails. *BMJ*. 2010;**344**:e2089.

The diabetic foot

Foot disease is common in type 1 and type 2 diabetes. The diabetic foot refers to a spectrum of diseases that include ulcers, bone or joint changes, and infection. The effect of peripheral neuropathy is to impair protective sensation in the foot, and abnormal pressure may lead to callosities and formation of ulcers. Healing is compromised by arterial and microvascular insufficiency.

Prevalence

• Fifteen to 20% of patients with diabetes develop foot ulcers.

Examination

• Overall shape of the foot and ankle.
• Bunions, pressure areas, callosities.
• Perfusion of the foot.
• Sensation.
• Movements (pain).
• Ulcers (clean or sloughy? Do they probe to bone?).
• Evidence of gangrene.

Regular monitoring and diabetic MDT are key to successful management. Remain vigilant for features of an acute diabetic foot (termed a 'diabetic foot attack'); this is a severe presentation of diabetic foot disease—an acutely inflamed foot, with rapidly progressive skin and tissue necrosis (± systemic features). Can rapidly (over hours) progress and become limb-threatening, resulting in amputation if untreated.

Investigations

These should include:
• Radiographs
• Doppler USS
• ABPI
• MRI—to establish if there is osteomyelitis and, if so, the extent.

Management

Guided by various classifications (including Wagner stage, SINBAD score, and Brodsky depth–ischaemia scale).

Non-operative

• Optimize diabetic control.
• Regular inspection and careful chiropody.
• Well-fitting footwear with deep, wide toe-box and custom-moulded insole.
• Prompt antibiotics for infection.
• Total contact casting may be needed.

Operative

• Debridement and active wound management (microbiology and appropriate antibiotic treatment).
• Local excision of osteomyelitis.
• Ray amputation.
• Partial calcanectomy.

- Partial foot amputation (Lisfranc or Chopart amputation).
- Below-knee amputation.

All patients with complications as a result of diabetes require multidisciplinary care by GPs, physicians, surgeons, nurse practitioners, and community healthcare professionals.

Further reading

National Institute for Health and Care Excellence (2015). *Diabetic foot problems: prevention and management.* NICE guideline [NG19]. Available from: ℘ www.nice.org.uk/guidance/ng19/

Rathur HM, Boulton AJM. Recent advances in the diagnosis and management of diabetic neuropathy. *Journal of Bone and Joint Surgery (British Volume)*. 2005;**87**:1605–10.

Vas PR, Edmonds M, Kavarthapu V, *et al*. The diabetic foot attack: ''tis too late to retreat!'. *International Journal of Lower Extremity Wounds*. 2018;**17**(1):7–13.

Entrapment syndromes of the lower limb

Structures causing entrapment
- Congenital osseous/fibrous bands.
- Benign tumours (e.g. exostosis, ganglion).
- Iatrogenic (e.g. scar tissue, surgical implants).

Types of entrapment
- Nerve—commonest.
- Vascular.
- Tendon.

Spinal nerve root entrapment
- From intervertebral disc prolapse or degenerative lateral recess stenosis.

Meralgia paraesthetica
- An entrapment syndrome of the lateral femoral cutaneous nerve—results in pain and paraesthesiae in a variable area of the lateral thigh.
- May be compressed as it enters the thigh from the abdomen or as it courses superficially below and medial to the ASIS.

Piriformis syndrome
- Compression of the sciatic nerve or its contributing parts by the piriformis in the gluteal region.
- Causes pain on sitting.
- Symptoms may be confused with spinal nerve root entrapment.

Popliteal artery entrapment
- Variant anatomy may cause extrinsic compression of the artery.
- Leads to pain and claudication in young patients.

Tarsal tunnel syndrome
(See ⮎ Tarsal tunnel syndrome, pp. 506–507.)

Peripheral nerve injuries in the lower limb

Peripheral nerve injuries in the lower limb are less common than their counterparts in the upper limb. May be traumatic or iatrogenic.

Anatomical classification of peripheral nerve injuries

(See ➲ Chapter 18, Peripheral nerve injuries, pp. 577–579.)

- Neurapraxia.
- Axonotmesis.
- Neurotmesis.

Specific at-risk lower limb injuries and peripheral nerves

- *Posterior hip dislocation.* The sciatic nerve lies posterior to the proximal femur and may undergo a traction injury as the hip dislocates or a compression injury as the hip is relocated. This highlights the importance of assessing neurological status on initial assessment of an injured limb and again following an intervention.
- *Pavlik harness.* Complications of Pavlik harness in the management of developmental dysplasia of the hip include compression of the femoral nerve by prolonged and excessive hip flexion.
- *Iliac crest bone harvesting.* The lateral femoral cutaneous nerve usually exits the pelvis, inferior and medial to the ASIS, but its course is variable and it is therefore prone to iatrogenic damage when harvesting bone graft.
- *Below-knee casting.* The fibular head, as well as other bony prominences, should be padded prior to applying the cast, in order to prevent pressure sores and direct compression of the common peroneal nerve as it courses around the fibular neck.
- *Saphenous vein cannulation.* The saphenous nerve lies adjacent to the vein at the ankle and is easily damaged, resulting in sensory loss to the medial border of the foot.
- *Compartment syndrome.* This surgical emergency occurs when the intracompartmental pressure rises to within 30mmHg of the systemic diastolic BP. This results in loss of tissue perfusion to the affected compartment, with the contents becoming increasingly ischaemic. Peripheral nerves are poorly tolerant of ischaemic damage.
- *THR.* During THR, injury to the femoral, sciatic, or superior gluteal nerves can occur with excessive retraction. The nerves usually recover over several weeks, but a few persist.
- *Achilles tendon repair.* The surgical approach should be on the medial border of the Achilles tendon, to avoid damaging the sural nerve, which runs near the lateral border of the tendon.

Adult orthopaedics: spine

Cervical spine in adults

Epidemiology

Neck pain is common, occurring in 10% of the population at any time. Modern-day technology has caused a rapid ↑ in the proportion of symptomatic neck pain, with 'text neck syndrome' being defined to describe repeated stress injury and pain in the neck resulting from excessive watching or texting on handheld devices over a sustained period.

Aetiology

Neck pain can represent a wide array of cervical spine disorders that can be divided into traumatic and atraumatic types.

Traumatic neck pain

Common after high-energy mechanisms of injury such as road traffic collisions:

- Soft tissue injuries—tendinous/ligamentous injury, whiplash injury
- Intervertebral disc herniation, annulus rupture
- Vertebral body fractures
- Facet subluxations or dislocations.

Atraumatic neck pain

- *Degenerative*—cervical spondylosis, degenerative disc disease, facet degeneration, synovial cyst.
- *Inflammatory*—RA, AS, polymyalgia rheumatica, polymyositis.
- *Infection*—osteomyelitis, spondylodiscitis, meningitis.
- *Tumour*—vertebral body tumours, metastatic tumours, intradural tumours, nerve sheath tumours.
- *Shoulder disorders*—subacromial impingement, adhesive capsulitis, tennis elbow, repetitive strain disorder, impingement syndrome.
- *Miscellaneous*—fibromyalgia, myofascial syndrome, torticollis, Paget's disease.
- *Referred pain*—cardiac, cholecystitis, lymph nodes, temporomandibular joint problems.

Clinical

Cervical assessment should focus on local or regional tenderness, ROM, and neurological assessment (UMN or LMN signs). In traumatic neck pain, the neck must be immobilized until it is confirmed that there is no instability and it has been documented that there is no neurological deficit.

Three main patterns of presentations clinical presentation

1. Axial neck pain

- Degeneration, facet joint pain, or ligamentous strain.
- Neck stiffness, headache.
- Referred pain to shoulder, chest, and face.
- Atlanto-occipital and atlanto-axial pain radiating to the neck, often exacerbated by neck rotation.

2. Radiculopathy

Clinical symptoms vary, depending on specific nerve root involvement.

Nerve root	Clinical presentation
C2	Pain over occipital region
C3	Pain in back of neck and mastoid area, pinna, and trapezius
C4	Pain and numbness in lower end of neck and top of shoulder girdle
C5	Pain in side of neck to lateral aspect of arm, weak deltoid, no reflex change, Epaulet sign, regimental badge sign
C6	Pain in lateral arm, forearm, and thumb, weak biceps and biceps reflex
C7	Pain in middle forearm and middle finger, weak triceps and triceps reflex
C8	Pain in medial forearm/little finger, intrinsic hand atrophy, normal reflexes
T1	Pain in armpit and anterior chest wall, intrinsic hand atrophy

- *Spurling's test*: reproduction or exacerbation of radicular arm pain on extension and ipsilateral rotation of the neck, due to forced foraminal narrowing on the affected side.

3. Myelopathy

- In contrast to radiculopathy, pain is not a common presenting feature of myelopathy. Symptoms include:
  - Gait disturbance (typically ataxic and broad-based, stooped and spastic)
  - ↑ tone and spasticity.
  - Paraesthesiae, sensory disturbance, and weakness (upper > lower limb)
  - Myelopathic hand—↓ dexterity, intrinsic muscle weakness
  - Hyperreflexia, Babinski sign
  - Positive Hoffman's test (long finger DIP tapped into extension and thumb flexion occurs)
  - Lhermitte's sign is present in 25% of patients (neck flexion causes electric shock-like symptoms going down the leg)
  - Paradoxical or inverted brachial reflex (tapping the brachialis tendon causes paradoxical finger flexion to occur)—this is the only positive sign of C6 involvement
  - Urinary disturbance (retention/frequency).
- Ask patient about functional impact (e.g. difficulty with doing up buttons, change in handwriting, unsteadiness on feet).

Box 17.1 shows grading of myelopathy.

> **Box 17.1 Grading of myelopathy**
> - Grade I: no neurological deficit
> - Grade II: subjective motor symptoms (weakness)
> - Grade IIIA: objective motor signs but ambulatory
> - Grade IIIB: objective motor signs and non-ambulatory

Investigations
- *Radiographs:*
  - Often show non-specific changes
  - Spinal canal can be seen in both AP and lateral views
  - Assessment of spinal alignment in lateral view
  - Oblique views used to assess neural foramina
  - Open mouth view to assess C1 and C2 fractures, and flexion/extension views to assess stability.
- *MRI:* demonstrates ligament injuries, nerve root compression, spinal cord compression, disc herniations, annular tears, foraminal stenosis, intrinsic changes, and cord oedema.
- *CT:* useful to assess bony abnormalities, detailed fracture patterns, and degenerative cervical osteophytes.
- *EMG and NCS:* provide useful information about nerve root involved and degree of neural involvement, as well as the location of nerve lesion.

Management
Non-operative options
- Axial neck pain due to degenerative disease is managed non-operatively in most cases.
- NSAIDs form the first line of analgesic treatment.
- Neuropathic medications are added for neurogenic pain.
- Physiotherapy is of prime importance—manual therapy, McKenzie exercises, ergonomic training, workplace adaptations, and postural rehabilitation form part of neck rehabilitation programme.
- Patients with severe, acute neurogenic pain with an identified root compression may benefit from a nerve root block, and those with facet joint pain may benefit from facet joint injections.
- Cervical collars can ease pain, but prolonged use should be avoided to prevent deconditioning of cervical musculature.

Operative options
- Indications for surgery include unstable fractures, neurological deficit, and persistent pain with identifiable focal cause.
- Myelopathy warrants early operation to prevent further neurological deterioration.
- Severe radicular pain not improved with conservative treatment may necessitate surgical decompression.
- Axial neck pain secondary to degeneration is generally not treated surgically, but if there are significant changes at a single segment, then fusion may be indicated.
- Approach for surgery can be anterior, posterior, or combined, based on the exact pathology. Procedures may involve decompression with or without fusion.

Lower back pain

Epidemiology

Back pain affects 8 out of 10 adults at some stage in their lives. The incidence of low back pain in developed countries is 15–20%; it is lower in developing countries. In 90% of patients with low back pain, it resolves within 6 weeks.

Aetiology

The causes of low back pain vary with age.

Children

- Trauma.
- Spondylolysis and spondylolisthesis.
- Intervertebral disc herniation.
- Scoliosis.
- Vertebral tumours—osteoid osteoma, benign osteoblastoma, Ewing's sarcoma, lymphoma.
- Infection.

Young adults

- Acute fractures.
- Acute disc herniation.
- Spondylolisthesis.
- Scheuermann's disease.
- AS.
- Metabolic bone disease.
- Spinal instability.

Older adults

- Degenerative disc disease and facetal arthropathy.
- Spinal stenosis.
- Osteoporotic fractures.
- Metastatic disease.
- Infection.

Risk factors associated with low back pain are obesity, smoking, manual labour, and traumatic events.

Common types of back pain

- *Discogenic back pain:* pain from disc degeneration, innervated layer of the annulus fibrosus.
- *Radicular back pain:* pain secondary to nerve root irritation, inflammation, or compression. Most commonly due to disc herniation, spinal stenosis, spondylolisthesis, or intraspinal pathology. Pain classically radiates to the buttock and/or leg along the dermatome of the nerve involved.
- *Referred back pain:* aortic aneurysm, visceral disease (peptic ulcer, pelvic inflammatory disease, endometriosis, gall bladder disease, pancreatic disease, renal disease, and pleural disease), infection, urinary tract infection (UTI), and arthritis of the hip.
- *Iatrogenic back pain:* dural adhesions, post-operative instability, post-operative discitis, arachnoiditis.
- *Psychogenic back pain:* organic pathology must be excluded.

Waddell's signs

Waddell's signs are used to describe non-organic or psychogenic back pain:

1. *Tenderness tests:* superficial and diffuse tenderness and/or non-anatomical tenderness
2. *Simulation tests:* these are based on movements which produce pain, without actually causing that movement, such as axial loading and pain on simulated rotation
3. *Distraction tests:* positive tests are rechecked when the patient's attention is distracted such as the SLR test
4. *Regional disturbances:* regional weakness or sensory changes which deviate from accepted neuroanatomy
5. *Overreaction:* subjective signs regarding the patient's demeanour and reaction to testing.

If there are more than three out of five signs present, then there is a high probability that the patient has a non-organic component to their pain. Non-organic signs in isolation should not be equated with the presence of a psychological component.

Clinical features

- Symptoms include back pain and stiffness and there may be altered sensation or motor deficits. There may be paravertebral muscle spasm, reduced movements of the spine, loss of normal thoracolumbar profile, and signs of a neurological deficit.
- Low back pain with radicular leg pain occurs with nerve root entrapment due to intervertebral disc prolapse (commonest cause), spinal stenosis, spondylolisthesis, and tumour infiltration into the canal.
- A thorough history is essential to elucidate the cause of the back pain, aggravating and alleviating factors, quality of pain, radiation, associated symptoms, weight loss, fever, night pain, and associated morning stiffness or other systemic symptoms.
- Examination findings: gait, posture, truncal balance, spinal movements, sites of tenderness, provocative movements, and a full neurological examination, including assessing for reduced SLR, nerve root tension signs, motor weakness, sensation loss, loss of deep tendon reflexes (LMN-type lesion); clonus, hyperreflexia, and positive Babinski signs (UMN-type lesion).
- Examine other systems from where the pain may be referred.
- Serious pathology may be heralded by so-called 'red flags':
  - <20 years of age or >50 years of age at onset
  - Non-mechanical pain
  - Nocturnal pain
  - Fever, night sweats, or weight loss
  - Thoracic pain
  - Severe or progressive neurological deficit
  - Sphincter disturbances
  - Immunosuppression
  - IV drug use (IVDU)
  - History of infection or malignancy
  - Significant trauma or deformity.
- Patients with these signs and symptoms must be assessed as a matter of urgency.

- *Cauda equina syndrome (CES)* (see ⮕ Chapter 20, Cauda equina syndrome, pp. 640–641).

Further reading

Abdu WA, Sacks OA, Tosteson AN, *et al*. Long-term results of surgery compared with nonoperative treatment for lumbar degenerative spondylolisthesis in the Spine Patient Outcomes Research Trial (SPORT). *Spine*. 2018;**43**(23):1619.

Weinstein JN, Tosteson TD, Lurie JD, *et al*. Surgical vs nonoperative treatment for lumbar disk herniation: the Spine Patient Outcomes Research Trial (SPORT): a randomized trial. *JAMA*. 2006;**296**(20):2441–50.

Back pain: investigations and management

Investigations

No investigations are indicated in most patients. However, patients with persistent pain or those who have signs suggesting serious underlying pathology need to be investigated.

- *Radiographs:*
  - AP and lateral radiographs of the spine may be useful in assessing spinal alignment, and assessing for acute fractures, destructive/lytic lesions, spondylolisthesis, and infective changes.
  - Certain particular radiographic signs are of importance—'*winking owl sign*' in destructive pedicle lesions, '*inverted napoleon hat sign*' in high-grade spondylolisthesis, and '*romanos lesions*' in AS.
  - Whole-spine radiographs may be indicated to assess overall spinal alignment and define scoliosis and/or kyphotic alignment.
- *MRI:* examination of choice. Detailed images include those of discal pathology, annular tears, disc herniation, ligamentum flavum hypertrophy, spinal stenosis, subacute fractures, ligamentous injuries, facetal arthropathy, tumour infiltration, metastatic lesion, spondylodiscitis involvement and destruction, prevertebral and epidural abscess, intraspinal lesion, spinal cord dysraphism and intrinsic abnormalities, congenital segmentation, and fusion abnormalities.
- *CT:* useful for detecting bone abnormalities (fractures, osteoid osteomas) and also used when patients cannot have MRI (cardiac pacemaker, metallic vascular clips).
- *Bone scan:* technetium bone scans are used for detecting early infection or localizing metastatic bone lesions.
- *Discography:* the painful segment can be investigated with provocative discograms to outline the architecture of the disc, and one can see if pain is reproduced with injection of dye into the disc. A normal disc is not usually painful when injected. Uncommonly performed now.
- *Laboratory tests:* no specific test. If infection or neoplasm is suspected, FBC, ESR, and CRP should be requested. In patients >50 years, there is a case for doing a workup to evaluate for any metastatic tumour, as well as a myeloma screen. In patients with marked stiffness or signs of CTD, a rheumatological screen and HLA-B27 testing may be requested.

Management

Non-operative

- Avoid rest—only very short periods are advised in the acute phase.
- Simple analgesics and anti-inflammatory medications are the usual first-line analgesic therapy for back pain, especially for periods of 4–6 weeks.
- Active approaches such as the McKenzie regime, and strength and conditioning of the core and back muscles may be helpful.
- For patients needing passive therapies, spinal mobilization techniques, including Maitland, mobilization with movement, and Kaltenborn techniques, are utilized, collectively labelled as 'passive physiological intervertebral movements'.

- Postural awareness and lifestyle modification are important in resolving mechanical neck and back pain.
- Active patient advice and education led by physiotherapists and all clinicians involved in the patient's care are of prime importance in long-term rehabilitation from back pain.
- NICE guidelines.

Operative
- Accurately defining the pathology is important in surgical planning and in determining the choice of surgery, levels of surgery, and approach.
- The ideal patient is one who is a non-smoker, has exhausted a comprehensive programme of non-operative treatment and rehabilitation, and has an identifiable source of their pain.
- Surgical options are multiple: decompression alone, decompression + fusion, posterolateral fusion, interbody fusion, stabilization only, tumour resection, abscess evacuation and biopsy, deformity correction, and disc replacement.
- The approach can be all posterior or can be combined anterior and posterior, or anterior alone. Anterior or lateral approaches include anterior lumbar interbody fusion (ALIF), extreme lateral interbody fusion (XLIF), and oblique lateral interbody fusion (OLIF).
- Minimally invasive and endoscopic surgical techniques allow surgical intervention without ↑ approach-related morbidity. However, these methods are indicated for select indications and have a steep learning curve associated with the surgical technique.
- Failure of surgery can be due to inappropriate patient selection, wrong-level surgery, unrealistic patient expectations, problems related to surgery, and secondary pathology contributing to low back pain.

Spondylosis

A degenerative disorder affecting the vertebrae, facet joints, intervertebral discs, and surrounding ligaments. It produces osteophytes, disc degeneration, narrowing of disc space, and facet joint degeneration, and can cause nerve root or cord compression.

Epidemiology

Degenerative changes of the spine are present in as many as 65% of patients aged >50 years. Of these, only a small number become symptomatic. It occurs more often in men than in women.

Clinical features

- Spondylotic changes can result in spinal canal, lateral recess, and foraminal stenosis. Spinal canal stenosis can result in myelopathy due to cord compression, whereas stenosis that occurs more laterally can cause radiculopathy due to root compression.
- Degenerative changes sometimes result in a painful and tender spine with reduced mobility.

Pathophysiology

Dehydration and ↓ elasticity of the intervertebral disc occur with age, and cracks and fissures appear in intervertebral discs. Surrounding ligaments also have less elasticity and thicken. There is collapse of intervertebral discs. The annuli of these discs bulge outward; uncinate processes over-ride and hypertrophy (compromising the ventrolateral portion of the foramen), and facets over-ride and hypertrophy (compromising the dorsolateral portion of the foramen). Marginal osteophytes develop.

Cervical spondylosis

Neck pain from cervical spondylosis is common. It affects men and women equally, although onset is usually earlier in men. Incidence rises with age.

Clinical features

- *Radiculopathy*: pain develops in the arms and fingers, with reduced reflexes. Dermatomal sensory loss and LMN weakness can be found.
  - There are eight cervical nerve roots and only seven cervical vertebrae. The cervical roots exit above their vertebrae. Thus, the lower nerve root at a given level is usually affected (e.g. C5/C6 pathology affects the C6 nerve root). The intervertebral joints involved (in ↓ order of frequency) are C5/C6 (thumb sensation, inverted supinator reflex—fingers flex on eliciting the reflex, but there is no other movement, and biceps muscle), C5/C6/T1 (little finger sensation and interossei), C6/C7 (middle finger sensation, triceps, triceps reflex), and C4/C5 (elbow sensation, biceps reflex, and deltoid). NB rare T1 radiculopathy is sometimes caused by this disease but usually arises due to a Pancoast tumour at the lung apex.
- *Myelopathy* (see ➲ pp. 535–536).
- *Other UMN signs*: include hyperreflexia, Hoffman's reflex, clonus, and Babinski sign. Lhermitte's sign: neck flexion/extension produces a sensation of electric shock through the upper and lower extremities and the trunk (25% of patients with cervical spondylotic myelopathy).

- *Differential diagnosis:* multiple sclerosis, acute disc prolapse, neurofibroma of nerve root, and subacute combined degeneration of the cord.

Thoracic spondylosis

Pain often triggered by flexion (disc pain) and hyperextension (facet joint pain). Thoracic roots exit below their vertebrae (unlike in the cervical spine).

Lumbar spondylosis

Usually asymptomatic. It is present in 27–37% of the asymptomatic population. It appears to be a non-specific ageing phenomenon.

Spondylosis occurs as a result of new bone formation in areas where the annular ligament is stressed. If symptomatic: the lumbar spine carries most weight, and therefore pain on activity. Sitting for long periods may cause symptoms because of pressure on the lumbar spine. Repetitive movements (e.g. lifting, bending) can also precipitate or aggravate the pain. Patients with spondylosis may become symptomatic if they develop nerve root impingement, disc disease, or spinal stenosis. Lumbar nerve roots exit below their vertebrae, producing symptoms in the same-level nerve root.

Investigations

- Plain radiographs, including obliques, CT, and MRI. There is poor correlation between findings of spondylosis on MRI and symptomatology.

Management

- *Medical:* analgesics, anti-inflammatories, muscle relaxants.
- *Non-operative options:* soft cervical collar (only for short periods) or lumbosacral orthosis, physiotherapy (core strengthening), TENS, acupuncture, weight loss, and lifestyle changes.
- *Operative:* seldom required.

Osteoporosis of the spine

(See ➲ Chapter 11.)

Clinical features

For most of its course, osteoporosis is silently progressive. End-stage osteoporosis culminates in fracture. Symptoms due to associated spinal fractures include back pain, loss of height of vertebral bodies, and *de novo* deformity in sagittal and/or coronal planes (kyphosis and scoliosis, respectively).

Diagnosis

- Plain radiographs of spine for fractures (Fig. 17.1).
- MRI of spine to exclude metastases as the cause of fractures.

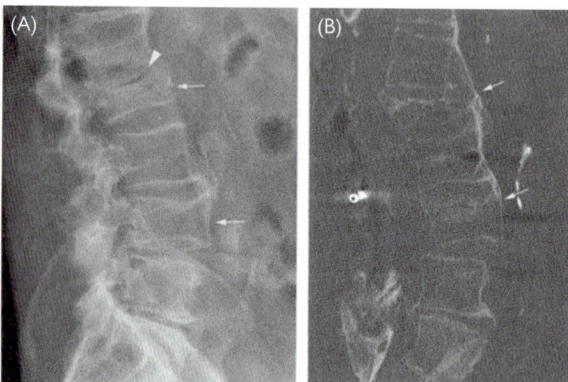

Fig. 17.1 Osteoporotic compression fracture. (A) Lateral radiograph of the lumbar spine in a 57-year-old man showing osteoporosis. There are superior end plate compression fractures of the lumbar spine at L2 and L4 (arrows). There is near-vertebra plana at the L2 level with intravertebral vacuum phenomenon (arrowhead), highly suggestive of an osteoporotic compression fracture. (B) Sagittal reformatted CT image redemonstrating the fractures (arrows) and showing significant osteopenia and accentuation of vertical trabeculae caused by osteoporosis. Prominent anterior ossifications may indicate underlying diffuse idiopathic skeletal hyperostosis.

Management

- *Non-operative* (see ➲ pp. 363–368).
- *Surgical treatment:* percutaneous vertebroplasty/balloon kyphoplasty with augmentation of body with PMMA cement. Balloon kyphoplasty also restores height.

Rheumatoid arthritis of the spine

RA is the commonest inflammatory disorder affecting the spine. It has a predilection for affecting the cervical spine, with involvement seen in up to 86% of patients and neurological effects noted in up to 58% of patients (see ⊃ Chapter 11).

Pathology

The pathogenesis of rheumatoid joint involvement is based on the theory of autoimmune response to antigenic expression by synovial cells, which leads to generation of RhF and immunoglobulin M (IgM) antibodies within the joint synovium. The inflammatory process leads to the development of the characteristic 'pannus', primarily composed of inflammatory cells and fibroblasts, amidst chronic granulation tissue, which elucidates proteolytic enzymes, including collagenases, resulting in local destruction of cartilage, ligaments, tendons, and bone. Inflammatory destruction leads to ligamentous laxity and bony erosion, which predisposes the cervical spine to instability, subluxation, and settling, most marked in the craniocervical junction, due to pure synovial facet joints, as well as axially oriented joints with no bony interlocking.

Pannus-borne inflammatory destruction of tissues leads to three major patterns of clinical involvement:

- *Atlanto-axial instability:*
  - Commonest, occurs in 50–80% of patients with RA of the cervical spine.
  - The transverse and apical ligaments, which prevent displacement of C1 on C2 vertebral bodies, are destroyed by pannus, causing most commonly anterior subluxation. The space available for the cord behind the dens is insufficient, causing pressure on the cord.
  - Radiographs show an ↑ space between the arch of the atlas and the front of the dens (<3mm normal).
- *Basilar settling ('pseudobasilar invagination', 'atlanto-axial impaction', 'superior migration of the odontoid'):*
  - Occurs in 20–40% of patients
  - Erosion of craniocervical osseo-tendinous-ligamentous structures leads to reduction in vertical distance between the brainstem and the odontoid
  - Can result in direct compression on the brainstem and foramen magnum, and can cause neurological injury or even death.
- *Subaxial instability:*
  - Occurs in 15–20% of patients
  - Classic 'stepladder' type of cervical deformity with multilevel subluxations and kyphosis
  - Excessive intervertebral movement becomes possible, and the cord or nerve roots can be compressed.

Risk factors for ↑ cervical spine involvement

- ♀ gender
- Younger age
- Peripheral joint erosions or severe polyarthritis
- Long RA duration
- Long-term corticosteroid treatment
- Rheumatoid factor positive
- Higher disease activity markers (ESR, CRP, DAS8 (disease activity score for Rheumatoid Arthritis))

Clinical features

Patients have varying clinical manifestations from the disease process:
- *Localized neck pain*—commonly over the occiput and craniocervical region
- *Radiculopathy*—neural tissue inflammation or dysfunction can manifest as pain radiating along the involved dermatome, which may be accompanied by weakness. Occipital headache, mastoid pain, ear pain, and facial pain may be manifestations of involvement of the C2 nerve, greater auricular nerve, greater occipital nerve, or spinal nucleus of the trigeminal tract
- *Myelopathy* (see ➲ pp. 535–536)
- *Vertebrobasilar insufficiency*—commonly associated with basilar invagination; may manifest as tinnitus, vertigo, loss of equilibrium, visual disturbance, diplopia, and dysphagia.

Investigations

- *Radiology:* plain radiographs of anterior, lateral, and odontoid peg views of the cervical spine. Flexion and extension lateral views are important to assess for dynamic instability. These should be 'patient-controlled' active, rather than passive, movement to prevent neurological injury. Several parameters are defined on radiographs to diagnose and prognosticate disease involvement. To achieve greater sensitivity, three or more parameters need to be considered together.
- *MRI:* mandatory to examine the soft tissues, extent of pannus, status of the spinal cord, space available for the cord (SAC) within the craniocervical junction, and cervicomedullary angle.

Parameter	Measurement	Reference values
Anterior atlanto-dens interval (AADI)	From the posterior aspect of the anterior ring of C1 to the anterior aspect of the dens	Normal: <3mm (adult)
Posterior atlanto-dens interval (PADI)	From the posterior aspect of the dens to the anterior aspect of C1 lamina	<14mm: ↑ neurological injury risk
McGregor line	Line drawn on lateral plain radiograph from the hard palate to the base of the occiput	Vertical settling of the occiput is defined as migration of the odontoid >4.5mm above the McGregor line

Parameter	Measurement	Reference values
Ranawat index	Line from the pedicles of C2 superiorly along the vertical axis of the odontoid until it intersects a line connecting the anterior and posterior arches of C1	A Ranawat value of <13mm is diagnostic of vertical settling
Redlund–Johnell measurement	Distance between the midpoint of the caudal end plate of C2 to the McGregor line	<34mm in men and <29mm in women are considered abnormal
Clark station	Determined by dividing the odontoid process into three equal parts in the sagittal plane	If the anterior ring of the atlas is level with the middle third (station II) or the caudal third (station III) of the odontoid process, basilar invagination is present

Management

Non-operative
- Analgesia and NSAIDs.
- MDT management for optimal medical treatment of underlying RA.
- Soft collar or firmer orthosis may relieve some symptoms.
- Close observation and follow-up to assess for early signs of deterioration.

Operative
- Surgical intervention may be required for pain, neurological compromise, or significant radiological cord compression.
- Surgery is possibly indicated in patients with grade II and IIIA disease. Patients with grade IIIB do not do as well following surgery.

Indications for surgery
1. Neurological deficit with spinal instability—absolute indication for posterior decompression and stabilization.
2. Neurologically intact patient:
   a. With basilar invagination and cord compression on MRI—cervical traction and posterior occipitocervical stabilization
   b. With radiological instability with SAC <13mm, cervicomedullary angle <135°, or cord diameter in flexion <6mm—posterior occipitocervical decompression and stabilization
   c. Subaxial instability with SAC <13mm—posterior subaxial cervical decompression and stabilization
   d. Neurological deterioration or persistent symptoms with basilar invagination and anterior cervicomedullary compression—anterior odontoid excision
   e. Unresponsive occipital pain with facetal arthropathy with or without radiographic instability—posterior stabilization only.

Other spinal problems

- ↑ risk of degenerative spinal pathology.
- Osteoporosis from primary disease, as well as from long-term steroid use.
- ↑ risk of pseudoarthrosis.
- Cervical spine involvement reflects advanced rheumatoid disease status; thus, patients have ↑ long-term mortality.

Further reading

Nguyen HV, Ludwig SC, Silber J, et al. Rheumatoid arthritis of the cervical spine. *Spine Journal.* 2004;**4**(3):329–34.

Ranawat CS, O'Leary P, Pellicci P, et al. Cervical fusion in rheumatoid arthritis. *Journal of Bone and Joint Surgery (American Volume).* 1979;**61A**:1003–10.

Zhu S, Xu W, Luo Y, Zhao Y, Liu Y. Cervical spine involvement risk factors in rheumatoid arthritis: a meta-analysis. *International Journal of Rheumatic Diseases.* 2017;**20**(5):541–9.

Ankylosing spondylitis: spinal manifestations

For an overview of AS, see ⊃ Chapter 11. Although AS affects any joint, it has profound effects on the vertebral column. The other *seronegative spondyloarthropathies* (enteropathic, psoriatic, Reiter's syndrome, and undifferentiated) may have similar manifestations in the spine.

Spinal features

- SIJ involvement is a hallmark of AS and appears early in the course of the disease.
- Pathogenesis consists of sequential or juxtaposed stages of active inflammation, bone erosion, osteophyte formation, and eventually bony ankylosis.
- Syndesmophytes, ossification around the intervertebral discs, result in the formation of a solid column of bone. Advanced cases may show a fused spinal column—'*bamboo spine appearance*' on radiographs.
- Progressive loss of spinal flexibility, bony fusion, loss of normal lumbar lordosis, and progressive thoracic kyphosis, due to multiple microfractures occurring over time, result in significant forward stooping, marked sagittal imbalance, and difficulty with mobilization.
- With progressive kyphotic deformity, forward gaze is affected—initially it is compensated by hyperlordosing the cervical spine, but with ↑ deformity and syndesmophyte fusion involving the cervical vertebrae, it becomes difficult.
- Involvement of one or both hips is common. Advanced cases present with hip flexion deformities and ankylosed hip joints, which exacerbate postural imbalance and mobility.
- Osteoporosis is commonly associated with AS.
- Chronic destructive discovertebral lesions, called Andersson lesions, found in 1.5–28% of AS cases.

Clinical presentation of spinal manifestations

- Classical early presentation is mild 'inflammatory' lower back pain, which is differentiated from the more ubiquitous degenerative back pain by peculiar characteristics: age at onset <40 years, duration >3 months, insidious onset, morning stiffness >30min, no improvement with rest, improvement with exercise, and awakening pain particularly in second half of the night and alternating with deep, dull buttock pain.
- Back pain is associated with stiffness, which improves with movement.
- Atypical symptoms include thoracic back pain, chest pain, chest wall stiffness, peripheral small joint stiffness, and visual symptoms.
- Rarely, neurological injury may occur with fractures. Osteoporosis in association with fused long spinal columns, presents a high risk of spinal fractures with low-energy trauma and devastating spinal cord injury.
- Acute-onset neck or back pain in a known patient of AS should mandate a search for a fracture, even in the absence of recognizable trauma. AS patients have a 3.5 times higher fracture risk than healthy adults.

Spine examination

- Chest expansion is restricted <2cm measured at the level of the nipples (normal is >7cm).
- Schober's test is positive (<5cm lumbar spine motion).
- FABER's test to assess the SIJ.
- Assessment of hip flexion contractures may be positive.
- In advanced cases, inspection from the side reveals the '*question mark*' deformity due to kyphosis and hip flexion deformities, as well as the '*chin on chest*' deformity secondary to progressive fixed cervical kyphosis, with loss of horizontal gaze.
- Assessment of severity of deformity:
    - *Gaze length*—as deformity ↑, the patient struggles to see in front of themselves. Measuring how far they can see provides a useful measure for disease progression.
    - *Wall–tragus distance (WTD)*—patients should be able to stand with the heels, buttocks, shoulders, and occiput flat against a wall. This may not be possible in AS. The measurement is from the wall to the tragus of the ear.
    - *Chin–brow vertical angle (CBVA)*—measured between the line vertical to the floor and the line joining the brow to the chin, normally 0°, giving the horizontal gaze.

Investigations of suspected spinal pathology

- *Plain radiographs:*
    - Recommend full-length spinal radiographs to assess for occult fractures, as well as to assess global spinal alignment.
    - Spinal radiographs may show shiny corners (romanus lesions), bridging syndesmophytes, disc space ossification, and appearance of a '*bamboo spine*' in advanced cases.
    - Pelvic radiographs may sacroiliitis or fused SIJs.
- *CT:*
    - Clearly outlines the bony anatomy
    - Typically, three patterns of spinal fractures can be identified:
        - Fresh 'shear'-type fractures
        - Stress fractures or pseudoarthrosis (Andersson lesion)
        - Vertebral compression fractures
    - Highly sensitive investigation for identifying occult or low-energy fractures in AS patients.
- *MRI:*
    - If AS is suspected, MRI is a highly sensitive modality of choice for early diagnosis as it demonstrates sacroiliitis.
    - Allows assessment of neurological elements and recognizes frequently associated intraspinal haematoma.
    - Investigation of choice to diagnose discovertebral pseudoarthrosis lesions (Andersson lesions).

Management

- *Non-operative* (see ➲ Chapter 11).
- *Operative:* depending on the pattern of spinal involvement, surgical options are as follows:

- *Traumatic fractures:* usually highly unstable injuries (equivalent of long bone fractures), and instrumented posterior spinal fusion is indicated. Long length of stabilization with multiple points of fixation without attempting correction of deformity are golden pearls to remember. Concomitant decompression is indicated in the presence of progressive neurological deficit or epidural haematoma.
- *Pseudoarthrosis or Andersson lesions:* mechanical stabilization is usually sufficient in the absence of neurological deficit. Anterior reconstruction is usually not indicated, as the pathogenesis is due to stress fractures and micromotion. Approach can be anterior or posterior.
- *Spinal deformity:* an opening wedge Smith–Peterson osteotomy (SPO) or a closing wedge pedicle subtraction osteotomy (PSO), with anterior reconstruction combined with an instrumented posterior fusion, may be required for severe kyphotic deformities to restore sagittal spinal alignment and horizontal gaze. These are high-risk procedures, with potential complications of neurological deficit and dural tear. Thus, careful patient selection, counselling, and accurate surgical planning are of utmost importance to affect a successful outcome.
- *Hip flexion contractures or ankylosis:* THA, combined with soft tissue releases, may be beneficial to improve overall truncal balance, postural alignment, and mobility. There is an ↑ risk of heterotopic ossification and post-operative dislocation in patients with AS.

Further reading

Bron JL, de Vries MK, Snieders MN, van der Horst-Bruinsma IE, van Royen BJ. Discovertebral (Andersson) lesions of the spine in ankylosing spondylitis revisited. *Clinical Rheumatology.* 2009;**28**(8):883–92.

Sieper J, Braun J, Rudwaleit M, Boonen A, Zink A. Ankylosing spondylitis: an overview. *Annals of the Rheumatic Diseases.* 2002;**61**(Suppl 3):iii8–18.

Zhang W, Zheng M. Operative strategy for different types of thoracolumbar stress fractures in ankylosing spondylitis. *Journal of Spinal Disorders and Techniques.* 2014;**27**(8):423–30.

Kyphosis in adults

Kyphosis is excessive curvature of the spine in the sagittal plane. With normal sagittal balance, a plumb line from C7 should fall through S1, allowing a wide variation in cervical and lumbar lordosis and thoracic kyphosis to achieve balance. The normal range for thoracic kyphosis is 10–40°, and for lumbar lordosis 30–80°, varying with age and gender.

Epidemiology

The incidence of kyphosis varies according to the underlying pathology—occurs in 15% of Caucasian ♀ with osteoporosis ('dowager's hump') and in 5% of patients with spinal TB.

Risk factors

These include family history of kyphosis, OP, spinal fracture, infection, and malignancy.

Aetiology

- Congenital.
- Developmental: Scheuermann's disease, developmental roundback, and spondylolisthesis.
- Acquired: inflammatory (AS), metabolic (OP), chondrodystrophic, neoplastic, post-traumatic, and iatrogenic (post-laminectomy, post-instrumentation).

Clinical features

Kyphotic deformities presenting in adults may develop from disorders of childhood. History must include family history of kyphosis, progression of the deformity. and other congenital abnormalities. It is important to ask about constitutional symptoms (e.g. weight loss, fevers, night sweats), as well as neurological symptoms. Previous medical history must include medication (steroids) and history of trauma or previous surgery. Examine with the patient standing in a neutral position and bending forward. Assess global coronal and sagittal alignment, with ROM of the spine and other joints. Flexibility of kyphosis can be assessed in the erect patient by extension and, with the patient lying down, by prone hyperextension. Complete neurological examination is necessary.

Investigations

Aimed at establishing the aetiology and evaluating the alignment of the spine to allow planning for surgery.

- *Plain radiographs:* AP and lateral views of the whole spine, including the pelvis (pelvic parameters influence thoracic and lumbar alignment). The patient must be standing, with their knees fully extended.
- *CT:* helpful in defining bony structures.
- *MRI:* shows soft tissues and neural elements and their relationships to bony structures.

Management

Surgery is indicated when non-operative measures fail or when the patient develops intractable pain, worsening kyphosis, or deteriorating neurology.

- *Non-operative:* analgesia, NSAIDs, physical therapy, and regular exercise. Bracing is not normally effective.
- *Operative:* anterior or posterior procedures, or a combination of these. Posterior fixation alone is usually sufficient for flexible deformities. Segmental vertebral fixation improves the chances of successful correction. To correct the deformity, several osteotomies may be needed: multiple facet osteotomies, closing wedge osteotomy, PSO, or vertebral column resection. Large deformities, especially those with short, sharp angular malalignments, ↑ the risks associated with surgery.

Ankylosing spondylitis

(See ⊃ Ankylosing spondylitis: spinal manifestations, pp. 326–327; ⊃ Chapter 11.) AS is a common cause for adult progressive thoracic kyphosis. Usually affects ♂ patients aged 20–40 years.

Post-traumatic kyphosis

Kyphosis following burst fractures is common, especially following thoracolumbar burst fractures. Surgery to stabilize and correct these deformities is associated with high complication rates. Kyphosis from osteoporotic fractures is also common and is usually treated non-operatively. NICE guidelines recommend vertebroplasty in patients:

- Who have severe ongoing pain after a recent, unhealed vertebral fracture despite optimal pain management, *and*
- In whom the pain has been confirmed to be at the level of the fracture by physical examination and imaging.

Scoliosis in adults

Abnormal curvature of the spine in the coronal plane of >10° (Fig. 17.2).

Epidemiology

Incidence of adult scoliosis is between 3% and 5%. The prevalence is ↑ with an ageing population. Disability caused by adult spine deformity in the elderly population is no different to that due to medical conditions such as cancer, heart disease, and diabetes.

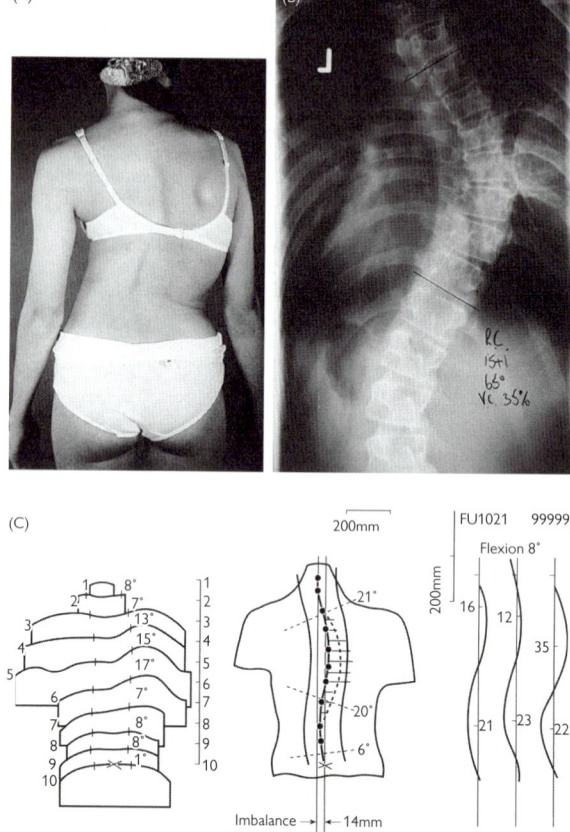

Fig. 17.2 (A) Patient with adolescent idiopathic scoliosis. (B) Radiograph of the patient. (C) Surface topography.

Reproduced from Bulstrode et al., Oxford Textbook of Orthopaedics and Trauma, with permission from Oxford University Press.

Aetiology

The commonest causes in adults are:
- Degenerative disease, often with osteoporosis
- Paediatric causes noted in adulthood (see ➲ Chapter 22)—progressive congenital, idiopathic, or neuromuscular curves
- Post-traumatic.

Clinical

Small curves are usually asymptomatic. Worsening pain and disability are common presenting symptoms in adults. Other symptoms are neurological symptoms, asymmetrical waistline, poorly fitting clothing, and prominence of one side of the chest. With scoliosis, there may be truncal asymmetry, a rib hump, loss of spinal movements, shoulder or pelvic imbalance, and signs of neurological deficits due to cord or nerve root compression. Multiple recent studies have highlighted the importance of sagittal spine alignment and its correlation with health-related quality of life (HRQoL) measures.

Investigations

- *Scoliosis view radiographs:* AP and lateral views of whole spine and pelvis. These are used to establish the cause of scoliosis, type of curve, and effects of the deformity on pelvic balance. The size of the curve is measured by determining the Cobb angle.
- *Lateral bending radiographs:* AP views with bending to each side to determine flexibility. Used in surgical planning.
- *CT:* used to assess bony structures and spinal canal. It is better than MRI in showing details of the vertebrae.
- *MRI:* used to image the spinal column and neural elements. It is better than CT in assessing soft tissues.
- *Bone densitometry:* depending on the age of the patient, bone densitometry may be necessary to check for osteopenia.

Management

In adults, the most important consideration in deciding on the type of treatment is severity of the patient's symptoms, rather than the size of the deformity. Aetiology plays a significant role. Treatment options include:
- Expectant management (observation)
- Orthosis
- Surgery.

Non-operative
- Analgesics, NSAIDs, physical therapy, and use of orthoses.

Operative

Indications for surgery are intractable pain, progressive deformity, and neurological compromise. Anterior, posterior, and a combination of anterior and posterior instrumented fusions are used.

Spondylolisthesis in adults

This is forward slippage of one vertebra relative to another. It usually occurs at L4/5 or L5/S1.

Aetiology (Newman and Stone)

Spondylolisthesis can be congenital, developmental, or acquired:
- Congenital or dysplastic (20%)—often marked slippage
- Isthmic (50%)—secondary to spondylolysis (fatigue fracture)
- Degenerative (25%)—arthritis of the lumbar facet joints
- Trauma—bilateral fractures
- Pathological—tumours, Paget's disease
- Iatrogenic—post-operative.

Clinical

May be asymptomatic. Usually have an insidious onset of low back pain and muscle spasm in the second to third decade. Flattening of the back, with a spinous process step-off on palpation. Symptoms of claudication (leg pain and weakness) may signal lateral recess stenosis.

Investigations

- Confirmed with standing lateral and oblique plain radiographs.
- CT provides detailed bone anatomy and is used in surgical planning.

Classification

- *Meyerding classification:* percentage of slip of the AP diameter of the vertebrae.
- *Spondyloptosis:* slippage >100%.
- *Slip angle:* the degree of tilting forward of the L5 body on the sacrum. Good correlation with clinical deformity and rate of progression. On a lateral radiograph, the angle is normally >0°.

Risk factors for slip progression

Young age at presentation, ♀, slip angle >10°, high-grade slip, dome-shaped sacrum, and inclined sacrum (>30° beyond vertical). Slip progression is less likely after skeletal maturity.

Management

- *Non-operative:* reduce sports and other high-impact activities, brace, and arrange physiotherapy. Serial plain radiographs are used to monitor the deformity.
- *Operative:* surgery is indicated if the slip is >50%, tilt angle is >30°, or there is progression, failure of non-operative treatment, or development of significant neurology.

Grade	I	II	III	IV	V
Percentage slip	<25	25–50	50–75	75–100	>100

- *Surgery*: grade I or II—*in situ* fusion with decompression. Repair of the pars defects with lag screws for slips <25%. Grade III or IV—extended *in situ* fusion and decompression. Decompression without fusion can be considered for elderly degenerative spondylolisthesis. A failed posterior fusion may require anterior interbody fusion.

Further reading

Matz PG, Meagher RJ, Lamer T, *et al*. Guideline summary review: an evidence-based clinical guideline for the diagnosis and treatment of degenerative lumbar spondylolisthesis. *Spine Journal*. 2016;**16**(3):439–48.

Schulte TL, Ringel F, Quante M, Eicker SO, Muche-Borowski C, Kothe R. Surgery for adult spondylolisthesis: a systematic review of the evidence. *European Spine Journal*. 2016;**25**(8):2359–67.

Infections of the spine: pyogenic infections and tuberculosis

Pyogenic infections

Pyogenic infections of the vertebral body are relatively uncommon, and are either frequently missed or diagnosed late. Diagnosis requires a high index of suspicion. *Spondylitis* affects the vertebrae. *Discitis* affects the intervertebral disc space. *Spondylodiscitis* involves both. Facet joints and the epidural space may also be affected.

Site
- The lumbar spine is most commonly involved (50–60% cases).
- Thoracic and cervical infections, although less common, are associated with a higher incidence of neurological deficit.

> **Risk factors for pyogenic spinal infections**
> - Older age (note bimodal distribution: <20 years and 50–70 years)
> - Intravenous drug abuse
> - HIV/acquired immune deficiency
> - Diabetes mellitus
> - Immunocompromised status
> - Long-term use of steroids
> - Multiple medical comorbidities
> - Morbid obesity
> - End-stage renal disease
> - Penetrating trauma
> - Urinary tract infection, infective endocarditis
> - Iatrogenic (previous spinal intervention)

Spread
- The haematogenous route is commonest, with the infective pathogen entering from a distant source and lodging in the spinal column via the bloodstream.
- Of particular interest is Batson's venous plexus—a system of valveless venous channels freely communicating the vertebral venous plexus to the pelvic and thoracic venous plexuses, and can form a route of blood-borne spread to the spine, especially from the pelvic organs (genitourinary system).
- Other rarer routes include direct inoculation, penetrating trauma, CSF seeding, and local infiltration.

Organisms
Identification guides treatment. Not identified in up to a third of cases:
- *Staphylococcal aureus* is the commonest causative organism.
- Others include *Staphylococcus epidermidis* (second commonest cause), β-haemolytic *Streptococcus*, and Gram-negative organisms (including *Escherichia coli*, *Salmonella* (in sickle-cell disease), *Pseudomonas* spp. (in IVDUs), *Proteus*, and *Pasteurella*).
- Fungal infection if immunocompromised. Parasites rare.

Complications

Paravertebral and/or epidural abscess, vertebral collapse, and neurological sequelae.

Clinical features

- Onset of symptoms is often insidious.
- (Lumbar) back pain is the commonest presentation. Rest pain and night pain are also common.
- Look for the classic triad: fever, back pain, and focal tenderness.
- Incidence of neurological affection of up to 10–20% is noted, most commonly due to compression from infected granulation or epidural abscess, direct infectious involvement of neural elements, spinal instability secondary to bony destruction, and vascular infarct of the cord due to thrombosis. Higher risk of neurology if cervical/thoracic.

Differential diagnosis

- Degenerative spinal disease.
- Tumours—primary or metastatic.
- Chronic granulomatous infections such as TB.
- Langerhans cell histiocytosis.
- Modic-type spinal changes (bone marrow signal changes on MRI).
- Inflammatory spondyloarthropathy.
- Schmorl's nodes (protrusions of the nucleus pulposus through the vertebral body end plate).

Investigations

- Radiographs may be normal for several weeks, with earliest change being loss of mineralization followed by progressive disc space narrowing, end plate and vertebral erosion, necrosis and destruction, sclerosis, and eventually new bone formation and intervertebral fusion by 6–12 months. Radiographs provide assessment of spinal alignment, and dynamic films are used to diagnose spinal instability.
- *MRI:* gold standard investigation. Allows early diagnosis and detects subtle inflammation; the modality is highly sensitive and specific. Allows differentiation from other differential diagnosis.
- *CT:* less sensitive than MRI. Allows detailed assessment of bone anatomy and extent of vertebral destruction, as well as surgical planning, especially when planning instrumentation.
- *Blood tests:* WCC, ESR, CRP, blood cultures, antistreptolysin O titre, and tuberculin test.
- *PET/99m-technetium bone scan:* high sensitivity after 48h. Can detect even low-grade infections, especially if there is presence of metalwork or scar tissue from previous operations.
- *Tissue biopsy:* to gain source sample and culture to grow pathogenic organism. May be CT-guided (radiology) or X-ray-guided (operating theatre).

Management

> **Principles of management of spinal infection**
>
> 1. Identification of the infective pathogen blood culture or tissue biopsy)
> 2. Microbe – sensitive antibiotic therapy
> 3. Restoring spinal stability
> 4. Eliminating dead space, necrotic tissue, abscess and infected granulation tissue and reducing infective load

Non-operative

- Infection itself is primarily a medical disease, and is successfully treated with antibiotics if there is a known pathogen and sensitive antibiotic(s).
- The usual recommended regimen is IV antibiotics for at least 2–4 weeks followed by oral antibiotics for 4–8 weeks. The total duration of treatment is usually 6–12 weeks. Duration and antibiotic regimen are based on the infective pathogen, as well as on multidisciplinary input from the infectious diseases and microbiology teams.
- Response to treatment is usually monitored by observing symptoms, blood tests (leucocyte count, CRP, and ESR), repeating blood cultures, and radiological evidence of healing or fusion.
- Favourable outcomes are usually noted in young, healthy individuals, without significant comorbidities or immunocompromised states, with a drug-sensitive pathogenic organism and good compliance to antibiotic dosage.

Operative

There are six main indications for surgery in spinal infections:
1. Neurological deficit
2. Spinal instability or progressive spinal deformity
3. Necessity to establish the diagnosis with open surgical biopsy from the affected site
4. Severe intractable pain or to permit early rehabilitation
5. Failure of medical management—to achieve source control
6. Fulminant sepsis—to reduce acute bacterial load.

Usual surgical treatment includes debridement, decompression, posterior instrumentation and stabilization, and anterior column reconstruction, in either combination as per the site, extent, and clinical involvement of the spinal column.

Tuberculosis

Fifteen per cent of patients with TB have extra-pulmonary involvement; the spine is the commonest extra-pulmonary site. Spinal involvement is seen in 50% of patients with musculoskeletal TB. At-risk groups in the developed world include: recent immigrants (African and South East Asian), those with HIV (TB is commonest HIV-related opportunistic infection worldwide), the homeless, and those with alcohol and drug abuse.

Pathology
- The common mode of spread is haematogenous or secondary to direct extension from infected viscera.
- Anatomical blood supply of the disc space comes from adjacent vertebral end plates, and this arrangement results in the classical '*paradiscal*'-type lesion in TB. Other types are '*central*', '*posterior*', and '*non-osseous abscess only*'.
- There is lymphocyte infiltration, along with macrophages and Langerhans-type giant cells, and eventual granulation tissue formation leads to the formation of a '*cold abscess*'. Subsequent erosion of bony structures and the intervertebral disc leads to vertebral collapse, instability, and deformity.

Clinical features
- Patients present with an insidious onset of back pain with systemic signs such as fever, malaise, night sweats, weight loss, and loss of appetite.
- Neurological symptoms may develop either from direct compression from a tubercular abscess or sequestrum (early stage), spinal instability (early stage), or vascular thrombosis with spinal cord infarction or from bony compression from severe spinal deformity (late stage).
- In advanced disease, advanced bony destruction may lead to spinal deformity. The clinical appearance of the deformity depends on the number of vertebrae involved: 'knuckle' (one vertebra); 'gibbus' (two vertebrae); and 'rounded kyphosis' (>3 vertebral collapse).

Investigations
- *Bloods:* high ESR/CRP ± WCC, serum IgM and immunoglobulin G (IgG) antibodies; purified protein derivative (PPD) of tuberculin. *Interferon-gamma (IFN-γ) release assay (IGRA)*. *QuantiFERON Gold assay*. Mantoux (tuberculin skin test).
- *Microbiology:*
  - Gold standard for diagnosis is culture-proven TB, with a biopsy sample from the infective site. Acid-fast bacilli (AFB) cultures were formerly done in Löwenstein–Jensen medium, but now BACTEC radiometric cultures are used, which provide results faster. In addition, polymerase chain reaction (PCR) and GeneXpert are the other tests useful for an accurate diagnosis (IGRA is becoming more widely available).
  - Histopathological evidence of Langerhans giant cells, as well as caseous necrosis or 'soft tubercle', is added value in diagnosis.
- *Radiographs:* two-thirds are abnormal. Spine radiographs demonstrate anterior body involvement and disc sparing initially, progressing to disc space narrowing, vertebral collapse, kyphosis, and spondylolisthesis; soft tissue thickening or signs of spinal instability. However, radiographs play little role in early diagnosis.
- *MRI:* most sensitive investigation (with contrast). Can show the extent of infection, necrosis, skip lesions, location of abscess, and compression of the spinal cord or nerve roots.
- *CT:* very useful to demonstrate the extent of bony destruction, to assess junctional areas such as craniocervical and cervicothoracic

regions, to assess for posterior column involvement, and to aid in biopsy and surgical planning.
- *Biopsy PCR*: quicker than Ziehl–Neelsen staining for AFB.

Management
- Initially, the anterior and inferior parts of the vertebral body (metaphysis) are affected, then the central part, leading to collapse (vertebra plana). The disc space is spared due to avascularity (except in the young). Multiple contiguous vertebrae are affected due to spread under ALL/PLL and segmental arteries (but 15% have skip lesions).
- Multidrug antitubercular chemotherapy is the mainstay of treatment of spinal TB. The commonest 'first-line' drugs are 'RIPES': rifampicin, isoniazid (with pyridoxine), pyrazinamide, ethambutol, and streptomycin. 'Second-line' drugs used in resistant cases include kanamycin, amikacin, capreomycin, and levofloxacin.
- Spinal orthosis are commonly used to maintain spinal alignment as part of conservative treatment.
- Surgery may depend on those with or those without neurological deficit, including to stabilize (anterior decompression/corpectomy, strut graft ± posterior instrumented stabilization) and correct kyphosis (halo, osteotomy).

Patients without neurological deficit	Patients with neurological deficit
Confirmation of diagnosis—biopsy	New or progressive neurological deficit
Evacuation of large paraspinal abscess	
Failure to respond to ATT	Worsening deficit despite ATT
Mechanical instability, bony destruction, impending kyphosis	Spinal tumour syndrome
	Cord compression secondary to spinal deformity in late TB

- Anterior, posterior, and combined approaches to the spine are used, depending on the extent of infection, compression of neural elements, and stability of the spine.
- Surgery may vary from simple decompression to global reconstruction of the spinal columns with debridement and 360° fusion. Global reconstruction is now possible via an all-posterior approach itself, obviating the need for morbid anterior procedures.
- In healed or late stages of spinal TB, PSO or internal gibbectomy may be needed through the healed or fused tuberculous vertebral column, to correct spinal alignment and achieve sagittal, as well as coronal, balance or to reduce pressure on the cord draped over the kyphotic hump.

Complications
- Cold abscesses are pathognomonic infected exudates—can become very large and track to form a retropharyngeal abscess (cervical), paravertebral abscesses (thoracic), or groin (femoral triangle) abscesses (lumbar).

- Later in the disease course, the disc space and vertebral bodies are destroyed, leading to anterior wedging (kyphys) and a palpable deformity (gibbus) ± neurological deficit (reported in 23–76% of cases).
- Formation of mycotic aortic aneurysm (pseudoaneurysm).
- Respiratory or renal complications with disseminated disease.
- Sinus formation.
- Pott's paraplegia.
- Drug-resistant TB—becoming an ↑ hazard with resistant strains of *Mycobacterium* not responding to first-line medications. Based on the extent of resistance demonstrated, they are labelled as: multidrug-resistant (MDR-TB); extensively drug-resistant (XDR-TB); and recently totally drug-resistant (TDR-TB).

Further reading

Garg RK, Somvanshi DS. Spinal tuberculosis: a review. *Journal of Spinal Cord Medicine*. 2011;**34**(5):440–54.

Hadjipavlou AG, Mader JT, Necessary JT, *et al*. Hematogenous pyogenic spinal infections and their surgical management. *Spine*. 2000;**25**:1668–79.

Lener S, Hartmann S, Barbagallo GMV, Certo F, Thomé C, Tschugg A. Management of spinal infection: a review of the literature. *Acta Neurochirurgica*. 2018;**160**(3):487–96.

National Institute for Health and Care Excellence (2016). *Tuberculosis*. NICE guideline [NG33]. Available from: ℅ www.nice.org.uk/guidance/ng33

Disc lesions: anatomy and pathology

Anatomy

Intervertebral discs make up a quarter of the spinal column's length. There are no discs between C1 and C2 and within the coccyx. They are avascular and rely on diffusion across vertebral end plates for nutrition. Discs are fibrocartilaginous structures serving as a shock-absorbing system to protect the spine. Movement at each disc is very small. They allow extension, flexion, and limited rotation.

Intervertebral discs are composed of an outer annulus fibrosus, which is a strong radial-like structure made up of type II collagen orientated at various angles (Fig. 17.3). It contains water and a proteoglycan matrix containing chondrocytes. The nucleus pulposus contains more water and proteoglycans in a hydrated gel-like matrix that resists compression. Vascular and neural elements are found only within the outer layer of the annulus fibrosus.

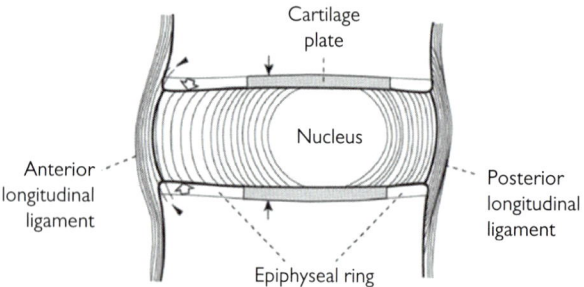

Fig. 17.3 Intervertebral disc.

Pathology

Age-related changes occur within the disc. Proteoglycan synthesis is reduced and less water is retained. Collagen levels ↑. The discs become stiffer and the annulus fibrosus transmits more load. The discs are able to withstand large forces (10,000N). With excessive loads, the first structure to fail is normally the bony vertebral end plate.

Disc lesions: herniated disc and disc prolapse

Herniated disc

Aetiology

The cause of disc herniation is related primarily to normal degenerative processes that occur with ageing. End plate fractures cause disruption of nuclear homeostasis and trigger autoimmune processes. Repetitive stresses across the discs may accelerate the process. Disc degradation leads to re-sorption or herniation.

History and examination

A thorough history should include onset, nature, and course of the pain, changes in bladder or bowel function, previous medical history, history of trauma, risk factors, and constitutional symptoms. Neurological examin-ation for patients with suspected nerve root compression should include careful assessment of motor and sensory functions, and nerve root tension signs must be elicited if present.

Investigations

Diagnosis is confirmed with MRI.

Management

Initial management is non-operative—rest, use of NSAIDs, and physio-therapy. If symptoms worsen (or do not resolve) over a few weeks, or progressive neurological deficit develops, then imaging and investigation are warranted.

Disc prolapse

Cervical disc

- Commonest in the third to fourth decade. More frequent in women (~60% of cases).
- Most commonly occur between C5–C6 and C6–C7 (i.e. causing C6/C7 nerve root radiculopathy).
- Provocative tests (e.g. Spurling's test, Hoffman's test, and Lhermitte's sign) can help with diagnosis.
- If non-operative management fails, nerve root blocks may be tried (less common than with lumbar disc pathology), followed by surgery. Anterior (anterior cervical discectomy with fusion) or posterior decompression may be performed.

Thoracic disc

- Thoracic disc herniation is rare, occurring in only 0.5% of all prolapsed discs. Peak in the fourth decade. Approximately 75% of cases occur below T8 and largely at the T11/T12 level.
- They present with thoracic back pain and there may be UMN signs involving the lower limbs. Thoracic disc herniation may produce chest, abdominal, or even groin pain, mimicking cardiac, GI, or urogenital problems.
- If pain persists despite non-operative treatment, surgery may be indicated. Costotransversectomy or a transthoracic approach is used to minimize cord handling, and a vertebral fusion may be added.

Lumbar disc

- Lumbar disc prolapse occurs commonly in patients aged 30–50 years. The lumbar spine is the spine region most commonly affected, and the L4, L5 disc herniates most often, followed by the L5, S1 disc.
- Lumbar disc herniations are a major cause of acute and chronic back and lower limb symptoms. Patients present with radiating lower limb pain (radiculopathy). The distribution of the pain is related to the level and position of disc prolapse, as these determine which nerve root is involved. Most disc prolapses that result in compression of neural elements occur in the posterolateral position. Far lateral disc prolapses comprise 6–10% of disc prolapses.

Classification

- By morphology:
  - Protruded—localized bulge with the annulus and posterior longitudinal ligament (PLL) intact
  - Extruded—protrudes through the annulus but is in continuity with the disc space
  - Sequestrated—protrudes through the annulus and there is a free fragment of the disc in the epidural space.
- By location:
  - Central—often associated with back pain only
  - Posterolateral—commonest. Usually affects the ipsilateral nerve root of the lower lumbar vertebrae
  - Far lateral—usually affects the ipsilateral nerve root of the upper lumbar vertebrae.

Disc lesions: discogenic pain

Discogenic pain can be defined as back pain without a radicular component and with no evidence of neural compression or segmental instability.

Aetiology

Discs have sensory nerve endings in the outer third of the annulus. Pressure within the disc can produce back pain by stimulating nociceptors in the PLL.

Clinical

Diagnosis is one of exclusions. Patients usually have a long history of back pain, often with radiation to the buttocks and posterior thighs. There is usually significant paravertebral spasm. There are no focal neurological signs.

Investigations

- *Radiology:* plain radiographs are normal or show degenerative changes.
- *MRI:* used to establish there is degenerative disc disease—loss of signal on T2-weighted images, annular tears, loss of disc height, and associated end plate changes.
- *Discography:* altered disc architecture and a positive provocative test (pain reproduced with injection of contrast under pressure) constitute a positive response. A positive test should also include a normal level as a reference.

Causes

Infection (discitis), torsional injury (circumferential tear of the annulus), and internal disc disruption.

Classification

- *Grade 0:* no disruption.
- *Grade 1:* disruption to inner third.
- *Grade 2:* middle third.
- *Grade 3:* outer third.

Management

- *Non-operative:* physiotherapy and epidural injection of local anaesthetic and steroid.
- *Operative:* fusion (anterior or posterior), usually with instrumentation or disc replacement for persistent, severe pain.

Spinal stenosis

Epidemiology

The incidence is 2–8%. Symptoms usually develop in the fifth and sixth decades.

Pathology

Disc dehydration leads to loss of disc height, which ↑ loading of the facets. The facets hypertrophy and this, together with a bulging annulus and thickening of the ligamentum flavum, leads to stenosis of the spinal canal. Spinal stenosis is narrowing of the spinal canal or neural foramina, producing root ischaemia and neurogenic claudication.

Types of stenosis

- *Central*—causes: medial encroachment, congenitally narrow canal ('trefoil' shape), spondylolisthesis; central disc herniation, and trauma or surgery.
- *Lateral*—causes: compression of the nerve root by lateral disc herniation, thickening of the ligamentum flavum, and hypertrophy of the superior articular process. Lateral recess stenosis often affects the traversing nerve root.
- *Foraminal*—causes: loss of disc height, disc herniation, and osteophyte formation. The exiting nerve root is compressed in the foramen.

Clinical

Patients, who are usually aged ≥60 years, present with unilateral or bilateral leg pain with or without back pain on walking upright (↑ spinal stenosis). It is often preceded by long-standing low back pain. The walking distance that precipitates the pain is unpredictable and is relieved by sitting or leaning forward (leaning on a walker/shopping trolley). Phalen provocation test—leg pain brought on by extension of the spine.

It is important to differentiate between neurogenic and vascular claudication (Table 17.1). Neurogenic claudication (spinal stenosis) causes pain, tightness, and numbness, as well as subjective weakness, in the lower limbs.

On examination, there is often loss of lumbar lordosis and ↓ lumbar movements, and occasionally there may be nerve root tension signs or evidence of a motor or sensory deficit.

Natural history

Symptoms remain unchanged in 60–70%, worse in 15–20%, and improve in 15–20% of patients.

Investigations

- *Plain radiographs*: degenerative changes are seen but are poorly defined.
- *CT*: look for lateral and central stenosis. Cross-sectional dural area of <100mm^2 denotes stenosis. Dural sac with AP diameter of <10mm is consistent with lumbar stenosis.
- *MRI*: gold standard. Allows visualization of the vertebral discs, neural elements, ligamentum flavum, and thecal sac.

Table 17.1 Comparison of vascular and neurogenic claudication

	Vascular	Neurogenic
Walking distance to onset of pain	Constant	Variable
Pain	Calf	Proximal to mid-thigh
Relieved	Standing	Sitting, bending forward
Lying flat	Relieves	May worsen
Uphill walking	Symptoms soon	Symptoms late
Cycling	Symptoms soon	Unaffected

Management

Patient selection is key to successful treatment.
- *Non-operative:* analgesia, physiotherapy, epidural or nerve root injections, treatment in the setting of a rehabilitation programme or pain clinic.
- *Operative:* indications—CES compression, progressive or severe neurological deficit, intractable leg pain, failed non-operative treatment, and worsening deformity/function. Procedures include a posterior approach with laminotomy or laminectomy and decompression of nerve roots. Resection of a facet joint is sometimes necessary to ensure nerve root decompression. Fusion with autogenous or synthetic bone added to decompression if spinal instability or spondylolisthesis demonstrated.
  - Problems with surgery—selecting the correct level (pre- and intraoperative), persistent pain (insufficient decompression, preoperative neuropraxia), recurrent pain (scar tissue), post-operative instability, non-union of fusion, and degenerative changes can develop at other levels.

Further reading

Amunsden T, Weber H, Nordal H, *et al*. Lumbar spinal stenosis: conservative or surgical management? A prospective 10-year study. *Spine*. 2000;**25**:1424–36.

Jolles BM, Porchet F, Theumann N. Surgical treatment of lumbar spinal stenosis: five-year follow up. *Journal of Bone and Joint Surgery (British Volume)*. 2001;**83**:949–53.

Katz JN, Harris MB. Lumbar spinal stenosis. *New England Journal of Medicine*. 2008;**358**(8):818–25.

Lurie JD, Tosteson TD, Tosteson A, *et al*. Long-term outcomes of lumbar spinal stenosis: eight-year results of the Spine Patient Outcomes Research Trial (SPORT). *Spine (Phila Pa 1976)*. 2015;**40**(2):63–76.

Coccydynia

Anatomy

The coccyx is the terminal-most part of the axial skeleton, composed of 3–5 fused rudimentary vertebral segments. The work 'coccyx' is derived from the Greek word for the cuckoo bird due to the similarity in appearance when viewed from the side, and it represents a human analogue of a vestigial tail. The bone articulates cranially with the sacrum through a vestigial disc, an articular process called the cornua, and coccygeal ligaments. Functionally, the coccyx serves several important functions: first, it primarily acts as an attachment site for sacro-pelvic muscles, ligaments, and tendons; second, along with the two ischial tuberosities, it provides weight-bearing support *(three legs of a tripod)*; and lastly it also provides positional support to the anus.

Epidemiology

- Up to five times commoner in ♀—coccyx rotated and facing backwards, which makes it more susceptible to trauma. The ♀ broader pelvis places sitting pressure on the coccyx, in addition to the ischial tuberosities.
- Commoner in adults. Obesity is a proven risk factor.

Aetiology

- External local trauma—usually fall backwards (direct impact).
- Minor trauma due to repetitive or prolonged sitting on hard surface— usually termed '*idiopathic coccydinia*'.
- Internal trauma—childbirth, baby's head rides over the coccyx.
- Infection (rare)—coccygeal spondylitis, pilonidal sinus.
- Tumours (rare)—involving the sacrum, can mimic coccydynia.

Clinical features

- '*Tailbone pain*' aggravated by prolonged sitting or leaning backwards while sitting. One-third of patients may present with overlapping back pain. Typically worsening of pain on standing.
- Some may report exacerbation with defecation.
- Focal coccygeal tenderness is the commonest examination finding. Examination should include pelvic and rectal palpation to feel for a mass and coccygeal mobility.
- If negative, look for referred causes of pain (disc herniation, degenerative disc disease, Tarlov cysts).
- Additional history to identify causes—recent trauma, weight loss, alteration of bowel habit, other signs of systemic diseases.

Investigations

- *Radiographs of the sacrum and coccyx:* to assess the coccygeal configuration and rule out a fracture or large tumour.
- *Dynamic radiographs* (sitting and standing): to check for sacrococcygeal instability (present in 70% of cases, associated with a positive outcome to coccygectomy).
- *MRI:* to look for infection/tumour/lumbar disc degeneration.
- *Bone scan and CT:* in refractory cases/preoperative planning.

Management

- *Non-operative:* conservative treatment effective in 90% of cases, but the patient must understand that improvement is often not rapid:
  - Oral and/or topical analgesics and NSAIDs
  - Doughnut/wedge-shaped pillow to ease pressure on the coccyx
  - Physiotherapy—pelvic floor exercises, local hot or cold packs
  - TENS
  - Local anaesthetic injection in/around the sacrococcygeal joint
  - Direct rectal manipulations indicated for persisted pain—acute correction of coccygeal alignment, breaking musculo-ligamentous adhesions, and pelvic floor spasms.
  - If pain persists, exclude sinister pathology (tumour, infection).
- *Operative:* failure of conservative treatment, particularly in those who have radiographic sacrococcygeal instability or subluxation.
  - Coccygectomy outcome needs careful patient selection. Discomfort may persist for some time. Functional recovery can take up to 12–24 months.
  - High complication rates, including wound infection, dehiscence, persistent drainage, and rectal injury. Complications occur if the plane of dissection is not strictly subperiosteal. Rectal perforation may lead to serious infection, and a diverting colostomy may be required. The commonest post-operative problem is ongoing or worsening coccygeal pain.

Adult trauma: upper limb

Brachial plexus injuries

The brachial plexus is derived from the anterior rami of the roots of C5, C6, C7, C8, and T1 (Fig. 18.1). Injuries to the brachial plexus are an uncommon but often life-changing event, with significant long-term sequelae.

Aetiology and anatomy

Injuries may be open or closed. Closed injuries are most commonly traction injuries (e.g. RTCs involving a motorcyclist or obstetric traction injuries due to shoulder dystocia in the second stage of labour). Other causes include lacerations, gunshot injuries, tumours, and irradiation.

Pathology

- Neurapraxia—good prognosis, complete recovery should occur.
- Rupture—post-ganglionic, may recover if continuity is restored.
- Lesion in continuity—stretching of large segment, no rupture, but peri- and intraneural fibrosis leads to poor prognosis.
- Avulsion—preganglionic root avulsion, poor prognosis.

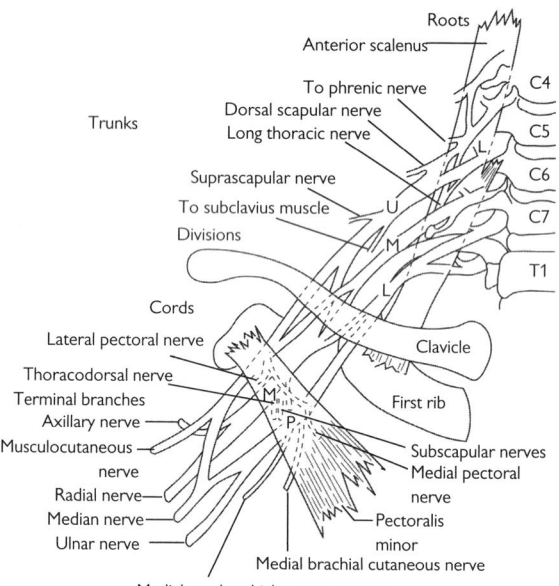

Fig. 18.1 The brachial plexus.

Reproduced from Bulstrode et al., *Oxford Textbook of Orthopaedics and Trauma*, with permission from Oxford University Press.

Classification

- *Anatomical:* upper trunk, lower trunk, complete, mixed.
- *Physiological:* degenerative (Wallerian), non-degenerative.

Assessment

- Broadly categorize lesions by whether: (1) the whole arm is involved; (2) the proximal upper limb (shoulder) is functional while the distal upper limb (hand) is dysfunctional; or (3) vice versa.
- Usually a history of high-energy injury to the upper limb with/without polytrauma.
- Patient complains of a painful (deafferentation), weak, or insensate upper limb.
- Look for position of the arm, bruising, or swelling (particularly in the supraclavicular fossa) if acute; muscle wasting and scars if chronic. Horner's syndrome (ptosis, miosis, anhydrosis, and enophthalmos) associated with lower root avulsions.
- Feel for brachial/radial pulse, Tinel's sign in supraclavicular fossa, sensation and motor power, muscle function, and sensory loss (Table 18.1).

Investigations

- *CXR:* first rib injury, raised hemidiaphragm (C3, 4, 5 injury).
- *MRI:* of cervical spine (? avulsion injury) to look for myelomeningocele.
- *Neurophysiology:* little value in acute injury; denervation changes are seen after 2–3 weeks. Sensory action potentials preserved in preganglionic avulsions, and absent in post-ganglionic ruptures.
- *MRA:* to assess for associated subclavian or vertebral artery injuries.

Management

- Resuscitation according to ATLS guidelines.
- Discuss early with a specialist nerve injury centre.
- Treat associated musculoskeletal and vascular injuries.
- Early treatment: may involve nerve repair, grafting, or transfer.
- Late treatment: functional splinting, tendon transfers, arthrodesis, amputation.

Table 18.1 Muscle function and sensory loss

Root injured	Functional loss	Sensory loss
C5/C6	Shoulder external rotation, flexion and abduction, elbow flexion, possibly wrist extension	Thumb and index finger
C5/C6/C7	Additionally elbow, wrist, finger, and thumb extension	Additionally middle finger
C8/T1	Finger and thumb flexion, median and ulnar intrinsics	Ring and little fingers
C5/T1	All arm function	All arm sensation

Reproduced from Bulstrode *et al.*, *Oxford Textbook of Orthopaedics and Trauma*, with permission from Oxford University Press.

Prognosis

Variable overall, dependent on degree and location of injury (better if low energy and close to motor end point) and on age of patient (younger do better). Poor prognosis in pan-plexus lesions, those with severe neuropathic pain secondary to nerve avulsion, supraclavicular sensory loss, or presence of Horner's syndrome.

Obstetric brachial plexus palsy

- Traction injury, usually from shoulder dystocia during labour.
- *Narakas classification:* group I, C5–6; group II, C5–7; group III, C5–T1; group IV, total plexus with Horner's syndrome.
- Many show spontaneous recovery. Exploration considered if no biceps function at 3 months (a prognostic marker).
- Careful observation of the shoulder is needed as may show subluxation or dislocation that can develop, even after neurological recovery.

Further reading

Narakas AO. The treatment of brachial plexus injuries. *International Orthopaedics*. 1985;**9**(1):29–36.

Peripheral nerve injuries

Peripheral nerves may be injured by different mechanisms, including laceration (knife, glass, sharp bone edge, scalpel), pressure (hard surface, tourniquet), traction, and ischaemia (tourniquet, arterial injury, burn eschar, compartment syndrome).

Classification

Two anatomical classifications are commonly quoted.

Seddon

- *Neurapraxia:* temporary conduction block. The nerve is intact. No Wallerian degeneration occurs distally, and no distal muscle denervation. Diagnosis of exclusion. Recovery within 6 weeks usual.
- *Axonotmesis:* discontinuity of the axon, but the supporting connective tissue tube remains intact and the nerve recovers slowly (1mm/day) as the axon regrows. Distal Wallerian degeneration and muscle denervation.
- *Neurotmesis:* the nerve is completely divided, and chances of recovery are slight without repair or nerve grafting.

Sunderland

- *I:* neurapraxia.
- *II:* loss of endoneurium.
- *III:* loss of endoneurium and perineurium.
- *IV:* loss of endoneurium, perineurium, and epineurium.
- *V:* neurotmesis.

Clinical

History should include:

- Mechanism of injury—sharp or blunt
- Duration since injury—prognostic, injuries >18 months old have poorer prognosis
- Development of neurological symptoms—onset and severity (immediately after injury, later, or after an intervention), sensory/motor deficiencies
- Progression—any improvement (more proximally innervated muscles recover first)
- Past medical history—if surgery has been performed, get a copy of the operation note; a history of diabetes/vascular disease may affect prognosis.

On *examination*, look for:

- Specific distribution of sensory loss
- Loss of autonomic function (e.g. loss of sweating)—this is useful in those who cannot explain sensory loss, particularly in children
- Pattern of muscle involvement—what muscles are not working and what muscles are still working (could be used for transfers)
- Advancing Tinel's sign—tapping on a peripheral nerve from distal to proximal, pain felt at point where regeneration has reached
- Associated vascular injury.

Common associated injuries include:
- Shoulder dislocation—axillary nerve
- Distal humeral shaft fractures—radial nerve
- Supracondylar distal humerus fractures—anterior interosseous nerve
- Finger lacerations—digital nerve
- Hip dislocation—sciatic nerve
- Knee dislocation—common peroneal nerve.

Investigations
- *Plain radiographs:* to establish if there is an associated fracture and to look for radio-opaque foreign bodies.
- *Neurophysiology tests* (see ⊃ Chapter 2, Neurophysiological tests, pp. 55–58): NCS and EMG can assess grade of nerve injury after 3–6 weeks.
- *Angiography:* useful if concomitant vascular injury suspected.

Management
Indications for exploring a nerve injury include:
- Penetrating injuries
- Open fractures
- When nerve injury follows an intervention such as surgery or manipulation of fracture
- When no recovery has occurred—the timing for this is controversial. It should be noted that motor end plates are unlikely to recover if not reinnervated within 18 months. This includes time to nerve repair or grafting, as well as time for recovery at 1mm/day.

Which injuries can be left?
- If there is a motor deficit, the joints affected should be passively mobilized and splinted in a safe position to prevent contractures while awaiting recovery. Sensory deficits should be protected from injury such as burns.
- Closed or incomplete injuries.
- Patients with paraesthesiae associated with closed crush injury or low-energy fracture patterns and no evidence of compartment syndrome.

Principles of repair
- Repair must not be under tension—transposition of the nerve may reduce tension (e.g. ulnar nerve injuries). Graft can span the defect to reduce tension.
- Oppose fascicles anatomically, motor to motor, sensory to sensory. Surface blood vessels aid in orientation.
- Use least traumatic method for repair—small sutures (8/0 to 10/0) and microinstruments.
- Place repair in healthy, vascularized bed of tissue.

Sources for nerve grafts
Autologous nerve graft material can be taken from any source where there will not be a functional deficit. Patients should be warned of areas of anaesthesia, although these should not include areas where protective sensation is vital such as the sole of the foot. In major, multiple nerve lesions, some of

the damaged nerves may be considered beyond the possibility of repair and can thus be used for graft. Sources include:

- PIN from the dorsum of the wrist (supplies wrist joint only)
- Sural nerve
- Medial cutaneous nerve of the arm
- Vein or artery interposition—provides a tube for nerve regeneration
- Synthetic tubes.

Salvage procedures include nerve transfers or tendon transfers.

Post-operative care

As for injuries awaiting recovery (see earlier). Tension can be reduced temporarily by splinting in an advantageous position (e.g. slight wrist flexion with wrist median nerve injuries).

Further reading

Seddon HJ. A classification of nerve injuries. *British Medical Journal*. 1942;**2**(4260):237.
Sunderland SS. The anatomy and physiology of nerve injury. *Muscle and Nerve*. 1990;**13**(9):771–84.

Adult hand injuries

The hand is critical to normal function. Post-traumatic stiffness can be devastating, so a core principle in managing injuries is to commence and maintain early range of motion.

Initial assessment

- Key factors in assessment are age, hand dominance, occupation, function (including hobbies), comorbidities, and treatment goals, as all impact the management decision.
- Examine for open injury, neurovascular deficit, shortening, rotational and angular deformity, and ROM.

Digital nerve block

A useful technique of regional anaesthesia, which allows for more thorough assessment and management of finger (or toe) injuries despite initial pain:

- Assess and document neurovascular status of the finger.
- Clean the area with antiseptic solution.
- Inject LA:
  - Volar anaesthesia: a single-injection, subcutaneous, volar digital block technique, using a fine-gauge needle and 2–3mL of LA agent—less painful than the traditional ring block
  - Dorsal anaesthesia: may require a dorsal ring block, as the single-injection volar technique does not always cover the dorsal nerves (1–2mL of LA in each webspace).
  - Commonly, LA without adrenaline is used (supplemented by a digital tourniquet), although evidence suggests adrenaline can be safely used in digits.

Soft tissue injuries to digits

- Injuries with minimal tissue loss or contamination, without neurovascular deficit, may be cleaned and closed primarily in ED.
- Soft tissue loss of <2cm without exposed bone or tendon may be allowed to heal via secondary intention with dressings.
- Larger defects, or those with exposed bone or tendon, are likely to require surgical debridement and coverage via flaps or grafts.
- Nail bed injuries are important, yet often neglected (common paediatric injury; finger crushed in a drawer or car door) (Fig. 18.2).
  - Failure to treat may result in deformed nail growth.
  - If associated with a phalanx fracture, treat as per BOAST open fracture guidelines (see ➜ Further reading, pp. 81–82).
  - Seymour fractures can occur in children: these are displaced distal phalangeal physeal fractures, with associated nail bed injury; they usually require operative intervention (Fig. 18.3).
  - Nail bed injuries usually require accurate repair with either a fine absorbable suture (e.g. Vicryl Rapide). The choice of whether to splint open the eponychium by suturing the (trimmed) nail plate back into place or using a substitute spacer (e.g. foil, sterile saline plastic), is debatable and lacks clear evidence.

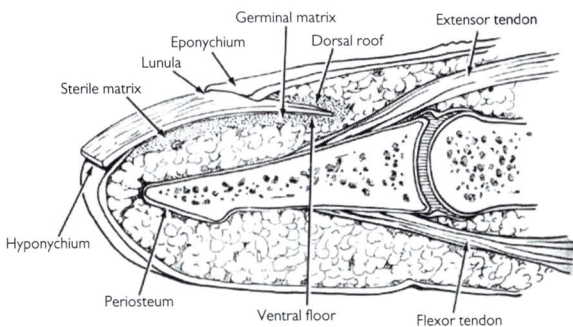

Fig. 18.2 Nail anatomy.

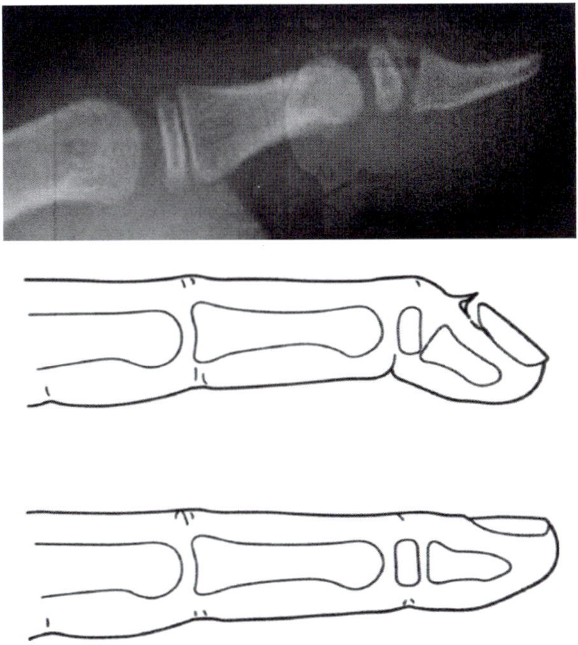

Germinal matrix · Eponychium · Lunula · Dorsal roof · Extensor tendon · Sterile matrix · Hyponychium · Periosteum · Ventral floor · Flexor tendon

Fig. 18.3 Dislocation of the nail base. This can occur if there is a bone or joint injury underneath, in this case a Salter–Harris type 1 epiphyseal fracture (Seymour fracture).

Distal phalanx injuries

- *Tuft injury:* results from a crush to the distal phalanx.
  - Closed distal phalanx fractures rarely require surgery, unless associated with an open soft tissue injury, in which case washout +/- repair of the soft tissue defect is usually necessary to prevent infection. Non-operative management to allow soft tissues to heal by secondary intention (e.g. semi-occlusive dressings) is usually possible.
- *Mallet finger:* results from forcible flexion of an extended finger.
  - Unable to fully extend the finger at the DIPJ.
  - The deformity is caused by bony or tendinous rupture of the extensor tendon insertion at the base of the distal phalanx.
  - The majority of cases can be managed in an extension splint (mallet splint), worn full time for 6–8 weeks. Surgery is considered for large bony fragments (>50% of the articular surface), with >2mm displacement or volar subluxation of the phalanx.
  - Untreated injuries can lead to an extensor lag at the DIPJ and swan neck deformity.
- *Jersey finger:* avulsion fracture of the FDP (so-called due to the common mechanism of forced extension of a flexed DIPJ when grasping an opponent's rugby jersey).
  - Commonest in the ring finger. Require surgical repair.
  - Classified by Leddy and Packer according to the level of retraction of the tendon; bony avulsions often stop marked retraction. Marked retraction requires prompt repair.

Other phalangeal and metacarpal injuries

- Most closed phalangeal and metacarpal fractures can be treated with buddy strapping and early mobilization.
- A useful method of assessment of rotation is to flex the fingers and ensure they all roughly point towards the scaphoid tubercle (comparing with the normal contralateral side) (Fig. 18.4).
- *MCPJ dislocations:* usually easily reduced and stable following reduction. A block to reduction usually results from volar plate entrapment in the joint and requires surgical open reduction.
- In general, consider surgery if >10° angulation (particularly in the coronal plane), 2–5mm shortening, any rotational deformity, or intra-articular extension. Greater angular tolerances are permitted for metacarpal neck/shaft fractures in the ulnar digits (see below).
- *Metacarpal neck fractures:* commonly following a punching injury.
  - Fracture of fifth metacarpal is 'boxer's fracture'.
  - Angulation of up to 60° well tolerated (treat with buddy strap ± volar slab or metacarpal brace), but check rotation.
  - Reduce and fix if rotated or multiple metacarpals fractured; isolated fractures usually stable due to intermetacarpal ligaments.
  - Less angulation is acceptable in second and third metacarpals (*aide-memoire*: 20–30–40–50, i.e. 20° for the second metacarpal neck, 30° for the third, etc.).

Thumb injuries

- *Bennett's:* partial intra-articular fracture of the base of the first metacarpal (Fig. 18.5).
  - Small ulnar fragment remains in place (due to attached beak ligament), with a subluxed radial fragment at the CMCJ (Fig. 18.5)

- Usually requires closed reduction and pinning (±ORIF) as rarely able to maintain reduction in plaster.
- *Rolando:* complete intra-articular fracture of the base of the first metacarpal with >2 fragments (T or Y shape).

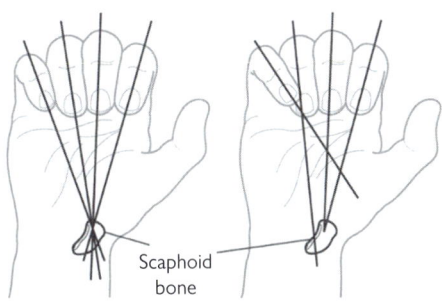

Scaphoid
bone

Fig. 18.4 Assessing for rotational deformities. With the fingers semi-flexed, all the fingernails should normally point towards the scaphoid.

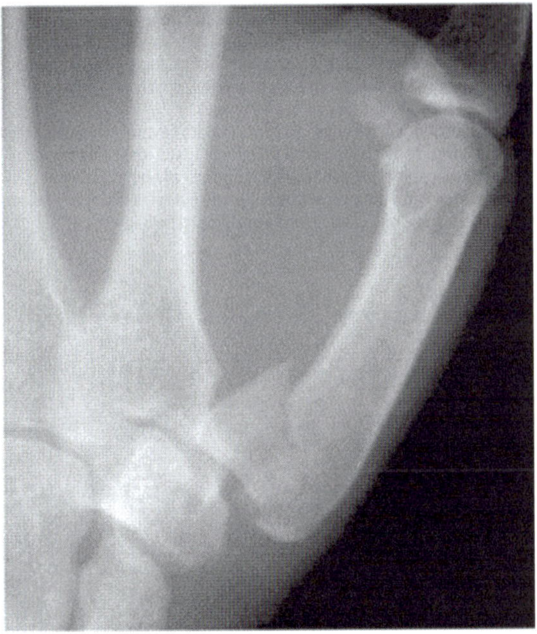

Fig. 18.5 Bennett's fracture.

- Treated with either closed reduction and pinning or ORIF.
- *Thumb CMCJ dislocation:*
  - Closed reduction and immobilization in extension and pronation.
- *MCPJ ulnar collateral ligament (UCL) rupture:*
  - May be purely ligamentous or associated with bony avulsion
  - 'Skier's thumb'—acute forced abduction
  - 'Gamekeeper's thumb'—chronic attrition of the UCL
  - Missed injuries result in weak pinch grip and impaired function
  - Diagnosed by stress testing with MCPJ in: (1) full extension (accessory ligament); and (2) 30° flexion (proper UCL)
  - Treat with thumb spica immobilization or reconstruction if grossly unstable or Stener lesion (adductor aponeurosis interposition).

Compartment syndrome

- Rare (probably underdiagnosed), but may be present after any injury.
- Treatment is surgical decompression of all 10 compartments (×4 dorsal interossei, ×3 palmar interossei, hypothenar, thenar, adductor pollicis) through five incisions (including carpal tunnel release) (Fig. 18.6).

Traumatic amputation

- The goal is to restore function.
- Considerations: patient, mechanism, level (based on flexor zones), cold/warm ischaemia time, associated structure injury.
- Replant indications: vary, but always consider reimplantation for the thumb, any digital amputation in a child, and multiple-digit amputation; some surgeons pursue a more aggressive approach of 'replant all' (provided microsurgical expertise available).
- Contraindications/challenges to replantation: severe soft tissue trauma (crush injury/mangled limb with functional tissue loss), segmental amputation, prolonged ischaemia time, medically unfit patient.
- Transport the amputated part by covering in a saline/Ringer's lactate-moistened gauze and placing into a sealed plastic bag on ice.

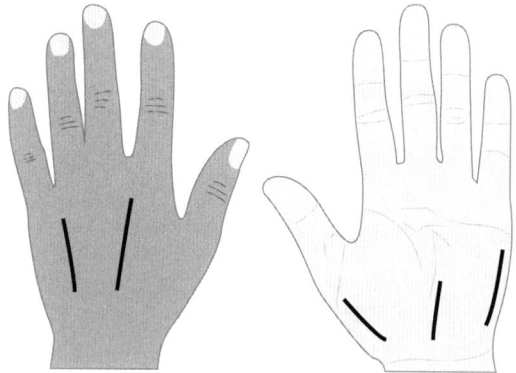

Fig. 18.6 Skin incisions for compartment releases within the hand.

- Ischaemia time:
  - Zone 1–2 digital amputations (no muscle; hence low level of metabolites produced): warm 12h, cold 24h
  - Zone 3–5 (more proximal) amputations: warm 6h, cold 12h
- More proximal: may require vascular shunting first.

Further reading

British Orthopaedic Association. *BOAST 4 open fracture guidelines*. Available from: ℗ www.boa. ac.uk/resources/boast-4-pdf.html

British Society for Surgery of the Hand. *Guidelines*. Available from: ℗ www.bssh.ac.uk/profession als/guidelines.aspx

Harbison S. Transthecal digital block: flexor tendon sheath used for anesthetic infusion. *Journal of Hand Surgery (American Volume)*. 1991;**16**:957.

Adult wrist injuries

Scaphoid fractures

- Most fractured carpal bone in young/active adults.
- Mechanism is usually a fall with forced wrist hyperextension.
- Simplest anatomical classification includes the distal pole, waist (middle 60%, commonest fracture site), and proximal pole.
- Primary blood supply is retrograde, arising from the distal pole through an end artery; the more proximal the fracture, the greater the risk of non-union and osteonecrosis.
- ♂ sex, sporting injury, anatomical snuffbox pain on ulnar deviation (early feature, <72h), and scaphoid tubercle tenderness (later feature, at 2 weeks) are independent predictors of fracture; may also have weakness of pinch and pain on thumb axial compression.
- Scaphoid series radiographs include PA without or with ulnar deviation, lateral, semi-pronated oblique, and posteroanterior 20° beam (elongated scaphoid) views (Fig. 18.7).
- Fractures are easily missed at presentation, risking sequelae.
- *Investigations:*
  - If clinical suspicion, but non-diagnostic radiographs: below-elbow cast (wrist in neutral, thumb free) and arrange further review and/or imaging.
  - Historically, repeat radiography was performed at 2 weeks but is not adequately sensitive/specific. NICE recommends prompt MRI.
  - CT may be a more rapidly available alternative, which also helps surgical planning (but is best for evaluating union).
- *Management:*
  - Distal pole fractures: usually below-elbow cast (~6 weeks).
  - ≤2mm displaced waist fractures: the SWIFFT RCT advocates for initial cast, with repeat clinical assessment at 6 weeks; if uncertainty about union, get a prompt CT. Partial union warrants a further period of cast immobilization, whereas no evidence of healing warrants surgical fixation.
  - >2mm displaced waist and proximal pole fractures: higher risk of non-union if untreated; the majority warrant surgical fixation.

(A)   (B)

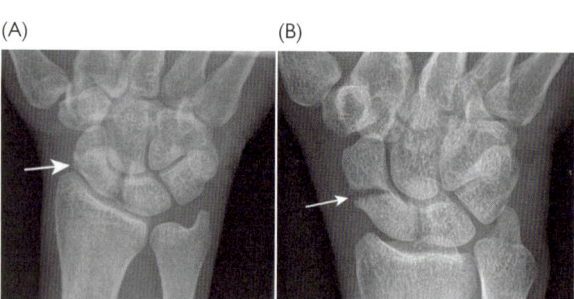

Fig. 18.7 Scaphoid radiographs: comparison between standard posteroanterior (A) vs posteroanterior view with ulnar deviation (B).

- *Complications:* Scaphoid non-union advanced collapse (SNAC) describes a recognised and progressive pattern of arthritis following scaphoid non-union, although the timing of its development is variable.

NB fractures of the other carpal bones are uncommon and can usually be managed in cast. Beware easily missed fourth/fifth metacarpal base fracture dislocations, with associated hamate fractures.

Carpal dislocations

- Carpal dislocations represent significant soft tissue injuries to the wrist, yet may be missed as 'sprains', with disastrous consequences.
- The scaphoid bridges the proximal and distal carpal rows; dislocation of either row causes rotation or fracture of the scaphoid.
- *Lunate and perilunate dislocations:*
  - Result from forced dorsiflexion of the wrist. The lunate remains attached to the radius, and the rest of the carpus dislocates (*perilunate* dislocation).
  - If the carpus spontaneously reduces, it may lever the lunate out anteriorly (*lunate* dislocation; can cause median nerve compression in the carpal tunnel).
  - The forces directed through the scaphoid can result in a (usually waist) fracture (*trans-scaphoid perilunate* dislocation).
  - Mayfield *et al.* described the sequential pattern of disruption as the injury force passes around the lunate (although injuries do not always follow this pattern) (Fig. 18.8):
    - I = scapholunate dissociation
    - II = + luno-capitate
    - III = + luno-triquetral
    - IV = lunate dislocated from the fossa.
  - *Gilula's lines* on a PA wrist radiograph may aid in diagnosis: the proximal and distal carpal row joint spaces should be separate, distinct parallel arcs; disruption suggests pathology (Fig. 18.9).
  - Other radiographic signs: triangular lunate ('piece of pie sign') and 'spilt tea cup' sign.
- *Management:*
  - Urgent reduction. May be achieved closed (traction to the wrist in extension, e.g. in Chinese finger traps, followed by palmar flexion with simultaneous pressure over the displaced lunate) or open.
  - Fix/repair bone/soft tissue disruption, as required, to restore stability to the wrist.
  - Maintain a low threshold for acute carpal tunnel release in the presence of any neurological symptoms.
  - If hand surgeon expertise is not immediately available, perform carpal tunnel decompression as a minimum, then promptly refer.
- *Complications:* osteonecrosis (AVN) of the lunate, median nerve injury, wrist stiffness, and ongoing instability.

Distal radial fractures

- One of the commonest orthopaedic injuries.
- Two main groups:

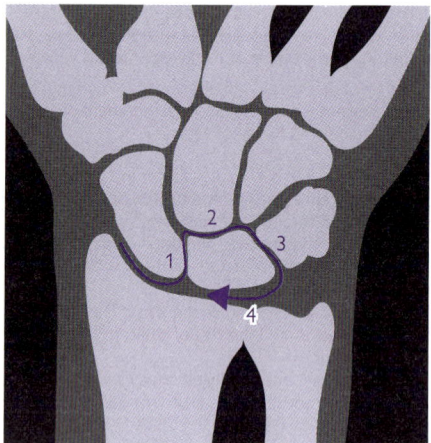

Fig. 18.8 Classically described direction of force in perilunate injuries.

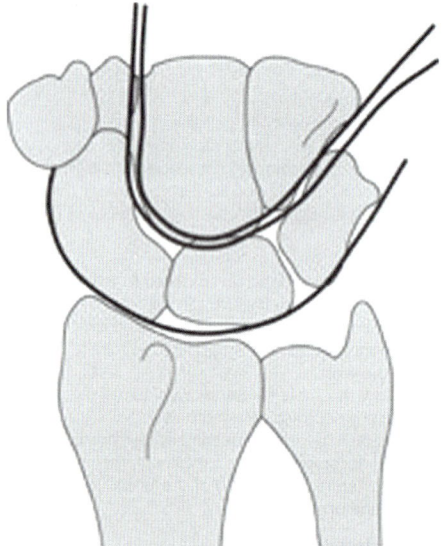

Fig. 18.9 Gilula's lines are defined by the proximal (A) and distal (B) articular surfaces of the proximal carpal row, in addition to the proximal (C) articular surface of the distal carpal row.

Reproduced from Evans *et al.*, *Operative Plastic Surgery*, 2019, with permission from Oxford University Press.

- Low-energy fragility fractures in older patients (particularly with osteoporosis)
- High-energy trauma in younger patients.
- Overall incidence ↑ with age; fragility fractures 'herald' other fragility fractures and are a marker of poor bone density. Secondary prevention as recommended by UK BOAST guidance.
- Comment on: (1) whether fractures are extra- or intra-articular; (2) angulation; (3) translation; (4) associated ulnar/other fracture; (5) comminution; (6) congruency of the DRUJ; (7) closed/open injury.
- Common eponyms (avoid these):
  - Colles': dorsally angulated extra-articular fracture
  - Smith's: volarly angulated extra-articular fracture
  - Barton's: intra-articular fracture with dislocation of the radiocarpal joint—can be volar or dorsal.
- As with any fracture, thorough assessment and documentation of the neurovascular status are vital.
- A clear understanding of the mechanism, alongside the patient's age, handedness, functional demands, and comorbidities, will influence management.
- Radiological assessment is based on PA and lateral radiographs of the wrist, paying particular attention to the '11–12–23' rule: volar tilt (~11°, lateral), radial height (~12mm, PA), and radial inclination (~23°, PA), although there is variation in these values between individuals (Fig. 18.10).
- Most displaced fractures should have reduction and plaster cast application at initial presentation, ideally under portable image intensification, to take pressure off the soft tissues, reduce the risk of carpal tunnel syndrome, and potentially avoid surgery if satisfactory reduction is achieved. Latest BOAST guidance recommends this is carried out by using regional anesthesia, such as a Bier's block, although many units still utilize haematoma block and Entonox®/Penthrox®.

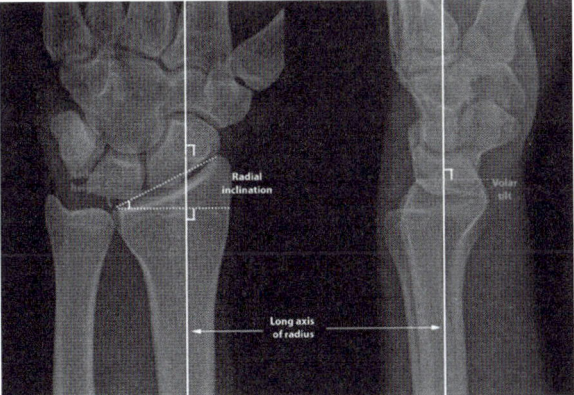

Fig. 18.10 Posteroanterior and lateral views of the wrist demonstrating radial inclination, height, and volar tilt.

- The decision for surgery is complex and controversial. There are no universally used parameters to determine who needs surgery and who does not, so this decision should be made on a case-by-case basis between surgeon and patient.
  - Generally, younger patients (<65 years), displaced fractures (any dorsal angulation, <5mm radial shortening, >2mm intra-articular step), or unstable patterns will benefit from surgery. Criteria such as those described by Lafontaine in 1989 (age >60 years, dorsal comminution, ulnar fracture, intra-articular, dorsal angulation >20°) suggest a higher risk of instability.
  - In those aged >65 years, with lower functional demand, there is some evidence that non-operative management with 4 weeks' cast immobilization and early movement yields satisfactory results, even in the presence of displacement, although each patient should be considered as an individual; a tennis playing, fit and active 70 year old with a displaced fracture may benefit from surgery, whereas in a bed-bound 50 year old with multiple medical co-morbidities, the risks of surgery may not outweigh the benefits. Similarly, in older patients with polytrauma (e.g. proximal femur fracture), wrist fracture fixation may aid mobilisation and functional recovery, thereby reducing overall morbidity and mortality.
- Where surgery is indicated, the choice of operative technique remains the subject of debate.
  - In recent years, there has been an ↑ trend towards ORIF by using a more anatomical volar locking plate (VLP) to achieve an anatomically reduced, stable construct that enables early mobilization.
  - However, several studies, most prominently the Distal Radius Acute Fracture Fixation Trial (DRAFFT), suggested that if dorsally displaced fractures requiring surgery can be satisfactorily reduced by closed means, stabilization with percutaneous wires achieves equivalent results to VLP and is more cost-effective; while the findings of such studies are debated and are not generalisable to all patient populations, this is now reflected in UK BOAST guidance.

Further reading

British Orthopaedic Association (2017). *BOAST 16: the management of distal radius fractures.* Available from: 🔗 www.boa.ac.uk/resources/boast-16-pdf.html

Costa ML, Achten J, Caroline P, et al. UK DRAFFT: a randomised controlled trial of percutaneous fixation with Kirschner wires versus volar locking-plate fixation in the treatment of adult patients with a dorsally displaced fracture of the distal radius. *Health Technology Assessment.* 2015;**19**(17):1–124, v–vi.

Costa, M.L., Achten, J., Ooms, A., Png, M.E., Cook, J.A., Lamb, S.E., Hedley, H. and Dias, J., 2022. Surgical fixation versus casting in adults with fracture of distal radius: DRAFFT2 multicentre randomised clinical trial. *bmj*, 376.

Dias, J.J., Brealey, S.D., Fairhurst, C., Amirfeyz, R., Bhowal, B., Blewitt, N., Brewster, M., Brown, D., Choudhary, S., Coapes, C. and Cook, L., 2020. Surgery versus cast immobilisation for adults with a bicortical fracture of the scaphoid waist (SWIFFT): a pragmatic, multicentre, open-label, randomised superiority trial. *The Lancet*, 396(10248), pp. 390–401.

Kulkarni K, Asif A, Dias J. Wrist pain that should not be missed. *BMJ.* 2021;**373**:n1067.

Lafontaine M, Hardy D, Delince P. Stability assessment of distal radius fractures. *Injury.* 1989;**20**(4):208–10.

Mackenney PJ, McQueen MM, Elton R. Prediction of instability in distal radial fractures. *Journal of Bone and Joint Surgery (American Volume).* 2006;**88**(9):1944–51.

Mayfield JK, Johnson RP, Kilcoyne RK. Carpal dislocations: pathomechanics and progressive perilunar instability. *Journal of Hand Surgery (American Volume).* 1980;**5**:226–41.

National Institute for Health and Care Excellence (2016). *Fractures (non-complex): assessment and management.* NICE guideline [NG38]. Available from: 🔗 www.nice.org.uk/guidance/ng38

Adult forearm injuries

The forearm is made up of the radius and ulna bound together by the interosseous membrane. Its primary function is pronation and supination, which require the radius to rotate around the ulna; injury to either can block rotation.

Isolated injury to either bone is uncommon, as the two form a closed ring. This ring encompasses the distal and proximal radioulnar joints (DRUJ and elbow joints, respectively). If only one forearm bone is fractured, look critically at the joints at either end for signs of disruption and associated injuries (e.g. Monteggia, Galeazzi, and Essex-Lopresti patterns of injury).

Maintenance of reduction through closed means can be difficult—3-point moulding of a well-fitting above-elbow cast may be sufficient. Disruption and interposition of soft tissues and tendency of the forearm to swell often mandate ORIF to reduce fractures. Fixation also allows early rehabilitation to prevent/avoid joint stiffness and muscle atrophy.

Sensory and motor function of each of the median (especially the anterior interosseus branch), ulnar, and radial nerves must be carefully tested and documented prior to any intervention. Compartment syndrome is rare, but also possible in the forearm, particularly with higher-energy injuries, so remain vigilant for this.

Combined fractures of radius and ulna shafts

- Fractures usually occur at about the same level in each bone.
- Injury usually clinically and radiologically obvious.
- Treatment is invariably operative (ORIF with plate fixation in adults/ older children; flexible elastic nailing in younger children) for anything other than minimal displacement, to achieve anatomical reduction. Note that greater deformity is tolerated in younger children (particularly <10 years) due to greater remodelling potential (see ➜ Chapter 23).

Galeazzi fracture–dislocation

- Radius (distal third) fracture in association with dislocation of the DRUJ; injury forces pass out through bone and soft tissue in the closed forearm ring.
- Mechanism is usually axial load with forced rotation.
- Always examine the wrist and elbow with any forearm injury, and order true PA and lateral wrist radiographs if isolated radius fracture to avoid missing a DRUJ injury.
- Operative treatment to restore length and rotation of the radius; if this is achieved, the DRUJ dislocation often reduces but may require temporary pinning to restore stability and allow soft tissues to heal. In experienced hands, concomitant acute TFCC reconstruction may be achievable if instability.
- Variant with distal ulnar physeal injury is easily missed, with a high rate of subsequent physeal arrest. Needs reduction ± wiring.

Monteggia fracture–dislocation

- Displaced (usually proximal third) ulnar fracture in association with radiocapitellar (radial head) dislocation (*aide-memoire:* 'Monteggi*A* = uln*A*').

- Usually results from fall on an outstretched arm in forced pronation.
- Examine for tenderness over the radial head.
- On any elbow radiograph, a line up the long axis of the radial neck should pass through the centre of the capitellum in adults/capitellar ossification centre in children (radiocapitellar line; Fig. 18.11). If it runs eccentrically, there is subluxation; if it misses, there is dislocation.
- Beware mistaking this injury for congenital radial head dislocation (radial head is small and convex, and capitellum is hypoplastic).
- Examine for PIN function, as this nerve winds around the radial neck as a branch of the radial nerve proper and can be injured.
  - Weakness of APL, EPB, EPL, EDC, EIP, ECU, and EDM.
- *Bado* classified these injuries based on the direction of radial head dislocation (Fig. 18.12):

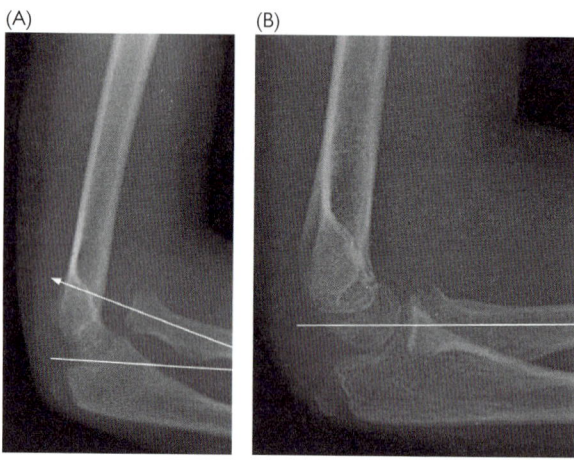

(A)   (B)

Fig. 18.11 Disrupted radiocapitellar line indicating radial head dislocation (A, arrowed) and realignment following reduction. Wrist radiographs should be taken to look for a second injury more distally.

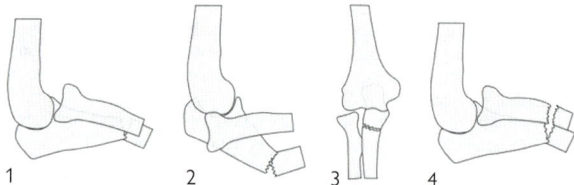

1   2   3   4

Fig. 18.12 Bado classification of Monteggia fractures based on the direction of radial head dislocation.

Reproduced from Bulstrode et al., *Oxford Textbook of Orthopaedics and Trauma*, 2011, with permission from Oxford University Press.

- I: anterior dislocation
- II: posterior dislocation
- III: lateral dislocation
- IV: both ulnar and radius fracture, together with radial head dislocation in any direction.
- In some paediatric cases, closed reduction and casting may be appropriate. Most cases are managed surgically to anatomically reduce and stabilize the ulna (flexible nailing in some younger children, plate fixation in most patients). This should achieve closed reduction of the radial head, unless the soft tissues (capsule and annular ligament) are disrupted and interposed, which may then require open reduction. Accurate reduction of the ulna is key to relocating the radial head.
- Complications include malreduction or redislocation of the radial head (careful radiographic follow-up is essential until union) and compartment syndrome.
- If radial head dislocation is missed, subsequent reduction is much harder and may be impossible, mandating either ulnar osteotomy or excision of the radial head.

Isolated ulnar shaft fracture ('night stick')

- A direct blow to the arm, classically raised in self-defence (hence the name).
- Management depends on patient and injury factors; minimally displaced injuries may be managed non-operatively in cast, although delayed or non-union is not uncommon and ORIF is often undertaken, particularly if significant displacement.

Adult elbow injuries

Most result from a fall either onto an outstretched hand or with direct trauma to the elbow. (Also see ➲ Chapter 13, Elbow instability, pp. 421–422).

A positive fat pad sign on a lateral radiograph indicates lipohaemarthrosis and a likely undisplaced fracture, which may otherwise be occult.

Elbow injuries are associated with marked stiffness, so avoid prolonged immobilization (a period of >3 weeks is rarely indicated).

Elbow dislocation

- Ninety per cent posterior or posterolateral.
- Examination reveals disruption of the equilateral triangle formed by the olecranon and epicondyles (this positional relationship is typically preserved in supracondylar fractures).
- Simple = dislocation without associated fracture.
- Complex = dislocation with associated fracture.
- O'Driscoll coined the phrase 'fortress of elbow stability', highlighting the key primary and secondary stabilizers of the elbow, some of which must be disrupted to allow for dislocation:
  - *Primary stabilizers:* ulno-humeral articulation, LUCL, anterior bundle of the MCL
  - *Secondary stabilizers:* radio-humeral articulation, common extensor origin, and common flexor–pronator mass
- The Horii circle describes the pattern with which the injury is thought to progress around the joint:
  - LUCL disruption allows posterolateral instability and radial head dislocation.
  - Anterior and posterior capsular disruption allows subluxation/dislocation of the ulna
  - Medial structures disrupt to varying degrees, allowing for complete dislocation and varus instability.
- Wrightington subsequently produced a further classification system that aims to encompass all types of elbow dislocation, and adopts a 3-column concept to guide management.
- *Terrible triad* = elbow dislocation + radial head fracture + coronoid fracture.
- *Management:*
  - Simple elbow dislocation may be managed with closed reduction and plaster cast application in ED.
  - Reduction can usually be achieved with:
    - Traction to improve coronal displacement
    - Forearm supination to shift the coronoid under the trochlea
    - Elbow flexion while placing direct pressure on the tip of the olecranon.
  - If the patient is sedated/under anaesthesia, it can be helpful to test stability prior to cast application, although this can also be done in 1–2 weeks after initial pain/swelling has settled in the clinic.
  - Surgery is indicated in complex dislocations where either reduction cannot be achieved or there is persistent instability. This typically involves repair/reconstruction of the LUCL, ORIF/replacement of

the radial head, and coronoid fixation ± MCL repair (depending on the personality of the injury).
* *Complications:* stiffness, neurovascular injury, compartment syndrome, chronic instability, and myositis ossificans.

Olecranon fracture
* Two common types:
  * Oblique traction injury resulting from a fall onto the hand (lower energy)
  * Multifragmentary fracture from a fall onto the elbow (higher energy)
* *Management:*
  * Undisplaced fractures may be treated in cast for 2 weeks followed by gentle mobilization
  * Displaced fractures generally require ORIF (tension band wire, screws, or plate)
  * Evidence that in older (>75 years), low-demand patients, even displaced fractures achieve equivalent outcomes with non-operative management (plaster cast)
* *Complications:* ulnar nerve injury, stiffness, non-union, and development of secondary OA.

Radial head fractures
* Often associated with ligamentous injury to the elbow (see ⟩ Chapter 18, Adult elbow injuries, p. 594).
* Classified by Mason (Fig. 18.13):
  * I: minimally displaced (<2mm) and no block to rotation (pronation/supination)
  * II: >2mm displaced and possible block to rotation
  * III: comminuted and displaced, with mechanical block to rotation
  * IV: concomitant elbow dislocation.

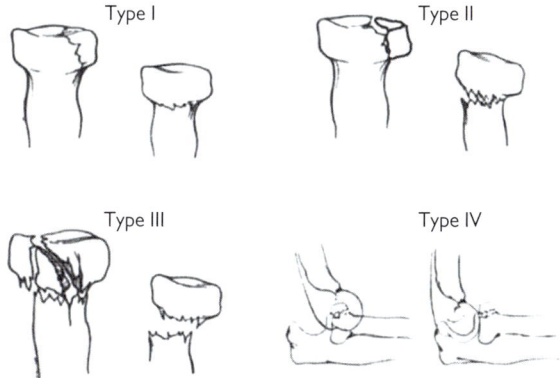

Fig. 18.13

- Assessment of elbow rotation in the context of acute trauma can be difficult to achieve due to pain and may therefore necessitate EUA. Alternatively, aspiration of elbow haemarthrosis and injection of LA will relieve pain and facilitate assessment of motion and stability.
  - *Safe window for aspiration/injection:* either directly posteriorly (soft spot proximal to the olecranon) or at the soft spot within the triangle formed by the lateral epicondyle, radial head, and olecranon.
- Remember to assess the wrist for associated soft tissue injury (Essex-Lopresti injury— damage to the interosseous membrane and DRUJ).
- *Management:*
  - Treatment for small/undisplaced fractures with no block to elbow rotation is collar and cuff for comfort, with early mobilization.
  - Larger, displaced fragments or those with a block to rotation may require ORIF with mini-screw/plate fixation; severe fragmentation mandates either radial head replacement or excision (latter not preferred in younger patients/those with ligamentous instability). CT helpful in decision-making and operative planning.
- *Complications:* stiffness, chronic wrist pain, and secondary elbow OA.

Further reading

O'Driscoll SW, Jupiter JB, King GJ, Hotchkiss RN, Morrey BF. The unstable elbow. *Journal of Bone and Joint Surgery.* 2000;**82**(5):724.

O'Driscoll SW, Jupiter JB, King GJ, et al. The unstable elbow. *Instructional Course Lectures.* 2001;**50**:91.

Savvidou OD, Koutsouradis P, Kaspiris A, Naar L, Chloros GD, Papagelopoulos PJ. Displaced olecranon fractures in the elderly—outcomes after non-operative treatment: a narrative review. *EFORT Open Reviews.* 2020;**5**(7):391–7.

Watts AC, Singh J, Elvey M, Hamoodi Z. Current concepts in elbow fracture dislocation. *Shoulder and Elbow.* 2021;**13**(4):451–8.

Adult humerus injuries

Proximal humeral fractures

- Common lower-energy fractures associated with osteoporosis (or higher-energy trauma in younger patients).
- *Clinical assessment:* assessment should include function of the axillary nerve, as determined by sensation in the 'regimental badge' area (motor function is often difficult to ascertain in the context of acute trauma, but the patient can be asked to attempt to move the shoulder forward, sideways, and backward, feeling for contraction of the anterior, lateral, and posterior deltoid, respectively).
- *Imaging:*
  - Obtain AP, scapular Y, and axillary/axial views (latter helpful in confirming GHJ congruity). In the trauma setting, alternative projections, such as the Velpeau or Nottingham views (modified trauma axials), may be easier to obtain.
  - Low threshold for CT, particularly in those patients for whom surgery is being contemplated.
- *Classification:*
  - *Neer's:* fracture lines tend to occur through the greater and lesser tuberosities, proximal humeral shaft (surgical vs anatomical neck), and humeral head, creating four potential 'parts', as described by Neer's classification. A part is considered to be a separate entity if it is >1cm displaced or >45° angulated.
  - *Hertel:* identifies key predictors of humeral head ischaemia, which include: <8mm calcar length attached to the articular surface, disrupted medial hinge, ↑ fracture complexity, displacement >10mm, and angulation >45°.
- *Management:*
  - The Proximal Fracture of the Humerus: Evaluation by Randomisation (ProFHER) trial suggested that where there is uncertainty about the need for surgery in cases of displaced proximal humerus fractures in adults, equivalent results could be achieved with non-surgical vs surgical (ORIF and hemiarthroplasty) management, which may have led to a trend towards non-operative management.
  - Most fractures in older patients can be managed non-operatively in the first instance, as fixation into osteoporotic bone yields poor results. Provide a collar and cuff sling to allow the weight of the arm to maintain soft tissue tension and aid in fracture alignment.
  - In younger patients, ORIF may be indicated in 2-, 3-, or 4-part fractures and in GT fractures with >5mm displacement.
  - With significant displacement or poor bone stock, shoulder arthroplasty may be indicated; 4-part fractures have a higher risk of developing AVN (an important determinant of outcome), making this a relative indication for arthroplasty.
  - There is an ↑ role for acute reverse shoulder arthroplasty in older patients with presumed rotator cuff deficiency.
- *Complications:* neurovascular injury (brachial artery, axillary nerve, brachial plexus), shoulder stiffness, non-union, secondary arthritis, and AVN.

Humeral shaft fractures

- *Fracture patterns:* may be transverse, spiral, or comminuted.
- *Assessment:* check and document radial nerve function.
- *Management:*
  - Most can be managed in a coaptation splint followed by functional brace, as moderate degrees of malalignment (<20° AP angulation and 30° coronal) or shortening (up to 3cm) are functionally well tolerated.
  - Indications for surgery are detailed in Box 18.1. Fixation options include ORIF with plate or IM nail, depending on fracture configuration. When performing an ORIF, the radial nerve should be visualized to avoid iatrogenic injury. The operative note should state where the nerve passes in relation to the metalwork (e.g. "over 3rd most proximal screw hole)".
  - Radial nerve palsy may be associated with up to 18% of humeral shaft fractures, but it is not in itself an indication for surgery, as 90% of cases are reported to improve with observation over 3 months; in their systematic review, Giannoudis *et al.* proposed a treatment algorithm, which includes the use of US to assess nerve integrity and relation to fracture, although the value of this is yet to be definitively validated.
  - Holstein–Lewis fracture: spiral fracture of the distal third of the humeral shaft. Has a higher rate of association with radial nerve palsy (~22%). This pattern serves a greater relative indication for surgical management, due to difficulty in controlling the fracture in a brace without extended periods of joint immobilization and the close proximity of the fracture to the nerve.

Distal humeral fractures

- *Patterns:*
  - Unicondylar, bicondylar, supracondylar, or intercondylar.
  - Also commonly described according to the AO classification: A, extra-articular; B, partial articular; and C, complete articular.
  - Supracondylar fractures are rare in adults; they represent unstable injuries which generally require fixation.

Box 18.1 Indications for open reduction and internal fixation of humeral shaft fractures

- Open injury
- Polytrauma
- Floating elbow (associated with both bone forearm fracture)
- Floating shoulder (rare)
- Associated elbow or shoulder dislocation to facilitate early mobilization
- Lower limb injury mandating use of crutches
- Radial nerve palsy occurring after manipulation of fracture
- Pathological fracture (usually metastases)
- Segmental fracture (relative indication for nailing if middle third)
- Delayed or non-union.

- Intercondylar fractures are the commonest: a fall (axial load) drives the coronoid into the trochlea, splitting the condyles apart.
- *Management:*
  - Intra-articular fractures require anatomical reduction. Principles are to reconstruct the articular surface (lag condylar fragments back together with screws) and reattach both to the diaphysis (with one or two orthogonal plates). An extensive procedure may require a posterior approach ± olecranon osteotomy to provide greater exposure.
  - It can be technically challenging to achieve stable fixation, allowing for early range of motion in such fractures. O'Driscoll described eight technical objectives for the surgeon:
    - Every screw in the distal fragments should pass through a plate.
    - Engage a fragment on the opposite side that is also fixed to a plate.
    - As many screws as possible should be placed in the distal fragments.
    - Each screw should be as long as possible.
    - Each screw should engage as many articular fragments as possible.
    - The screws in the distal fragments should lock together by interdigitation, creating a fixed-angle structure.
    - Plates should be applied, such that compression is achieved at the supracondylar level for both columns.
    - The plates must be strong and stiff enough to resist breaking or bending before union occurs at the supracondylar level.
  - If highly comminuted and/or poor bone quality precludes surgical management, treatment ranges from early mobilization ('bag of bones philosophy') to primary hemiarthroplasty or total elbow replacement.

Further reading

Arora S, Goel N, Cheema GS, Batra S, Maini L. A method to localize the radial nerve using the 'apex of triceps aponeurosis' as a landmark. *Clinical Orthopaedics and Related Research.* 2011;**469**(9):2638–44.

Duckworth AD, Clement ND, McEachan JE, White TO, Court-Brown CM, McQueen MM. Prospective randomised trial of non-operative versus operative management of olecranon fractures in the elderly. *Bone and Joint Journal.* 2017;**99-B**(7):964–72.

Hertel R, Hempfing A, Stiehler M, Leunig M. Predictors of humeral head ischemia after intracapsular fracture of the proximal humerus. *Journal of Shoulder and Elbow Surgery.* 2004;**13**(4):427–33.

Neer C. Displaced proximal humeral fractures: part I. Classification and evaluation. *Clinical Orthopaedics and Related Research.* 1970;2006;**442**:77–82.

O'Driscoll SW. Optimizing stability in distal humeral fracture fixation. *Journal of Shoulder and Elbow Surgery.* 2005;**14**(1 Suppl S):186S–94S.

Ostermann RC, Lang NW, Joestl J, Pauzenberger L, Tiefenboeck TM, Platzer P. Fractures of the humeral shaft with primary radial nerve palsy: do injury mechanism, fracture type, or treatment influence nerve recovery? *Journal of Clinical Medicine.* 2019;**8**(11):1969.

Rangan A, Handoll H, Brealey S, et al. Surgical vs nonsurgical treatment of adults with displaced fractures of the proximal humerus: the PROFHER randomized clinical trial. *JAMA.* 2015;**313**(10):1037–47.

Shao YC, Harwood P, Grotz MRW, Limb D, Giannoudis PV. Radial nerve palsy associated with fractures of the shaft of the humerus. *Journal of Bone and Joint Surgery (British Volume).* 2005;**87**(12):1647–52.

Adult shoulder injuries

Clavicle fractures

- *Mechanism:* direct blow to the clavicle or fall onto an outstretched arm.
- *Anatomy:*
  - Commonest site of fracture is junction of middle and outer third
  - Proximal fragment elevated by pull of the sternocleidomastoid.
- *Assessment:* examine to exclude neurovascular injury, pneumothorax, or ipsilateral limb/rib injury.
- *Management:*
  - Controversy remains on operative vs non-operative management of mid-shaft fractures.
  - Majority of mid-shaft fractures can be managed non-operatively with a broad arm sling and early motion as comfort allows; non-union rates are higher with non-operative management, but surgery carries a risk of complications that are not insignificant.
  - RCT evidence shows that mid-shaft fractures with ≥100% displacement may do better with ORIF, achieving higher union rates and improved early function (UK Clavicle Trial and Canadian Orthopaedic Trauma Society). However, treating all mid-shaft clavicle fractures with ORIF is not cost-effective; Nicholson et al. recommend assessment at 6 weeks, with three key predictors of non-union (≥2 factors associated with 60% non-union risk and should prompt consideration of surgery), including:
    - Quick-DASH functional score >40
    - No visible callus on the radiograph
    - Fracture movement on examination.
  - Early surgery may also be appropriate for those needing rapid return to function (self-employed, manual/physical occupation).
  - Other useful tools aid in shared decision-making/prognostic calculators—for example, Robinson's calculator (available from: ✇ www.cambridgeorthopaedics.com), which estimates the probability of union at 6, 12, and 24 weeks, based on simple patient and fracture data.
  - Displaced lateral and medial third fractures (the former are commoner) often require operative intervention, as a higher risk of non-union/injury to surrounding structures, respectively. Neer's classification of lateral third fractures is based on the fracture relationship to the coracoclavicular ligaments.

Scapula fractures

- *Mechanism:* uncommon injury resulting from high-energy trauma, and therefore often associated with other injuries (head, neck, chest, brachial plexus, vascular).
- *Classification:* described according to the anatomical structure involved (i.e. glenoid, neck, body, coracoid, acromion).
- *Imaging:* CT usually required to confirm fracture pattern (often obtained as part of trauma CT series). Maintain a high index of suspicion for scapulothoracic dissociation, which carries high rates of associated vascular and neurological injury (90%). Can be recognized based on a laterally displaced scapula on the AP radiograph or on CT.

- *Management:*
  - Majority managed non-operatively with sling immobilization, followed by early range of motion as comfort allows.
  - Intra-articular extension involving >25% of the glenoid and/or a significant articular step should prompt consideration of surgery.

Sternoclavicular dislocation

- Acromioclavicular dislocation (see ⮑ Chapter 13, Acromioclavicular joint disruption, pp. 408–410).
- Shoulder dislocation (see ⮑ Chapter 13, Acute shoulder dislocations, pp. 400–402).

Further reading

Ahrens PM, Garlick NI, Barber J, Tims EM; Clavicle Trial Collaborative Group. The Clavicle Trial: a multicenter randomized controlled trial comparing operative with nonoperative treatment of displaced midshaft clavicle fractures. *Journal of Bone and Joint Surgery (American Volume).* 2017;**99**(16):1345–54.

Canadian Orthopaedic Trauma Society. Nonoperative treatment compared with plate fixation of displaced midshaft clavicular fractures. A multicenter, randomized clinical trial. *Journal of Bone and Joint Surgery (American Volume).* 2007;**89**:1–10.

McKee M, Pelet S, McCormack RG, et al. Multicenter randomized clinical trial of nonoperative versus operative treatment of acute acromio-clavicular joint dislocation. *Journal of Orthopaedic Trauma.* 2015;**29**(11):479–87.

Nicholson JA, Clelland AD, MacDonald D, Clement N, Simpson H, Robinson CM. Displaced midshaft clavicle fracture union can be accurately predicted with a delayed assessment at six weeks following injury: a prospective cohort study. *Orthopaedic Proceedings.* 2020;**102**(Supp 4):5–5. Bone & Joint.

Nicholson JA, Clement N, Goudie E, Robinson CM. Routine fixation of displaced midshaft clavicle fractures is not cost-effective. *Bone and Joint Journal.* 2019;**101-B**(8):995–1001.

Robinson CM, Court-Brown CM, McQueen MM, Wakefield AE. Estimating the risk of nonunion following nonoperative treatment of a clavicular fracture. *Journal of Bone and Joint Surgery (American Volume).* 2004;**86-A**(7):1359–65.

Robinson's prognostic calculator. Available from: ✎ http://www.cambridgeorthopaedics.com /easytrauma/classification/clavicle/prognostic%20index%20diaph.htm

Adult trauma: lower limb

Fractures of the pelvic ring in adults

These represent 3% of all fractures. Typical mechanism is high-energy trauma in young adults (e.g. RTAs, falls from height, crush injuries). Can also present following low-energy falls in the elderly, osteoporotic population (fragility fractures). Important in a significant proportion of patients presenting with polytrauma, and the potential for associated life-threatening injuries should be anticipated and assessed. Significant mortality; evidence suggests up to 15% in closed injuries and up to 60% in open fractures.

Classification

Multiple systems exist, including Tile (Fig. 19.1) and Young and Burgess (Fig. 19.2). The Tile classification is based on stability of the posterior sacro-iliac complex (think of the pelvis as a ring; a disruption in two places makes it unstable):

- Type A—pelvic ring stable. Include iliac wing fractures, pubic rami fractures, and avulsion injuries around the periphery of the pelvis
- Type B—rotationally unstable, but vertically stable ring disruption. Include the anterior–posterior compression or 'open-book' and lateral compression-type fractures, in which the posterior part of the ring is usually at least partially stable in the vertical plane
- Type C—vertically and rotationally unstable ring disruption. Include the vertical shear or 'Malgaigne' fractures, with fractures of the pubic rami and sacrum or SIJ, and superior displacement of the hemipelvis. Typically associated with massive bleeding.

Management

- As per BOA's BOAST guidance. Patients with pelvic fractures and signs of haemodynamic instability should be managed in major trauma centres.
- Team-based ATLS approach to identify and address associated immediate life-threatening injuries.
- AP pelvic radiograph as part of primary survey—trauma CT increasingly rapidly available and often supersedes plain radiographs.
- Haemodynamic instability is present in ~15%. Resuscitation includes early use of pelvic binder (if not applied pre-hospital) and blood transfusion according to massive transfusion protocols. Early administration of tranexamic acid is advised and can reduce mortality.
- Call for senior input early.

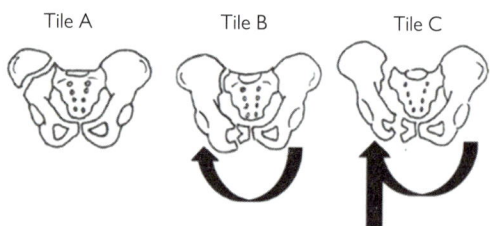

Tile A   Tile B   Tile C

Fig. 19.1 Tile classification.

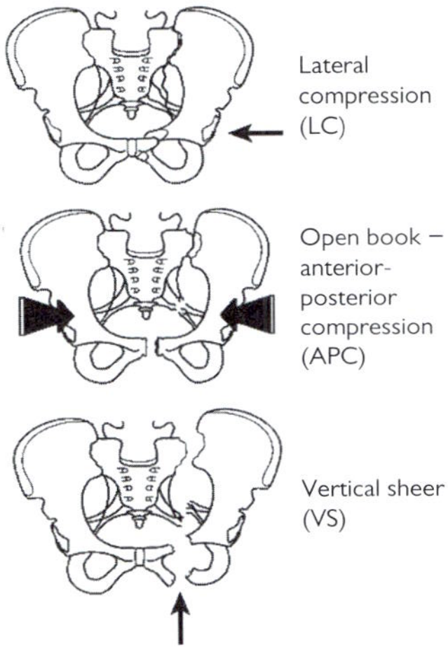

	Classification	Description	Stability
Lateral compression (LC)	LC 1	Pubic ramus and ipsilateral sacral ala compression fractures	Stable
	LC 2	Crescent iliac fracture	Rotationally unstable
	LC 3	Ipsilateral lateral compression and contralateral APC	Unstable
Open book – anterior-posterior compression (APC)	APC 1	Pubic symphysis diastasis <2.5 cm	Stable
	APC 2	Pubic symphysis diastasis <2.5 cm (anterior SIJ diastasis)	Rotationally unstable
	APC 3	Pubic symphysis diastasis >5 cm (anterior and posterior SIJ diastasis)	Unstable
Vertical sheer (VS)	VS	Fractures of pubic ramus and SIJ, with hemipelvis vertical displacement	Unstable
	Combined	Complex pattern	Varies

Fig. 19.2 Young and Burgess classification.

Important to appreciate that patients with unstable pelvic fractures presenting with haemodynamic instability may have alternative sources for haemorrhage (e.g. thoracic and/or abdominal cavity bleeding), which must not be missed. Associated injuries may require emergency surgery in conjunction with the general surgical team. If no other injuries are found and ongoing haemodynamic compromise, emergency interventions include interventional radiological angiographic embolization or surgical preperitoneal packing with external fixation of the unstable pelvis.

Open fractures of the pelvis require multidisciplinary management, including general and urological surgical input.

Once stabilized, definitive workup includes pelvic inlet and outlet views ± CT to plan operative fixation according to fracture type by experienced pelvic surgeons in specialist centres.

Associated pelvic injuries

- Urethral injury occurs in up to 15% of ♂. Blood at the urethral meatus is suggestive. A single attempt at catheterization is permissible (for BOAST guidelines, see ➲ Further reading, pp. 92–94). If bloodstained urine, then perform retrograde cystography; if unable to pass a catheter, perform retrograde urethrography and the urology team should be involved.
- Bladder rupture in up to 15% of major fractures.
- Vaginal laceration.
- Rectal injury (rare: <1%).

Complications

- Mortality up to 15% in closed fractures, depending on associated injuries and blood loss. Can be up to 60% in open pelvic fractures.
- Neurological deficit: up to 33%, predominantly with major posterior injuries, usually lumbosacral plexus (L5, S1) or femoral nerve.
- VTE: DVT (30–50%), PE (5–7%).
- Infection.
- DIC.
- ARDS/fat embolus.
- Chronic pain.
- Gait abnormality.
- Sexual dysfunction.

Further reading

British Orthopaedic Association (2016). *BOAST: the management of urological trauma associated with pelvic fractures.* Available from: ⌘ www.boa.ac.uk/resource/boast-14-pdf.html

British Orthopaedic Association (2018). *BOAST: the management of patients with pelvic fractures.* Available from: ⌘ www.boa.ac.uk/resource/boast-3-pdf.html

Gray A, Chandler H, Sabri O. Pelvic ring injuries: classification and treatment. *Orthopaedics and Trauma.* 2018;**32**(2):80–90.

Mi M, Kanakaris NK, Wu X, Giannoudis PV. Management and outcomes of open pelvic fractures: an update. *Injury.* 2021;**52**(10):2738–45.

Tosounidis TI, Giannoudis PV. Pelvic fractures presenting with haemodynamic instability: treatment options and outcomes. *The Surgeon.* 2013;**11**(6):344–51.

Adult acetabular fractures

The acetabulum is a concavity in the bony pelvis, conceptually viewed as an 'inverted Y', supported by the anterior and posterior columns. These fractures involve the hip joint and can represent some of the most challenging injuries treated by orthopaedic surgeons. Bimodal distribution: high-energy trauma in the young population; low-energy trauma in the elderly population. Given the significant force required to fracture an acetabulum, have high suspicion for associated injuries (e.g. spine, extremity, abdomen, thorax).

Classification

Judet and Letournel classification

Five *elemental* types in which a single column or wall is affected; five *associated* types which are a combination of a minimum of two of the elemental patterns and are, by definition, more complex injuries.

Elemental (or simple) fracture types

- Posterior wall.
- Anterior wall.
- Posterior column—involvement of strut running from posterior superior iliac spine (PSIS) to ischium.
- Anterior column—involvement of strut running from ASIS to pubis.
- Transverse—fracture line traverses the acetabulum, creating a ring disruption with superior and inferior fragments.

Combination (or associated) fracture types

- Posterior column and wall.
- Posterior wall and transverse.
- T-shaped—combination of transverse and a vertical fracture through the inferior fragment.
- Associated both columns (ABC)—disruption of both pelvic struts.
- Anterior column and posterior hemitransverse.

Investigations

- AP pelvis radiograph.
- Judet view radiographs—45° iliac oblique and obturator oblique views:
  - Iliac oblique view shows the posterior column and anterior wall.
  - Obturator oblique view shows the anterior column and posterior wall.
- CT with 3D reconstruction helps to further define fracture patterns and intra-articular fragments—most frequently used.
- Pelvic angiography may be necessary in an unstable patient.

Management

- Significant incidence of associated injuries—assess as per ATLS protocols, with resuscitation and identification of other injuries prior to definitive management of the acetabular fracture.
- Principles of management are to restore congruency between the femoral head and the acetabulum, with a stable reduction of the fracture.

- For minimally displaced fractures or peripheral wall fractures without intra-articular fragments, conservative management may be indicated.
- In fracture–dislocations of the hip joint, reduction of the femoral head is an emergency; skeletal traction can maintain reduction until definitive surgery can take place (e.g. if need to transfer to specialist centre).
- When the column(s) are significantly disrupted, operative reduction and stabilization are increasingly indicated.
- Primary arthroplasty has emerged as a treatment option in some fracture patterns, particularly in elderly patients.
- These injuries should be treated by experienced surgeons in specialist centres. Studies show good long-term outcomes in ~80% of patients treated operatively.

Complications

- Infection (2–5%).
- DVT and PE (5%).
- Sciatic nerve injury (2–6%).
- Femoral head AVN (3–9%).
- Heterotopic ossification.
- Secondary OA.

Further reading

Briffa N, Pearce R, Hill AM, Bircher M. Outcomes of acetabular fracture fixation with ten years' follow-up. *Journal of Bone and Joint Surgery (British Volume)*. 2011;**93**(2):229–36.
Ziran N, Soles GL, Matta JM. Outcomes after surgical treatment of acetabular fractures: a review. *Patient Safety in Surgery*. 2019;**13**(1):16.

Adult hip (proximal femur) fractures

The commonest reason for admission to an acute orthopaedic bed in the UK. Risk of hip fracture ↑ with age. The majority of patients are aged >65 years (mean age 84 years), with low-energy falls from standing height in elderly patients (i.e. fragility fractures) predominating over higher-energy trauma in younger patients (those aged <40 years account for <3% of all cases). The 30-day mortality is ~6%. Comorbid and frail patient populations require multidisciplinary management, including orthogeriatricians and occupational therapists/physiotherapists to optimize outcomes.

Classification

The term 'hip fracture' refers to all proximal femoral fractures (from the femoral head to ~5cm distal to the lesser trochanter).

The simplest classification divides fractures into *intracapsular* and *extracapsular* anatomical regions. The hip capsule covers the acetabulum to the intertrochanteric line anteriorly and to the intertrochanteric crest posteriorly. Fractures proximal to this are intracapsular, and those distal are extracapsular. The main blood supply to the adult femoral head is retrograde via 'retinacular' vessels, which run within the capsule—can be damaged in displaced intracapsular fractures, predisposing to AVN and non-union if fixation is attempted.

Intracapsular fractures can be further subclassified by the Garden classification (Fig. 19.3):
- *Type I*: incomplete fractures (including valgus impacted)
- *Type II*: undisplaced complete fractures

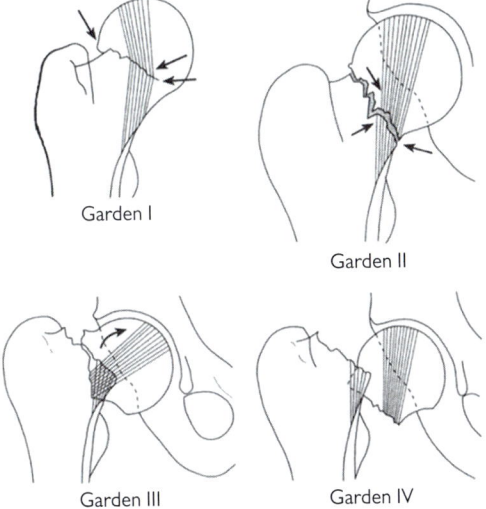

Garden I

Garden II

Garden III

Garden IV

Fig. 19.3 Garden classification.

- *Type III:* complete and partially displaced
- *Type IV:* complete and fully displaced.

The Pauwels classification, based on the orientation of the fracture line relative to the horizontal, also guides stability—more vertical patterns are more unstable, with a higher risk of AVN and non-union (type 1 = <30°; type 2 = 30–50°; type 3 = >50°).

Extracapsular fractures are typically further divided into intertrochanteric (normal and reverse obliquity) and subtrochanteric fractures (extending distal to the lesser trochanter). Several classifications exist (e.g. AO, Evans) but are complicated to remember.

Diagnosis

- *Radiographs:* AP and lateral views.
- *CT/MRI:* helpful in occult cases/unclear diagnosis.

Management

Significant work has been undertaken, including development of the NHFD, to improve hip fracture care in the UK in recent years. Management should be coordinated and multidisciplinary in nature, following a 'hip fracture programme' (for NICE guideline, see ➔ Further reading, pp. 212–213; see also ➔ Chapter 7, Best Practice Tariff, p. 216. Surgery should ideally be performed within 36h. Bone health assessment and management of osteoporosis should be part of the management, alongside a standardized clerking proforma, rapid medical optimization, and assessment of cognitive function.

Intracapsular fractures

- *Garden 1 and 2 (i.e. minimally displaced or undisplaced):* in younger patients, anatomical reduction and fixation of the fracture should be considered to preserve bone. Commonly used options include three cannulated screws (in an 'inverted pyramid' configuration) vs a 2-hole DHS (± anti-rotation screw). The evidence base does not clearly confirm either technique to be superior in terms of outcomes or reoperation rate.
- *Garden 3 and 4 (displaced):* particularly in the over-65 population, treatment is arthroplasty (via a lateral approach) due to significant risk of non-union and AVN (40%) with fixation as a result of interruption in the femoral head's blood supply. Hemiarthroplasty is suitable for most patients, compared with THR (for fitter, more active individuals. In younger patients, fixation can be considered, but anatomical reduction must be achieved and open reduction techniques may be required. There is evidence to suggest more vertical fracture patterns may be better treated with a DHS over cannulated screws.

Extracapsular fractures

Femoral head blood supply is relatively unaffected and fixation is indicated. Options include a sliding (dynamic) hip screw (SHS/DHS), cephalomedullary (intramedullary) nail fixation, and fixed-angle devices such as locking plates and blade plates. The evidence base, alongside NICE guidance, suggests a DHS should be used for intertrochanteric fractures and an intramedullar nail for subtrochanteric fractures. For stable (intact posteromedial cortex, calcar) intertrochanteric fractures, there is no difference in functional outcomes with either implant. Unstable fractures typically have large posteromedial displaced fragment (i.e. the lesser trochanter/calcar is displaced) and/or thin lateral wall thickness, or significant subtrochanteric extension, or a reverse oblique fracture pattern. In these unstable patterns, an intramedullary nail should be considered. (See ➲ Adult femoral injuries: subtrochanteric, shaft, and supracondylar fractures, p. 613 for subtrochanteric fractures.)

Complications
- Thromboembolic complications (DVT and PE).
- Lateral hip pain.
- Infection.
- AVN.
- Non-union and failure of fixation.
- Mortality (6.1% at 30 days).

Further reading
AO Foundation. *Proximal femur*. Available from: ℘ https://surgeryreference.aofoundation.org/orthopedic-trauma/adult-trauma/proximal-femur

Fixation using Alternative Implants for the Treatment of Hip fractures (FAITH) Investigators. Fracture fixation in the operative management of hip fractures (FAITH): an international, multicentre, randomised controlled trial. *The Lancet*. 2017;**389**(10078):1519–27.

National Institute for Health and Care Excellence (2011). Hip fracture: management. Clinical guideline [CG124]. Available from: ℘ www.nice.org.uk/guidance/CG124

Nuffield Department of Orthopaedics, Rheumatology and Musculoskeletal Sciences. *WHiTE Study*. Available from: ℘ www.ndorms.ox.ac.uk/clinical-trials/current-trials-and-studies/the-white-study

Royal College of Physicians. *NHFD*. Available from: ℘ https://www.nhfd.co.uk

Adult femoral injuries: subtrochanteric, shaft, and supracondylar fractures

Subtrochanteric fracture

- Located between the lesser trochanter and 5cm distally.
- Bimodal incidence; young-adult high-energy trauma (initial management ATLS protocol) or older-adult pathological fracture (osteopenia, metastatic disease, and atypical fractures related to prolonged bisphosphonate use—the latter classically present with a transverse fracture with associated cortical beaking/thickening).
- Psoas and abductors typically pull the proximal fragment strongly into flexion and abduction—needs to be corrected to achieve reduction— open reduction may be necessary.

Management

Typically, anterograde cephalo-medullary (intramedullary nail) device used—especially in elderly patients. These devices have a biomechanical advantage (shorter lever arm and load-sharing device) over a lateral plate device. Fixed-angle device (contoured proximal femoral locking plate/blade plate) is another option, but more technically challenging, often reserved for revision surgery or more comminuted fractures involving the greater trochanter. In atypical fractures associated with bisphosphonate use, strong consideration should be given to stopping bisphosphonates; radiograph of the contralateral femur is mandatory. Higher rates of delayed/non-union seen in atypical fractures.

Femoral shaft fracture

- Common injury; frequently seen with high-energy trauma. ↑ incidence of low-energy 'fragility fractures' in the elderly, osteoporotic population. ATLS management principles should be followed and associated injuries identified, and the patient resuscitated and stabilized.
- Open injuries uncommon and associated with high-energy trauma.

Definition

- >5cm below the lesser trochanter and >8cm above the knee joint.

Assessment

ATLS protocol. Up to 1500mL of blood may be lost from a single femoral fracture. Ensure patient adequately resuscitated. Radiographs should include whole femur to assess for ipsilateral femoral neck fracture (incidence 2–6%) or distal supracondylar fractures. CT angiography if ABPI <0.9 (neurovascular injury uncommon).

Management

Thomas splint in ED—provides haemostasis and analgesia. Gold standard surgical treatment for femoral shaft fractures is reamed, locked intramedullary nail, with union rates of >95% and low incidence of complications. Debate regarding timing of definitive surgical fixation, especially in setting of polytrauma. Studies demonstrate ↓ incidence of thromboembolism and pulmonary complications, and reduced length of stay if femoral shaft fractures treated definitively within 24h. 'Damage control' strategy with external fixation and delayed definitive internal fixation considered in patients with persistent metabolic derangement despite resuscitation (i.e. not meeting the following criteria: pH ≥7.25, base excess ≥−5.5mmol/L, or lactate <4.0mmol/L) (see ⭢ Chapter 3, Polytrauma, p.70).

Relative indications for considering retrograde nailing technique
- Distal extra-articular fracture (i.e. distal to the femoral isthmus).
- Ipsilateral femoral neck and shaft fracture; allows separate implant for optimal neck fixation. Nail reconstruction as further option.
- Associated acetabular or pelvic fracture which requires alternative proximal incision.
- 'Floating knee'—can use same incision for tibial intramedullary nail.
- Shaft fracture above knee replacement or below hip replacement.

Supracondylar (distal femoral) fracture

Extends from distal diaphyseal–metaphyseal junction to articular surface of distal femur. Represents <1% of all fractures; ~5% of all femur fractures. Bimodal distribution: ~80% of these are 'fragility fractures' in elderly patients. Majority of these fractures are extra-articular, and many are significantly comminuted. Risk of vascular injury due to proximity of popliteal artery. Neurovascular assessment mandated. Low threshold for ABPI or CT angiography indicated if <0.9.

Management
- *Non-operative:* typically only indicated if patient has unacceptably high anaesthetic risk or is non-ambulatory. Hinged knee brace or cast brace.
- *Operative:*
  - Anatomical angular stable locking plate: minimally invasive plate osteosynthesis (MIPO) techniques increasingly popular to encourage biological healing of fracture.
  - Retrograde intramedullary nail. Specifically designed nails have multiple distal locking options to allow reduction and fixation of comminution.
  - External fixation. Temporizing measure in polytrauma/open fractures with contamination/soft tissue injury precluding incisions.
  - Distal femoral replacement. Increasingly considered an option in comminuted fractures with poor bone stock to allow the patient to rapidly return to weight-bearing.

Further reading

Byrne JP, Nathens AB, Gomez D, Pincus D, Jenkinson RJ. Timing of femoral shaft fracture fixation following major trauma: a retrospective cohort study of United States trauma centers. *PLoS Medicine*. 2017;**14**(7):e1002336.

Hoskins W, Sheehy R, Edwards ER, et al. Nails or plates for fracture of the distal femur? Data from the Victoria Orthopaedic Trauma Outcomes Registry. *Bone and Joint Journal*. 2016;**98**(6):846–50.

Moore TA, Simske NM, Vallier HA. Fracture fixation in the polytrauma patient: markers that matter. *Injury*. 2020;**51**:S10–14.

Panteli M, Mauffrey C, Giannoudis PV. Subtrochanteric fractures: issues and challenges. *Injury*. 2017;**48**(10):2023–6.

Adult femoral injuries: periprosthetic fractures

Rising frequency due to ↑ in number of arthroplasty procedures performed and an ageing population. Challenging injuries to manage; 20-year post-operative fracture probability of 3.5% following THR. CT imaging helpful to delineate fracture pattern. *Unified Classification System (UCS)* provides a guide for treating all periprosthetic fractures—irrespective of bone affected:

- Types A/B/C are similar to the Vancouver system (see below).
- Type D involves one bone supporting two implants (e.g. femur between a hip and a knee replacement).
- Type E involves two bones supporting one replacement (e.g. acetabulum and femur after a hip replacement).
- Type F involves an unreplaced joint surface, but articulated with the implant (e.g. acetabulum after a hemiarthroplasty).

Hip

For periprosthetic hip fractures, the *Vancouver classification* is commonly used and helps to guide treatment:

- *A:* trochanteric (greater or lesser trochanter) fracture: non-operative if undisplaced. Cables or plating system if significantly displaced.
- *B:* around stem:
  - *B1:* prosthesis well fixed, ORIF; consider strut graft
  - *B2:* prosthesis loose, good bone stock; revise to long-stemmed prosthesis which bypasses the fracture
  - *B3:* prosthesis loose, poor bone stock, requires careful individual case planning; options are proximal femoral replacement or long-stemmed revision prosthesis, with low threshold for augmentation of bone stock with allograft
- *C:* fracture well distal to stem, ORIF.

Knee

Undisplaced fracture, stable prosthesis
- Non-operative.

Displaced fracture, prosthesis stable
- Locking plate as for supracondylar fracture ± grafting.
- Retrograde femoral nail as option if prosthesis design allows entry.

Loose prosthesis
- Revision to long-stem prosthesis.
- Distal femoral replacement.

Further reading

Abdel MP, Watts CD, Houdek MT, Lewallen DG, Berry DJ. Epidemiology of periprosthetic fracture of the femur in 32 644 primary total hip arthroplasties: a 40-year experience. *Bone and Joint Journal.* 2016;**98**(4):461–7.

Duncan CP, Haddad FS. The Unified Classification System (UCS): improving our understanding of periprosthetic fractures. *Bone and Joint Journal.* 2014;**96**(6):713–16.

Masri BA, Meek RM, Duncan CP. Periprosthetic fractures evaluation and treatment. *Clinical Orthopaedics and Related Research.* 2004;**420**:80–95.

Adult hip dislocation

Native hip dislocation

Rare injury, associated with high-energy trauma—RTA, fall from height, etc. Hip joint is inherently stable; high degree of bony conformity and strong stabilizing ligaments—large force required to cause dislocation. Significant incidence of associated injuries (e.g. fractures of femoral head, neck, and acetabulum, and other systems due to high-energy trauma). Manage initially as per ATLS guidelines; identify associated injuries and resuscitate as necessary.

Definitive management
- Emergent reduction after resuscitation—an orthopaedic emergency. Reduction within 6h reduces the risk of subsequent AVN of the femoral head.
- Typically performed in the operating theatre under general anaesthesia—low threshold for muscle relaxation.
- Numerous eponymously named techniques (like shoulder reduction) (e.g. Bigelow manoeuvre). Commonly, in-line traction with the hip and knee flexed—assistant stabilizes the pelvis. Assess stability following reduction with fluoroscopy.
- Distal femoral skeletal traction pin required in unstable injuries to maintain reduction prior to definitive surgical treatment (e.g. if unable to reduce closed and not in a specialist centre).
- Preoperative CT useful for:
  - Locating acetabular rim fractures (± intra-articular fragments requiring removal), which may require fixation for capsular reattachment and stability
  - Delineating associated femoral head or neck fractures
  - If preoperative CT not performed, post-operative CT is mandatory (evaluates for fracture, bony fragments, and congruity of reduction)
  - Open surgical management required for irreducible dislocation, dislocation associated with femoral neck fracture, intra-articular fragments within joint, head-splitting fractures, incongruent reduction, and instability following reduction. Surgical management should be undertaken in specialist centre by specialist pelvic and acetabular surgeon. Pipkin classification for associated fractures.

Complications
- AVN of femoral head.
- Thromboembolism.
- Sciatic nerve injury.
- Retained bone fragments in joint.
- Heterotopic ossification; consider prophylaxis.
- Joint incongruence ± instability.
- Secondary OA.

Prosthetic hip dislocation

Incidence varies in the literature, but modern techniques typically <2% after primary hip replacement.

Classification
- Timing in relation to surgery: early (<12 weeks) vs late.
- Direction of dislocation: anterior, posterior (commonest), or multidirectional.
- Aetiology: component malposition (CT needed to assess version of cup and stem), abductor insufficiency, impingement, late wear of polyethylene, spinopelvic imbalance, unknown aetiology.

Management

In uncomplicated dislocation (i.e. without periprosthetic fracture or displaced components, e.g. dual mobility liner), closed reduction by manipulation can be performed. This can be attempted in the ED with safe sedation and patient consent. If this fails, then reduction under general anaesthesia and muscle relaxant is warranted. Intraoperative fluoroscopy can be used to perform EUA to guide future potential treatment. Post-reduction, the patient is allowed to fully weight-bear, with hip precautions. Hip brace or knee immobilizer (to prevent hip flexion by keeping the knee straight) can be considered, but often not tolerated well by patients.

Open reduction rarely required but may be necessary for displaced components (e.g. 'intraprosthetic' dislocation in dual mobility constructs)—arthroplasty surgeon should be involved.

Recurrent dislocation will likely require revision surgery if the patient is medically fit, to address the identified aetiology.

Adult knee injuries

Knee (tibio-femoral) dislocations

Rare, but significant and potentially limb-threatening injury; typically, high-energy injury (road traffic collisions), but low-energy injuries can occur in patients with significantly high BMI. Dislocation can self-reduce before presentation. Identification of patients, and timely and detailed examination are necessary to reduce complications from associated vascular and neurological injuries. Significant rate of associated popliteal vessel injury ~5–10%; intact pulses do not exclude injury—measure ABPI (<0.9 requires vascular imaging and vascular surgery referral). Rate of neurological damage of 25%, usually the common peroneal nerve.

Classification
- Kennedy (direction of tibial displacement), most commonly anterior.

Management
- Emergent closed reduction. Irreducible joint uncommon but mandates open reduction. Spanning external fixator recommended if unable to hold knee reduced with splint. If concomitant vascular injury requiring repair, external fixator is necessary to protect vascular repair. Prophylactic fasciotomy should be considered in vascular injury to prevent compartment syndrome.
- Definitive management remains debatable—options include repair of ligaments ± reconstruction in an acute or staged manner.

Proximal tibio-fibular joint dislocation

Less than 1% of knee injuries, typically sports injury. Manage with closed reduction. Surgical repair/reconstruction considered for chronic pain or symptomatic instability.

Acute patellar dislocation

Typically non-contact twisting injury. Dislocation ruptures the MPFL. Anatomical factors can predispose: trochlear dysplasia, patella alta (high-riding patella), ↑ tibial tubercle to trochlea groove distance (TT-TG), ↑ Q angle. Need to rule out osteochondral lesion—consider skyline view radiographs to visualize the patellofemoral joint, and early MRI if high suspicion. First-time dislocation typically treated with physiotherapy. Surgical treatment for recurrent dislocation and high-level sports players—treatment should address anatomical factors.

Traumatic ligamentous injuries

Medial collateral injuries

Commonest ligamentous knee injury. *Mechanism:* typically excessive valgus stress to the loaded knee. *MRI:* diagnostic and can identify associated injuries (e.g. meniscus, cruciate ligaments). Majority of injuries can be treated conservatively with rehabilitation ± bracing. Surgical repair or reconstruction uncommon, considered for multi-ligament knee injuries and chronic instability.

Lateral collateral injuries

Isolated injury uncommon, associated with injuries of other structures (e.g. PLC). *MRI:* diagnostic and identifies injuries to other structures. Isolated injuries typically managed conservatively. LCL has been demonstrated to heal less well than MCL; surgical repair/reconstruction increasingly used for multi-ligament injury and grade 3 isolated injury.

Cruciate ligaments
(See ➲ pp. 480–482; see also ➲ Chapter 15.)

Extensor mechanism injuries

- *Quadriceps tendon rupture:* typically ♂ aged >40 years, eccentric loading of knee with planted foot. Injury can be partial or complete—imaging helpful to delineate (USS or MRI). Non-operative treatment in brace considered for partial injury (ability to SLR maintained). Surgical repair if complete with loss of extensor mechanism; suture anchors increasingly popular, but traditionally managed with transpatellar drill holes and suture fixation. Chronic injuries with retraction of tendon may require tendon lengthening procedure ± allograft.
- *Patellar tendon rupture:* less common injury, typically younger patients. Injury associated with long-standing tendon degeneration. Usually complete tear requiring surgical intervention. Location of tear dictates repair technique—suture anchor repair for avulsions from bone surface; mid-substance tear less common; end-to-end repair may require autograft augmentation (e.g. gracilis or semitendinosus graft).
- *Patellar fractures:* typically ♂ aged 20–50 years, following direct blow or eccentric load to flexed knee. Treatment guided by status of extensor mechanism; if clinically intact (able to SLR), can be treated conservatively in brace or cylinder cast. Fixation indicated if extensor mechanism not intact; tension band constructs for simple 2-part fractures; comminuted fractures may require screw fixation combined with cerclage techniques or new specific angular stable plates.

Haemarthrosis

- *Primary (spontaneous) non-traumatic:* consider bleeding disorders, anticoagulant, vascular tumours/malformations (e.g. PVNS). Recurrent haemarthroses can cause secondary OA. Correct underlying clotting abnormality ± acute aspiration; consider synovectomy.
- *Traumatic:* differentials—ligament injury, patella dislocation, meniscal tear, osteochondral injury. MRI can usually differentiate. Treatment dependent on lesion.

Adult leg injuries

Tibial plateau fractures

~2% of all fractures. Associated with high-energy trauma, can be low-energy falls in elderly population. Intra-articular injuries frequently associated with significant injury to soft tissue envelope, especially in high-energy injuries. Wide spectrum of injury patterns. Increasingly managed with surgical intervention.

Classification

Schatzker classification commonly used:

- *Type I:* lateral split
- *Type II:* lateral split depression
- *Type III:* pure lateral depression
- *Type IV:* medial split or split depression
- *Type V:* bicondylar (both plateaus involved)
- *Type VI:* tibial condylar fragments separated from shaft by metaphyseal fracture.

However, this only considers fractures on the AP radiograph. The 'three-column' concept of Luo *et al.* appreciates these injuries can involve 3D coronal shear patterns (involving the medial, lateral, and posterior columns), with ↑ appreciation that these necessitate reduction and fixation to improve outcome.

Management

High-energy injuries should be managed as per the ATLS protocol.

Plain film radiographs and CT allow assessment of fracture pattern. Thorough vascular and neurological assessments are mandatory—a higher incidence of neurovascular injury in medial plateau injuries. Consideration of, and assessment for, compartment syndrome, particularly in high-energy injuries. Open fractures with significant contamination, fracture dislocations, vascular injuries, and compartment syndrome require emergent treatment, typically with temporizing spanning external fixator (with vascular repair and fasciotomy as necessary).

- *Non-operative:* considered in low-energy injuries if fracture is minimally displaced or undisplaced or if patient medically unfit or non-ambulatory. Early full ROM in hinged knee brace, with minimal weight-bearing, aims to prevent stiffness and displacement.
- *Operative:* indications for surgical fixation are controversial. Open fractures, fractures with vascular injury, or compartment syndrome are definite indications. Typically, articular step of >2mm, condylar widening >5mm, coronal plane instability, angular deformity, medial condyle fractures, and bicondylar fractures are indications for surgical treatment, but no consensus in the literature. High-energy injuries with significant soft tissue envelope trauma are typically treated with temporizing external fixation, with staged definitive fixation when soft tissue condition allows. Definitive treatment options include:
  - ORIF with elevation of joint surface, restoration of alignment, and stable fixation—fixation with pre-contoured locking plates, bone substitutes to fill voids, and specific fixation of coronal shear fragments increasingly common
  - External fixation with tensioned, fine-wire ring fixators.

Tibial shaft fractures

Commonest long bone fracture. Up to 25% will be open injuries. Commoner in ♂, younger patients more likely to have higher-energy injuries. Tibial fracture is the commonest cause for compartment syndrome, which must be assessed for thoroughly and managed emergently if present. ATLS principles for high-energy injuries.

Management

- No definite consensus on optimal treatment of closed, minimally displaced shaft fractures. The decision is based on multiple factors, including premorbid condition, ambulatory status, fracture pattern, fracture location, skin condition, presence of risk factors (e.g. smoking, diabetes), and surgical preference.
- *Cast treatment* is considered for low-energy fractures with acceptable alignment (typically <5° varus/valgus, <10° AP angulation, minimal rotation, and simple fracture pattern). MUA is occasionally required to obtain a good closed reduction and apply a plaster. A POP cast can be wedged to correct low-level angulation in certain circumstances. Patella tendon-bearing plaster (Sarmiento) can allow a patient to weight-bear during fracture healing. Complications of cast treatment include malunion, delayed union, pressure sores, stiffness, and thromboembolism.
- *Locked intramedullary nailing* is suitable for most diaphyseal fractures; aims of treatment are to correct rotation, length, and alignment. Main arguments for intramedullary nailing are faster union rates and ↓ time to weight-bearing without the need for plaster cast application.
- *Plating* has a role in periarticular fractures and intra-articular extension. Contoured locking plates are increasingly popular. Skin condition, smoking, diabetes, and PVD are potential contraindications.
- *Circular frames* provide an alternative option in some centres. Fractures can be reduced and stabilized without large incisions and internal fixation. It provides an option for patients with poor healing potential, extensive soft tissue insults, open fractures, and bone loss. Certain centres may use this as a standard choice of treatment.
- Open fractures require early IV antibiotics, timely and thorough debridement, and stabilization. BOA/British Association of Plastic Reconstructive and Aesthetic Surgeons (BAPRAS) guidelines advocate for treatment in specialist centres with access to orthopaedic and plastic surgeons when possible. Primary definitive internal fixation is safe if there is minimal contamination and soft tissue coverage can be achieved. Spanning external fixation is indicated when this cannot be achieved, and early exchange to definitive fixation is advocated for. External fixation with tensioned, fine-wire circular fixators should be considered in significant contamination, bone loss, and multilevel fractures.
- Absolute indications for surgery: open fracture, vascular injury, compartment syndrome, polytrauma.

Complications

- Delayed or non-union (high-energy injury, displacement, fragmentation, infection).

- Malunion.
- Compartment syndrome (3–20%).
- Infection (<2% after intramedullary nail, ↑ in open injury with severity).

Tibial pilon (plafond) fractures

Involve weight-bearing articular surface of distal tibia. Mechanism of injury typically high-energy axial compression (driving talus into tibial plafond); low-energy rotational injuries also exist. Associated soft tissue injury typically severe, and careful management is needed to optimize outcome.

Management

ATLS protocol if high-energy mechanism—identify and treat life-threatening injuries. CT delineates fracture pattern and allows surgical planning—often performed after initial ex-fix ('span, scan, and plan' approach). Degree of injury to soft tissue envelope determines timing of definitive surgical management; higher risk of infection and wound breakdown if definitive open reduction performed on a fragile soft tissue envelope. Staged management approach with temporizing ex-fix common to allow soft tissues to improve before considering definitive fixation. Open fractures should be managed as per BOA/BAPRAS guidelines. Principles of treatment are to re-establish articular congruency, correct alignment, and reduce risk of soft tissue complications.

Options are:
- ORIF, typically with anatomically contoured locking plates
- External fixation with tensioned ring fixators
- Primary arthrodesis (typically considered when reconstruction of the joint surface is non-viable in elderly patients).

Complications

- Wound breakdown and infection.
- Malunion/non-union, pain, stiffness, instability.
- Secondary OA.

Further reading

Bear J, Rollick N, Helfet D. Evolution in management of tibial pilon fractures. *Current Reviews in Musculoskeletal Medicine*. 2018;**11**(4):537–45.

Jeelani A, Arastu MH. Tibial plateau fractures: review of current concepts in management. *Orthopaedics and Trauma*. 2017;**31**(2):102–15.

Luo CF, Sun H, Zhang B, Zeng BF. Three-column fixation for complex tibial plateau fractures. *Journal of Orthopaedic Trauma*. 2010;**24**(11):683–92.

Nanchahal J, Nayagam S, Khan U, *et al*. *Standards of the Management of Open Fractures of the Lower Limb*. London: Royal Society of Medicine Press, 2009.

Adult ankle injuries

The ankle joint comprises articulations, with associated ligaments (Fig. 19.4), between the distal tibia and the fibula (interosseus syndesmosis), the talus and the tibia (medial and lateral ligament complexes), and the calcaneum/talus and the fibula (CFL and ATFL).

Relatively small disturbances of the articular contours and soft tissue constraint can adversely affect transmission of load; ↑ joint contact stresses (same load over a reduced area of contact) lead to OA.

Injuries are divided into those that directly disrupt the load-bearing surface of the distal tibia (pilon) and those that compromise the stability and alignment of the ankle (medial, lateral, and posterior malleolar fractures and ligament ruptures).

Ankle fractures

One of the commonest orthopaedic injuries worldwide. Refers to injury in which one of medial, lateral, or posterior malleolus is fractured.

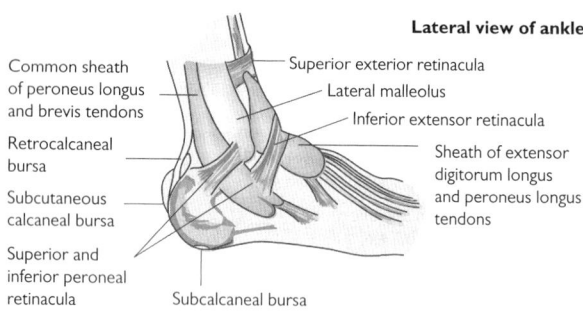

Lateral view of ankle

Common sheath of peroneus longus and brevis tendons

Retrocalcaneal bursa

Subcutaneous calcaneal bursa

Superior and inferior peroneal retinacula

Subcalcaneal bursa

Superior exterior retinacula

Lateral malleolus

Inferior extensor retinacula

Sheath of extensor digitorum longus and peroneus longus tendons

Medial view of ankle

Tibia

Sheath of flexor digitorum longus

Posterior tibial artery

Posterior tibial nerve

Flexor retinaculum

Sheath of flexor digitorum longus

Posterior tibial tendon end sheath

Fig. 19.4 Ankle anatomy.

Reproduced from Hakim, Clunie, and Haq, *Oxford Handbook of Rheumatology*, with permission from Oxford University Press.

Key treatment principle is to restore stability and alignment to the injured ankle—to prevent development of post-traumatic OA.

Classification/stability

The *Danis–Weber classification* is commonly used. This suggests the higher the fibula fracture, the greater the energy transfer and soft tissue disruption, with a greater propensity for instability.

* *Level of fibula fracture relative to tibiofibular syndesmosis:*
  * A: below
  * B: at the level of
  * C: above.

However, this system is based totally on the lateral column. It does not take into account medial column injuries of bone or ligament, which have been demonstrated to determine the overall stability of an ankle more than the lateral column. Also, the posterior malleolus is increasingly gaining importance in ankle stability. In reality, the Weber classification is an oversimplified method to assess a potentially complex injury.

The *Lauge–Hansen classification* (Table 19.1) is based on the mechanism of injury and relates the position of the foot at the time of injury (first word) and the direction of the deforming force (second word) to the fracture pattern with a predicted sequence of injuries to the structures. It is a more complex classification system and aids in recognizing what anatomical structures may have been damaged.

Neither of these classifications can definitively guide treatment. The key to decision-making is to ascertain whether a fracture pattern is stable or unstable. Unstable injuries include bimalleolar fractures, trimalleolar fractures, lateral malleolar fractures with talar shift or tilt, and fracture–dislocations. If stability is equivocal, weight-bearing X-rays within 1 week can demonstrate talar shift in unstable injury patterns.

Imaging

AP, mortise (15° internal rotation), and lateral views. Additional radiographs of the whole lower leg are required when clinical examination suggests a more proximal fracture of the fibula (Maisonneuve injury). Consider CT to delineate fracture in complex injuries when the posterior malleolus is involved.

Management

* *Initial:* protect soft tissue envelope—a clinically dislocated or grossly deformed ankle mandates reduction and splintage. Manage open fractures as per BOA/BAPRAS guidelines (see ➲ Adult leg injuries, pp. 81–82).
* *Definitive:* goal is to achieve a congruent and stable joint, with early return to function.
* *Non-operative:* treatment in cast or suitable brace/orthosis for stable injury patterns; patients should be allowed to weight-bear as tolerated.
* *Operative:* ORIF to achieve reduction and stabilization of the ankle mortise. The syndesmosis should be assessed and stabilized as necessary.

Table 19.1 Lauge–Hansen classification

Supination–adduction	1. Transverse fibular fracture or tear of lateral ligaments
	2. Vertical medial malleolus fracture
Supination–external rotation (of talus in mortise)	1. Disruption of anterior tibiofibular ligament ± avulsion of anterolateral tibia (Tillaux fragment)
	2. Spiral/oblique fracture of distal fibula at syndesmosis
	3. Disruption of posterior tibiofibular ligament or fracture of posterior malleolus
	4. Fracture of medial malleolus or deltoid ligament rupture
Pronation–abduction	1. Transverse fracture of medial malleolus or deltoid ligament disruption
	2. Rupture of syndesmotic ligaments or avulsion fracture
	3. Short horizontal/oblique fibular fracture above syndesmosis
Pronation–external rotation	1. Transverse fracture of medial malleolus or deltoid ligament disruption
	2. Disruption of anterior tibiofibular ligament ± avulsion fracture
	3. Short oblique fracture of fibula above syndesmosis (if proximal = Maisonneuve fracture)
	4. Rupture of posterior tibiofibular ligament or avulsion of posterolateral tibia
Pronation–axial compression (pilon)	1. Fracture of medial malleolus
	2. Fracture of anterior margin of tibia
	3. Supramalleolar fibula fracture
	4. Transverse fracture of posterior tibial surface

Increasingly, it has been appreciated that posterior malleolus fractures impact syndesmosis stability and clinical outcome. There is ↑ evidence that these fractures should be reduced and fixed—CT can help plan the surgical approach.

If surgery is delayed by >24h from time of injury, swelling may mandate a prolonged period of rest and elevation before safe surgery. Severe, highly unstable injuries may require temporary external fixation to hold reduction, while allowing soft tissues to settle.

Further reading

Haraguchi N, Haruyama H, Toga H, Kato F. Pathoanatomy of posterior malleolar fractures of the ankle. *Journal of Bone and Joint Surgery*. 2006;**88**(5):1085–92.

Lampridis V, Gougoulias N, Sakellariou A. Stability in ankle fractures: diagnosis and treatment. *EFORT Open Reviews*. 2018;**3**(5):294–303.

Lauge-Hansen N. Fractures of the ankle: II. Combined experimental-surgical and experimental-roentgenologic investigations. *Archives of Surgery*. 1950;**60**(5):957–85.

Mason LW, Kaye A, Widnall J, Redfern J, Molloy A. Posterior malleolar ankle fractures: an effort at improving outcomes . *Journal of Bone and Joint Surgery*. 2019;**4**(2):e0058.

Adult spine emergencies

Soft tissue disorders of the neck

Whiplash

In 1995, whiplash-associated disorder (WAD) was defined by the Quebec Task Force as an acceleration–deceleration mechanism of energy transfer to the neck. It may result from rear-end or side-impact motor vehicle collisions but can also occur during diving or other mishaps. The impact may result in bony or soft tissue injuries (whiplash injury), which in turn may lead to a variety of clinical manifestations called 'Whiplash-Associated Disorders'.

Legal definition

'Whiplash injury' is defined in UK legislation as a sprain, strain, tear, or rupture of one or more of the muscles, tendons, or ligaments in the neck or back, which has been caused by the backward, forward, or sideway movement of the neck beyond the limit of its normal range of motion.

Epidemiology

The incidence of WAD varies across countries. In the UK, it is ~9 per 1000 people—the highest in Europe.

Mechanism

The commonest mechanism is a rear-end, low-impact collision. The trunk is forced backwards on the seat, and the neck hyperextends, then recoils forward.

Clinical features

Affected individuals most commonly complain of neck pain and stiffness. Other symptoms include interscapular, shoulder, and back pain, alongside occipital headache. Limb paraesthesiae or weakness may occur, rarely related to a particular dermatome or myotome. Symptoms usually develop within 48h of the injury. Psychological symptoms (depression, anxiety) are commonly associated.

Clinical signs are often absent. Spinal tenderness, muscle spasm, reduced ROM, and neurology are occasionally found.

Based on the severity of symptoms, WAD is classified into five grades:
- Grade 0: no neck complaints or physical sign(s)
- Grade I: neck pain, stiffness, or tenderness only; no physical sign(s)
- Grade II: neck complaint AND musculoskeletal sign(s) (including ↓ range of motion and point tenderness)
- Grade III: neck complaint AND neurological sign(s) (including ↓ range of motion and point tenderness)
- Grade IV: neck complaint AND fracture/dislocation.

Investigations

Usually none is required. Lateral and AP radiographs or CT of the cervical spine at the time of the injury may be requested if clinically indicated. MRI is useful if persistent neurology.

Prognosis

Symptoms largely stabilize within 3 months, but there is significant fluctuation in symptom severity between 3 months and 2 years. This suggests that the outcome cannot be accurately assessed during that time. ~12% of patients describe improvement of symptoms between 2 and 7.5 years; 29% complain of continuing pain, and 33% report ↑ severity of symptoms following the trigger accident.

Management

- Whiplash injuries are quite difficult to treat because of the interaction of several factors, including patient psychology, socio-economic factors, legal issues/compensation, and physical health.
- Reassurance, early mobilization, and physiotherapy are important.
- Analgesia, NSAIDs, and muscle relaxants can be used acutely.

Medico-legal reporting

At their peak, whiplash injuries cost the UK economy well over £3 billion per annum, with their frequency ↑ by 25% since 2002, constituting over three-quarters of motor insurance claims. However, the UK government is implementing statutory instruments to set defined maximum tariff levels for damages following soft tissue injuries after road traffic collisions.

Further reading

Spitzer WO, Skovron ML, Salmi LR, et al. Scientific monograph of the Quebec Task Force on whiplash-associated disorders: redefining 'whiplash' and its management. Spine. 1995;**20**(8 Suppl.):8S–58S.

Tameem A, Kapur S, Mutagi H. Whiplash injury. Continuing Education in Anaesthesia, Critical Care and Pain. 2014;**14**(4):167–70.

Tomlinson PJ, Gargan MF, Bannister GC. The fluctuation in recovery following whiplash injury: 7.5-year prospective review. Injury. 2005;**36**:758–61.

Watkinson A, Gargan MF, Bannister GC. Prognostic factors in soft tissue injuries of the cervical spine. Injury. 1991;**22**:307–9.

Cervical spine trauma

General principles

History

Mechanism of injury is important, as this can guide underlying fracture patterns.

Examination

Spinal tenderness—thorough neurological examination, including perianal sensation and rectal tone. Use of the NEXUS low-risk criteria can help to decide whether imaging is required:

- GCS score 15/15 (and no evidence of intoxication)
- No distracting injury (e.g. ankle fracture–dislocation)
- No neurological deficit (moving all four limbs, normal sensation, not complaining of paraesthesiae)
- No posterior midline cervical tenderness—ask someone else to stabilize the neck from the front while you palpate the spine.

If all above criteria are met, then active movements may be checked as per the Canadian C-Spine Rule (Fig. 20.1) (see ➲ Further reading, p. 631).

Imaging

Plain radiography has historically been the first imaging modality. The standard series includes AP and lateral (visualizing C1 to T1), and open mouth views of the C-spine. Tracing lines (Fig. 20.2) on the lateral images can suggest potential injury (a formula advocated by ATLS). Open mouth views are used to assess the odontoid peg (C2). If significant injury is suspected, then cross-sectional imaging is warranted; CT remains the most sensitive and readily available imaging modality. MRI is helpful to evaluate soft tissue integrity, especially of the posterior ligamentous complex, particularly in unconscious patients (for clearance of the spine, see BOAST guidelines in ➲ Further reading, p. 647).

Cervical injuries

In adult blunt trauma, cervical spine injuries represent 2–6% of all cases and one-third of all spinal injuries. They occur in a bimodal distribution: young patients in the setting of high-energy trauma, and older patients in the setting of low-energy falls.

Upper cervical spine

Occipital condyle fractures

Most injuries to the occipital condyles are caused by high-energy trauma. Incidence is reported to range from 3% to 16%. Three subtypes are described by Anderson and Montesano:

- *Type 1:* impaction fracture of condyle from axial loading. These tend to be comminuted. Unilateral type 1 fractures are stable, but bilateral fractures may be unstable.
- *Type 2:* part of a more extensive basioccipital fracture that involves one or both occipital condyles. The commonest mechanism of injury is a direct blow to the skull. The fracture is usually stable.
- *Type 3:* avulsion fracture near the alar ligament insertion. The mechanism of injury is forced rotation of the head combined with

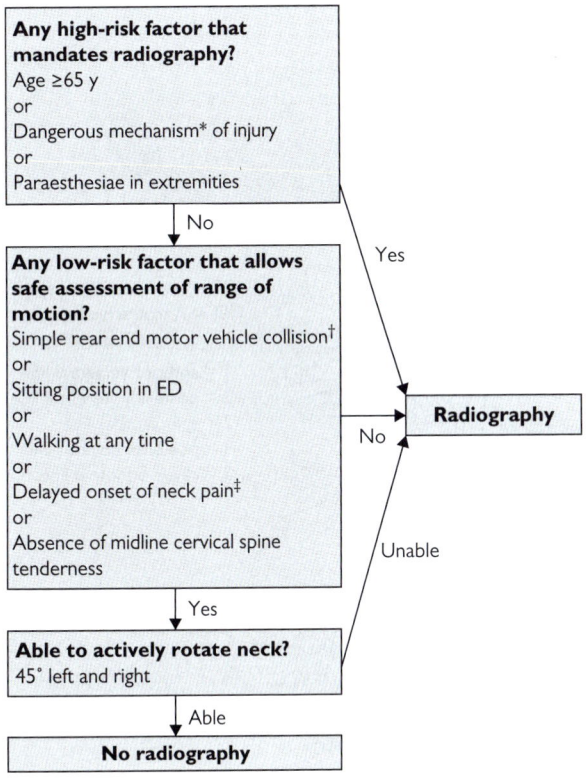

Fig. 20.1 Canadian C-Spine Rule.

lateral bending. Potentially unstable injuries owing to avulsion of the alar ligament.

Type 1 and 2 fractures can be treated with a rigid cervical orthosis. Type 3 injuries can be treated initially with an orthosis or a halo vest, but may require occipito-cervical fusion.

Atlas (C1) fracture
- First described by Jefferson in 1921. Comprise 2–13% of all cervical spine fractures, and ~25% of all injuries to the atlanto-axial complex. Caused by axial loading.
- Treatment depends on the extent of fracture displacement and the integrity of the transverse ligament. Options include 12–16 weeks of external immobilization in a halo jacket and internal instrumentation

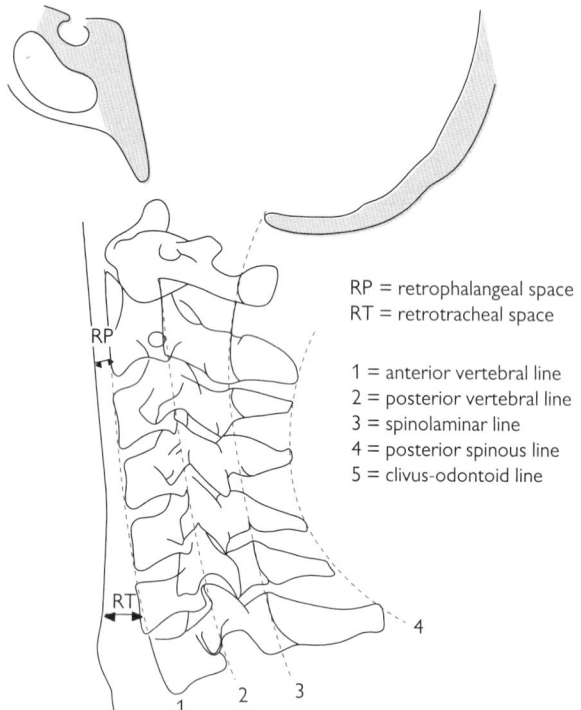

RP = retrophalangeal space
RT = retrotracheal space

1 = anterior vertebral line
2 = posterior vertebral line
3 = spinolaminar line
4 = posterior spinous line
5 = clivus-odontoid line

Fig. 20.2 Anatomy of the cervical spine.

if unstable (>6.9mm combined overhang of lateral masses on open mouth view).

C1/C2 rotary subluxation (torticollis)

- *Aetiology:* upper respiratory tract infection, trauma, inflammatory arthritis.
- Common cause of childhood torticollis.
- Grisel's syndrome is a condition of atraumatic C1/C2 subluxation following a respiratory infection or retropharyngeal abscess.
- Treatment includes a soft collar, NSAIDs, and an exercise programme if presentation is <1 week from onset. (Halter) traction or a halo jacket for 8–12 weeks if subluxation onset is >2–4 weeks from onset. If closed reduction fails, open reduction ± posterior C1–C2 fusion.

C2 (odontoid peg) fracture
- Fractures of the dens constitute 7–13% of all cervical spine injuries, with a high incidence in older patients.
- Usually visualized on open mouth and lateral C-spine radiographs.
- Commonest classification described by Anderson and D'Alonzo:
  - *Type 1:* avulsion injuries at the tip of the dens
  - *Type 2:* base of the dens; non-union rate reported to be about 32%
  - *Type 3:* extends into the body of C2.
- Type 1 may be treated non-operatively (rigid cervical collar). Types 2 and 3 can be treated either non-operatively or operatively (individualized treatment for each patient). Type 2 fractures in older patients are often managed with a rigid collar and allowed to go on to (painless) fibrous non-union; emerging evidence suggests collars confer more morbidity than non-immobilization. In younger patients, a halo vest may be a good option for an undisplaced type 2 fracture or an undisplaced/minimally displaced type 3 fracture in a patient with few or no risk factors for non-union. Surgical intervention for displaced type 2/3 fractures performed either with anterior odontoid screw fixation or posterior atlanto-axial arthrodesis.

Traumatic spondylolisthesis of the axis (hangman's fractures)
May be caused by a variety of mechanisms, including combinations of extension, flexion, distraction, and axial loading of the cervical spine. The fracture line passes through the neural arch of the axis. Best classified by using a modified Effendi classification.

Treatment depends on type; most can be managed non-operatively. There are three subtypes:
- Type 1: through the pars interarticularis bilaterally, with <3mm translation and no angulation
- Type 2: bi-pedicular fractures, with >3mm displacement and angulation of C2 on C3
- Type 3: unstable injuries with severe displacement and angulation, associated with unilateral or bilateral facet dislocation of C2 on C3.

Isolated type 1 fractures may be treated in a rigid cervical collar for 8–12 weeks. Type 2 fractures are treated with a halo vest. All type 3 fractures should be treated with surgical reduction and posterior C2–3 fusion.

Lower cervical spine
Injuries in the subaxial spine from C3–C7 account for two-thirds of all cervical injuries. The mechanism of injury is most commonly from vehicular trauma in many cases (high-energy), followed by falls.

Mechanism of injury
- Vertical compression leads to compression or burst fractures.
- Distraction injuries (posterior/anterior tension band injuries).
- Translation injuries.
- Facet injuries (fracture/dislocation)—flexion–distraction injuries (Fig. 20.3).

Management principles
- *Facet injuries:* <50% subluxation on lateral radiographs usually suggests a uni-facet dislocation, with >50% suggesting bi-facet dislocation (more likely to be associated with a significant cord injury). The former are

	Points
Morphology	
No abnormality	0
Compression	1
Burst	+1 = 2
Distraction (e.g., facet perch, hyperextension)	3
Rotation/translation (e.g., facet dislocation, unstable teardrop or advanced staged flexion compression injury)	4
Disco-ligamentous complex (DLC)	
Intact	0
Indeterminate (e.g., isolated interspinous widening, MRI signal change only)	1
Disrupted (e.g., widening of disc space, facet perch or dislocation)	2
Neurological status	
Intact	0
Root injury	1
Complete cord injury	2
Incomplete cord injury	3
Continuous cord compression in setting of neuro deficit (Neuro Modifier)	+1

Fig. 20.3 (A) Sagittal MRI scan showing C4–5 dislocation, with cord impingement caused by displacement of the spinal column and a retropulsed C4–5 disc. (B) Treatment consisting of emergency anterior C4–5 discectomy, with interbody fusion and plate fixation.

Reproduced from Hakim, Clunie, Haq, *Oxford Textbook of Rheumatology*, with permission from Oxford University Press.

harder to reduce, but more stable once reduced. In most cases, MRI is recommended pre-intervention to determine if there is associated disc herniation. Treatment options include closed reduction (Gardner–Wells tongs or halo brace) vs open reduction (anterior approach—single-level ACDF if a disc is present, with a posterior approach for reduction and instrumented stabilization—lateral mass screws).

• *Vertebral fractures*: the aim is to protect neurological function and maintain stability. The Subaxial Cervical Spine Injury Classification (SLIC) score can help to guide management of fractures (Fig. 20.4).

(A)   (B)

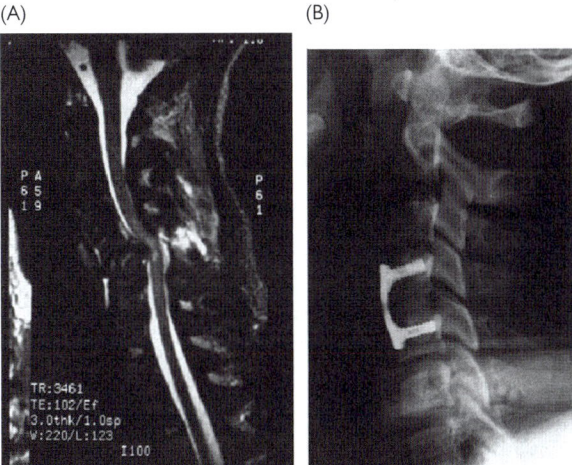

Fig. 20.4 Subaxial Cervical Spine Injury Classification (SLIC) score. 1–3 = non-surgical; 4 = either; 5–10 = surgical management.

Further reading

Anderson LD, D'Alonzo RT. Fracture of the odontoid process of the axis. *Journal of Bone and Joint Surgery (American Volume)*. 1974;**56**:1663–74.

Bellabarba C, Kandziora F, Gomes Vialle LR (eds). *AOSpine Master Series, Volume 6: Thoracolumbar Spine Trauma*. New York, NY: Thieme Medical Publishers, 2015.

British Orthopaedic Association (2015). *BOAST: spinal clearance in the trauma patient*. Available from: ℞ www.boa.ac.uk/resource/boast-2-pdf.html

Levine AM, Edwards CC. The management of traumatic spondylolisthesis of the axis. *Journal of Bone and Joint Surgery (American Volume)*. 1985;**67**:217–26.

Panacek EA, Mower WR, Holmes JF, Hoffman JR; NEXUS Group. Test performance of the individual NEXUS low-risk clinical screening criteria for cervical spine injury. *Annals of Emergency Medicine*. 2001;**38**(1):22–5.

Patel AA, Dailey A, Brodke DS, *et al*. Subaxial cervical spine trauma classification: the Subaxial Injury Classification system and case examples. *Neurosurgical Focus*. 2008;**25**(5):E8.

Garfin SR, Eismont FJ, Bell GR, Fischgrund JS, Bono CM (eds). *Rothman-Simeone and Herkowitz's The Spine*, 7th edn. Philadelphia, PA: Elsevier, 2018.

Stiell IG, Clement CM, McKnight RD, *et al*. The Canadian C-Spine rule versus the NEXUS low risk criteria in patients with trauma. *New England Journal of Medicine*. 2003;**349**:2510–18.

Thoracolumbar spine trauma

The thoracolumbar junction is the commonest injury site for thoracic and lumbar trauma. Patients are mostly young ♂ following high-energy trauma. Road traffic collisions are the commonest cause of thoracolumbar fractures, followed by falls.

The spectrum of injuries is related to the type and severity of the forces, and to the direction in which they are applied to the spine. Distraction, flexion, extension, rotation, shear forces, or a combination of these forces may be applied. If sufficient force is applied, bone and/or ligaments or joints fail, and fractures and dislocations occur.

Initial clinical assessment

- Patients with known or suspected spinal injuries should be evaluated as per ATLS protocol (see ➲ Chapter 3, pp. 64–66). Spinal injury precautions should be maintained, provided there is suspicion of spinal injury.
- Associated injuries are common, and may include head, chest, abdomen, pelvis, and long bone injuries. Bear these in mind during primary and secondary surveys, particularly in obtunded patients.
- The back is then inspected (after a log-roll into the lateral decubitus position) for bruises, abrasions, swellings, local tenderness, and deformity.
- Serial neurological examinations (as per the ASIA chart) are critical, including testing motor and sensory functions, and reflexes. Rectal examination should be considered, assessing perianal sensation and tone.

Imaging

Suspected spinal trauma requires radiological evaluation. The primary goal is to identify any spinal injury, and the secondary goal is to assess the stability of that injury to guide subsequent treatment. It includes:

- *Radiographs:* initial investigation—should include AP and lateral views of the thoracic and lumbar spine.
- *CT:* to exclude or define bony injuries. Many trauma centres now use a spiral CT trauma series (head, neck, chest, abdomen, pelvis) as part of the standard trauma evaluation protocol, which provides coronal and sagittal views of the spine
- *MRI:* useful in documenting soft tissue (posterior ligamentous complex) and neurological (cord or nerve root) injuries, and distinguishing old vs new (insufficiency) fractures.

Fig. 20.5 shows the three columns of the thoracic and lumbar spine.

Types of fractures

Compressive flexion (wedge fracture)
Results from axial compression through the vertebral body, with failure through the anterior column. The fracture may involve the superior or inferior end plates alone, or both. Plain radiographs are usually diagnostic, but CT may be necessary to confirm the diagnosis.

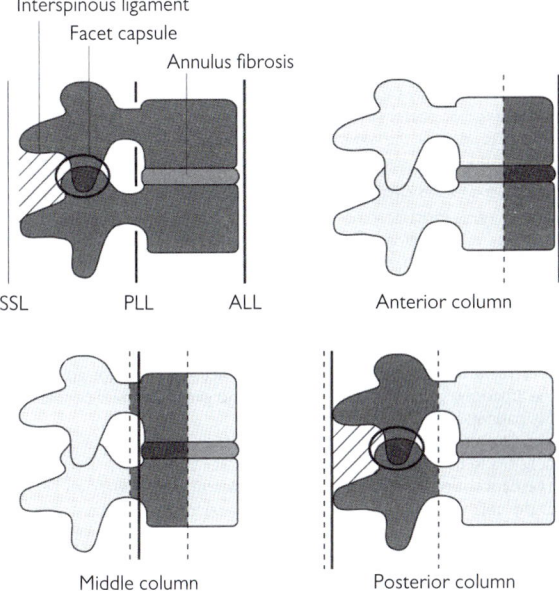

Fig. 20.5 The three anatomic columns. SSL, supraspinous ligament; PLL, posterior longitudinal ligament; ALL, anterior longitudinal ligament.

Reproduced from Bulstrode *et al.*, *Oxford Textbook of Orthopaedics and Trauma*, with permission from Oxford University Press.

Burst fracture

Results from axial compression through the vertebral body. The generally accepted differentiation of compression and burst fractures is involvement of the middle column, which is present in burst fractures and spared in compression fractures. Plain radiographs are usually diagnostic, but CT may be required to confirm diagnosis.

Flexion–distraction injuries (Chance fracture)

Result from distractive forces on the spine rather than from axial compression forces like in compression and burst fractures. All three columns may fail as a result of flexion about an axis at, or anterior to, the anterior longitudinal ligament. The injury may be purely osseous, purely ligamentous, or a combination of both. Diagnosis can be made with plain radiographs, but CT is needed to assess the precise anatomy of the osseous and facet injuries. MRI is particularly helpful in identifying the extent of the ligament and disc involvement.

Fracture–dislocations

Caused by a variety of mechanisms, including shear, rotation, distraction, flexion, and extension. All three spinal columns are disrupted. The hallmark is unilateral or bilateral facet disruption. Diagnosis can be made by plain X-ray. The AP view may show lateral translation, whereas the lateral view may show anterior or posterior translation (>50% suggests bi-facet dislocation). CT helps to identify the extent of bony and facet injuries, and MRI to assess the condition of soft tissue structures, including the disc and ligaments.

Extension and extension–distraction injuries

Relatively rare. Most commonly seen in patients with an ankylosed spine (e.g. AS or diffuse idiopathic skeletal hyperostosis (DISH)). Conventional radiography may highlight the injury. CT will help to confirm the diagnosis. MRI can help to assess the neural elements (including any haematoma) and the disco-ligamentous complex.

Management principles

- Treatment of thoracic and lumbar spine fractures should be guided by the anatomy, spinal stability, neurology, and overall medical condition of the patient, including other injuries.
- The aim is to achieve neural decompression in the case of neurological deficit, and to maintain or restore spine stability.
- The concept of 'stability' was classically described by White and Panjabi as the ability of the spine under physiological loads to limit patterns of displacement so as not to damage/irritate the cord and nerve roots and to prevent incapacitating deformity/pain due to structural changes. Acute or chronic instability is excessive displacement of the spine that can result in neurological deficit, deformity, or pain.
- The decision to treat a fracture operatively or non-operatively depends on several parameters. Indications for surgery include spinal mechanical instability, significant spinal deformity, or neurological deficit.
- Several surgical techniques are available for treatment of thoracolumbar fractures such as isolated posterior, isolated anterior, and combined anterior–posterior approach.
- The thoracolumbar injury classification and severity score (TLICS) moves away from decision-making based solely upon the 3-column concept and emphasizes the 'posterior tension band' (posterior ligamentous complex) in maintenance of stability (Fig. 20.6). This can therefore help to determine management.

Morphology

- Compression fracture (1 point)
- Burst fracture (2 points)
- Translational/rotational injury (3 points)
- Distraction injury (4 points)

Posterior ligamentous complex integrity

- Intact (0 points)
- Suspected or indeterminate injury (2 points)
- Definite injury (3 points)

Neurologic involvement

- Intact (0 points)
- Nerve root injury (2 points)
- Incomplete spinal cord/conus medullaris injury (3 points)
- Complete spinal cord/conus medullaris injury (2 points)
- Cauda equina injury (3 points)

Fig. 20.6 TLICS (thoracolumbar injury classification and severity score). <3 = non-surgical; 4 = either; >5 = surgical management.

Further reading

Bellabarba C, Kandziora F, Gomes Vialle LR (eds). *AOSpine Master Series, Volume 6: Thoracolumbar Spine Trauma.* New York, NY: Thieme Medical Publishers, 2015.

Garfin SR, Eismont FJ, Bell GR, Fischgrund JS, Bono CM (eds). *Rothman-Simeone and Herkowitz's The Spine,* 7th edn. Philadelphia, PA: Elsevier, 2018.

Lee JY, Vaccaro AR, Lim MR, *et al.* Thoracolumbar injury classification and severity score: a new paradigm for the treatment of thoracolumbar spine trauma. *Journal of Orthopaedic Science.* 2005;**10**(6):671–5.

White AA, 3rd, Johnson RM, Panjabi MM, Southwick WO. Biomechanical analysis of clinical stability in the cervical spine. *Clinical Orthopaedics and Related Research.*1975;**109**:85–96.

Cauda equina syndrome

Introduction

CES is a rare, but devastating, condition caused by compression of the terminal spinal nerve roots (i.e. usually after L1), usually due to an acutely prolapsed lumbar disc herniation. If undiagnosed and untreated, it can result in permanent neurological deficit, including weakness, alongside bowel, bladder, and sexual dysfunction. While litigation costs remain high, clinical presentation varies and the evidence base to guide management remains limited, with no consensus on diagnosis, when to image, or timing of intervention.

Spectrum of pathology

One of the reasons for this is that CES comprises a spectrum, rather than a distinct entity, with continuous (rather than stepwise) progression from CESE (early/suspected), to CESI (impending), to CESR (with retention), to CESC (complete), with no clear transition point between stages. The aim is to intervene certainly before a permanent neurological deficit develops (i.e. before CESR, and ideally early in CESI) (Table 20.1).

Epidemiology

Reported incidence varies between <1 and 2 per 100,000; 1–10% lumbar disc prolapse. ♂ > ♀. Fourth decade. Commonest at L4–5.

Causes

- Lumbar disc prolapse (commonest).
- Tumours.
- Trauma (retropulsion of vertebral fragment).
- Epidural haematoma/abscess.
- Spondylolisthesis (developmental).
- Iatrogenic (spinal surgery).

Clinical features

Classic 'red flag' features are severe lower back pain, (bilateral) radicular pain ('sciatica'), perianal (saddle)±genital sensory loss, bladder/bowel/

Table 20.1 Spectrum of cauda equina syndrome

Stage	Clinical features
CESE (early)	(Bilateral) radicular pain Low back pain
CESI (impending)	Urinary neurogenic symptoms (poor stream, need to strain, altered sensation, loss of desire to void)
CESR (retention)	Neurogenic urinary retention (painless retention, overflow incontinence)
CESC (complete)	Loss of cauda equina function, loss of perianal sensation, paralysed/insensate bladder/bowel

sexual dysfunction. Note that not all patients with true CES will have a 'classic' presentation.

Diagnosis

Time-sensitive; this is an orthopaedic emergency. While CES has previously been regarded as a clinical diagnosis, poor correlation of clinical findings with CES and ready access to MRI have meant that prompt imaging is now the established standard.

- *Bloods:* FBC, CRP—to exclude infection.
- *Pre- and post-void bladder scan:* document the residual volume. No consensus on what residual volume correlates with CES, but >100–200 is considered abnormal and warrants further imaging. One study demonstrated <200mL to have a high negative predictive value.
- *Imaging:*
  - *MRI:* gold standard modality; 24/7 access to a scanner and a reporting radiologist must be available in centres that manage CES. MRI should be performed as an emergency scan as soon as there is any clinical concern.
  - *CT myelography:* alternative if patient is unable to have MRI (e.g. certain pacemakers, MRI-incompatible implants).

Management

Prompt surgery if high suspicion/confirmed CES (discectomy or decompression). No consensus on optimal timing or what delay will result in permanent loss of neurological deficit, although intervention should be 'at the earliest opportunity', with the British Association of Spinal Surgeons suggesting 'nothing is to be gained' by delay.

Further reading

British Association of Spine Surgeons (2018). *Standards of care for investigation and management of cauda equina syndrome (CES).* Available from: ℘ https://spinesurgeons.ac.uk

Eames N, Golash A, Birch N. Cauda equina syndrome: a graphical representation of a time-sensitive condition. *Bone and Joint 360.* 2019;**8**(1):3–7.

Todd NV, Dickson RA. Standards of care in cauda equina syndrome. *British Journal of Neurosurgery.* 2016;**30**(5):518–22.

Venkatesan M, Nasto L, Tsegaye M, Grevitt M. Bladder scans and postvoid residual volume measurement improve diagnostic accuracy of cauda equina syndrome. *Spine.* 2019;**44**(18):1303–8.

Sacral trauma

The sacrum acts as a keystone at the junction of the pelvis and spinal column. It forms the posterior part of the pelvic ring, along with the SIJs. Forces transmitted through the lumbosacral junction into the upper sacrum pass laterally through the SIJs to the pelvis.

Sacral trauma occurs in two distinctly different patient groups, as a result of either high- or low-energy trauma. Sacral fractures can affect the stability of the pelvic ring and/or the spinopelvic junction, and may lead eventually to bladder/bowel/sexual dysfunction and lower extremity weakness and pain.

AP pelvis radiographs allow for detection of sacral fractures. However, with the use of plain radiographs alone, sacral fractures can be easily missed; CT and MRI may help to identify fractures and guide management.

Anatomical considerations

The sacrum is a triangular bone composed of five kyphotically oriented vertebral segments. The sacral promontory is the ventral part of the S1 body that projects anteriorly into the pelvis. The sacral ala are the lateral portions that articulate with the ilium, through the SIJs. Medial to the ala are four paired ventral and dorsal neural foramina, through which ventral and dorsal nerve root rami pass, respectively.

Fracture classification

The sacrum may be divided into three zones. In zone 1, the fractures remain in the sacral ala, lateral to the neural foramina. In zone 2, fractures occur in the neural foramina area, lateral to the spinal canal. In zone 3, the fractures involve the spinal canal.

Management

- Decision-making is dependent on several factors, including fracture anatomy, pattern, neurological status, and the patient's general health.
- *Non-operative:* for minimally displaced, unilateral fractures without associated neurological deficit. Consists of a period of recumbency followed by protected weight-bearing with crutches or a frame.
- *Operative:* performed with the aim of neurological decompression in cases of neurological deficit and stabilization in cases of instability.

Further reading

Garfin SR, Eismont FJ, Bell GR, Fischgrund JS, Bono CM (eds). *Rothman-Simeone and Herkowitz's The Spine*, 7th edn. Philadelphia, PA: Elsevier, 2018.

Spinal cord injury

Spinal cord injury (SCI) is a catastrophic, devastating event that can markedly impact many facets of a patient's life. It is defined as an injury to the spinal cord that partially or completely affects the sensory, motor, and reflex functions of the spinal cord. Suspect unstable spinal injuries after significant blunt trauma; incidence of up to 34% in unconscious patients. Protect and perfuse the cord.

Epidemiology

According to the National Spinal Cord Injury Statistical Center (NSCISC) 2020 SCI data sheet:
- *Incidence:* ranges from 12–16 per million per year (UK) to 54 per million per year (USA)
- *Age:* average age at injury has ↑ from 29 (during the 1970s) to 43 years (since 2015)
- *Gender:* ~78% of new SCI cases are ♂.

Aetiology

SCI has both traumatic and non-traumatic causes. Trauma accounts for the majority (75%), with road traffic collisions the commonest, followed by falls, acts of violence (e.g. gunshots, stabbing), and sporting injuries.

Anatomy

(Fig. 20.7)
- *Dorsal column tracts:* afferent—fine touch (tactile sensation), vibration, and proprioception.
- *Spinothalamic tracts:* afferent—pain, temperature, and crude touch.
- *Corticospinal tracts:* efferent—voluntary motor.

Spinal and neurogenic shock

- *Spinal shock:* may feature initially following severe SCI. Often presents as a transient ↑ in BP (catecholamine release), followed by hypotension, flaccid paralysis/sensory loss below the injury level, urinary retention, and faecal incontinence. May last for a few hours to several days/weeks. The end of spinal shock is described as either the return of the bulbocavernosus reflex (catheter tug/squeeze of glans penis or clitoris→observe contraction of anal sphincter) or the return of deep tendon reflexes and/or reflexive detrusor function.
- *Neurogenic shock:* may be present, manifested as haemodynamic instability (hypotension, bradyarrhythmia, and temperature dysregulation) resulting from sudden loss of autonomic tone due to SCI (commonly seen with an injury level above T6). Management involves IV fluid resuscitation, alongside vasopressors/inotropes to address hypotension and prevent secondary injury. Reflex bradycardia (due to loss of β receptor activity) augments the already unopposed vagal tone; noradrenaline (has both α and β activity) treats both hypotension and bradycardia.

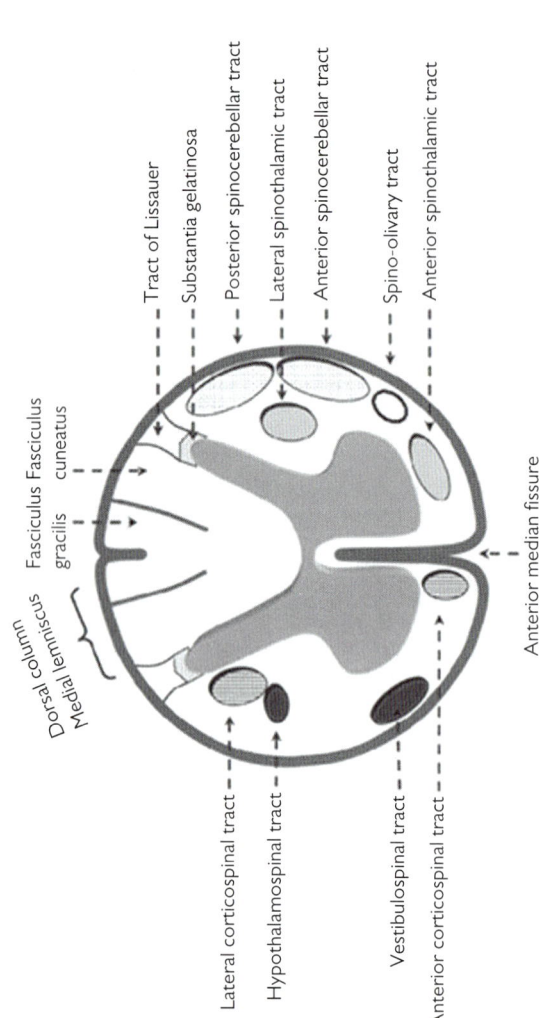

Fig. 20.7 Spinal cord pathways.

Documentation and severity grading

An established, standardized system is the ASIA Impairment Scale, which enables objective serial documentation of neurological status and concludes a final grade that is similar to the Frankel system (Table 20.2).

Classification

SCI may be broadly classified into 'complete' and 'incomplete':
- *Incomplete:* some motor or sensory function below level of injury
- *Complete:* no cord function below level of injury. Confirm by loss of voluntary anal contraction and S4–5 sensation (no sacral sparing).

Common syndromes

Fig. 20.8 shows the major spinal cord syndromes.

Incomplete

Central cord syndrome
- Commonest type of incomplete SCI.
- Characterized by disproportionately greater motor deficit in the upper than in the lower extremities.
- Usually occurs as a result of hyperextension with pre-existing acquired stenosis due to osteophytic spurs or hypertrophied ligamentum flavum (i.e. older patients).
- Most patients have moderate (but incomplete) recovery.

Brown-Séquard syndrome
- First described by Brown-Séquard in 1849.
- Cord hemisection secondary to penetrating trauma.
- Presents with ipsilateral loss of motor and posterior column (proprioception and vibration) functions and contralateral loss of pain and temperature sensation below the level of the lesion.
- Best prognosis of all of the incomplete lesions.

Table 20.2 American Spinal Injury Association (ASIA) Impairment Scale grading system

ASIA grade	Clinical status below the level of injury
A	Complete: no preservation of function below level of injury and no sacral sparing ('complete' Frankel)
B	Incomplete: sensory, but not motor, function is preserved below the neurological level and includes the sacral segments S4–S5 ('sensory only' Frankel)
C	Incomplete: motor function is preserved below the neurological level, and more than half of key muscles below the neurological level have a muscle grade <3 ('motor useless' Frankel)
D	Incomplete: motor function is preserved below the neurological level, and at least half of key muscles below the neurological level have a muscle grade of 3 or more ('motor useful' Frankel)
E	Normal: motor and sensory function are normal ('recovery' Frankel)

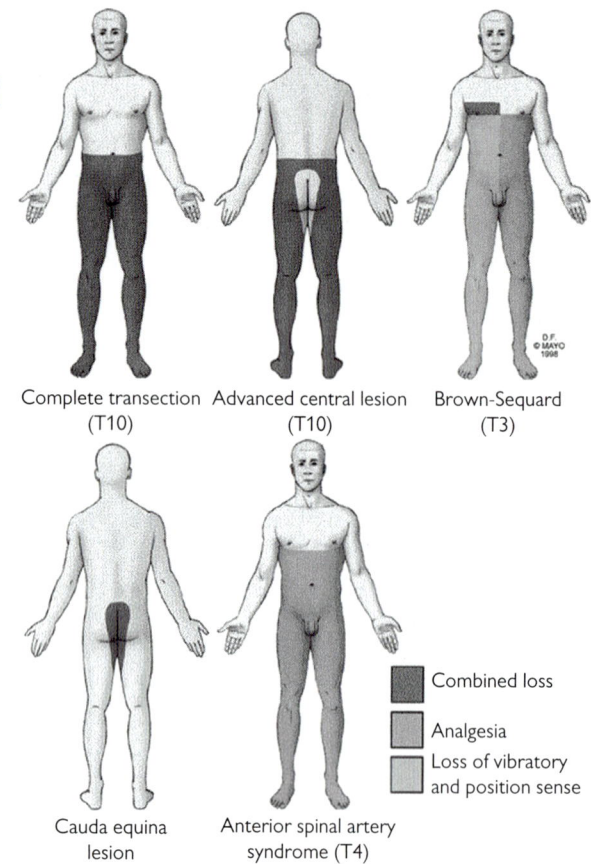

Complete transection (T10)   Advanced central lesion (T10)   Brown-Sequard (T3)

Cauda equina lesion   Anterior spinal artery syndrome (T4)

■ Combined loss

■ Analgesia

□ Loss of vibratory and position sense

Fig. 20.8 The major spinal cord syndromes.

Posterior cord syndrome
- Relatively rare.
- Presents with ipsilateral loss of proprioceptive sensation, fine touch, pressure, and vibration below the lesion, alongside deep tendon areflexia.
- Poor prognosis.

Anterior cord syndrome
- Cord infarction in territory supplied by the anterior spinal artery, often via flexion/compression injury.
- Presents with paraplegia or tetraplegia, based on the location of the injury in the spinal cord. Loss of pain and temperature sensation, and preservation of 2-point discrimination and joint position sense (posterior column function).
- Poorest prognosis of all incomplete syndromes.

Complete
- No motor or sensory function is preserved.

Management

In the UK, the BOAST guidelines make recommendations on the principles of management of traumatic SCI. Comprehensive multidisciplinary initial management improves outcomes and prevents complications. Principles of management include the following:
- *ATLS approach:* clear protocols for protecting and clearing the neck/spine following trauma; immobilize the C-spine with semi-rigid collar, sandbags, and straps. Log-roll the patient until spinal injury is excluded.
- *Adequate resuscitation:* consider neurogenic shock (injury above T6→lose sympathetic outflow→vasodilatation, hypotension, bradycardia.
- *ASIA chart:* document examination (secondary survey). Palpate the whole spine.
- *Urinary catheter and rectal examination:* assess sensation of catheter tug or bulbocavernosus reflex (when returns=spinal shock over).
- No indication for steroids.
- Local or regional 24/7 access to CT (2–3mm, helical) and MRI (suspected cord injury, neurology).
- Management of cases at, or with the support of, recognized SCI centres, with early transfer or specialist review if appropriate.
- Defined protocols for resuscitation and acute management (including skin care, bowel/bladder care, neuroprotection, and psychological support).

Cervical spine clearance
- *CT C-spine* if patient unreliable (intoxicated) or if unable to assess (patient unconscious) >48h (with CT head if consciousness impaired). Include thoracic/lumbar spine CT (or plain X-ray) if concerns.
- *Canadian C-Spine Rule* or *NEXUS criteria:* if conscious, helps to decide whether imaging is required to clear the C-spine.

Further reading

British Orthopaedic Association (2022). *BOAST: the management of traumatic spinal cord injury.* Available from: www.boa.ac.uk/resource/boast-the-management-of-traumatic-spinal-cord-injury.html
Garfin SR, Eismont FJ, Bell GR, Fischgrund JS, Bono CM (eds). *Rothman-Simeone and Herkowitz's The Spine,* 7th edn. Philadelphia, PA: Elsevier, 2018.
Greenberg MS. *Handbook of Neurosurgery,* 9th edn. New York, NY: Thieme Medical Publishers, 2020.
National Spinal Cord Injury Statistical Center. Available from: www.nscisc.uab.edu
Roberts TT, Leonard GR, Cepela DJ. Classifications In Brief: American Spinal Injury Association (ASIA) Impairment Scale. *Clinical Orthopaedics and Related Research.* 2017;**475**(5):1499–504.

Metastatic spinal cord compression

MSCC is spinal cord or cauda equina compression by either direct pressure and/or vertebral fracture/collapse or instability by metastatic spread or direct extension of malignancy, resulting in actual/impending neurological compromise. The spine has a valveless venous plexus (Batson's plexus) ideal for metastatic spread. Patients may present with acute cervical/thoracic spine or progressive lumbar spine pain (may be unremitting or aggravated by straining), local spinal tenderness, night pain preventing sleep, and acute neurological disturbance (cord/cauda equina compression, altered bladder or bowel function, altered peripheral neurology, perianal anaesthesia, gait disturbance).

Management: key principles

- Refer to MSCC coordinator for admission (within cancer network).
- MRI: <24h (altered neurology), <1 week (pain suggests metastases).

Table 20.3 Tokuhashi scoring

Characteristic		Score
General condition (performance status)	Poor	0
	Moderate	1
	Good	2
Number of extraspinal bone metastases	>2	0
	1–2	1
	0	2
Number of metastases in vertebral body	>2	0
	1–2	1
	0	2
Metastases to major internal organs	Unremovable	0
	Removable	1
	None	2
Primary site of the cancer	Lung, osteosarcoma, stomach, bladder, oesophagus, pancreas	0
	Liver, gall bladder, unidentified	1
	Others	2
	Kidney, uterus	3
	Rectum	4
	Thyroid, breast, prostate, carcinoid	5
Palsy	Complete (Frankel A/B)	0
	Incomplete (Frankel C/D)	1
	None (Frankel E)	2

Criteria of predicted prognosis—total score: 0–8, <6 months; 9–11, 6–12 months; and 12–15, >1 year.

	Score
Location	
Junctional (occiput-C2, C7–T2, T11–L1, L5–S1)	3
Mobile spine (C3–C6, L2–L4)	2
Semirigid (T3–110)	1
Rigid (52–55)	0
Pain	
Yes	3
Occasional pain but not mechanical	1
Pain-free lesion	0
Bone lesion	
Lytic	2
Mixed (lyticiblastic)	1
Blastic	0
Radiographic spinal alignment	
Subluxation/translation present	4
De novo deformity (kyphosisiscoliosis)	2
Normal alignment	0
Vertebral body collapse	
>50% collapse	3
<50% collapse	2
No collapse with >50% body involved	1
None of the above	0
Posterolateral involvement of spinal elements	
Bilateral	3
Unilateral	1
None of the above	0
Total score	
Stable	0–6
Indeterminate	7–12
Unstable	13–18

Fig. 20.9 SINS (Spinal Instability Neoplastic Score) system.

- Dexamethasone loading 16mg (except lymphoma) → 16mg OD with PPI (5–7 days, then taper) if not for surgery/radiotherapy.
- Flat bed rest (neutral spine alignment), log-roll (significant pain/neurology), regular inspection for pressure sores, VTE prophylaxis.
- Urinary catheter (bladder dysfunction); laxatives (constipation).
- Start treatment before further neurological deterioration (ideally within 24h of confirmed MSCC diagnosis).
- Assess life expectancy (*Tokuhashi score*) (Table 20.3); anaesthetic risk (ASA).
- *Management options:* radiotherapy, kyphoplasty/vertebroplasty, spinal stabilization (assess with Spinal Instability Neoplastic Score (SINS)) (Fig. 20.9). Surgery after 24h of paraplegia/tetraplegia for pain relief.

Further reading

British Orthopaedic Oncology Society. Available from: ℘ https://boos.org.uk/services/educational-resources

Fisher CG, DiPaola CP, Ryken TC, *et al.* A novel classification system for spinal instability in neoplastic disease: an evidence-based approach and expert consensus from the Spine Oncology Study Group. *Spine (Phila Pa 1976).* 2010;**35**(22):E1221–9.

National Institute for Health and Care Excellence (2008). *Metastatic spinal cord compression in adults: risk assessment, diagnosis and management.* Clinical guideline [CG75]. Available from: ℘ www.nice.org.uk/guidance/cg75

Patchell RA, Tibbs PA, Regine WF, *et al.* Direct decompressive surgical resection in the treatment of spinal cord compression caused by metastatic cancer: a randomised trial. *The Lancet.* 2005;**366**(9486):643–8.

Tokuhashi Y, Matsuzaki H, Oda H, *et al.* A revised scoring system for preoperative evaluation of metastatic spine tumor prognosis. *Spine.* 2005;**30**(19):2186–91.

Paediatrics

Paediatric orthopaedics

Cerebral palsy: introduction

Heterogeneous group of multisystem disorders caused by a non-progressive insult (static encephalopathy) to the developing brain. Conventionally defined as syndrome secondary to a brain injury that occurred before 2 years of age.

Incidence

- The commonest cause of physical disability in children.
- 2–3 per 1000 live births.
- In children weighing <1500g at birth, the rate is 70 times higher than those weighing >2500g.

Aetiology

- *Prenatal:* maternal infection (toxoplasmosis, rubella, CMV, herpes, syphilis); maternal exposure to alcohol/drugs; congenital brain malformations.
- *Perinatal:* birthweight <2500g with prematurity; anoxia.
- *Postnatal:* meningitis, head injury, immersion, intracerebral haemorrhage.

Systemic manifestations

- Neurological: developmental delay, behavioural problems, epilepsy.
- GI: feeding difficulties, gut motility problems, immobility contributing to constipation.
- Respiratory: aspiration, recurrent lower respiratory tract infections, sleep apnoea.
- Cardiac abnormalities.
- Vision/hearing/communication difficulties.

Musculoskeletal manifestations

- Weakness, poor motor control, early onset of fatigue.
- Spasticity (velocity-dependent resistance to passive stretch) is a feature of all lesions of the pyramidal system. Spasticity in a muscle is mediated via the stretch reflex that is hyperactive.
- Contractures: muscle growth is dependent on normal stretch of muscles as bone grows. Abnormal stretch reflex leads to abnormal muscle growth; the muscle–tendon unit shortens, and contractures develop with growth.
- Abnormal movement of joints (secondary to spasticity and/or weakness) can lead to development of deformities.
- Deformity negatively impacts function and exaggerates weakness and fatigue.
- Over time can lead to degenerative joint disease and intractable pain.

Classification

Physiological

- *Spastic* (commonest, 60%): ↑ muscle tone, hyperreflexia, slow and restricted movement. Contractures typical.
- *Dystonic* (20%): basal ganglia involvement. Slow, writhing involuntary movements. Choreiform athetosis. Movements ↑ with emotional tension and disappear in sleep.

- *Ataxic* (10%): involvement of the cerebellum. Weakness, coordination difficulties, tremor, difficulty with fine or rapid movements.
- *Hypotonic*.
- *Combined* (spasticity occurs in 30% of CP types other than spastic).

Topographical
- *Diplegia:* predominantly both legs, but upper limbs may be affected to variable degree.
- *Hemiplegia:* unilateral upper and lower limb involvement.
- *Total body involvement:* previously known as quadriplegia, but also involves truncal imbalance.

Functional

Gross Motor Function Classification System (GMFCS)
A validated and reliable 5-level functional grading system based on the ability to sit and walk (Fig. 21.1). Better describes and predicts motor function than topographical categorization:
- *Level I:* near-normal level of gross motor function
- *Level II:* ability to walk independently, but limitations in activities such as running or jumping; stairs with handhold
- *Level III:* requiring assistive devices to walk and using a wheelchair for longer distances
- *Level IV:* ability to stand for transfers, minimal walking ability, depending mainly on wheelchair for mobility
- *Level V:* lacking head control; inability to sit independently, stand, or walk; dependent for all aspects of care.

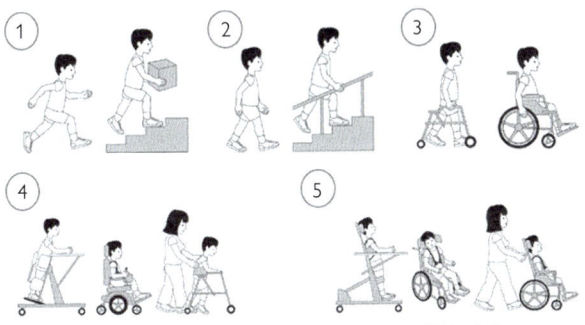

Fig. 21.1 Gross Motor Function Classification System (GMFCS) levels (at age 6–12 years).

Cerebral palsy: general management principles

Diagnosis

Diagnosis may be anticipated in the context of known ante/peri/postnatal insult. Unexpected cases can present as failure to meet developmental milestones, gait abnormalities, and joint contractures (e.g. toe-walking, early hand dominance).

Clinical features

- Delayed motor milestones.
- Gait abnormalities: toe-walking, scissoring, foot drop.
- Dystonic, choreoathetoid movements, dyspraxia.
- Spasticity: clonus, positive Babinski reflex, hyperreflexia.

Investigations

- Referral to paediatrician/neurologist for review.
- MRI of the brain classically demonstrates periventricular leucomalacia.

Management: general principles

- MDT care of child and family involves multiple agencies, including primary care practitioner and community medical teams (paediatrics, physiotherapy, occupational therapy, psychology, social care, school authorities), to ensure holistic care.
- Involvement of specialist care as required by clinical manifestations.
- Focus of care according to the 'six Fs' of childhood disability: Function, Family, Fitness, Fun, Friends, and Future.
- As the child grows and develops, priorities change:
  - In early years, focus on enhancing and encouraging development requires close family engagement, supported by therapists and community teams.
  - Moving from infancy to childhood, ↑ focus on function and social integration. Maximizing functional potential is key.
  - Moving from childhood to adolescence and early adulthood, the aim is to maintain functional level, maximize potential for independence, and ensure long-term comfort.
- Orthopaedic intervention has an essential role, particularly in childhood and adolescence when secondary manifestations of impaired muscle activity lead to problems with deformity and anatomical development, which may impair function and lead to later pain.

Management: musculoskeletal

Spasticity management

- *Botulinum toxin A:* irreversible competitive inhibitor of presynaptic cholinergic receptors. Inhibits release of acetylcholine at the neuromuscular junction; 2- to 3-months' duration of action. Injections (blind or US-guided) can provide local reduction in spasticity; helpful if tone (rather than contractures) is problematic.
- *Antispasmodic agents:* include baclofen (probable γ-aminobutyric acid (GABA) agonist, central and peripheral effects). Enteral dose often used

in evenings as has a sedative effect. The intrathecal route is an option in non-ambulant patients and avoids systemic effects.
- *Selective dorsal rhizotomy (SDR)*: neurosurgical resection of dorsal rootlets that do not show a myographic or clinical response to stimulation. Aims to reduce spasticity. Specific indications only (stable gait pattern in spastic diplegia, limited by spasticity, age ideally 4–8 years). Unclear if beneficial in the longer term, but evidence is growing. Offered in specific specialist centres only.

Orthoses
- Primary focus is on optimizing function. Their role in preventing development of deformity is unproven. Specific goals are individualized:
  - To address weakness and poor motor control (e.g. foot drop splint in hemiplegia—weak ankle dorsiflexion); rigid AFO provides stability in stance (poor distal motor function)
  - Spinal bracing: arrest/slow progression of scoliosis.

Orthopaedic surgery
- Focus is on addressing the secondary effects of CP on the growing musculoskeletal system, so that they do not impair achieving maximal functional potential.
- Important that expectations are realistic; maximal functional potential is preordained by the extent of the brain injury.
- General principles:
  - *Soft tissue rebalancing*. Early deformity that remains partially flexible can be addressed by lengthening short muscles. There is generalized weakness in CP, so overall muscle strength must be preserved; hence, intramuscular tendon lengthening is the preferred technique. Must consider function of specific muscles being lengthened (e.g. over-lengthening of anti-gravity ankle plantar flexors weakens them excessively and may contribute to 'crouch gait'). Muscle transfers should be of split tendons to avoid overcorrection.
  - *Correction of fixed bone deformity*. Fixed deformity can be more effectively addressed with corrective procedures on bone and joints. Usually not required until late childhood (>8 years), but if the deformity is expected to be progressive, early correction can improve long-term outcomes (e.g. varus derotation osteotomy (VDRO) of the femur in hip subluxation; growth rods in progressive spinal deformity).
  - *Salvage procedures*. Arthrodesis, excision arthroplasty, hip replacement.

Further reading
Graham HK, Selber P. Musculoskeletal aspects of cerebral palsy. *Journal of Bone and Joint Surgery (British Volume)*. 2003;**85**:157–66.
Rosenbaum P, Gorter JW. The 'F-words' in childhood disability: I swear this is how we should think! *Child: Care, Health and Development*. 2012;**38**(4):457–63.

Cerebral palsy: clinical assessment

History

- Consider the diagnosis if not already made (abnormal gait is often referred to orthopaedics first).
- Perinatal history, growth and developmental history, associated medical problems (respiratory, GI, neurological—epilepsy/behavioural, metabolic).
- General functional status: use of aids, sitting posture, upper and lower limb function, mobility, independence, education, and recreational engagement.
- Assess functional trajectory—deteriorating? What is the functional problem? Is there pain? Importantly, is the problem related to the anatomical abnormality—is it surgically treatable? For example, slow gait velocity (a functional problem) is unlikely to be due to only ankle equinus contracture (the anatomical abnormality)—rather it is a multifactorial issue.
- Is there a progressive anatomical problem likely to deteriorate without intervention (e.g. spinal deformity, hip subluxation, joint contractures)?
- Essential to appraise ideas, concerns, and expectations of patient and family (may not align).

Examination

- *General assessment:* observe gait/seating posture, general tone, associated medical issues (percutaneous endoscopic gastrostomy (PEG), secretion clearance, respiratory support).
- *Lower limb examination:*
  - Leg length discrepancy (common in hemiplegia, usually static and inconsequential); may indicate hip subluxation
  - Joint movement range:
    - Hip: flexion (>90° for sitting), Thomas' test for flexion contracture (impairs gait mechanics if excessive), abduction (important for perineal care), and rotational range (indicates hip dysplasia)
    - Knee extension (popliteal angle–hamstring length), knee flexion contracture, patella height
    - Ankle dorsiflexion (Silfverskiöld test)
    - Foot posture: hindfoot varus/valgus, forefoot equinus, supination/pronation (flexible vs fixed)
  - *Muscle strength and control:*
    - Anti-gravity muscle power—stand from chair (gross assessment), hip stability in gait (Trendelenberg)
    - Confusion test (resisted hip flexion causes ankle dorsiflexion)—confirms poor motor control.
- *Upper limb examination:*
  - Passive movements of shoulder, elbow, forearm, wrist, fingers, and thumb
  - Active motor control: hand to mouth, forearm rotation, grip strength
  - Assess access for dressing, hygiene, and skin care; function can be enhanced with simple orthoses; cosmesis is a concern for some.

- *Spine assessment:* scoliosis, initially flexible, later structural, but rare in ambulant CP (cf. non-ambulant)—Adam's forward bending test differentiates postural vs structural curve (see ⊃ Chapter 22).
- *Non-ambulant patients—seating comfort:* pelvic obliquity (due to spinal deformity, asymmetrical hip deformity), hamstring length, joint ranges for therapeutic (non-weight-bearing) standing.

Examination tips

- *Popliteal angle:* supine, flex hip to 90° and extend knee—measure angle between vertical and tibia position: 0° = full knee extension.
- *Thomas' test:* supine, hyperflex contralateral hip to remove any anterior pelvic tilt, then extend ipsilateral hip to assess hip extension (do with lower legs off end of couch if knee flexion contracture).
- *Duncan–Ely test:* prone, rapidly flex knee up to 90° from extension and watch whether and when the buttocks rise, indicating quadriceps spasticity.
- *Thigh–foot axis:* prone, flex knee to 90°; assess angle between heel bisector and midline of thigh = tibial torsion.
- *Silfverskiöld test:* to compare ankle dorsiflexion range, with knee flexed (gastrocnemius relaxed) and knee extended; reveals extent of gastrocnemius contracture vs contribution of soleus/tendoachilles to equinus.
- *Trendelenberg test:* to assess pelvic stability in single-leg stance (hip abductor strength).

Investigations

- *Imaging:* hip radiographic surveillance; MRI of the brain confirms diagnosis (often with input from neurologist/paediatrician).
- *3D gait analysis:* objective, standardized, reproducible, and quantifiable method to evaluate gait patterns—aids in decision-making.
- *Cerebral Palsy Integrated Pathway (CPIP):* annual review with community physiotherapy team assessing joint ranges and hip surveillance—enables early detection of any deterioration and referral for specialist review.

Further reading

Krigger KW. Cerebral palsy: an overview. *American Family Physician.* 2006;**73**:91–100.
Vitrikas K, Dalton H, Breish D. Cerebral palsy: an overview. *American Family Physician.* 2020;**101**:213–20.

Cerebral palsy: ambulant (GMFCS I–III)

Patterns of involvement

- *Hemiplegia:* predominantly unilateral upper and lower limb involvement; usually normal intelligence and high function level (typically GMFCS level I or II).
- *Diplegia:* bilateral involvement, usually lower limb > upper limb, may be asymmetrical, more variable functional level (GMFCS levels I–III).

Table 21.1 highlights the differences between these patterns of involvement.

Typical clinical features

- *Upper limb:* elbow flexion, forearm pronation ('folded wing' posture seen, especially as the child walks), wrist flexion/ulnar deviation, thumb in palm; posture may be exaggerated in times of excitement/stress.
- *Lower limb:* distal involvement commonest with foot drop ± equinus at ankle, cavovarus or planovalgus foot deformities. More proximal involvement with hamstring ± psoas overactivity, leading to knee and hip flexion contractures. Hip abductor weakness and proximal femoral anteversion lead to internal hip rotation and apparent adducted leg position, with scissoring in gait.
- *Gait pattern:* typical patterns.
- *Hip subluxation:* rare but does occur.

Gait analysis

- Undertaken by specialist groups that include orthopaedic surgeons, clinical scientists, and therapists.
- Evaluates the following data:
  - Physical examination findings
  - 2D video recording of gait (can be paused, played back, and slowed down)
  - 3D kinematics (graphical mapping of limb movements in coronal, sagittal, and axial (rotational) planes)
  - 3D kinetics examining the moments acting across lower limb joints

Table 21.1 Different patterns of involvement

Hemiplegia	
Type 1	Weak or paralysed/silent dorsiflexors (=foot drop)
Type 2	Type 1 + triceps surae contracture
Type 3	Type 2 + hamstrings and/or rectus femoris spasticity
Type 4	Type 3 + spastic hip flexors and adductors
Diplegia	
Type 1	True equinus
Type 2	Jump gait (with/without stiff knee)
Type 3	Apparent equinus (with/without stiff knee)
Type 4	Crouch gait

- Dynamic EMG from superficial or needle electrodes to establish which/whether muscles firing inappropriately out of phase
- Pedobarography: to evaluate pressure fields acting between the plantar surface of the foot and the ground
- Energy cost of walking by using calorimetry or oxygen consumption.

Management

Principles

- Optimize functional achievements according to GMFCS level, in the face of anatomical problems arising in a growing child with abnormal neuromuscular function.
- MDT approach involving the physiotherapists, occupational therapists, neurologists, paediatricians, orthotists, and orthopaedic surgeons.

Medical management

- Targeted spasticity management (botulinum toxin) of overactive muscle groups effective in younger child—may reduce functional effect of spasticity.
- Limited evidence that botulinum toxin injections can prevent development of contractures and/or deformity.
- Botulinum toxin irreversibly inhibits the neuromuscular junction. Effects subside when new connections are made. Diminishing effect over repeated injections. Theoretically weakens already weak muscle groups.
- Systemic spasticity management (e.g. baclofen)—in more severe diplegia, can help general hypertonicity, but side effects (somnolence) may limit daytime use.
- Regional spasticity management (intrathecal baclofen)—usually reserved for severe spasticity in non-ambulant patients as significant risks.

Orthoses

- Orthoses can accommodate for deformity (for comfort) and/or compensate for weakness/poor motor control—historically thought to prevent deformity, but this is no longer an accepted indication.
- Orthosis must improve function and/or comfort (otherwise discard).
- In ambulant CP, orthoses are commonly used to compensate for poor distal motor control (both upper and lower limbs).
- *Neoprene or dynamic Lycra/neoprene 'second skin' splints:* for upper limb. Wrist splints enhance hand function by maintaining a functional position for the wrist.
- *Posterior leaf spring (PLS) AFO:* compensates for weak ankle dorsiflexion and resists ankle plantar flexion (no varus/valgus control).
- *Solid AFO:* wider calf shell extends anterior to malleoli, providing varus/valgus control, as well as preventing foot drop.
- *Hinged AFO:* adjustable ankle hinges allow uniplanar movement (usually permit dorsiflexion) but provide control.
- *Ground reaction force (GRF) AFO:* orthosis extends proximally over anterior pretibial area, converting GRF to knee extension moment; indicated for crouch gait pattern of the hip, knee, and ankle flexion.

Surgical options

- Goal: to address contractures/deformity/muscle imbalance limiting achievement of appropriate functional goal and/or comfort.

- Ideally address muscle imbalance and bone deformity at all anatomical levels (foot/ankle, knee and hip, spine) simultaneously—avoids the 'birthday syndrome' (isolated distal correction reveals proximal involvement requiring another operation in the following year, i.e. single-event multilevel surgery (SEMLS)).
- Avoiding overcorrection is essential; easy to do at the ankle if more proximal contributions are not understood and addressed.
- 3D instrumented gait analysis is useful before major surgical intervention in unpicking primary from secondary abnormalities.
- SEMLS, which may be staged into bony and soft tissue procedures, followed by intensive physiotherapy rehabilitation, is best performed by expert teams with a paediatric anaesthetist and intensive care facilities available.

Lower limb surgery
- *Hip:* psoas (intramuscular) tendon lengthening at pelvic brim; adductor lengthening; femoral derotation osteotomy for persistent anteversion (±varus for hip dysplasia); containment procedures for subluxation.
- *Knee:* hamstring lengthening; rectus femoris transfer (indicated if reduced knee flexion in swing phase with out-of-phase contraction on EMG); anterior distal femoral-guided growth/distal femoral extension osteotomies for knee flexion contractures.
- *Foot and ankle:* plantar flexor lengthening (gastrocnemius aponeurosis recession if isolated contracture ± soleus ± tendoachilles lengthening as per Silverskiöld's test); tibialis posterior recession ± split transfer and/or split tibialis anterior tendon transfer for flexible equinovarus deformity (lateralizing calcaneal osteotomy if fixed deformity); calcaneal lengthening osteotomy and tibialis posterior advancement for flexible planovalgus deformity (subtalar arthrodesis for fixed deformity correction).

Upper limb surgery
- Less commonly indicated on functional grounds but may be required for cosmesis and modest functional gains.
- Options include: tendon releases (pronator teres, biceps), tendon transfers (FCU to ECRB for weak wrist extension), tendon lengthening (long flexors), and wrist arthrodesis, thumb-in-palm release, and humeral derotation osteotomy.

Further reading

Renshaw TS, Deluca PA. Cerebral palsy. In: Morrissy RT, Weinstein SL, eds. *Lovell and Winter's Pediatric Orthopaedics*, 6th edn. Philadelphia, PA: Lippincott Williams & Wilkins, 2006; pp. 1–99.

Cerebral palsy: non-ambulant (GMFCS IV and V)

Patterns of involvement
- Usually all four limbs involved, with impaired spine/trunk control.
- Some function at GMFCS level III, but vast majority at levels IV and V.

Problems
- Primary challenges are maintaining seating comfort and posture, and preventing development of painful contractures or joint displacement.
- For some individuals, maintaining ability to assist with standing transfers helps to preserve some independence—otherwise most are hoist-dependent.
- Common problems:
  - Scoliosis
  - Hip displacement—90% of GMFCS level V (Table 21.2)
  - Hamstring contractures affecting seating
  - Foot posture affecting shoe-wear and skin integrity.

Clinical assessment
- General considerations (essential in preoperative workup): cardiorespiratory health, GI function, epilepsy management.
- Evaluate wheelchair comfort and posture: popliteal angle >90° can compromise seating comfort; a moulded chair can accommodate for fixed spinal/lower limb deformity.
- *Hip examination:* supine (stabilize the pelvis) to conduct Galeazzi test (hip subluxation) and assess ROM (asymmetry in range can indicate early subluxation)—late dislocation may be painful; limited hip abduction compromises perineal care.
- *Spinal assessment:* neuromuscular scoliosis is typically C-shaped (cf. adolescent idiopathic scoliosis). Can be rapidly progressive with growth, so annual review is mandatory. Forward bend/traction under arms when seated can differentiate a flexible vs a fixed curve. This can impact seating comfort and GI/respiratory function.
- *Knee:* flexion contractures/hamstring length (popliteal angle).

Table 21.2 Correlation between GMFCS level and hip displacement

GMFCS level	Incidence of hip displacement (%)
I	0
II	15
III	41
IV	69
V	90

From Soo B, Howard JJ, Boyd RN, *et al.* Hip displacement in cerebral palsy. *Journal of Bone and Joint Surgery.* 2006;88(1):121–9.

- *Foot and ankle:* equinus/cavovarus/planovalgus postures can prevent comfortable AFO wear (often useful for therapeutic standing) and become stiff, compromising skin over bony prominences.
- *Upper limb:* assessment usually focused on flexibility to allow dressing and hygiene, but also consider active function (e.g. for powered wheelchair/independent feeding).

Investigations

- *Hip surveillance:*
  - CPIP protocol establishes a framework for radiological evaluation of hips in CP—the goal is to identify hip subluxation early, so smaller intervention has greater success.
  - Risk is greatest in GMFCS levels III, IV, and V—hence annual pelvic radiographs recommended until age 16 years (Table 21.2).
  - Hip migration measured according to Reimer's Migration Index (percentage of femoral head uncovered by acetabular roof)—>30% is the CPIP threshold for orthopaedic review.
  - Other features: acetabular dysplasia (shallow—global deficiency, often posterior vs DDH usually anterolateral), coxa valga (hard to assess as often very anteverted proximal femur), gracile bones (not true osteoporosis, but weak secondary to limited weight-bearing and ↑ fracture risk).
- *Preoperative assessment:* respiratory review (sleep studies), gastroenterology review, anaesthetic, dietary, coagulation (the antiepileptic sodium valproate inhibits platelets).

Management

Medical

- Local and systemic tone modification, analgesia.

Orthoses

- Rigid AFOs to accommodate foot deformity and provide some stability for assisted standing.
- Standing frames for emotional well-being and GI and respiratory function.
- Bracing for spinal deformity does not prevent progression but may slow it down.
- Custom-moulded (wheel)chair that supports the trunk, accommodates pelvic obliquity, and avoids pressure points.

Surgical options

- Soft tissue release (hip adductors ± hamstrings, psoas) for early-detected hip displacement may slow progression (Fig. 21.2).
- Established subluxation requires reconstruction VDRO of the femur (often bilateral) ± pelvic osteotomy for acetabular dysplasia (Dega).
- Long-standing dislocation with painful femoral head ulceration is difficult to salvage; salvage with hip resection and interposition myoplasty is an option if intractable pain. Prevention is much better.
- For severe spinal curves (>40–50°), a long instrumented posterior fusion (down to the pelvis) ± anterior release may be indicated.

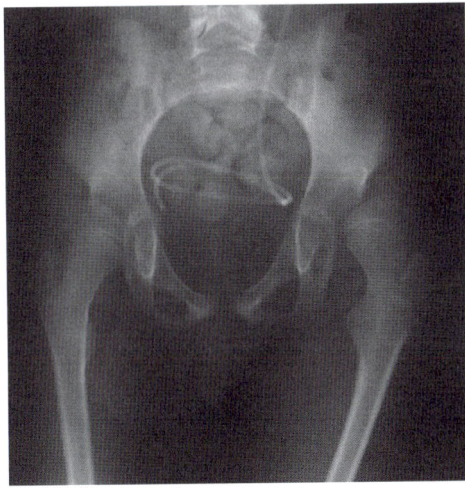

Fig. 21.2 Radiograph showing a migrating left hip.

- These are major procedures requiring careful preoperative assessment and optimization of respiratory, GI, and other comorbidities (seizures, poor nutrition, anaemia, etc.).

Further reading

Flynn JM. Management of hip disorders in patients with cerebral palsy. *Journal of the American Academy of Orthopaedic Surgeons.* 2002;**10**:198–209.

Renshaw TS, Deluca PA. Cerebral palsy. In: Morrissy RT, Weinstein SL, eds. *Lovell and Winter's Pediatric Orthopaedics*, 6th edn. Philadelphia, PA: Lippincott Williams & Wilkins, 2006; pp. 1–99.

Developmental dysplasia of the hip

DDH is the commonest (1–3%) abnormality in newborn infants. It is a spectrum disorder, ranging from mild hip dysplasia to hip dislocation. It is 'developmental' due to the potential progressive nature. The congenital or teratologic form represents dislocated, non-reducible hip joint(s) and is often part of more complex problems or syndromes. The exact causes of DDH are unknown, but there are known risk factors.

Major risk factors
- First-degree positive family history.
- Breech position.
- Birthweight >5kg.
- Congenital calcaneovalgus.

Minor risk factors
These may include:
- Firstborn child
- Multiple birth
- ♀ gender
- Oligohydramnios
- Prematurity
- Postnatal positioning (swaddling).

Associations
- 'Packaging' disorders (torticollis, knee hyperextension).
- Foot deformities (metatarsus adductus, clubfoot).

Types of DDH
- *Dysplasia:* morphological changes of the acetabulum and sometimes the proximal femur, but articular surfaces are concentrically in contact.
- *Subluxation:* there is contact between both articular surfaces of the acetabulum and proximal femur, but not concentrically reduced.
- *True dislocation:* there is no contact between the articular surfaces of the proximal femur and acetabulum.

Natural history
Residual DDH or dislocation into adulthood has been associated with pain and early development of OA. DDH is the main cause of THR in young people.

Screening
The UK Newborn and Infant Physical Examination (NIPE) programme guidelines determine that clinical screening (instability manoeuvres of Barlow and Ortolani tests) should be done universally as part of the physical examination of the newborn within 72h of birth.

Clinical screening
- *Ortolani test:* abduction and gentle elevation of dislocated femoral head results into a 'clunk' of reduction.
- *Barlow 'provocation' test:* gentle depression of adducted hip results in palpable subluxation or dislocation of unstable hip.

- *Klisic test:* the line drawn from the greater trochanter to the ASIS points below the umbilicus if the hip is dislocated.
- *Galeazzi test:* hips flexed at 90° and feet placed on the table, and the femur will appear shortened on the unilateral dislocated side.
- *Hip abduction:* dislocated hips have limited abduction in flexion, which is the most important clinical sign after 3 months of life, as both Barlow and Ortolani tests become unreliable after 3 months.

If clinical instability is found, then specialist hip US screening should be performed at 2 weeks of age.

If primary risk factors of first-degree family history and/or breech position at, or after, 36 weeks of pregnancy are identified without hip instability at NIPE, then US screening can be postponed to 6 weeks of age.

Investigations

Neonatal hip ultrasound
Visualizes the hip joint during the first 6 months of life, before the femoral head ossifies. Reinhard Graf described the most popular and widely used US screening technique in neonatal hip screening by using the α angle (osseous acetabular development) and β angle (cartilaginous acetabular development) on static views (Fig. 21.3).

Generally performed when:
- Positive family history
- Breech presentation
- Clinical evidence of instability
- Associated conditions identified
- 'Packaging' disorder found.

Dynamic hip US screening has also been described, but with reportedly reduced reproducibility. Some countries practise universal screening (Austria, Germany, and Switzerland), but well-designed studies have not shown a reduction in incidence of late hip dysplasia.

Anteroposterior radiograph of the hips
- Can be used from 4 months, as the femoral epiphysis becomes visible.
- Perkin's (P) and Hilgenreiner's (H) lines are drawn through triradiate cartilages and vertically down from the acetabular edge, respectively. In

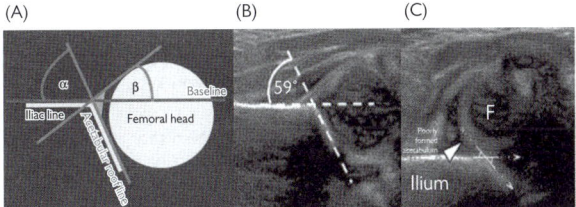

Fig. 21.3 (A) Graf (α and β) angles. Normal: α >60° and β <55° in a mature infant hip. (B) Ultrasound scan of a normal hip. (C) Ultrasound scan of a dysplastic, dislocated hip (α = 43).

physiological hips, the ossific nucleus should be found in the lower inner quadrant made by the P and H lines.
- Acetabular index (AI) is a measure of ongoing acetabular dysplasia.
- Shenton's line: restoration is a key end point in reduction of dislocation or subluxation.

Management

Aim is to achieve and maintain a concentric reduction of the femoral head in the acetabulum to allow for continued normal hip development.

0–6 months

- High rate of spontaneous resolution (90%) of transient instability in the first 6 weeks of life.
- Clinically unstable hips with sonographic confirmation of DDH at 2 weeks of life need abduction harness treatment.
- Clinically stable hips with primary risk factors and sonographic confirmation of DDH at 6 weeks of life also need harness treatment.
- Most popular and widely used is the Pavlik abduction harness, which is loosely applied and regularly checked (to minimize the rate of AVN, femoral nerve palsy, and pressure sores). Aim is to abduct both legs in hip flexion. Harness treatment lasts typically 6–12 weeks. If the harness fails to maintain sonographic reduction of unstable hips 1–2 weeks after application, then it needs to be discarded as it can worsen the dysplasia (Pavlik harness disease).

6–12 months

- 'Delayed' presentation or failed harness treatment requires general anaesthesia, hip arthrography, a trial of closed reduction, and a hip spica application in practical reality (90–100° flexion and 50–70° abduction). An adductor tenotomy can also be performed to ↑ the Ramsey 'safe abduction arc' of maintained reduction. 'Open assisted closed reduction' can also be attempted by releasing the tight iliopsoas tendon. If a concentric hip reduction is seen on the hip arthrogram, then a hip spica is applied for 3 months (spica changed at 6 weeks), followed by another 3 months of weaning hip abduction brace.
- If a concentric reduction cannot be achieved, then need to proceed with an open reduction of the dislocated hip (Fig. 21.4).
- There is strong evidence in the literature to suggest that open reduction does not have to be delayed until the ossific nucleus has ossified, as previously believed. Open reduction can be achieved via either a medial or an anterior approach. Medial open reduction is indicated in children aged <1 year, as otherwise it carries a high risk of AVN.

1–2 years

- Closed reduction is now unlikely to succeed, even after adductor tenotomy/iliopsoas release. Anterior open reduction is the preferred procedure in this age group to release and remove obstacles to reduction of the femoral head into the acetabulum (Table 21.3).
- An anterior open reduction can be combined with a pelvic and/or femoral osteotomy followed by a hip spica for 6–12 weeks. Various pelvic osteotomies have been described (including Salter innominate, reorientation osteotomy, and incomplete pericapsular Dega and Pemberton osteotomies (Fig. 21.5).

(A)   (B)

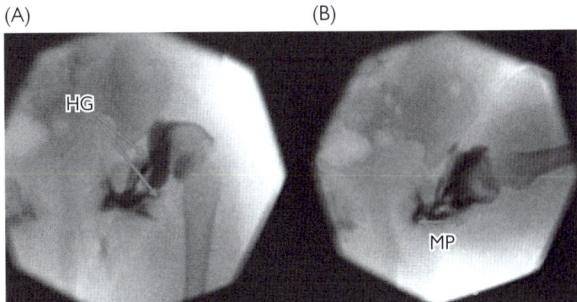

Fig. 21.4 Arthrogram showing a dislocated left hip, with the leg in neutral position (A) and an unsuccessful attempt of closed reduction with flexion, abduction, and internal rotation (B). Hourglass constriction (HG) develops via compression of the tight iliopsoas tendon to the hip joint capsule. Medial pooling (MP) is a sign of 'blocked' reduction.

Table 21.3 Extra- and intracapsular obstacles to hip reduction

Extracapsular	Intracapsular
Iliopsoas	Teres ligament
Adductors	Transverse acetabular ligament
Anteromedial capsule	Pulvinar (acetabular fibrofatty tissue)
	Limbus (everted labrum)
	Neolimbus (hypertrophied joint cartilage)

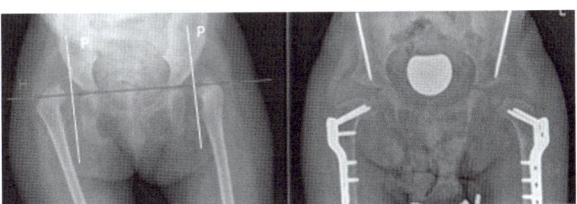

Fig. 21.5 Late-presenting bilateral dislocated hips in a 2-year-old girl. Both ossific nuclei are found to be on the upper outer quadrants made by the Hilgenreiner's line (H) and Perkin's line (P). Treatment consisted of staged bilateral hip reconstructions (open reduction, proximal femoral varus osteotomy, and Salter osteotomy).

2–8 years
- Open reduction is now inevitable. Preoperative traction to facilitate reduction is now largely abandoned in favour of femoral shortening osteotomy.

>8 years
- Controversial whether hip reconstruction should be attempted or whether to wait instead for eventual hip arthroplasty when needed.
- Untreated dislocation produces an abnormal gait, and is associated with a risk of ipsilateral knee symptoms and hip pain from the fourth decade of life requiring THR.
- Symptomatic residual hip dysplasia in adolescents is subject to arthroscopic or open hip preservation surgery (peri-acetabular osteotomy (PAO)) to reduce symptoms and delay early OA.

Further reading

NHS England (2024). *Newborn and infant physical examination (NIPE) screening programme handbook.* Available from: ℘ www.gov.uk/government/publications/newborn-and-infant-physical-examination-programme-handbook/newborn-and-infant-physical-examination-screening-programme-handbook

Sewell MD, Rosendahl K, Eastwood DM. Developmental dysplasia of the hip. *BMJ.* 2009;**339**:b4454.

Yang S, Zusman N, Lieberman E, Goldstein RY. Developmental dysplasia of the hip. *Pediatrics.* 2019;**143**(1):e20181147.

Perthes' disease

Perthes' disease is a childhood hip condition in which blood supply to the capital femoral epiphysis is interrupted, causing AVN (more generically termed 'osteonecrosis'). This leads to progressive deformity of the femoral head and secondary degenerative OA in later life. Over a century, following the first reports, the condition has remained challenging, with ongoing debate and no established consensus on aetiology and treatment.

Perthes' disease affects four times as many boys, at an average of 4–9 years, with an incidence of 5 in 100,000 (20% bilateral, but almost never simultaneously). It is a self-limiting disease, with complete revascularization of the epiphysis over a period of 2–4 years.

Perthes' disease is believed to be caused by a combination of genetic and environmental factors (maternal smoking and socio-economic deprivation), repeated subclinical trauma, and possible coagulation problems (e.g. factor V Leiden mutation, protein C and S deficiency).

Presentation and imaging

- Children present with groin and/or knee pain, a limp, leg length discrepancy, and restricted ROM of the hip.
- *Hip radiographs:* AP and frog lateral views (hips flexed, abducted, and externally rotated) are needed to establish the diagnosis and extent of epiphyseal involvement.

Classifications

Waldenström *et al.* graded Perthes' disease into four stages: initial, fragmentation, reossification, and healed. Joseph *et al.* further modified the first three stages into early and late sub-stages, with an impact on both treatment decisions and patient outcome. During the early fragmentation stages, the epiphysis is 'biologically plastic', subject to remodelling and amenable to surgical treatment (containment theory), whereas once the disease has entered the late fragmentation stage, then irreversible changes to the femoral head have taken place. The modified Elizabethtown classification is modification of the Waldenström classification and helps with determining disease stage (Table 21.4).

Several other staging classification systems have been proposed to describe Perthes' disease. Herring described the lateral pillar collapse classification system (A, no collapse; B, <50%; B/C, 50%; C, >50%).

Catterall reported four stages according to the degree of epiphyseal involvement (>25%, 25–50%, 50–75%, and >75%). Both Herring and Catterall classification systems are based on the full extent of the fragmentation (questionable clinical usefulness of both classification systems, as established epiphyseal changes are no longer reversible), and concerns over reproducibility have also been raised with both systems.

Salter and Thompson classified Perthes' disease into two stages, based on the presence of a subchondral fracture in the initial stage (but only 50% of children with Perthes' disease will show this radiographic feature).

Finally, Stulberg rated hip joint congruence into five groups with prognostic significance at maturity (Table 21.5).

Table 21.4 Modified Elizabethtown classification

Stage	Description
Ia	Sclerosis of part or whole epiphysis; no loss of height
Ib	Sclerotic epiphysis and loss of epiphyseal height
IIa	Epiphyseal fragmentation started (one or two vertical fissures)
IIb	Fragmentation is advanced
IIIa	New bone is visible covering less than one-third of epiphysis width
IIIb	New bone has grown to over one-third of epiphysis width
IV	Healed femoral head

Table 21.5 Stulberg rating system at maturity

Group	Shape of femoral head and acetabulum	Congruence of hip joint	Prognosis
I	Spherical femoral head	Congruence	Excellent
II	Large, spherical head	Congruence	Excellent
III	Elliptical, mushroom-shaped femoral head	Incongruence	Late arthritis
IV	Flattened femoral head and round acetabulum	Incongruence	Early arthritis
V	Flattened femoral head and flattened acetabulum	Congruent incongruence	Early arthritis

Prognostic signs

There are several factors contributing to a poorer outcome.
- Catterall described several 'head at risk' signs (horizontal growth plate, lateral calcification, femoral head extrusion, metaphyseal cysts, and V-shaped radiolucency of the lateral epiphysis and adjacent metaphysis— the Gage sign).
- Clinical signs for poor prognosis are ♀ gender, late presentation (>8 years), progressive stiffness, a heavier child, and a longer duration from onset to healing.

Management

Early stages

The concept of 'containment' attempts to maintain the femoral head within the acetabulum throughout the entire evolution of Perthes' disease, thereby protecting the epiphysis from deforming forces at the acetabular margin.

Containment can be applied via both conservative and operative methods, and aims to prevent both the femoral head from getting extruded or the reversal of extrusion of the femoral head.

Non-operative containment consists traditionally of protected or non-weight-bearing, maintenance of hip range of motion, and application of an abduction cast or brace. However, there is no high-quality evidence to support conservative treatment for Perthes' disease. Moreover, prolonged weight-bearing restrictions and/or conservative containment treatments can be associated with social and psychological problems in childhood.

Operative containment can be achieved by femoral and/or pelvic osteotomy. Proximal femoral varus osteotomy is the most widely used procedure. Redirectional innominate osteotomy (Salter), triple or peri-acetabular osteotomy, and labral support shelf acetabuloplasty are pelvic procedures performed to ↑ acetabular coverage of the femoral head.

Operative non-containment options are preferred when the femoral head is non-containable, as in the case of hinged abduction (the outer part of the femoral head hinges on the lateral lip of the acetabulum as the leg is abducted). This is a poor prognostic factor and progression to OA can be expected. Proximal femoral valgus osteotomy ± pelvic osteotomy has been recommended to overcome this extra-articular hinging and to bring a more congruent surface of the femoral head under the acetabulum.

Importance of early operative intervention

Operating at the initial and sclerotic stages, or at the early fragmentation stage, of Perthes' disease can bypass (or reduce the duration of) the fragmentation stage. Early surgery can result in a healed spherical femoral head in a large proportion of children.

Other facts about operative treatment include:
- Patients aged <6 years, or those with Herring group A hips, do well and do not need any specific operative treatment.
- In the lateral pillar B and B/C groups, the outcomes of operative treatment are superior in children aged >8 years, whereas there is no difference with surgery in children aged between 6 and 8 years.
- Group C hips frequently have poor outcomes unrelated to treatment modality.

Other procedures

Arthrodiastasis is an operative method that uses pins and an external fixator to unload the joint, which can improve healing—either in the early stages or in patients older than 8 years with advanced Perthes' disease. Core decompression has also been used to remove necrotic bone and induce revascularization. Both surgical techniques have been described in studies with small numbers of patients, no controls, and short follow-up periods; hence, these techniques are not widely accepted in UK practice.

Treatment in later stages

If a hip joint deformation is present after the healed stage, then arthroscopic or open hip preservation procedures can be utilized to treat residual intra- and/or extra-articular impingement. Hip arthroscopy for mild cases and open surgical hip dislocation with or without PAO for more severe cases can provide pain relief, improve abductor strength, and restore proximal femoral anatomy.

THR is the treatment of choice for degenerative OA changes in patients with healed Perthes' disease.

Pharmacological treatment

Bisphosphonates have been used to treat patients with Perthes' disease with the maintenance of Z-scores, but their application in clinical use is unproven. Use of BMPs or other anabolic agents is currently only experimental, and additional studies are required prior to their clinical use.

Further reading

Ibrahim T, Little DG. The pathogenesis and treatment of Legg–Calvé–Perthes disease. *Journal of Bone and Joint Surgery Reviews*. 2016;**4**(7):e4.

Joseph B, Varghese G, Mulpuri K, Rao KLN, Nair NS. Natural evolution of Perthes disease: a study of 610 children under 12 years of age at disease onset. *Journal of Pediatric Orthopaedics*. 2003;**23**(5):590–600.

Slipped capital femoral epiphysis

Also known as slipped upper femoral epiphysis (SUFE), this is a separation of the proximal femoral epiphysis and the femoral neck at the hypertrophic zone of the proximal femoral growth plate. The actual epiphysis is held in the acetabulum via the ligamentum teres, whereas the femoral neck rotates anteriorly, laterally, and superiorly.

It is the commonest hip disease in adolescence and, in severe cases, is the commonest reason for THR in this young age group. Early diagnosis is critical to prevent further slippage and its disastrous consequences. Unfortunately, diagnostic delays are still common due to the atypical presentation of most patients.

Aetiology

Incidence of 5 in 100,000. Affects more boys than girls ($\male$:$\female$ = 1.7:1). Typical age 10–14 years.

Limited understanding of the exact cause, but there is an association with obesity. Endocrine pathologies (mainly hypothyroidism) or comorbid disease (Down syndrome, renal osteodystrophy, GH replacement) are less common associations (<3%) but must be considered, particularly in bilateral disease.

Recent studies have focused on the various histological changes the proximal femoral growth plate undergoes, which are present in the pre-slip stages and likely cause consequent further slippage, and on the role of a bone prominence protruding down from the epiphysis (epiphyseal tubercle) and its association to growth plate stability.

Presentation

Symptoms are usually vague, often not located at the hip level, and may not even involve pain. A limp and/or groin, thigh, and knee ache might be present, whereas limited hip internal rotation and flexion are common clinical findings. Every child from early pre-adolescence through to skeletal maturity is at risk.

Classifications

Classified according to the duration of symptoms (acute <3 weeks; chronic >3 weeks; acute-on-chronic→exacerbation of chronic symptoms), stability (stable/unstable, as defined by ability or not to weight-bear with or without crutches), and severity of slip percentage or slip angle (mild, 0–30; moderate, 30–60; and severe, >60) (Fig. 21.6).

Contralateral slip has an incidence of 40% in healthy individuals and up to 80% in children with pre-existing conditions (metabolic, endocrine, and syndromic diseases), and is less frequent after the triradiate cartilage closes.

Imaging

Plain AP and lateral hip radiographs confirm the diagnosis. Klein's line (drawn proximally up the superior femoral neck) in both views should pass through the edge of the epiphysis but will miss with SCFE (Fig. 21.7). Other signs visible on plain radiographs include widening of the epiphysis and blurring of the proximal femoral metaphysis. MRI may be used for diagnosis in situations where the radiographs are negative. This is often termed a 'pre-slip' when indicative of SCFE.

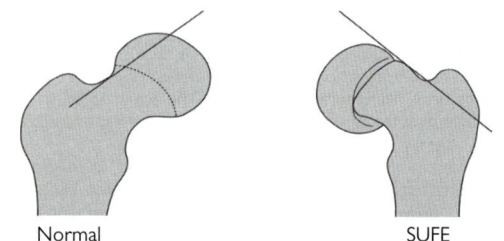

Fig. 21.6 Trethowan or Klein's line revealing how a slip alters the relationship of the femoral neck to the epiphysis. SUFE, slipped upper femoral epiphysis.

Reproduced from Bulstrode *et al.*, *Oxford Textbook of Orthopaedics and Trauma*, with permission from Oxford University Press.

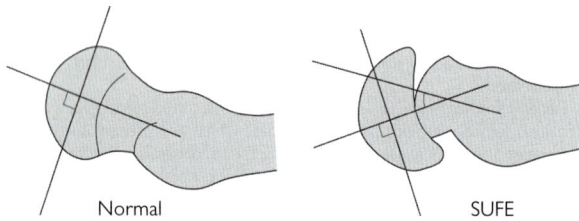

Fig. 21.7 The extent of epiphyseal displacement expressed in degrees or as a proportion of femoral head displacement on the neck. SUFE, slipped upper femoral epiphysis.

Reproduced from Bulstrode *et al.*, *Oxford Textbook of Orthopaedics and Trauma*, with permission from Oxford University Press.

Management

Pinning *in situ* with a single cannulated screw, positioned in the central epiphysis in both AP and lateral hip views, is the gold standard treatment for mild and some moderate SCFEs. Avoidance of forced closed reduction (associated with AVN) is essential, and hip decompression via aspiration prior to pinning of acute SCFEs is also encouraged to prevent AVN.

Most moderate or severe SCFEs can be treated acutely with gentle open reduction and stabilization (Parsch technique) or with a sub-capital osteotomy (ideal procedures to treat SCFE as they restore hip ROM, relieve symptoms, and minimize OA development). Osteotomies can be performed anteriorly (Fish osteotomy) or via Ganz surgical hip dislocation (modified Dunn osteotomy). Both have a steep learning curve and can be associated with a higher risk of complications than pinning. NICE guidelines have therefore been published with regard to surgical hip dislocation, suggesting it should only be performed in specialist centres (Fig. 21.8). These procedures aim to avoid tension on critical posterolateral vessels to the

(A) (B)

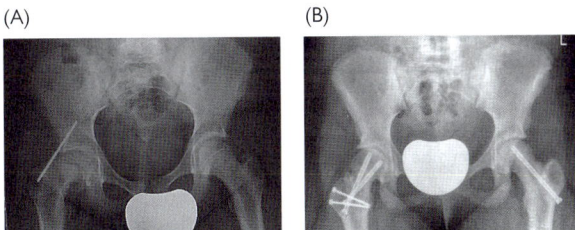

Fig. 21.8 Severe, acute, unstable right slipped capital femoral epiphysis in a 12-year-old girl. Klein's line (red) does not transect the right proximal femoral epiphysis (A). The patient underwent open reduction and subcapital osteotomy on the right hip and contralateral pinning (B).

femoral head but carry risks, including AVN, in particular when performed for moderate or severe, unstable SCFEs.

Residual femoroacetabular impingement can be treated with arthroscopic techniques to debride any CAM deformities. These can be performed in combination with intertrochanteric osteotomies.

Complications

- *AVN:* associated with unstable slips, and attempts to force a closed reduction, usually after treatment.
- *Chondrolysis:* aetiology unknown, usually seen (but not exclusively) following joint penetration from screw fixation.
- *Non-union or hip instability:* associated with sub-capital osteotomies.
- *Secondary OA:* proportional to severity of the slip.

Further reading

Georgiadis AG, Zaltz I. Slipped capital femoral epiphysis: how to evaluate with a review and update of treatment. *Pediatric Clinics.* 2014;**61**(6):1119–35.

Mahran MA, Baraka MM, Hefny HM. Slipped capital femoral epiphysis: a review of management in the hip impingement era. *SICOT-J.* 2017;**3**:35.

National Institute for Health and Care Excellence (2015). *Open reduction of slipped capital femoral epiphysis.* Interventional procedures guidance [IPG511]. Available from: www.nice.org.uk/guidance/ipg511

Perry DC, Metcalfe D, Costa ML, Van Staa T. A nationwide cohort study of slipped capital femoral epiphysis. *Archives of Disease in Childhood.* 2017;**102**(12):1132–6.

Femoral anteversion

This involves ↑ anteversion of the femoral neck, with compensatory internal rotation of the femur.

Epidemiology

Seen in childhood and twice as common in ♀ than in ♂. Can be hereditary and often asymmetrical in severity.

Presentation

The common presentation is intoeing, which is often more disturbing for parents than for the children themselves. The child often prefers to sit in the classical 'W' position on the floor. May be clumsy runners.

Other causes of intoeing gait
- Metatarsus adductus.
- Internal tibial torsion.

Examination

- Gait analysis reveals intoeing and an inward-facing patella.
- Hip ROM is tested in the prone position. The child will have excessive internal rotation of >70° (normal 20–60°). There will be a consequential reduction in external rotation of <20° (normal 30–60°).
- Tibial torsion is assessed for by looking at the thigh–foot angle in the prone position (varies with age, so check angles).

Imaging

Often not required, although CT/MRI can be used to objectively quantify femoral anteversion. If surgery is considered, then the rotational profile of the entire limb should be assessed by CT.

Management

The natural history is for excessive femoral anteversion to resolve by the age of 10 years; hence, observation and reassurance are all that is usually needed. If the child is older than 10 years and is more significantly affected, then derotational osteotomy of the femur can be performed.

Coronal plane deformities

Genu varum

A varus deformity of the knee. Common in children under 2 years of age. Between the ages of 12 and 24 months, there is a transition from physiological varus to neutral, and then onto physiological valgus, as highlighted by the Salenius curve (Fig. 21.9).

- *Causes:* include physiological varus, Blounts disease, rickets, osteogenesis imperfecta, skeletal dysplasia, and trauma to the physis (direct trauma, infection, tumour).
- *Management: non-operative*—observation, bracing in certain cases; *operative*—hemiepiphysiodesis (e.g. 8-plate), physeal bar resection, proximal tibial osteotomy.

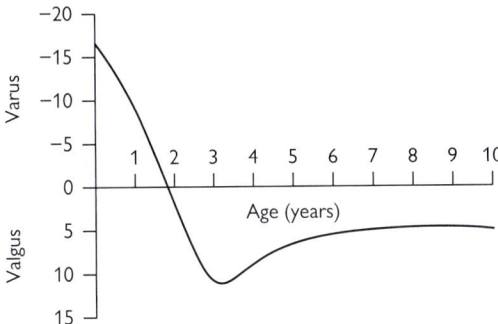

Fig. 21.9 Salenius and Vankka graph.

Genu valgum

A valgus deformity of the knee. There is a normal physiological valgus that occurs through childhood but should be <12° by age of 7 years. After this, pathological causes should be investigated for.

- *Causes: bilateral*—physiological, skeletal dysplasia (e.g. spondyloepiphyseal dysplasia), renal osteodystrophy. *Unilateral*—trauma, infection, vascular, benign tumours (osteochondromas, fibrous dysplasia).
- *Management: non-operative*—observation; *operative*—with significant skeletal growth remaining, hemiepiphysiodesis should be performed over the medial side of the knee (femur ± tibia). If there is insufficient growth remaining, then distal femoral osteotomy can be performed.

Further reading

Salenius P, Vankka E. The development of the tibiofemoral angle in children. *Journal of Bone and Joint Surgery (American Volume)*. 1975;**57**:259–61.

Osteochondritis dissecans

Idiopathic lesion of bone and cartilage, with a small, abnormal bone–cartilage (osteochondral) segment. OCD is a spectrum disorder, with very mild forms through to complete separation forming a detached loose body inside the joint and a residual osteochondral defect from its origin. The commonest site is the lateral aspect of the medial femoral condyle (70–80%) of the knee. Aetiology is unknown, but repetitive microtrauma and impaired local blood supply are implicated.

Clinical

Adolescents present with activity-related vague pain, swelling, catching, locking, and instability. A knee effusion is usually present. Extension may be blocked by a loose body. Bony tenderness can be elicited on direct palpation of the OCD defect. Pain from medial femoral condyle lesions may be reproduced when extending the fully flexed knee, with the tibia kept internally rotated (Wilson's test).

Investigations

Knee radiographs (AP, lateral, tunnel, and skyline views) can show the lesion. However, MRI is the gold standard to assess the size, extent, and instability of the lesion, as well as continuity of the articular cartilage.

Classification

Lesions classified according to the integrity of the articular cartilage and stability of the underlying subchondral bone. Final classification based on inspection at the time of surgical investigation and according to the International Cartilage Regeneration and Joint Preservation Society classification:

- *Grade I:* intact articular surfaces, but softening (underlying oedema)
- *Grade II:* articular cartilage breach, but stable on probing
- *Grade III:* fully detached lesion but remains *in situ*
- *Grade IV:* empty defect with loose body.

Management

Depends on the stage (subchondral stability, integrity of overlying cartilage) and skeletal age of the patient.

- *Non-operative:* indicated for stable lesions (activity modification, with or without use of crutches and anti-inflammatory drugs) for a period of 3–6 months. More likely to be successful for low-grade lesions in skeletally immature children.
- *Operative:* arthroscopic or open surgery if locked knee or symptomatic loose body (latter can be removed or reattached if suitable) (Fig. 21.10). OCD can be fixed or debrided, and the subchondral bone drilled with k-wires (improves vascularity, while the defect heals with fibrocartilage). With larger defects, chondral or osteochondral grafting may be considered.

Discoid meniscus

Round, rather than crescent-shaped, meniscus. A common finding (3–5% of the population), but not always symptomatic. Occasionally, it can form a complete disc. ~90% occur on the lateral side of the knee; 25% are bilateral. They often tear due to their large size and poorer-quality collagen within the meniscus (Fig. 21.11).

(A)   (B)   (C)

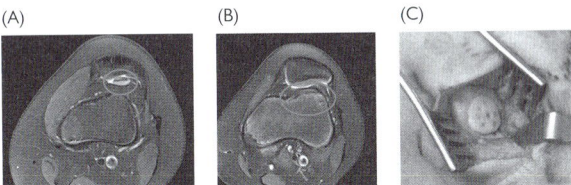

Fig. 21.10 Osteochondritis dissecans with a loose body (A) and an osteochondral defect of the lateral femoral condyle (B), and after open reduction and fixation with a central absorbable screw and peripheral nails (C).

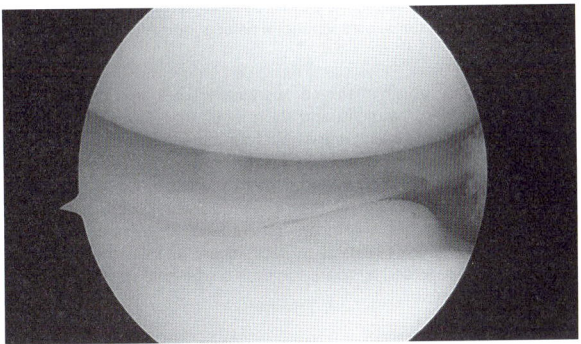

Fig. 21.11 Incomplete discoid meniscus with a radial tear in the meniscal body.

Clinical features
Pain is the commonest complaint, but clicking, swelling, and locking are other presenting symptoms. Findings on examination include joint line tenderness, clicking, effusion, loss of flexion or extension range, positive (Apley) grind test, and thigh muscle wasting.

Investigations
Plain radiographs of the knee may (albeit rarely) show widening of the lateral joint space, flattening of the lateral femoral condyle, and tilt of the lateral tibial condyle. MRI is the most appropriate investigation to diagnose and characterize the meniscus and any associated tear (with/without a bucket handle component).

Management
Asymptomatic discoid menisci do not require treatment. If symptomatic (due to a tear and/or instability), then arthroscopic meniscoplasty (partial meniscectomy) and repair of any tear may be necessary. Occasionally, these lesions require subtotal meniscectomy to obtain a stable rim. Meniscal allograft transplant may be considered for residual symptoms.

Meniscal tears

These injuries are increasingly seen in childhood due to ↑ participation in competitive contact sports.

Clinical

Most meniscal injuries occur with rotation motions of the partially flexed knee. Recurrent knee effusions, pain, locking, clicking, and instability are the main symptoms. McMurray test can be positive (a 'click' is felt when the internally rotated knee is extended from a fully flexed position).

Investigations

MRI is the gold standard to identify and confirm a meniscal injury in children and adolescents. It can also identify other concomitant pathologies, including physeal injuries, fractures, osteochondral defects, and ACL injuries.

Management

Meniscal tears are usually managed operatively. They are unlikely to heal with non-operative treatment, and the risk of tear propagation is high. Modern knee surgery is encompassed around meniscal preservation surgery over debridement or excision. Paediatric meniscal tears have great healing potential due to their ↑ vascularity over adults.

Most meniscal injuries are subject to 'all-inside' arthroscopic repair techniques using anchors placed arthroscopically. Anterior meniscal horn tears can be repaired by using 'outside-in' techniques, whereas the 'inside-out' technique is still regarded by some surgeons as the gold standard meniscal repair procedure.

Anterior knee pain

Description

Anterior knee pain (AKP) is common in adolescents. It can result from several musculoskeletal conditions, so diagnosis may be difficult. In the absence of a definable pathology, the condition is usually referred to as 'idiopathic AKP'. The term 'chondromalacia patella' is sometimes used interchangeably with AKP, although this is inaccurate as chondromalacia patella is a surgical finding rather than a diagnosis.

Aetiology

AKP is a diagnosis of exclusion, as in most cases, there is no true mechanical derangement of the knee. Aetiology is often unclear and likely multifactorial through a combination of genetic, developmental (e.g. dysplasia of the patellofemoral joint or joint laxity), and acquired factors (repetitive loading, direct trauma) resulting in symptoms.

Differential diagnosis

- *Mechanical:* maltracking, instability, chondral lesions, OCD, patellar tendinopathy, plicae.
- *Developmental:* Sinding–Larsen–Johansson, OS disease, bipartite patella.
- *Traumatic:* patellar stress fracture.
- *Rare:* CRPS, foreign body, neuroma, tumour, systemic arthritides (e.g. juvenile idiopathic arthritis (JIA)), non-organic causes.

Clinical features

Insidious onset with poorly localized pain, usually worse with physical activity (running, jumping, squatting) or prolonged sitting with the knee flexed. Occasional instability, usually from quadriceps inhibition. History should include activity limitations, previous treatment, and symptoms related to the other knee. Assess gait, lower limb alignment, patellar tracking (Q angle, lateral tilt, lateral tracking, rotational profile), stability, and movement of both knees (usually full range in idiopathic AKP). There may be patellar maltracking, crepitus, or quadriceps wasting. Also assess lumbar spine, hips, ankles, feet, and neurology.

Investigations

- *Radiology:* radiographs of the knee (AP, lateral, tunnel, skyline views). Coronal plane alignment can be assessed with Maquet views.
- *MRI:* may be helpful in excluding chondral and ligamentous lesions.
- *Dynamic CT:* to see if the patella is incongruent with quadriceps contraction.

Management

- *Non-operative:* idiopathic AKP managed by activity modification to reduce stress on the knee and exercises to improve flexibility and muscle strength. Knee braces and pain relief may help.
- *Operative:* targeted to defined pathology:
  - Instability: stabilize the patella with soft tissue ± bony procedures
  - Chondral lesion: stabilize with chondral regeneration surgery (chondroplasty, autologous cell techniques, osteochondral autografting)
  - Plicae: excision
  - Bipartite patella: excision or stabilization.

Congenital knee disorders

Congenital knee dislocation

Presents with a dramatic clinical appearance, with a notable hyperextension deformity of the knee at birth (Fig. 21.12). When bilateral, it is almost always syndromic (i.e. arthrogryposis, Larsen syndrome) and also highly associated with CTEV and DDH.

Classification

- *Hyperextension:* passive knee reduction, with flexion possible.
- *Subluxation:* knee does not bend beyond neutral, but there is tibiofemoral articular contact.
- *True dislocation:* knee flexion not possible, with the dislocated tibia lying anterior to the femur.

Management

Address the hyperextended form ASAP in infancy, with serial long leg weekly casting; reduction and 90° knee flexion are usually achieved after 3–5 weeks. Recurrence is unusual. The subluxed and dislocated forms can be treated successfully with less invasive procedures (including mini-open or percutaneous quadriceps tenotomies), compared with conventional extensive releases ± femoral shortening osteotomies.

Congenital patellar dislocation

Rare. Represents a hyperflexion deformity of the knee. The most severe form is an irreducible, laterally dislocated patella, already present at birth. It is caused by disruption of the normal internal rotation of the laterally placed thigh structures during embryogenic development. Clinically, there is a fixed flexion contracture of the knee, a valgus deformity, and external rotation of the tibia. Often missed or misdiagnosed, as radiographs fail to show the unossified patella in children aged <3 years (USS or MRI needed). Extensive surgical releases are often needed.

Congenital absence of anterior cruciate ligament

Rare. Usually coexists with other dysplastic conditions of the lower limb, including congenital knee dislocation, proximal femoral focal deficiency (PFFD), and fibular hemimelia. Often well tolerated but may become a problem if corrective treatment, such as leg lengthening, is undertaken.

Congenital talipes equinovarus

Common birth defect affecting 1 in 1000 live births (♂:♀ = 3:1). Majority are idiopathic but may be associated with additional malformations, chromosomal abnormalities, and genetic syndromes (e.g. arthrogryposis).

Characteristic appearance of hindfoot equinus and varus, and midfoot varus and cavus. Severity before and after treatment is graded (Pirani score) according to the appearance of the lateral foot border (straight or curved), extent of equinus ('empty heel pad sign'), and extent of uncovering of the lateral talar head. Affected foot and calf are always smaller (degree proportional to severity). Diagnosis is clinical; radiographs are not useful in early management.

Ponseti technique

In the 1950s, Ignatio V. Ponseti, an orthopaedic surgeon in Iowa, began reporting good results with a staged technique of serial manipulation and stretch followed by long leg casting with the knee flexed at 90° (usually 5- to 7-weekly casts). His technique was completed in two stages:

- Correction of deformity (stretch, cast ± Achilles tenotomy)
- Maintenance of correction (specialized boots with bar).

Ponseti suggested ideally starting serial casting in the first weeks of an infant's life, although we now know that it can still be as effective in older children. The first cast treats the first ray cavus deformity, and parents should be warned this usually makes the deformity appear worse. Subsequent casts treat the adduction and varus deformities. A percutaneous Achilles tenotomy is needed in about 90% of cases to treat the equinus deformity, taking place before a final cast is applied for 3 weeks. The central tenets of the technique are shown in Table 21.6. In reality, the Ponseti technique is a fluid and progressive elevation and abduction of the first ray about the talus, unlocking the midfoot and hindfoot as the first ray moves around. It is critical to correct each sequential deformity before moving on to the next step; otherwise correction will stall.

To prevent relapses, after the last cast is removed, an abduction brace ('boots and bar') must be worn full-time for 3 months, and thereafter at night for ideally 5 years. The brace consists of a bar with two boots attached to its ends, which are fixed in an externally rotated and abducted position.

While Ponseti's short-term results were initially considered inferior to extensive surgical releases, the long-term results in the 1990s were confirmed to be excellent—far better than for operative releases—and yielded comparable function to that of unaffected feet. Today, it is regarded as the gold standard technique worldwide.

Recurrence

For idiopathic clubfoot, the success rate of Ponseti's technique (in Iowa at least) approaches 100%, but there remains a strong tendency for relapse without good compliance with the daily 'boots and bar' regimen, as tolerance becomes difficult after the age of 2 years. Relapses usually respond to repeat manipulation, casting ± repeated tenotomy.

After the age of 2.5 years, transfer of the tibialis anterior tendon to the lateral cuneiform may be needed (in about 40% of cases) to correct residual

Table 21.6 Ponseti technique (mnemonic 'CAVE')

Deformity	Manipulation and position of cast	Pitfalls
Cavus	Elevate (supinate) first ray	Dorsiflexion is all that is required—first cast to correct cavus only
Adduction (midfoot)	Abduct first ray by using counter-thumb pressure against the uncovered lateral talar head	Avoid the cuboid as a fulcrum (kite's error), which will lock the hindfoot in varus
		Foot remains supinated—do not attempt to force into pronation
Varus (hindfoot)	Correction follows with further abduction of first ray, allowing the os calcis to abduct under the talus	If the midfoot cavus has not been corrected, the correction will stall at this point
Equinus (hindfoot)	Talar head now covered, hindfoot varus corrected (os calcis abducts into valgus under the talus), and foot elevated with the forepart in maximal abduction	15° ankle dorsiflexion must be achieved; otherwise percutaneous release of tendoachilles is indicated (in 70–80% of cases)

dynamic supination of the forefoot in the swing phase of gait. It is also an option for the non-brace-tolerant or older children with relapse of supination and in whom the foot remains supple.

Complex cases

Non-idiopathic CTEV stands out as the most difficult to treat. Both teratologic (associated with arthrogryposis) and atypical or complex clubfeet (shortened, stubby forefeet in severe equinus, and coexisting deep medial and posterior creases) need modified manipulation techniques and require repeated intervention, with a high risk of recurrence.

Further reading

Cooper DM, Dietz FR. Treatment of idiopathic clubfoot. A thirty-year follow-up note. *Journal of Bone and Joint Surgery (American Volume)*. 1995;**77**(10):1477–89.

Ferreira GF, Stéfani KC, Haje DD, Nogueira MP. The Ponseti method in children with clubfoot after walking age: systematic review and metanalysis of observational studies. *PLoS One*. 2018;**13**(11):e0207153.

Van Bosse HJ. Challenging clubfeet: the arthrogrypotic clubfoot and the complex clubfoot. *Journal of Children's Orthopaedics*. 2019;**13**(3):271–81.

Congenital vertical talus

An uncommon condition of fixed dorsal (and lateral) dislocation of the navicular on the talus. Produces a characteristic 'rocker-bottom' sole appearance, which comprises a hindfoot fixed in equinus and a dorsally dislocated midfoot. The majority have associated abnormalities (e.g. arthrogryposis, spinal dysraphism, myopathy in the teratologic form). Idiopathic congenital vertical talus (CVT) is therefore a diagnosis of exclusion.

Diagnosis

Usually made in the neonate. Confirmed by lateral radiographs taken in maximum dorsiflexion and plantar flexion (Fig. 21.12) The navicular ossifies between 3 and 5 years of age, so the line of the first ray is extrapolated to infer its long axis. Even in plantar flexion, the navicular remains dorsally dislocated; if it appears to partially reduce, the milder diagnosis of 'oblique' talus is made. In CVT, the maximum dorsiflexion view shows the os calcis to remain fixed in equinus.

Management

Consists of serial manipulation, stretching, and long leg casting by using a 'reverse Ponseti' technique. This has replaced prior extensive surgical releases. Now involves 4- to 6-weekly casts in progressive plantar flexion and adduction to relocate the talonavicular joint; in the final cast, the foot is positioned in extreme equinovarus, resembling a clubfoot. In the original technique description, temporary percutaneous pinning of the talonavicular joint and a percutaneous Achilles tenotomy were performed prior to application of the final cast. 'Boots and bars' are worn full-time for 2 months, and thereafter at night for 2 years to prevent relapse. Once patients start walking, daytime bracing with a solid AFO can also be used instead.

High recurrence rate of both idiopathic and teratologic CVT cases. Options include limited open capsulotomy and reduction of the talonavicular joint, with percutaneous Achilles tenotomy as an effective surgical treatment following serial casting (Fig. 21.13).

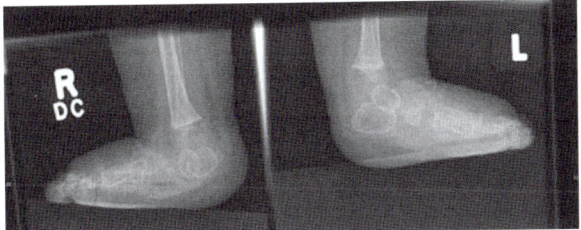

Fig. 21.12 Lateral radiographs of right congenital vertical talus in maximum dorsiflexion.

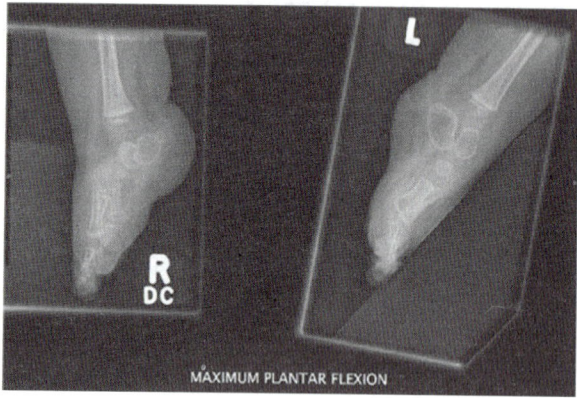

Fig. 21.13 Lateral radiographs of right congenital vertical talus in maximum plantar flexion.

Further reading

Dobbs MB, Purcell DB, Nunley R, Morcuende JA. Early results of a new method of treatment for idiopathic congenital vertical talus. *Journal of Bone and Joint Surgery.* 2006;**88**(6):1192–200.

Wright J, Coggings D, Maizen C, Ramachandran M. Reverse Ponseti-type treatment for children with congenital vertical talus: comparison between idiopathic and teratological patients. *Bone and Joint Journal.* 2014;**96**(2):274–8.

Tarsal coalition

Affects 13% of the population (up to 60% of cases are bilateral). Caused by failure of mesenchymal segmentation and differentiation, producing an abnormal bridge between the tarsal bones. Can be:

- Congenital (40% of first-degree relatives may have coalitions)
- Developmental (genetically programmed to develop)
- Acquired (traumatic, infective, degenerative)
- Associated with other pathologies (CTEV, fibular hemimelia).

Commonest are either calcaneonavicular coalition (CNC) or between the middle facet of the talocalcaneal joint (talocalcaneal coalition (TCC)), as they undergo metaplasia from fibrous syndesmosis to cartilaginous synchondrosis and bony synostosis during childhood and adolescence; affected joints usually become symptomatic between either 8 and 12 years (CNC) or 12 and 16 years (TCC) if motion causes pain (75% are asymptomatic).

Coalition is the commonest cause of a rigid flat foot. Pain is felt either in the medial hindfoot by the sustentaculum tali (felt as a prominence anteroinferior to the medial malleolus) for TCC or in the sinus tarsi (depression in front of the distal fibula) for CNC; both may produce lateral heel pain from fibular impingement if marked hindfoot valgus.

Imaging

- *AP foot weight-bearing radiograph* shows ↑ angle between the long axis of the talus and the calcaneum (planovalgus).
- *Lateral foot weight-bearing radiograph* shows a flattened/inverted angle between the talus and the first metatarsal long axis (absence of the medial longitudinal arch) and reduced calcaneal pitch (horizontal position of the calcaneus).
- *CNC* is usually seen on an oblique foot view, showing the characteristic 'ant-eater sign' (prolonged calcaneal beak).
- *TCC* is harder to be seen on radiographs. The characteristic 'C-sign' and dorsal beaking of the talus may be visible on lateral foot radiographs.
- *MRI* is the gold standard to diagnose fibrous or cartilaginous TCC and exclude other tarsal coalitions.

Management

- *Non-operative:* below-knee walking cast (4–6 weeks) should relieve pain; otherwise consider the possibility that coalition is incidental to another diagnosis. Follow with a moulded orthotic insole.

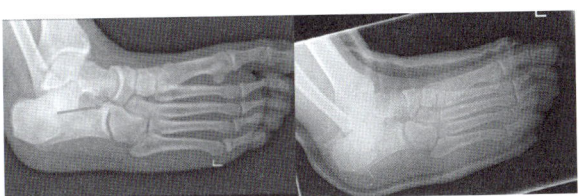

Fig. 21.14 CNC coalition with the characteristic 'ant-eater' calcaneal beak (red arrow) and after excision and interposition with autologous fat graft.

- *Operative:* if symptoms persist. Resect the coalition, and interpose bone wax, autologous fat, or adjacent tendon (Fig. 21.14). Caution if extensive TCC (the hindfoot may collapse further into valgus) and/ or severe flat foot deformity; consider lateral column lengthening osteotomy (especially if extreme, rigid planovalgus is present) or hindfoot fusion.

Further reading

Mosca VS, Bevan WP. Talocalcaneal tarsal coalitions and the calcaneal lengthening osteotomy: the role of deformity correction. *Journal of Bone and Joint Surgery*. 2012;**94**(17):1584–94.

Mosca VS, Sponseller PD. Flexible flatfoot and tarsal coalition. *Orthopaedic Knowledge Update: Pediatrics*. 2002;**2**:215–19.

Pes planovalgus (flat foot)

Loss of medial longitudinal arch with midfoot sag, valgus hindfoot, and abduction/supination of the forefoot in relation to the hindfoot (*plano-abductio-valgus*) (Fig. 21.15).

Flexible flat foot

- Characterized by mobility of the subtalar joint. Ask the child to stand on tiptoes; the hindfoot will invert when looking from behind, as the medial longitudinal arch reconstitutes.
- Associated with benign hypermobility and syndromal causes (Ehlers–Danlos syndrome, Marfan syndrome, osteogenesis imperfecta, Down syndrome).

Rigid flat foot

- Hindfoot maintained in valgus; stiffness often symptomatic on rough ground (loss of subtalar accommodation) or a cause of recurrent ankle sprains or foot stress fractures.
- Differential diagnosis includes tarsal coalition and CVT ('Persian slipper' appearance to foot, with os calcis in equinus and the navicular dorsally dislocated on the talus), accessory navicular, and neuromuscular disease.

Management

Most flexible flat feet in children require reassurance only and will resolve into adulthood. A few remain symptomatic in the area under the uncovered head of the talus and will respond to a moulded foot orthosis.

There is no indication for treatment of asymptomatic flexible flat feet. Orthotics will not change the shape of the foot in the longer term.

Examine for tightness of the tendoachilles, with the knee extended and flexed (Silfverskiold test). Failure to address this may lead to a 'midfoot break' (secondary midfoot abduction). Treat with stretching, serial casting, or botulinum toxin (Botox) injection to the calf.

Occasionally require surgical release of tendon Achilles ± corrective hindfoot or lateral column osteotomy. Arthroereisis (implant insertion

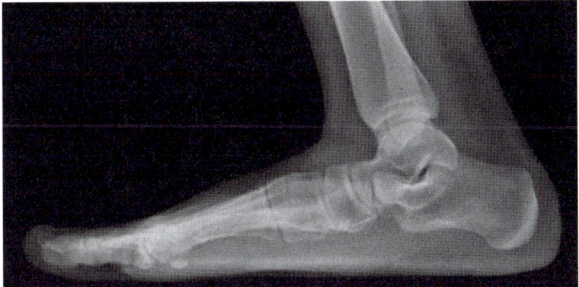

Fig. 21.15 Pes planovalgus.

into the sinus tarsi or the calcaneus to stop talocalcaneal impingement) has gained popularity, as newer devices have fewer complications than previously reported, but overall effectiveness remains controversial.

Rigid flat foot requires correction of the underlying cause, which is usually surgical.

Further reading

Bernasconi A, Lintz F, Sadile F. The role of arthroereisis of the subtalar joint for flatfoot in children and adults. *EFORT: Open Reviews*. 2017;**2**(11):438–46.

Carr JB, Yang S, Lather LA. Pediatric pes planus: a state-of-the-art review. *Pediatrics*. 2016;**137**(3):e20151230.

MacKenzie AJ, Rome K, Evans AM. The efficacy of nonsurgical interventions for pediatric flexible flat foot: a critical review. *Journal of Pediatric Orthopaedics*. 2012;**32**(8):830–4.

Pes cavus (high-arched foot)

A deformity characterized by a high (cavus) arch, hindfoot varus, plantar flexion of the first ray, and forefoot adduction (Fig. 21.16).

Aetiology

Unlike flexible pes planovalgus (PPV), the pes cavus deformity is fixed, progressive, and commonly (60–70%) associated with an underlying neurological abnormality. Fifty per cent of those with neurological abnormality have hereditary motor and sensory neuropathy (HMSN). This is also common with CP (classically hemiplegia) and myelomeningocele. Type I–III HMSN commonly present to orthopaedics; the hypertrophic (type I) and Dejerine–Sottas (type III) forms are demyelinating (with reduced or absent reflexes and slowing on NCS), but the axonal type (type II) is normal for these tests. Examine for first dorsal interosseous wasting, a common sign, and also ask about family history as most forms are inherited.

Clinical features

The plantar flexed first ray is associated with tight plantar fascia and a pronated forefoot. The hindfoot goes into secondary supination or varus, becoming fixed over time. The Coleman block test evaluates mobility of the subtalar joint and is critical to surgical planning; if plantar flexion of the first ray is accommodated by a block under the heel and lateral border, the hindfoot varus corrects to neutral/physiological valgus unless this secondary deformity has become fixed.

Management

- Establish or exclude an underlying abnormality.
- Appropriate orthotics: generally accommodative for fixed deformity to spread load and relieve pressure areas.
- Surgery may be inevitable—follow these principles:
  - *Correct fixed bony and soft tissue deformities while preserving joint motion* (e.g. first ray dorsiflexion osteotomy and plantar fascia release ± hindfoot dorsolateral displacement osteotomy, depending on results of the Coleman block test) (Fig. 21.17).
  - *Balance the muscle forces* (e.g. tibialis posterior transfer to the dorsum of the foot, extensor hallucis longus transfer to the first ray).
  - *Leave future options open:* pes cavus is a progressive deformity, so recurrence is highly likely. Avoid early resort to arthrodesis.

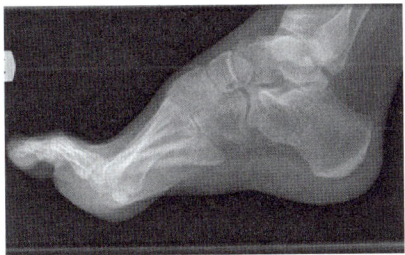

Fig. 21.16 Pes cavus deformity in a skeletally mature adolescent.

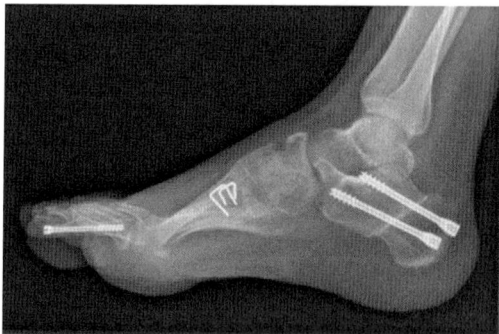

Fig. 21.17 Pes cavus treated with a first ray dorsal closing wedge osteotomy, extensor hallucis longus transfer to first ray, arthrodesis of hallux interphalangeal joint, and dorsolateral calcaneal displacement osteotomy.

Further reading

Sanpera I, Villafranca-Solano S, Muñoz-Lopez C, Sanpera-Iglesias J. How to manage pes cavus in children and adolescents? *EFORT Open Reviews.* 2021;**6**(6):510–17.

Calcaneovalgus foot

Classic 'packaging' defect secondary to a cramped intrauterine environment. Neonatal presentation with the dorsum of the foot touching the anterior surface of the tibia and apex anterolateral tibial bowing.

Management

Parental reassurance that bow will correct spontaneously in the first years of life and foot position will improve with/without simple stretching or splintage. Risk of fracture is very low (cf. higher risk with congenital pseudarthrosis of the tibia).

However, warn that residual limb length discrepancy is common. This is usually small, but not always, and needs follow-up to skeletal maturity in case a limb equalization procedure is needed.

Hallux valgus (bunion)

A common condition, occurring in up to 36% of the paediatric population. Characterized by lateral deviation of the first metatarsal, creating medial apex deformity at the first MTPJ. It has a multifactorial genetic basis and it is associated with pes planus or a long/varus first metatarsal. Commonly seen bilaterally; if unilateral, then other causes need to be excluded, including CP, spinal cord anomalies, and peripheral nerve lesions.

Management

Most children are asymptomatic. Non-operative management is focused on footwear modifications and orthotics, but has been shown to have a limited role in preventing progression. Surgical correction is indicated once conservative treatment has failed, and ideally after skeletal maturity to prevent recurrence. Surgical interventions (such as Scarf or basal osteotomy) show good clinical and radiological outcomes, with rates of recurrence and other complications lower than historically reported figures.

Further reading

Harb Z, Kokkinakis M, Ismail H, Spence G. Adolescent hallux valgus: a systematic review of outcomes following surgery. *Journal of Children's Orthopaedics*. 2015;**9**(2):105–12.

Idiopathic or habitual toe-walking

Tiptoe-walking is relatively common in toddlers aged up to 4–5 years. Habitual toe-walkers will have done so since their earliest steps; this should be sought in the history. Often a family history (in ~50%).

Diagnosis

A diagnosis of persistent or new-onset toe-walking beyond this age involves exclusion of underlying causes, primarily neurological disorders. Most frequent is CP (spastic diplegia), typically associated with a flexed knee during gait, followed by muscular dystrophy in boys, of which Duchenne muscular dystrophy (X-linked) is the commonest. Gower's sign is a useful test in clinic; ask also about delayed motor milestones.

Consider HMSN (Charcot–Marie–Tooth (CMT) disease), especially if later onset (>6 years of age) after previously normal walking. Ask for family history, and examine for cavovarus feet and first dorsal interosseous wasting. Always examine the spine for an underlying anomaly; a midline pit, hairy tuft, lipoma, or other abnormality should prompt MRI for underlying tethered cord, syrinx, or diastematomyelia.

Toe-walking may also be associated with learning disorders and autism.

Management

For confirmed idiopathic toe-walking, management can be challenging, with high recurrence rates and often considerable parental pressure to intervene. Reassurance is helped by the fact that persistence beyond skeletal maturity is rare, but there are theoretical concerns about the development of a secondary midfoot break and PPV for untreated calf contracture. There may be a particular issue with joint laxity; stabilize the midfoot when testing ankle dorsiflexion to avoid spurious motion through this region.

Dynamic tightness may respond to physiotherapy, botulinum toxin injections, and night splints. Fixed contracture ('congenital short tendoachilles') may require serial casting or surgery (percutaneous Achilles tendon release or lengthening of the gastrocnemius aponeurosis). Again, there is a high recurrence rate (30–60%) and a risk of (disastrous) overcorrection (weak push-off and no good surgical rescue option).

Further reading

Eastwood DM, Menelaus MB, Dickens DR, Broughton NS, Cole WG. Idiopathic toe-walking: does treatment alter the natural history? *Journal of Pediatric Orthopedics. Part B.* 2000:**9**(1):47–9.

Metatarsus adductus

Medial deviation of the forefoot (through the mid-tarsal joints) in isolation is a common (~1 in 1000 live births) neonatal foot deformity. Most forms are a '*packaging*', rather than a '*manufacturing*', defect, reflecting a tight intra-uterine environment; therefore, it is important to examine also for other packaging problems such as torticollis, plagiocephaly, and hip dysplasia.

Differentials and assessment

- As a purely forefoot condition, this does not affect the hindfoot; it should therefore be differentiated from both *clubfoot* (in which there is fixed hindfoot equinus and varus, with midfoot cavus) and *skew foot* (a less common congenital deformity of metatarsus adductus, combined with midfoot abduction and hindfoot valgus).
- As a cause of in-toeing (and tripping) in toddlers, metatarsus adductus should also be differentiated from persistent femoral neck anteversion and internal tibial torsion (using the Staheli rotation profile assessment).
- Progressive deformities ± cavus presenting in older age groups should prompt investigation for a more proximal spinal abnormality.
- The heel bisector line should pass through the second/third web but instead passes laterally in metatarsus adductus—a useful guide to severity, flexibility, and response to treatment.

Management

Non-operative

- Majority are flexible (90%) and resolve physiologically within the first year of life. Another 5% will resolve by 4 years without treatment.
- Radiographs are not usually helpful.
- Serial stretch, manipulation and casting, and/or application of a reverse counter shoe are still practised by some, albeit without robust evidence of their effectiveness (as most improve naturally).

Operative

Very rarely required for resistant feet. Options include:

- Tarso-metatarsal osteotomies—largely abandoned because of stiffness and recurrence
- Multiple basal metatarsal osteotomies
- 'Cut and shut' tarsal osteotomies— a closing wedge cuboid and opening wedge cuneiform osteotomy, transferring the bone wedge across the foot.

Further reading

Feng L, Sussman M. Combined medial cuneiform osteotomy and multiple metatarsal osteotomies for correction of persistent metatarsus adductus in children. *Journal of Pediatric Orthopaedics.* 2016;**36**(7):730–5.

Williams CM, James AM, Tran T. Metatarsus adductus: development of a non-surgical treatment pathway. *Journal of Paediatrics and Child Health.* 2013;**49**(9):E428–33.

Juvenile idiopathic arthritis

JIA is arthritis that persists for >6 weeks in children/adolescents (aged <16 years). Arthritis of a known cause must be excluded. ~1 in 1000 children will develop swelling of ≥1 joint; 50% of these will progress to JIA. Commoner in ♀; 25% have severe disease (degenerative arthritis, blindness), and 50% resolve without sequelae.

Diagnostic criteria

- A diagnosis of exclusion: must rule out infection.
- One of the following criteria must be present: rash, RhF positive, iridocyclitis. C-spine involvement, pericarditis, tenosynovitis, intermittent fever, and morning stiffness.

Associated conditions

- *Systemic (Still's disease):* acute-onset JIA with multiple joint involvement, rash, daily high fever, and splenomegaly; exclude infection; incidence ♂ = ♀; usually presents at age 5–10 years.
- *Ocular involvement:* typically iridocyclitis, a form of anterior uveitis. May be silent. Urgent ophthalmologic evaluation (slit-lamp) essential. May cause rapid visual loss if untreated. Positive ANA titre ↑ the risk (80% of cases of anterior uveitis in children are associated with JIA).
- *C-spine involvement:* risk of kyphosis, ankylosis, atlanto-axial instability.

Classification

- *Onset:* early (pre-teens) vs late.
- *Polyarticular (30%):* involvement of ≥5 joints (both large and small) in the first 6 months of the disease. May be RhF-positive; 60% remission rate.
- *Oligoarticular (pauciarticular) (50%):* commonest. Peak incidence between second and third year of life. ♀ > ♂. Usually involves a few large joints, commonly the knee/ankles; single hip joint rarely involved in isolation; asymmetrical; 70% remission; early onset more likely ocular disease.
- *Systemic (20%):* Still's disease.

Clinical findings

- *Symptoms:* joint inflammation (swelling, pain), morning stiffness, visual changes, systemic upset (fever).
- *Examination findings:* joint swelling (effusion acutely, synovial thickening later), stiffness, reduced range of motion (loss of full knee extension, finger flexion/extension—may be subtle). Severe disease may result in joint destruction with deformity, instability, and muscle wasting. Rash may be evident (Still's disease). Anterior uveitis evident on slit-lamp examination if ocular involvement.

Investigations

- *Laboratory:* RhF seropositive in <15%, associated with more severe disease and joint destruction, and greater likelihood of progression to adult RA. ANA positivity is diagnostic. Basic serology less helpful as often normal. CRP/WCC may help to exclude infection.
- *Radiology:*

- Plain radiographs often normal at presentation. In advanced disease, there are classically juxta-articular erosions, with osteopenia and joint destruction evident later.
- Flexion–extension neck radiographs help to rule out atlanto-axial instability (see ➔ Chapter 22).
- USS can confirm synovial inflammation and joint effusions. May be combined with joint aspiration ± injection.
- MRI can help to confirm diagnosis and exclude osteomyelitis/septic arthritis, although usually not required (helpful to rule out mechanical problems mimicking JIA).

Management

- Refer to paediatric rheumatology:
  - Immunomodulating medications
  - DMARDs, including TNF inhibitors (etanercept), monoclonal antibodies against B-cells (rituximab), and purine synthesis inhibitors (azathioprine)
  - Anti-inflammatories: NSAIDs, intra-articular steroid injections.
- Regular ophthalmological review.
- Orthopaedic involvement:
  - Less common in modern practice due to success of DMARDs
  - Joint aspiration/synovial biopsy sometimes needed for diagnosis
  - Joint washout for severe synovitis
  - Correction of secondary joint or growth deformity
  - Joint replacement for end-stage burnt-out disease—usually not until skeletal maturity
- Physiotherapy and occupational therapy input essential.

Further reading

Viswanathan V, Murray KJ. Management of children with juvenile idiopathic arthritis. *Indian Journal of Pediatrics*. 2016;**83**(1):63–70.

Juvenile spondyloarthropathy

Spondyloarthropathies are characterized by arthritis that affects the spine and other large joints. There are several subtypes in adults, with onset usually in the third decade of life; onset *before* the age of 16 years distinguishes the condition as juvenile spondyloarthropathy.

Introduction

- Heterogeneous group of HLA-B27-associated inflammatory syndromes, but in most cases, spine and SIJs are affected eventually.
- HLA-B27 status varies, but RhF is *absent* in all juvenile spondyloarthropathies—hence 'seronegative spondyloarthropathy'.
- Distinct subcategories, commonly: (1) enthesitis-related arthritis (ERA); (2) psoriatic arthritis; and (3) undifferentiated arthritis. Most have an adult-equivalent condition.
- Of all cases of JIA, 8% may be enthesitis-related arthritis, 6% psoriatic arthritis, and 20% undifferentiated arthritis.
- Diagnostic criteria for AS does not have a lower age limit; 11% of AS cases have an onset at age of between 5 and 16 years.

Clinical features

- Periods of mild to moderate inflammatory flares between times of disease quiescence.
- Peripheral arthropathy is the commonest presenting feature in children (vs back pain in the adult population); usually large joints in the lower limb. Asymmetrical pattern.
- Lack of back pain does not preclude sacroiliac involvement; 20% of those with juvenile spondyloarthropathy have 'silent' sacroiliitis (only seen on MRI).
- Anterior uveitis is the commonest extra-articular manifestation, presenting with redness, pain, and photophobia, most commonly in HLA-B27-positive patients.
- GI inflammation may be present in 60%.

Diagnostic criteria

Established by International League of Associations for Rheumatology (ILAR), with subtypes identified by the following:

- *ERA:*
  - *Presence of enthesitis* (inflammation of tendon/ligament insertions, commonly patella/Achilles tendon)—common first symptom, and/or
  - *Arthritis prior to age of 16 years*, plus
  - ≥2 of the following:
    - Sacroiliac tenderness
    - Inflammatory back pain
    - Presence of HLA-B27
    - History of anterior uveitis or acute uveitis
    - Family history of spondyloarthropathy
- *Psoriatic arthritis*—children rarely have skin findings and may only develop skin changes in adulthood; hence, the diagnostic criteria are:
  - Presence of arthritis at age <16 years, plus

- ≥2 of the following:
  - Psoriasis in a first-degree relative
  - Dactylitis
  - Nail pitting
  - Onycholysis
- *Undifferentiated spondyloarthropathy*—children who do not fit into any of the above two categories are defined by ILAR as having 'undifferentiated' spondyloarthropathy. ♀:♂ preponderance of 3:1.

Extra-articular manifestations are less common.

Investigations

Laboratory
- RhF negative.
- HLA-B27 status provides prognostic indication of severity.

Imaging
- *Radiography:* pelvis for SIJ involvement (sclerosis, erosions, widening, ankylosis). Spine shows syndesmophytes (ossification of deep fibres of the anterior longitudinal ligament) causing a 'bamboo spine' appearance in AS (symmetrical syndesmophytes), but not in others (asymmetrical syndesmophytes and skip distribution). Cervical spine for atlanto-axial instability.
- *MRI:* allows earlier detection of inflammatory changes (bone marrow oedema in SIJ).
- *USS:* enthesitis (tendon thickening, calcification, hypoechogenicity, and bony erosions at insertion).

Management

- Posture and range of motion exercises—physiotherapy essential.
- NSAIDs—positive response suggests DMARDs may be effective.
- Methotrexate and sulfasalazine help in reducing joint erosions and damage in chronic peripheral joint involvement, BUT limited use in axial skeleton disease management.
- Anti-TNF therapy is the mainstay of current treatment (etanercept, infliximab, adalimumab), and is both safe and efficacious in the paediatric population. Limits disease flares and can occasionally induce disease remission. Carries a risk of infections (e.g. TB, histoplasmosis) and autoimmune disease (e.g. lupus, multiple sclerosis).

Further reading

Scofield RH, Sestak AL. Juvenile spondylarthropathies. *Current Rheumatology Reports.* 2012;**14**:395–401.

Osteomyelitis in children

In children, bone pain + fever = osteomyelitis until proven otherwise.

Epidemiology

- Incidence 1:5000. Age <13 years; mean age 6.6 years; 2.5 times commoner in ♂.
- *Risk factors:* diabetes, haemoglobinopathy, RA, chronic renal disease, immune compromise, varicella infection.

Pathophysiology

- Bacteraemia ± local trauma (30% of cases) lead to ↑ susceptibility of bacterial seeding in paediatric metaphysis.
- Rich metaphyseal vascularity (and sluggish flow, and low pH and oxygen tension provide a favourable environment for growth). Common at age <10 years due to an underdeveloped immune system.

Microbiology

- *Staphylococcus aureus:* commonest in all children. Meticillin-resistant *S. aureus* (MRSA) associated with DVT and septic emboli. Community-acquired MRSA strains may have the Panton–Valentine leucocidin (PVL) cytotoxin (complex multifocal infections, prolonged fever, abscesses, DVT, sepsis).
- *Group B Streptococcus:* commonest in neonates.
- *Kingella kingae:* ↑ prevalence in the young (need enrichment).
- *Pseudomonas:* associated with foot puncture wounds.
- *Haemophilus influenzae:* less common due to vaccination.
- *Mycobacterium TB:* children often have extra-pulmonary disease.
- *Salmonella:* seen in patients with sickle-cell disease.

Classification

- *Acute haematogenous: bacteraemia* (skin graze, dental caries) seeds, then established metaphyseal infection travels in Haversian and Volkmann canals. *Osteonecrosis* occurs during the inflammatory response and *purulence* develops, which breaks through the cortex and leads to *subperiosteal collections*. Where the periosteum connects to a joint, *septic arthritis* can develop (e.g. shoulder, elbow, hip, ankle; not the knee). NB in children aged <1 year, infection can cross the physis for *direct epiphyseal/joint involvement.*
- *Chronic:* periosteal elevation impairs blood supply to bone, so a region of avascular bone develops. This *sequestrum* becomes a nidus for ongoing infection and new bone develops around this (*involucrum*). A more chronic abscess with sclerotic bone/fibrous margin is known a *Brodie's abscess.*

Clinical features

- *History:* limb pain, recent trauma or infection, immunization history (need Gram-negative cover if no *H. influenzae* vaccination).
- *Clinical signs:* limp, febrile (but rarely septic). Limb may be oedematous, warm, swollen, and tender (check the pelvis, spine, and limbs). Movement may be restricted if severe.

- *Radiographs:* may be normal. Subtle loss of tissue planes/oedema; 5–7 days, see new periosteal bone; 10–14 days, osteolysis; 1–2 weeks, abscesses and metaphyseal bone density loss.
- *CT:* useful in late disease to characterize bone loss.
- *MRI:* gold standard for early detection of marrow and soft tissue oedema, and the presence of subperiosteal collection—guides surgical decision-making if response to antibiotics is suboptimal.
- *Bone scan:* rarely used. Can help to localize pathology (whole-body MRI preferred). Technetium-99 can localize multifocal infection.
- *Laboratory:* WCC only elevated in 25% of cases and poor correlation with response to treatment. CRP elevated in 98% of cases within 6h of onset and is most sensitive to monitor response to treatment; usually normalizes within a week if treatment is successful. If no improvement after 48–72h, then change treatment. ESR is less available and declines too slowly to guide treatment.
- *Microbiological:* bone aspiration positive in 50–70%, so more helpful than blood cultures (30–50% positive).

Management—acute

- Empirical antibiotic treatment is appropriate in early disease with no periosteal/bone abscess. Commence immediately after blood is drawn for culture (no need to wait for bone aspiration to confirm pathogen).
- Choice of antibiotic depends on local guidelines (close liaison with microbiology team). Third-generation cephalosporins are often recommended. Flucloxacillin usually appropriate if low risk of MRSA. Multi-agent therapy in PVL *S. aureus.*
- Duration of IV therapy is controversial. Some evidence suggests shorter IV durations are suitable; tailor to response, and step-down to oral according to culture results, clinical response, and CRP.
- Failure to improve clinically in 48h indicates need for alternative treatment. Imaging is key to establishing if focus requires surgical drainage (evacuate purulence, debride, irrigate, drill bone to access and drain intraosseous collections, send tissue for culture/histology).

Management—chronic

- Children have excellent healing and remodelling capacity once infection is treated and can resorb extensive sequestra.
- However, infection is difficult to eradicate with a large sequestrum; surgical debridement improves the chance of clearing infection.
- Preservation of the periosteum provides the best remodelling potential, but extensive bone loss may require complex reconstructive techniques (bone transport; Masquelet—induced membrane with spacers).
- Numerous classifications. Cierny–Mader helps with stratification (Fig. 21.18).

Pitfalls and complications

- *DVT:* rare in children, but ↑ risk with MRSA, >8 years, surgical treatment. In those not responding to IV antibiotics and surgical drainage, consider infected embolus (especially MRSA-PVL).
- Infection near and across a physis carries a risk of growth arrest; warn parents and follow up for longitudinal or angular growth arrest.

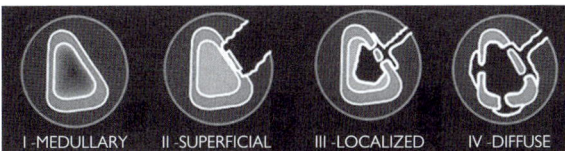

Fig. 21.18 Cierny–Mader classification.

- Thirty per cent of acute leukaemia patients present with bone pain secondary to osseous infiltration, many with elevated CRP/fever. Radiological features mimic infection; request blood film ± haematology review for bone marrow aspirate if FBC shows anaemia or neutropenia.
- Bone tumours can mimic the radiological appearance of osteomyelitis (e.g. eosinophilic granuloma (benign) or Ewing's sarcoma (malignant)). Essential to biopsy in chronic cases with established bone changes; send samples for microbiology and histopathology.

Chronic recurrent multifocal osteomyelitis

- Idiopathic inflammatory disease of the skeleton meeting these criteria:
  - Multiple sites of apparent osteomyelitis (typical radiological features)
  - Pathology and culture specimens negative
  - No improvement with antibiotics.
- Primarily children/adolescents, commonly girls, peak age 10 years.
- Tubular long bones and clavicle most affected.
- Pathophysiology poorly understood, but some associated conditions:
  - Pustulosis palmoplantaris syndrome: chronic relapsing palmo/plantar pustules, likely rheumatological
  - SAPHO syndrome: chronic recurrent multifocal osteomyelitis with synovitis, acne, pustulosis, hyperostosis, and osteitis.
- Remains a diagnosis of exclusion.
- Clinically: episodic/focal pain, malaise, localized swelling.
- Radiographs may show eccentric metaphyseal lesions with sclerosis. Bone scan can show other sites. MRI to check for soft tissue involvement and help to narrow the differential.
- WCC typically normal. ESR/CRP may be raised.
- Biopsy and bone cultures are negative.
- *Management:* in liaison with paediatric rheumatologist. Simple analgesics/NSAIDs. Also consider steroids and bisphosphonates.

Further reading

Dartnell J, Ramachandran M, Katchburian M. Haematogenous acute and subacute paediatric osteomyelitis: a systematic review of the literature. *Journal of Bone and Joint Surgery (British Volume)*. 2012;**94-B**:584–95.

Septic arthritis in children

Intra-articular infection in children is a surgical emergency requiring prompt diagnosis, urgent surgical management, and IV antibiotics.

Epidemiology

- Peak in first year of life; 50% in children aged <2 years.
- Hip in 35%; knee in 35%.
- Risk factors: prematurity (immunocompromised), caesarean section, neonatal intensive care unit (NICU) admission, invasive procedures.

Pathophysiology

- Inoculation (trauma, surgery) causes bacteraemia—seeding may be directly to the synovium or via metaphyseal osteomyelitis.
- The hip, shoulder, elbow, and ankle have intra-articular metaphyses (the knee does not), so osteomyelitis can spread into adjacent joints.
- Neonates have transphyseal vessels—direct spread to joint more likely.
- Inflammatory/infected synovial cells and bacteria release matrix metalloproteinases (proteolytic enzymes) that damage cartilage in <8h; joint pressure can cause AVN of the femoral head.

Microbiology

- *Neonates:* group B *Streptococcus* commonest in community-acquired (transvaginal delivery); *S. aureus* as cause of nosocomial infections in neonates.
- *Infants:* *S. aureus* commonest. Consider PVL variant if severe/multiple foci of infection.
- *Adolescents:* *Neisseria gonorrhoeae* commonest (atypical presentation—preceding migratory polymyalgia, multiple joints, small red papules); high-dose penicillin (no surgery) often successful.
- *Other:* group A β-haemolytic *Streptococcus* common following varicella infection (NB invasive group A *Streptococcus* is notifiable to public health); HACEK organisms (fastidious—*Haemophilus*, *Actinobacillus*, *Cardiobacterium*, *Eikenella*, *Kingella*).

Clinical features

- *History:* recent local trauma or infections, vaccination history important (e.g. *H. influenzae*). Recent antibiotics can mask signs.
- *Symptoms:* pain (usually more acute and severe than osteomyelitis), limp, avoidance of weight-bearing.
- *Signs:* pyrexia, tachycardia, sepsis (peripheral vasodilatation, high cardiac output, oliguria), localized swelling/effusion, tenderness, erythema, severe pain with passive motion (pseudoparalysis in infants). Joints rest in position, maximizing joint capsule volume: hip FABER; knee (30°) flexion.

Investigations

- *Radiographs:* may be normal if early. May see lateral subluxation of the hip (widened joint space caused by pus), subluxation, or dislocation. May see bone lesions if associated osteomyelitis.
- *USS:* essential in neonates (examination challenging and signs can be minimal). Compare with contralateral side. May detect effusion and guide aspiration, but cannot differentiate sterile vs infected effusion.

Table 21.7 Modified Kocher criteria for hip pain in a child

WCC	>12,000 cells/μl	**Likelihood of septic arthritis**
Refusal to weight-bear		Kocher (1999): 0 = 0.2%; 1 = 3%; 2 = 40%; 3 = 93%; 4 = 99%
Fever	>38.5°C	Caird: 0 = 17%; 1 = 37%; 2 = 62%; 3 = 83%; 4 = 93%; 5 = 98%
ESR	>40mm/h	
CRP	>2.5mg/L	

- *MRI:* often difficult to arrange quickly. May identify adjacent osteomyelitis.
- *Laboratory:* help to distinguish from transient synovitis (Caird's modified Kocher criteria) (Table 21.7). CRP most sensitive and rises rapidly; raised CRP and inability to weight-bear are sensitive in combination.

Differential diagnosis

- Transient synovitis is commonest differential.
- Other differentials include: inflammatory arthropathy (JIA), malignancy (including leukaemia), bleeding disorders, PVNS, acute rheumatic fever, Lyme disease, and Henoch–Schönlein purpura.

Management

- Joint aspiration for microbiology (usually under general anaesthesia in children, so often immediately prior to washout): Gram stain positive in 30–50% only (so negative aspirate microscopy does not exclude); culture positive in 50–80%; WCC >50,000/mm³ in aspirate (75% polymorphonuclear neutrophils), protein levels less than serum levels.
- Emergent surgical drainage and irrigation of the joint.
- Broad-spectrum IV antibiotics after aspiration, rationalized by culture results; multiple washouts may be required.
- MRI if not improving, to exclude osteomyelitis.

Complications

- Physeal destruction/bar (causing limb length discrepancy/deformity).
- Osteonecrosis—need follow-up and repeat imaging.
- Joint instability (immobilize the hip in spica after washout to prevent secondary dislocation).
- Secondary degenerative joint disease due to chondrolysis (causes stiffness/ankylosis).

Further reading

Caird MS, Flynn JM, Leung YL, Millman JE, D'Italia JG, Dormans JP. Factors distinguishing septic arthritis from transient synovitis of the hip in children. A prospective study. *Journal of Bone and Joint Surgery (American Volume)*. 2006;**88**(6):1251–7.

Kocher MS, Zurakowski D, Kasser JR. Differentiating between septic arthritis and transient synovitis of the hip in children: an evidence-based clinical prediction algorithm. *Journal of Bone and Joint Surgery (American Volume)*. 1999;**81**:1662–70.

McCarthy JJ, Dormans JP, Kozin SH, et al. Musculoskeletal infections in children. *Journal of Bone and Joint Surgery (American Volume)*. 2004;**86**:850–63.

Congenital myopathies

These are rare disorders presenting in infancy or childhood with diffuse muscle hypotonia, gross motor delay, poor coordination, and facial weakness. Orthopaedic considerations principally focus on developing joints, scoliosis, hip dysplasia, and foot deformities. Due to lacking definitive treatment, multidisciplinary management is essential.

Aetiology

- Over 20 genes are associated with congenital myopathy subtypes—underlying alterations distinguish each type.
- Commonest are central core myopathy, nemaline myopathies, centronuclear myopathies.

Clinical presentation

- Birth/early years—hypotonia, delayed milestones, myopathic facies.
- Severe forms have reduced fetal movement—need respiratory support at birth; mild forms present in adulthood.
- *Differential diagnosis:* spinal muscular atrophy, muscular dystrophy, metabolic problems, toxin exposure.

Examples

- *Core central myopathies—alterations in ryanodine receptor:*
  - Muscle biopsy for definitive diagnosis: dye-free cores in muscle fibres. Congenital hip dislocation, cavovarus feet, patellar subluxation, scoliosis. Associated with malignant hyperpyrexia following general anaesthesia. Facial and extraocular muscles are relatively spared.
- *Nemaline myopathies—alterations in nebulin, actin, and tropomysin:*
  - Muscle biopsy: nemaline rods at the level of muscle fibres
  - Associated with slender, but strong, muscles, facial weakness and nasal speech, cardiomyopathy, and respiratory failure.
- *Centronuclear myopathies:*
  - Muscle biopsy: central nuclei in muscle cells
  - May present early or late. Commonest is severe infantile myopathy with significant facial and limb weakness. Respiratory failure in infancy is common
  - May have muscle contractures in the hips, knees, feet, and ankles.

Diagnosis

- Muscle biopsy.
- Imaging with MRI/USS to assess for patterns of skeletal muscle changes to characterize myopathy.

Management

Primarily supportive. Deformities managed with stretching/bracing. Consider risks of general anaesthesia before considering surgical intervention.

Further reading

Lewis D. Weakness and hypotonia. In: Marcdante KJ, Nelson WE, eds. *Nelson Essentials of Pediatrics*, 6th edn. Philadelphia, PA: Saunders/Elsevier, 2011; Chapter 24, Section 182.

Muscular dystrophy

Myopathies due to inherited, non-inflammatory, progressive muscle disorders without a central or peripheral nerve abnormality.

Duchenne muscular dystrophy

Pathophysiology

- X-linked recessive: Xp21.2 dystrophin gene defect due to a point deletion and nonsense alteration (30% spontaneous alterations).
- Dystrophin absence→sarcolemma membrane instability→leak intracellular contents (high CPK level)→poor muscle fibre regeneration, resulting in progressive replacement of muscle with fibrous/fatty tissue (loss of skeletal/cardiac muscle elasticity/strength).

Clinical features

- Affected ♂ are normal at birth and generally walk by 18 months.
- All manifest features by age of 5 years.
- Intelligence quotient (IQ) reduced (average of 85), compared with normal population (100).
- Classic gait is waddling (due to gluteus weakness), wide-based with hyperlordosis, and toe-walking.
- Tendency to fall without tripping or stumbling.
- Test for Gower sign in any ♂ toe-walker aged under 5 years; weakness in proximal hip muscles uncovered when the child stands up from seated position by 'walking' hands up thighs.
- Iliopsoas/tendoachilles contractures develop.
- Scoliosis very common and progresses to compromise respiratory reserve.
- Lose walking ability by age of 7–13 years when contractures and scoliosis (usually rapidly) progress.
- Other findings: absent deep tendon reflexes (<30%), calf pseudohypertrophy resembling 'inverted champagne bottle' (60%), macroglossia (30%).
- Cardiopulmonary involvement makes Duchenne muscular dystrophy a terminal disease, with death typically by the third decade.

Investigations

- CPK level 50–300 times normal, but falls with ↓ in muscle mass over time. LDH and aldolase also raised.
- Genetic testing.
- *USS:* ↑ echogenicity in the affected muscles (and corresponding reduction from bone).
- *EMG:* short duration, polyphasic action potentials with ↓ amplitude.
- *Muscle biopsy* (not always required for diagnosis): variations in fibre size with focal areas of degeneration; absent dystrophin.

Management

- Aim is to keep the child ambulatory for as long as possible.
- Physiotherapy for gait training and transfer techniques; orthotics—AFOs and later KAFOs may support prolonged ambulation; spinal bracing may slow scoliosis progression.
- A wheelchair is needed in the later stages of the disease.

- Steroid therapy used to stabilize muscle strength and preserve pulmonary function; also slows progression of scoliosis.

Orthopaedic options
- *Foot deformities*: tendoachilles lengthening for ankle equinus, tibialis posterior transfer (through the interosseus membrane) for equinovarus deformity.
- *Scoliosis*: instrumented fusion while respiratory capacity permits. Cardiorespiratory complications rise dramatically once FVC falls below 30%.

Differential diagnosis—other muscular dystrophies

Myotonic dystrophy
- Autosomal dominant; second commonest muscular dystrophy.
- Classically myotonia (delayed muscle relaxation), muscular dystrophy, cardiac conduction abnormalities, cataracts, endocrine disorders.
- Seventy-five per cent are type 1 (MD1 = Steinert's disease), and most present in adulthood (a few have severe congenital form); MD2 is mild.
- Clinically: expressionless facies, delayed motor milestones, foot deformities, scoliosis.
- Management: therapy, orthoses, surgery for foot/spine deformities.

Fascioscapulohumeral muscular dystrophy
- Autosomal dominant (30% spontaneous). Affects both sexes (♂ more severely) during teens or early adulthood. Third commonest dystrophy.
- Progressive weakness in face, shoulder, and upper arm.
- No reduction in life expectancy.
- Classical 'flat' facies due to facial muscle weakness; unable to whistle or blow cheeks out; winging of scapulae, causing poor control of shoulder motion.
- Surgical fusion of the scapula to the thoracic wall may help with function.

Becker's muscular dystrophy
- Similar (same genetic defect) to Duchenne muscular dystrophy, but symptoms start later (age 10 years or even adulthood) and are less severe; slower progression; cardiomyopathy often significant.

Further reading

Canavese F, Sussman M. Orthopaedic manifestations of congenital myotonic dystrophy during childhood and adolescence. *Journal of Pediatric Orthopaedics*. 2009;**29**:208–13.

Sussman M. Duchenne muscular dystrophy. *Journal of the American Academy of Orthopaedic Surgeons*. 2002;**10**:138–51.

Spinal muscular atrophy

Genetic condition causing idiopathic degeneration of anterior horn motor neurons in the spinal cord, medulla, and midbrain. This results in denervation of muscle fibres and progressive muscle weakness, fasciculation, paralysis, deformities, and respiratory/gut problems.

Aetiology

- One in 10,000 newborns affected; 1 in 40 of the population are carriers. Autosomal recessive inheritance.
- Ninety-five per cent associated with a deletion in the survival motor neuron (SMN) gene on chromosome 5.

Classification

- Four types, based on age at onset and motor milestones achieved.
- Diagnosis of types I–III usually made before age of 3 years:
  - *Type I*: Werdnig–Hoffmann disease (most severe) presents at age <6 months
  - *Type II*: intermediate, presents at age >6 months
  - *Type III*: Kugelberg–Welander disease presents after age of 2 years
  - *Type IV*: adult onset, rare.

Investigations

- Genetic testing for absent/altered SMN gene.
- Muscle biopsy if genetic testing negative.
- EMG—to distinguish from other motor neuron diseases.
- Radiological imaging of hips and spine.

Clinical

- Severe proximal muscle weakness in lower limbs, absent reflexes.
- Fasciculations may be present; tongue fasciculations pathognomonic.
- Dysphagia, respiratory compromise, scoliosis, hip dislocations.
- Progressive loss of function; may be rapid at around time of accelerated growth spurt or intercurrent illness.

Management

- Genetic counselling.
- Physiotherapy and occupational therapy; orthoses (spinal brace).
- Prompt treatment of respiratory complications.
- Surgical treatment of scoliosis; growing rods in young, posterior instrumented fusion to pelvis in mature.
- Surgical treatment of hip dislocation and contractures controversial as high recurrence. Do not aid in ambulation but may prevent pain.
- Gene therapy has been proven to substantially improve survival in SMA type 1, and may reduce severity of other types
  - Disease modifying therapy (intra-thecal nusinersen, oral risdiplam) stimulate production of SMN2 protein
  - Gene replacement therapy (single IV infusion of onasemnogene abeparvovec) may benefit <2 yrs, replacing SMN1 gene
- Gene therapy more effective if started early before symptoms develop - now newborn screening in US

Further reading

Medline Plus. *Spinal muscle atrophy*. Available from: ℘ https://medlineplus.gov/genetics/condition/spinal-muscular-atrophy/

Mesfin A, Sponseller PD, Leet AI. Spinal muscular atrophy: manifestations and management. *Journal of the American Academy of Orthopaedic Surgery*. 2012;**20**(6):393–401.

Hereditary motor and sensory neuropathies

Charcot–Marie–Tooth disease

- CMT ('peroneal muscular atrophy') is the commonest inherited progressive peripheral neuropathy (1 in 2500 affected).
- Genetic alteration results in affected nerve structure. Commonly an autosomal dominant duplication on chromosome 17 coding for peripheral myelin protein 22 (PMP-22).
- Many forms. CMT I–III are the main forms with orthopaedic manifestations:
  - *CMT I (hypertrophic demyelinating neuropathy—types A, B, C):* autosomal dominant. Onset first/second decade. Slowed nerve conduction velocity, absent deep tendon reflexes. Normal life expectancy. Motor > sensory. Progressive cavovarus foot
  - *CMT II (axonal neuropathy—not demyelination):* variable inheritance. Later onset. Normal nerve conduction and reflexes. Results in a flaccid foot
  - *CMT III (Dejerine–Sottas disease):* point alteration of PMP-22. Autosomal recessive inheritance. Onset in infancy. Loss of deep tendon reflexes. Severe demyelinating disease. Delayed ambulation, pes cavus, foot drop, glove-and-stocking pattern of sensory change, and spinal deformity.

Clinical features

- *Symptoms:* motor deficits (distal weakness, atrophy, instability/clumsiness, frequent ankle sprains, stair climbing difficult). Variable sensory deficit.
- *Examination:* cavovarus foot, hammer/claw toes (usually symmetrical), unopposed pull of peroneus longus plantar flexes first ray—compensatory hindfoot varus (flexible, later stiff—check by using Coleman block test), intrinsic hand weakness, scoliosis, hip dysplasia.

Investigations

- *Genetic testing:* duplication on chromosome 17.
- *EMG:* low conduction velocities and amplitude.

Management

- *Non-operative:* accommodative shoe-wear. Orthotics—corrective (lateral hindfoot post if flexible varus), accommodative (recession for plantar-flexed first ray), or supportive (AFO to prevent sprains).
- *Operative:* soft tissue reconstruction (flexible feet—peroneus longus to brevis transfer, posterior tibial tendon transfer, tendoachilles lengthening, Jones transfer to correct toe clawing, calcaneal osteotomy, first ray osteotomies if rigid, triple arthrodesis once skeletally mature).

Friedreich's ataxia

- Commonest spinocerebellar degenerative disease (1 in 50,000)—lesions in dorsal root ganglia, corticospinal tracts, cerebellum, and peripheral sensory nerves.

- Autosomal recessive inheritance. GAA repeat alteration at 9q13 reduces the frataxin gene (mitochondrial protein, iron metabolism/ oxidative stress).
- Onset at age of between 7 and 25 years.

Clinical features

- Classically ataxia, areflexia, and positive plantar response; wide-based gait and nystagmus.
- Cardiomyopathy, cavovarus foot, and scoliosis may develop. Deformities may benefit from surgical management.
- Often wheelchair-bound by 30 years. Death occurs at age of between 40 and 50 years.

Further reading

Wilmshurst JM, Ouvrier R. Hereditary peripheral neuropathies of childhood: an overview for clinicians. *Neuromuscular Disorders*. 2011;**21**(11):763–75.

Hereditary connective tissue disorders

Marfan syndrome

- Autosomal dominant disorder: Alteration in fibrillin-1 (*FBN1*) gene on chromosome 15, multiple alterations (30% spontaneous).
- Disorder of fibrillin (glycoprotein, which is essential for the formation of elastic fibres found in connective tissue).

Clinical features

- Arachnodactyly (spider-like fingers—long and slender).
- High-arched palate.
- Arm span greater than height (dolichostenomelia).
- Pectus (chest wall) deformities.
- Scoliosis (50%—often first noted signs) and spondylolisthesis.
- Planovalgus foot deformities.
- Protrusio acetabulae.
- Cardiac valve abnormalities—aortic incompetence.
- Ocular—superior lens dislocation in 60% of patients.
- Dural ectasia and meningocele can occur.
- Striking joint laxity.

Investigations

- Cardiac, genetic, and ophthalmic, according to specialist expertise.
- Radiographs of spine.
- MRI prior to surgery to check for dural ectasia.
- Cardiac studies prior to anaesthesia.

Orthopaedic management

- Generally non-operative, with high recurrence rate after soft tissue correction and significant anaesthetic risks.
- Protrusio acetabulae usually requires hip replacement if symptomatic (once skeletally mature).
- Scoliosis and kyphosis may require anterior discectomy with posterior fusion and instrumentation.

Ehlers–Danlos syndromes

- Clinically and genetically heterogeneous group of heritable CTDs.
- The International Consortium on Ehlers–Danlos Syndromes proposed an updated classification in 2017: 13 subtypes, but with much clinical overlap. Genetic testing needed to show variant and characterize subtype.
- Autosomal dominant and autosomal recessive inheritance patterns across the subtypes.

Clinical features

- Classically (Villefranche major criteria):
  - Hyperextensibility of skin
  - Joint hypermobility
  - Tissue fragility—atopic scarring and bruising.
- Multiple other (minor) criteria with less diagnostic specificity:
  - Smooth and velvety skin, molluscoid pseudotumours, subcutaneous spheroids/spherules

- Complications of joint hypermobility (sprains, dislocations/subluxations, pes planus). Muscle hypotonia. Delayed gross motor development. Musculoskeletal pain
- Manifestations of tissue extensibility and fragility (e.g. hiatus hernia, anal prolapse in childhood, cervical insufficiency, vascular aneurysms); easy bruising
- Surgical complications (post-operative herniae)
- Positive family history.

Management
- *General:* skin care, avoid trauma, avoid sun exposure; plastic surgery for pseudotumours, careful wound closure.
- *Musculoskeletal:* physiotherapy for children with hypotonia and delayed development. Light, non-weight-bearing muscle-strengthening isometric training for hypermobile, painful joints. Avoid competitive sports with heavy lifting. Splints, orthotics, and bracing may help. Surgery may have a role, albeit with unpredictable results (spine/joint stabilization).

Homocystinuria

- Rare inherited metabolic disorder: ↑ blood and urine concentration of homocysteine, a sulfur-containing amino acid.
- Reduced cystathionine β-synthase (CBS) enzyme activity (conversion of methionine to cysteine; gene locus 21q22): homocysteine and methionine accumulate in tissues and impair cross-linking of collagen fibres.
- Incidence of 1 in 344,000 worldwide (higher in Ireland: 1 in 65,000); autosomal recessive inheritance. Usually presents by age of 4 years.
- Fifty per cent are responsive to pyridoxine (vitamin B6); milder disease.

Clinical features
- *Skeletal:* marfanoid habitus (main differential), with normal to tall stature (occasionally failure to thrive in infancy), fine and brittle hair, hypopigmentation, high-arched palate, crowded teeth, arachnodactyly, limited joint mobility, pectus excavatum/carinatum, and kyphoscoliosis.
- *Ophthalmological:* dislocation of the lens, usually downward and medially (ectopia lentis), myopia, glaucoma.
- *Neurological:* general learning disability (average IQ 80; 30% have normal IQ), seizures, cerebrovascular events, psychiatric disorders.

Investigations
- Homocysteine/methionine levels, urinary amino acids, CBS activity.

Management
- Pyridoxine (vitamin B6) is the drug of choice; patients may be divided into pyridoxine-sensitive and pyridoxine-insensitive (methionine-restricted diet).

Further reading

Shirley ED, Sponseller PD. Marfan syndrome. *Journal of the American Academy of Orthopaedic Surgeons.* 2009;**17**(9):572–81.

Chapter 22

Paediatric orthopaedics: spine

Chiari malformation

There are four types of hindbrain abnormalities, classified based upon the severity and nature of the anatomic defect. 'Chiari malformation' is the preferred nomenclature for Chiari type I malformation. The term 'Arnold–Chiari malformation' is used for the type II malformation. Types III and IV are more uncommon.

Chiari I

- A heterogeneous entity, with the common feature of impaired CSF circulation through the foramen magnum. Named after Hans Chiari, who described it in the 1890s. May be congenital or acquired. Least severe.
- The cerebellar tonsils (±medulla oblongata) herniate >5mm below the foramen magnum (below the McRae line, from the basion to the opisthion).
- Average age of presentation is 41 years. ♀ > ♂. Often found incidentally.
- MRI of the brain and cervical spine is the most useful investigation to make the diagnosis.
- Syringomyelia (fluid-filled cavity within the spinal cord) is present in 30–70% of the cases; can lead to neurological deficit.

Presenting symptoms
Variable but may include:
- Pain—commonest symptom; headache, particularly in the suboccipital region; or neck pain.
- Weakness, sensory disturbance, dysphagia, diplopia, tinnitus, vomiting, incoordination.

Associated abnormalities
- Syrinx.
- Scoliosis.
- Hydrocephalus.
- Basilar impression.

Chiari II (Arnold–Chiari malformation)

- Brainstem herniation; caudally dislocated cervico-medullary junction, pons, fourth ventricle, and medulla.
- Usually associated with myelomeningocele and hydrocephalus.
- Presents at birth or in childhood with brainstem and lower cranial nerves dysfunction.

Chiari III and IV

Type III is rare. The original description cited dislocation of the cerebellum below the foramen magnum into an occipital encephalocele. Prognosis is poor for most, as it is usually incompatible with life. Type IV is cerebellar hypoplasia without herniation, associated with a small posterior fossa.

Management

- Asymptomatic patients may be monitored and operated upon if they become symptomatic.
- Symptomatic and stable patients may be considered for observation, with surgery indicated in case of deterioration.

- Closure of spina bifida defects.
- CSF shunting to relieve hydrocephalus.
- Surgical decompression: relieves pressure on the neural elements and restores CSF flow, which can reverse hydrocephalus and syringomyelia:
  - Anterior (transoral clivus–odontoid resection)
  - Posterior (suboccipital craniectomy).
- Drainage of syrinx by direct aspiration or surgical myelotomy.

Myelodysplasia (spina bifida)

Congenital neural tube defect in which there is incomplete closure of the neural tube, resulting in prolapse of the dural sac containing the spinal cord and nerve roots. Typically affects the lumbosacral spine. Prevention by early prenatal administration of folic acid.

Description

- Spina bifida/myelodysplasia = any congenital defect involving insufficient closure of the spine (Fig. 22.1):
  - Spina bifida occulta: defect in the vertebral arch, but confined cord and meninges
  - Meningocele: protruding sac, but no neural elements
  - Myelomeningocele: protruding sac with neural elements; accounts for 75% of all cases of spina bifida aperta
  - Rachischisis: neural elements exposed, with no covering.

Incidence and aetiology

- Up to 15% for spina bifida occulta; incidence of 0.1–5 per 1000 births for other types.
- Risk factors: folate deficiency (supplementation ↓ the risk by 70%), maternal hyperthermia, maternal diabetes, sodium valproate.
- Up to 10% have chromosomal abnormality (trisomy 13/18/triploidy).

Risk factors

- Lack of prenatal folic acid, medications/drugs (folate antagonist, valproic acid, cocaine), mothers with 5,10-methylenetetrahydrofolate reductase (*MTHFR*) gene polymorphism, Maternal heat exposure in the form of hot tubs, saunas, or fever; obesity.

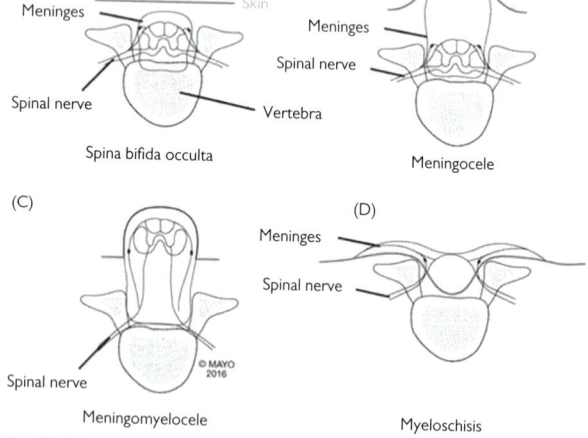

(A)

Skin

Meninges

Spinal nerve

Vertebra

Spina bifida occulta

(B)

Meninges

Spinal nerve

Meningocele

(C)

Spinal nerve

© MAYO 2016

Meningomyelocele

(D)

Meninges

Spinal nerve

Myeloschisis

Fig. 22.1 Spectrum of spina bifida.

Clinical manifestations

- Midline defect in posterior elements of vertebrae may be noted at birth (or antenatally), with protrusion of meninges and neural elements into the dural sac.
- Spina bifida occulta may be indicated by a tuft of hair overlying or dimpling of the sacrum.
- USS useful for confirmation.
- Prognosis: survival and neurological impairment depend on level of spinal segment involved: untreated = 90% mortality; L3 or above, confined to wheelchair; L5, good prognosis for ambulation.

Special considerations

- Immunoglobulin E (IgE)-mediated latex allergy—present in 20–70% of patients.
- Can result in profound anaphylaxis—usually first on any surgical list.

Neurological deficit

- Variable motor (including paraplegia) ± sensory deficit; functional motor level may not exactly correspond to anatomical level of defect.
- Neurogenic bladder can cause urinary incontinence, recurrent UTIs, and high-pressure renal impairment.
- Arnold–Chiari type II malformation; hydrocephalus is common; tethering of cord distally can cause cerebellar herniation.
- Seizures and meningitis.

Musculoskeletal problems

- Deformities related to functional level of lesion, including:
  - Scoliosis:
    - Congenital—associated with underlying vertebral anomaly
    - Acquired—related to muscle imbalance (40–60% of those with myelomeningocele)
  - Severe kyphosis (gibbus)
  - Hip subluxation/dislocation
  - Contractures: hip abduction and external rotation, fixed knee flexion, ankle equinus (often equinocavovarus).

Prenatal detection of neural tube defects

- *Serum α-fetoprotein (AFP)*: high maternal serum AFP level between 15 and 20 weeks' gestation carries a higher risk of neural tube defects.
- *USS*: prenatal USS will detect 90–95% of cases of spina bifida. It can be correlated with high AFP level to differentiate neural tube defects from other non-neurological causes of elevated AFP level.
- *Amniocentesis*: AFP level in amniotic fluid is elevated with open neural tube defects, with a peak between 13 and 15 weeks of pregnancy. The procedure carries a 6% risk of fetal loss.

Investigations (postnatal)

- MRI to image the spinal cord.
- Plain radiographs to assess for scoliosis and hip dysplasia/dislocation.
- CT of the brain/USS of the head to assess hydrocephalus.

Management

- *Functional:* physiotherapy, occupational therapy, orthoses.
- Orthopaedic goals must align closely with functional aims.
- *Neurosurgical:* repair of defect as indicated and release, or correction, of associated cord anomalies and hydrocephalus (survival rates dramatically improved with antibiotics and improvements in neurosurgical techniques).

Orthopaedic management

- *Scoliosis:* bracing is ineffective; fusion for severe curves, preserving lumbosacral motion in ambulant children to assist with gait.
- *Hip dislocation:* previously aggressive approach now has more functional focus; reconstruct unilateral hip dislocations in ambulators with low (sacral) level lesion; bilateral and higher lesions unlikely to cause disability, so left alone; muscle transfers no longer performed; contracture release alone indicated for unbalanced pelvis.
- *Knee disorders:* weak quadriceps treated with KAFO; flexion contracture impairs KAFO use, so may be corrected surgically; rotational abnormality correction restores lever arms for muscle function.
- *Foot disorders:* common (60–90%); incidence of 30% of clubfoot (talipes equinovarus) with myelodysplasia—rigid and insensate, so high complications with casting, lower threshold for surgical releases; dorsiflexion deformity with L5/sacral level patients due to unopposed tibialis anterior activity—anterior release and tendon lengthening; vertical talus also common—serial casting alone insufficient.
- *General principles for foot deformity:* high risk of pressure ulceration, so arthrodesis avoided. Supple, deformed, but braceable foot is always preferable; tendon releases preferable to transfers, and extra-articular bony procedures ideal to preserve motion.

Other considerations

- *Meningitis:* particularly if there is direct exposure of meninges or neural tissue.
- *Bladder/bowel dysfunction:* neurogenic bladder can lead to recurrent urinary sepsis.
- *Sensory loss:* predisposes to development of pressure sores.
- *Motor loss:* weakness and spasticity can lead to scoliosis, hip dislocation, lower limb contractures, and foot deformities.
- *Neurosurgical problems:* Chiari II malformation, syrinx formation, dermoid tumour, hydrocephalus, and tethered cord.
- *Psychological problems:* mild developmental difficulties, depression.

Outcome

- With no treatment, only 14–30% of spina bifida aperta infants survive infancy.
- With treatment, 85% of infants survive.
- The commonest cause of early mortality is complications from Chiari malformation (respiratory problems) where late mortality is related to shunt malfunction.
- Eighty per cent will have normal IQ. Learning difficulties are most closely related to shunt infection.

Further reading

Swaroop VT, Dias L. Orthopedic management of spina bifida. Part I: hip, knee, and rotational deformities. *Journal of Children's Orthopaedics*. 2009;**3**(6):441–9.

Swaroop VT, Dias L. Orthopaedic management of spina bifida. Part II: foot and ankle deformities. *Journal of Children's Orthopaedics*. 2011;**5**(6):403–14.

Poliomyelitis

Caused by viral destruction of the anterior horn cells of the spinal cord, classically resulting in motor weakness (flaccid paralysis) with preserved sensation.

Aetiology

- Caused by a high-infectivity enterovirus; main route of infection is via the GI tract (faeco-oral transmission) in humans.
- Three serotypes: P1, P2, and P3.
- Serotype P1 accounts for 85% of paralytic disease (prior to the introduction of vaccine).
- Ninety-five per cent of infections are asymptomatic (in an immunocompetent host) or result in minor flu-like illness; <1% of infections result in flaccid paralysis.

Vaccination

- Parenteral inactivated vaccine (Salk) introduced in 1956 for routine immunization. Reduced incidence of poliomyelitis by 90% in the USA.
- Enteral live attenuated vaccine (Sabin) replaced Salk in 1962; cheap, taken orally, and excreted in faeces, leading to herd immunity.
- However, with excretion of live virus, there is a small incidence of vaccine-induced paralytic poliomyelitis in non-immunized direct contacts.
- In the UK, children currently receive parenteral vaccination as part of the national immunization programme.
- The WHO aims to eradicate polio globally—currently only endemic in Pakistan and Afghanistan.

Clinical features

- *Acute poliomyelitis*—minor or major:
  - *Minor:* 1–3 days before paralysis, GI complaints, systemic manifestations (sore throat, fever, malaise, headache); duration 2–8 weeks
  - *Major:* all forms of CNS disease caused by poliovirus (aseptic meningitis (non-paralytic), polio encephalitis, bulbar polio, paralytic poliomyelitis, and combinations).
- *Clinical signs:* fever, nuchal rigidity (stiff neck), pleocytosis in CSF; asymmetrical muscle weakness; rarely transverse myelitis features.
- *Recovery/convalescent stage:* acute symptoms and myalgia resolve; paralysis starts to recover; duration 2 years.
- *Residual paralysis stage:* no further recovery of muscle power—deformities may progress.
- *Post-polio syndrome:* late manifestations occurring in patients aged 30–40 years after acute illness; 25–60% suffer this; cause unknown—not virus reactivation, probably degenerative disease in affected individuals.

Diagnosis

- Serological diagnosis. PCR is technique of choice for identifying serotype and differentiating between wild-type and vaccine-induced poliomyelitis.
- CSF: usually an ↑ in WCC and mildly elevated protein level.

Differential diagnosis
- Infection by other enteroviruses or flavivirus.
- Tickborne encephalitis.
- Guillain–Barré syndrome.
- Acute intermittent porphyria.
- HIV neuropathy.
- Diphtheria.
- Disorders of neuromuscular junction.

Management
- *Acute poliomyelitis:* strict bed rest and analgesia; physiotherapy/orthotics to prevent contractures; ventilatory support as required.
- *Recovery/convalescent/residual stage:* physiotherapy, including stretching, muscle retraining, and splintage of limbs to prevent deformity; orthoses may be used to compensate for loss of function and improve mobility; orthopaedic surgery may be needed to address deformities, typically:
  - External tibial torsion
  - Genu valgum
  - Genu recurvatum
  - Equinus deformities
  - Pes cavovarus
  - Toe clawing.

Further reading
Watts HG. Orthopedic techniques in the management of the residua of paralytic poliomyelitis. *Techniques in Orthopaedics*. 2005;**20**(2):179–89.

Torticollis

From Latin *torti* (twisted) and *collis* (neck). It arises from involuntary contraction of the neck muscles, leading to abnormal posture and movement of the head. It is a combined deformity of head tilt and rotation involving the cervical spine.

Epidemiology

Torticollis can occur at any age in children.

Congenital muscular torticollis (CMT) is the commonest form of torticollis. It is estimated to involve 0.3–2% of all newborns. It occurs because of trauma to the sternocleidomastoid (SCM) muscle and is often seen in the first 2 months after birth. There is an ↑ incidence following breech and forceps deliveries, as well as in first-born children. It can sometimes be associated with other packaging problems, including facial asymmetry (reduced facial growth on the affected side), plagiocephaly, and congenital foot and hip problems.

Atlanto-axial rotatory subluxation (AARS) is the commonest acquired form of childhood torticollis. It usually follows trauma or infection (upper respiratory tract infection—Grisel's syndrome) in up to 50% of cases. It may also occur following head/neck surgery (20% of cases).

Spasmodic torticollis is a type of dystonia affecting the muscles of the neck, resulting in involuntary muscle contraction. It often involves the trapezius and SCM muscles, which results in abnormal head posture.

Aetiology

- *Congenital:* occipito-vertebral bone anomalies, neck skin webbing. Commonest is CMT.
- *Acquired:* idiopathic, neurogenic (spinal cord and posterior fossa tumours, syringomyelia, bulbar palsies, tumours, ocular problems, drug-induced dystonia (e.g. phenothiazines), inflammatory (pyogenic, rheumatoid, tuberculous), or traumatic (AARS, fractures).

Congenital muscular torticollis

Clinical

The child presents with their head tilted towards the affected side (facing upwards or downwards), rotation of the chin to the contralateral side, and restricted passive and active neck movements. They may have neck pain, but this condition is usually painless. The head is typically held in a position flexed away from the pain. Movements may be intermittent or abnormal posture. The head and neck may be fixed by continuous muscle spasm. A small knot may be palpable in the involved SCM on the involved side—an SCM tumour (not a true malignancy, but a fibrous mass in one of the SCM muscles, representing a reaction to intrauterine or birth trauma).

Natural history

In most cases, torticollis resolves in several days to weeks. A few children develop neck problems lasting for months to years. Persistent neck muscle spasms may require referral to a neurologist or surgeon.

Investigations
- *Radiology:* plain cervical radiographs are indicated to ensure the deformity is purely due to a muscular problem, and not due to structural pathology of the base of the skull or cervical spine.
- *CT:* used to establish if there is fixed rotation and to define bony elements of the skull and cervical spine.
- *MRI:* used to detect brain, spinal cord, nerve root, and intervertebral disc abnormalities. Also useful when an inflammatory process, infection, or neoplasm is suspected. Will require general anaesthesia in younger patients.

Management
- *Non-operative:* gentle, daily manipulation of the neck with stretching exercises to try and tilt the head to the opposite side. Passive stretching is successful in resolving torticollis in 90–95% of cases, in the first year of life. Invasive, but non-operative, options aim to relax the contracted neck muscles and focus on preventing involuntary muscle contraction. These include local injection of botulinum toxin to paralyse affected muscles or ablation of the nerve supply to the affected muscles (selective denervation).
- *Operative:* surgery is reserved only for a few selected cases. SCM release is indicated for failure of non-operative treatment. It should be performed after 2 years of age. It involves division of the lower ends of the two heads of the SCM and overlying tight fascia. The incision is just superior to the clavicle. Structures at risk are the carotid vessels and jugular vein. Division of the proximal part of the SCM is more difficult and places the spinal accessory nerve at risk. Complications include persistent pain, scar tissue formation, recurrence (usually from inadequate release), and neurovascular injury. Operative measures resolve the torticollis in ~92% of patients selected for operative intervention.

Atlantoaxial rotatory subluxation

Clinical
The child presents with a 'cock robin' appearance—the head is rotated to the opposite side of the subluxation, whereas the SCM spasm is on the same side as the tilt; a left-sided subluxation therefore causes chin rotation to the right, with a right SCM spasm. This is the opposite to what happens in CMT, in which the ipsilateral SCM is shortened and spastic. Pain is a feature of this form of torticollis. The deformity may be mobile or fixed. If untreated, head and facial asymmetry may develop.

Investigations
- *Radiology:* plain radiographs should include AP, lateral, and open mouth views.
- *CT:* dynamic CT (with the head rotated maximally to each side) should be performed to confirm the diagnosis and determine any deformity. Dynamic CT is considered the gold standard in diagnosing AARS and differentiates this from positional asymmetry.

Management
- *Non-operative:* may resolve spontaneously, but if it does not, then it should be treated with a soft collar and physiotherapy if the patient presents within 1 week. If it does not reduce within 1 week, then halter traction is needed, followed by serial monitoring. Halo traction followed by a Halo vest can be tried if 2 weeks of halter traction fails or if the presentation is after 4 weeks from onset.
- *Operative:* surgery indicated for failed reduction after 2 weeks of Halo traction or if the patient presents after 3 months from onset. Neurological deficit is another indication for surgery. The subluxation should be corrected, and the C1/C2 vertebrae fused to prevent recurrent subluxation.

Further reading

Ghanem I, El Hage S, Rachkidi R, Kharrat K, Dagher F, Kreichati G. Pediatric cervical spine instability. *Journal of Children's Orthopaedics.* 2008;**2**(2):71–84.

Lustrin ES, Karakas SP, Ortiz AO, *et al.* Pediatric cervical spine: normal anatomy, variants, and trauma. *Radiographics.* 2003;**23**(3):539–60.

Scoliosis in children

Deformity of the spine in the coronal plane of >10°.

Classification

The two main groups are:
- Postural scoliosis
- Structural scoliosis.

The latter is further subclassified into congenital, idiopathic, neuromuscular, and miscellaneous groups.

Congenital scoliosis

Fig. 22.2 shows different types of vertebral anomalies that produce congenital kyphosis or kyphoscoliosis.

Classification

Failure of formation
- Complete hemivertebra: fully segmented.
- Semi-segmented or non-segmented: incarcerated or non-incarcerated.
- Incomplete or partial vertebra: wedge or butterfly vertebra.

Failure of segmentation
- Unilateral bar or bilateral bar (block vertebra).
- Mixed variety.

Description

Lateral curvature of the spine secondary to developmental vertebral anomalies producing imbalance of longitudinal growth. The hallmark is vertebral anomaly. There is a very high incidence of both intraspinal and extraspinal associated anomalies (VACTERL).

Investigations

MRI is essential. Intraspinal lesions include diastematomyelia, tethered spinal cord, syringomyelia, and low conus. Skin abnormalities (hairy patch, dimple in the midline) may herald a congenital vertebral anomaly. Neurological assessment is essential.

Management

Bracing is not usually successful. Surgical treatment is indicated if non-operative treatment measures fail. Operative options include: posterior *in situ* fusion, combined posterior hemiarthrodesis and anterior hemiepiphysiodesis to arrest growth on the convex side, instrumented stabilization (growing rods), and instrumented fusion.

Idiopathic scoliosis

Idiopathic scoliosis is the commonest type of scoliosis in children (Fig. 22.3).

Classification
- Infantile before age of 3 years.
- Juvenile between 4 and 9 years.
- Adolescent idiopathic scoliosis after 10 years of age.

These age distinctions have prognostic significance.

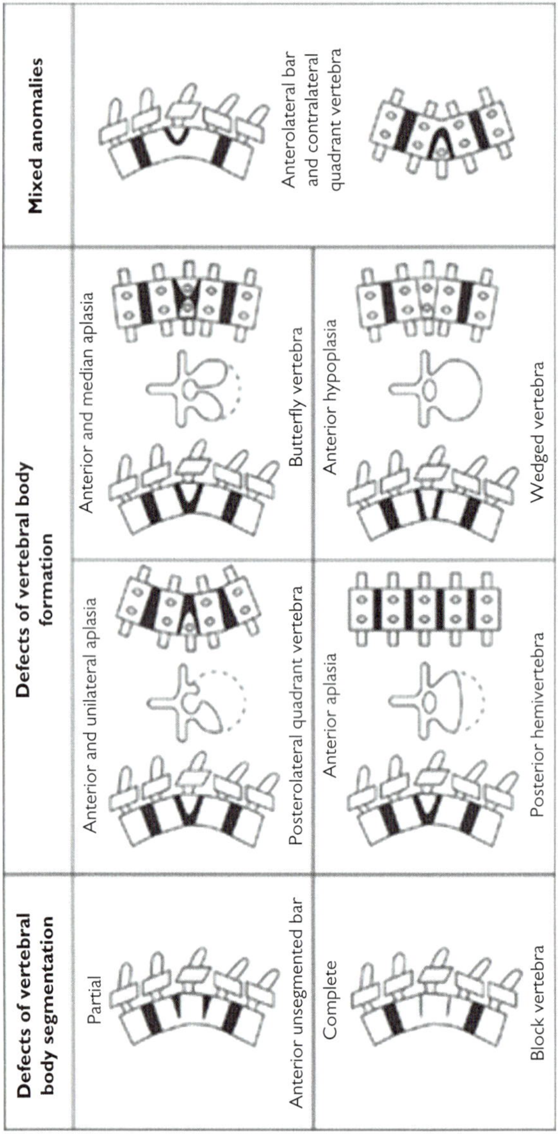

Fig. 22.2 Different types of vertebral anomalies that produce congenital kyphosis or kyphoscoliosis.

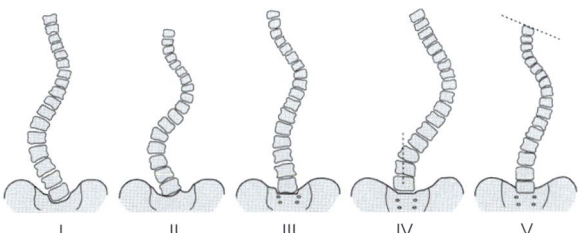

Fig. 22.3 King–Moe classification system for idiopathic scoliosis. Type I, primary lumbar curve greater than the compensatory thoracic curve; type II, primary thoracic curve with compensatory lumbar curve; type III, short pure thoracic curve; type IV, long C-shaped thoracolumbar curve; type V, double thoracic curve, with extension into the cervical spine and compensatory lumbar curve.

Reproduced from Bulstrode *et al.*, *Oxford Textbook of Orthopaedics and Trauma*, with permission from Oxford University Press.

Epidemiology

Prevalence of idiopathic scoliosis is 0.5%.

Aetiology

The aetiology is unknown and is likely multifactorial. Disorganized skeletal growth, hormonal factors (melatonin), and a neurological deficit (posterior column lesion) have been implicated in the development of idiopathic scoliosis.

Clinical

Most children present with a deformity of the trunk, different shoulder heights, asymmetrical chest or waist creases, or apparent limb length discrepancy. Obtain a detailed family history and birth history, and confirm developmental milestones (mental and physical) and neurological symptoms. On examination, look for shoulder height asymmetry, protruding scapulae, hip asymmetry, frontal asymmetry, abnormal creases, hairy patches, and café-au-lait spots. Palpate the curve. Drop a 'plumb line' (a straight line from the centre of C7 vertebral body in the sagittal plane should pass through the posterior–superior corner of S1) to assess spinal balance (line anterior = positive; line posterior = negative). Forward bending confirms whether the curve is postural (corrects) or structural (no correction), and establishes the degree of flexibility. In the commonest curve pattern (right thoracic), the right shoulder is rotated forward and the medial border of the right scapula protrudes posteriorly. A complete neurological assessment is required. Hamstring tightness should be established. Measure leg lengths; if there is a discrepancy, correct by using blocks to see if the curve disappears (suggesting compensatory curve due to leg length discrepancy). Skeletal maturity must be assessed—Risser staging commonly used (Fig. 22.4). Peak growth velocity occurs before Risser 1. Sander's classification, closure of the medial olecranon apophysis, and evaluation of hand radiographs with a Greulich and Pyle atlas are other useful radiological techniques to estimate skeletal maturity.

Risser stage

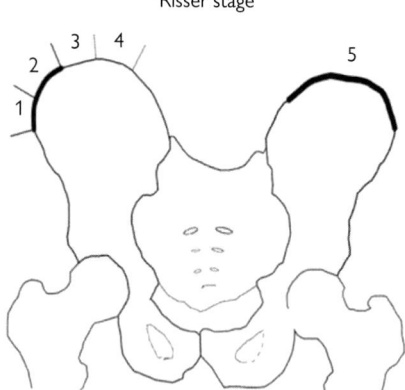

Fig. 22.4 Risser staging.

Infantile idiopathic scoliosis (under 3 years of age)

Description

Association with congenital cardiac pathologies, DDH, breech presentation, ↑ maternal age, inguinal herniae, and spinal cord anomalies. Some may resolve with time. ♂ tend to have left thoracic curves.

Investigations

Measurements of the curve is via the rib vertebral angle difference (RVAD) of Mehta or the Cobb angle (Fig. 22.5). All need MRI to rule out spinal dysraphism.

Management

Serial body casting is the mainstay of treatment in infantile idiopathic scoliosis. Curves are likely to deteriorate if they are >40° or if the rib vertebral angle difference is >20°.

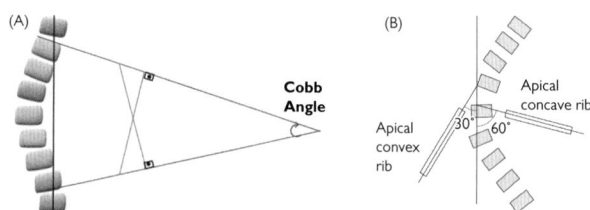

Fig. 22.5 (A) Cobb angle. (B) Rib vertebral angle difference of Mehta.

Juvenile idiopathic scoliosis (3–10 years of age)

Description

Commoner in ♀. The thoracic curve can be to the left or to the right. Lumbar curves are rare. About 70% of juvenile idiopathic curves progress and need some form of treatment; 50% require surgery. A high incidence of intraspinal pathology is reported.

Investigations

MRI is essential.

Management

Curves >40–45° will progress and need surgery. Surgery varies, depending on the type of curve. Growing rod constructs may be used, with other options including posterior fusion, anterior fusion, or combined anterior and posterior fusion. Beware the 'Crankshaft' phenomenon—(excessive) anterior growth after posterior fusion alone, which may result in spinal rotation.

Adolescent idiopathic scoliosis

Description

Curve patterns in adolescent idiopathic scoliosis can be classified using the King–Moe (Fig. 22.3) and Lenke's classification systems (the latter has gained popularity and is now more widely used). The likelihood of progression depends on the size of the curve and on skeletal and physiological maturity—more mature patients with smaller curves have a lower risk of progression. The Adam's forward bending test is a simple and effective screening tool to identify scoliosis.

Investigations

- *Plain radiographs:* AP and lateral standing views (including the pelvis) are used to characterize the deformity. Bending views are helpful in determining flexibility and to differentiate structural (inflexible) from compensatory curves (flexible). Assess the Risser stage, and measure the Cobb angle.
- *MRI:* used to exclude intraspinal pathology if this is suggested by clinical assessment.
- *Other tests:* perform pulmonary function testing in patients with moderate to large deformities.

Management

- *Non-operative:* either observation or orthotic use. Observation includes interval radiographs to evaluate progression. Electrical muscle stimulation, physiotherapy, manipulation, and nutritional therapies are ineffective. Children with curves as small as 20° and who are Risser 0 should be braced early. Bracing can also be effective in reducing curve progression in older children with modest curves (20–39°). It is recommended that bracing should be for 23h/day. Problems include pressure effects (local pain) and psychosocial issues, resulting in poor compliance.
- *Operative:* if non-operative measures fail or with curves >45°. Spinal fusion remains the gold standard. The goals are to safely correct the deformity and achieve a solid bony fusion. A posterior or anterior

approach can be used. An anterior release can be performed prior to posterior fusion. Modern instrumentation allows for adequate curve correction. Intraoperative monitoring during surgery can allow early recognition and treatment of spinal cord dysfunction. Somatosensory and motor evoked potentials (SSEPs) are commonly used to monitor spinal cord function. The Stagnara wake-up test may also be employed in certain cases. Complications include excessive bleeding, infections (including delayed), usually caused by low-virulence organisms such as *Propionibacterium acnes*, and spinal cord or nerve root injury. Other complications include pneumothorax, vascular or visceral injury, pseudarthrosis, persistent pain, progressive deformity, and broken instrumentation. Clinical outcomes are strongly linked with curve magnitude. Regardless of treatment, patients with scoliosis have a higher self-reported rate of arthritis and back pain, alongside poorer perceptions of their overall health and body image.

Neuromuscular scoliosis

Description

Typically long C-type curves that involve the entire thoracic and lumbar spine—may extend from the neck to the sacrum.

Classification

- *Neuropathic:* CP, spinocerebellar degeneration (Friedreich's ataxia), myelomeningocele, syringomyelia, cord tumour or trauma, spinal muscular atrophy, LMN problems (poliomyelitis).
- *Myopathic:* arthrogryposis, muscular dystrophy, myotonia, NF, mesenchymal, Marfan syndrome, Ehler–Danlos syndrome, homocystinuria.
- *Miscellaneous:* post-laminectomy, post-trauma.

Management

- *Non-operative:* bracing, wheelchair modification.
- *Operative:* spinal fusion with instrumentation. Aim for a balanced spine, with the head centred over the pelvis.

Further reading

King HA, Moe JH, Bradford DS, Winter RB. The selection of fusion levels in thoracic idiopathic scoliosis. *Journal of Bone and Joint Surgery (American Volume)*. 1983;**65**(9):1302–13.

Lenke LG, Betz RR, Harms J, *et al.* Adolescent idiopathic scoliosis: a new classification to determine extent of spinal arthrodesis. *Journal of Bone and Joint Surgery*. 2001;**83**(8):1169–81.

Sitoula P, Verma K, Holmes L, *et al.* Prediction of curve progression in idiopathic scoliosis. *Spine*. 2015;**40**(13):1006–13.

Kyphosis in children

Kyphosis is an excessive curvature of the spine in the sagittal plane. There is wide variation in normal range, but the average thoracic curve is 40°. There is an initial ↑ with age, with a peak at 14 years.

Classification

Congenital kyphosis
- *Type I:* failure of segmentation.
- *Type II:* failure of formation.
- *Type III:* mixed.

Acquired kyphosis
- Scheuermann's disease.
- Postural round back.
- Inflammatory.
- Metabolic.
- Post-traumatic.
- Iatrogenic.
- Neoplastic.

Congenital kyphosis

Description
Congenital deformities in the sagittal plane, similar to those in the coronal plane. Congenital deformities are rarely seen in the sagittal plane alone; they are associated with other vertebral anomalies, nervous system anomalies, or pathology related to other organ systems. There may be skin breakdown, abdominal viscera compression, pulmonary impairment (>100° thoracic region), and poor sitting posture. A severe angular deformity may develop with a gibbus at the apex. Congenital kyphosis often progresses rapidly if untreated and may lead to paralysis (type I).

Investigations
- *Radiographs:* AP and lateral erect and lateral hyperextension views are used to characterize the deformity.
- *CT:* used to define bony anatomy, especially in surgical planning.
- *MRI:* to evaluate the spinal canal and neural elements.

Management
- *Non-operative:* almost no role for non-operative treatment. Bracing is ineffective. Traction contraindicated due to risk of paralysis.
- *Operative:* posterior *in situ* fusion alone can be used to treat children aged <5 years with curves <50°, as some correction of kyphosis occurs with growth. Anterior fusion may be indicated for older children and those with modest curves. Anterior and posterior fusion is usually necessary for children aged >5 years with curves >50°. Instrumentation may aid in correction of the deformity. Children with secondary neurological deficits should have decompression of neural elements.

Scheuermann's kyphosis

The commonest cause of acquired kyphosis in children. Defined as a rigid thoracic hyperkyphosis >45°, with >5° wedging in three consecutive vertebrae.

Description

AVN of the ring apophysis occurs due to excess mechanical stress. Herniation of disc material occurs through end plates (Schmorl's nodes).

Epidemiology

The incidence of kyphosis due to Scheuermann's disease is 0.4–0.8%. ♂:♀ ratio is equal. Does not occur in children aged <10 years; peak incidence in boys aged 10–12 years.

Aetiology

Remains unknown. This is a defect of endochondral ossification (in the secondary ossification centres of vertebrae).

Clinical

Activity-related pain is a common complaint, usually at the apex of the curve; this is often self-limiting. The cosmetic effects of the kyphosis often concern adolescents. Examination reveals an adolescent with poor posture, ↑ kyphosis, and tight hamstrings. Backache or tenderness may be found. The deformity becomes more prominent with the Adam's forward bending test. Neurological deficits are rare.

Investigations

- *Radiographs:* erect AP and standing views, and a lateral hyperextension view are indicated. Criteria for diagnosis include irregular end plates, narrowing of disc spaces, three consecutive vertebrae with wedging of >5° each, and kyphosis >45°. Associated radiographic findings include disc space narrowing, end plate irregularities, spondylolysis, and scoliosis. Lumbar disease, which is less common, does not have wedging. There is an ↑ incidence of spondylolysis in Scheuermann's disease.

Management

Bracing or surgery can be used to correct the kyphosis.

- *Non-operative:* patients with curves <50° are treated with observation and physical therapies. In skeletally immature patients with significant kyphosis that is painful or deteriorating, bracing is used. It should be continued to skeletal maturity. Bracing is most effective where the apex of the kyphosis is below T7 or the curve is small.
- *Operative:* surgery is usually undertaken if the kyphosis is >75°. Posterior instrumented fusion might be needed, along with posterior corrective osteotomies ± anterior release.

Postural round back deformity

Modest kyphosis of 40–60° is usually found. It is correctable and vertebral morphology is normal. If diagnosed after 13 years, Scheuermann's disease needs to be excluded. Rehabilitation includes postural and hyperextension exercises. Bracing may be required.

Further reading

McMaster MJ, Singh H. The surgical management of congenital kyphosis and kyphoscoliosis. *Spine.* 2001;**26**(19):2146–54.

Spondylolysis and spondylolisthesis in children

Spondylolysis is a fatigue fracture of the pars interarticularis. The commonest level is L5. Bilateral superior articular processes are in continuity with the pedicles and vertebral body, but most of the lamina, spinous process, and inferior articular processes are detached. *Spondylolisthesis* is the anterior slippage of one vertebra on another.

Spondylolisthesis

Classification

Wiltse and Newman classification:
- Type I: congenital or dysplastic
- Type II: isthmic:
  - IIa: spondylolysis
  - IIb: isthmic elongation
  - IIc: acute fracture
- Type III: degenerative
- Type IV: traumatic
- Type V: pathological.

Aetiology

Spondylolysis is associated with prolonged erect posture and sports involving hyperextension. An inherited form has been identified.

Spondylolisthesis only affects humans; 90% of cases occur in the lumbar spine at L5. The majority are isthmic (i.e. associated with spondylolysis). Dysplastic spondylolisthesis is rare and occurs due to congenital changes in the upper sacrum. The disc below the listhesis is usually pathological, and the disc above may be degenerate. May be associated with lumbar scoliosis, primarily due to rotation with forward slippage of one vertebra on another.

Natural history

The vast majority settle as the slip stabilizes. Patients with some forms of isthmic spondylolisthesis develop back and leg pain symptoms. It is difficult to predict who will become symptomatic. Risk factors for progression are young age, ♀ sex, type of slip, degree of slip (>50%), and radiological evidence of instability.

Clinical

Most children with spondylolisthesis are asymptomatic. It is the commonest cause of back pain in adolescents and is associated with sporting activities and occasionally trauma. Back pain usually begins with walking or standing. It is activity-related. The pain can radiate to the buttock or lateral aspect of the thigh/calf. When severe, it can cause gait disturbance, numbness, or muscle weakness. Signs of cauda equina compression may develop. Claudication may signal lateral recess stenosis.

Examination

On examination, there is flattening of the back (loss of lordosis) and a spinous process step-off may be palpable. Hamstrings are usually tight. Examination must include assessment of distal neurology.

Investigations

- *Radiographs*: a lateral view will show the extent of the slip. The film should be centred on the lumbosacral junction. The percentage slip is calculated by measuring the relative displacement of one vertebra to an adjacent vertebra. The slip is graded as follows: grade I, <25%; grade II, 25–50%; grade III, 50–75%; grade IV, 75–100%; and grade V, >100% (spondyloptosis) (Fig. 22.6). The slip angle can also be measured on a lateral radiograph. The actual defect is to the pars interarticularis and can be seen in 80% of lesions (a proportion requires oblique views for better visualization—Scottie dog sign of La Chapelle).
- *CT*: can demonstrate lysis, but lesion may be missed if slices are not in the same plane.
- *MRI*: to assess compression of neural elements and state of the disc. With recent advances, this is also as sensitive as SPECT imaging, albeit without the risk of radiation.
- *Bone scans*: may be 'hot' in the acute phase and, if so, suggests a higher likelihood of union.

Management

- *Non-operative*: rest, analgesia, and (if symptoms do not settle) lumbosacral orthosis may be helpful.
- *Operative*: indications for surgery include slip >50% or progressing in adolescents, persistent back and/or leg pain unresponsive to non-operative treatment, and significant neurological deficit. L1–L4 pars interarticularis defects can be repaired primarily in most cases (when there is no or minimal listhesis). Grades I and II: *in situ* L5–S1 posterolateral fusion ± anterior fusion; decompression may be

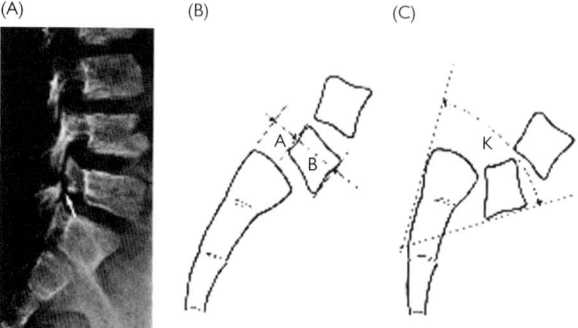

(A)   (B)   (C)

Fig. 22.6 (A) Spondylolysis (arrow) of L5 on a lateral radiograph. (B) Calculation of the amount of vertebral slip according to Laurent and Einola: slip (%) = A/B × 100. (C) Measurement of lumbosacral kyphosis as the angle between the posterior wall of S1 and the anterior (or posterior) wall of L5.

Reproduced from Bulstrode et al., *Oxford Textbook of Orthopaedics and Trauma*, with permission from Oxford University Press.

necessary if there is nerve root compression. Grades III–V: extended *in situ* fusion ± reduction and decompression ± anterior fusion.

Further reading

Crawford CH, Larson AN, Gates M, *et al.* Current evidence regarding the treatment of pediatric lumbar spondylolisthesis: a report from the Scoliosis Research Society Evidence Based Medicine Committee. *Spine Deformity.* 2017;**5**(5):284–302.

Laurent LE, Einola S. Spondylolisthesis in children and adolescents. *Acta Orthopaedica Scandinavica.* 1961;**31**(1):45–64.

Back pain in children: overview

Epidemiology

Back pain is uncommon in children aged <10 years. Only 20% of patients with back pain in this age group are diagnosed with an identifiable cause. Prevalence reaches that of the adult population by the age of 18 years.

Aetiology

The causes of back pain in children include: slipped vertebral apophysis and spondylolisthesis, disc herniation, osteomyelitis, TB, discitis, spinal cord tumours, eosinophilic granuloma, metastatic disease (neuroblastoma), rheumatological disease, and occasionally referred pain from visceral pathology.

All children aged under 12 years with pain for >1 month, night pain, a rigid spine, painful scoliosis, abnormal neurology, weight loss, fever, or a history of NF should be assessed and investigated as a matter of urgency.

Clinical

Children presenting with back pain require careful evaluation. The pain must be fully characterized. A full neurological history must be obtained. A history of trauma is important, in particular of any traumatic event related to recreational or sporting activities. The signs may be difficult to elicit in young children. Look for swelling, deformity, and skin lesions. Examine the gait carefully. Range of motion of the spine is important. Assess if there is any leg length discrepancy, and examine the joints for abnormality. Neurological examination must include power, tone, reflexes (deep tendon and abdominal), sensation (light touch, pin-prick, vibration sense, and proprioception), and nerve root tension signs.

Investigations

These are important in evaluating a child with back pain, especially if there are constitutional symptoms.

Laboratory
• FBC, ESR, CRP. Further studies may be necessary (e.g. RA screen or HLA B27 status).

Radiology
• *Plain radiographs:* should be obtained to look for spondylolisthesis, fractures, and erosions of end plates, and to assess the overall shape of the spine.
• *MRI:* used to look for discitis, disc degeneration, disc prolapse, and pathology involving the spinal cord (syrinx) or nerve roots. Requires general anaesthesia in younger children.

Back pain in children: presentation and treatment of specific disorders

Disc herniation

Clinical

Herniated discs occur less frequently in children than in adults. They often present with back pain radiating into the lower limbs. On examination, signs of radiculopathy may be elicited.

Investigations

The investigation of choice is MRI.

Management

- *Non-operative:* rest and pain control (analgesia and anti-inflammatory medication). Treated for up to 3 months in this way.
- *Operative:* if pain persists or if there is deterioration in neurology, surgery needs to be considered (usually discectomy ± fusion). In children with a congenitally narrow canal, decompression may be necessary.

Slipped vertebral apophysis

Description

Occurs in the lower lumbar spine when fusion between the vertebral ring apophysis and the central cartilage is incomplete. The ring apophysis with adjacent disc is displaced into the vertebral canal. Associated with heavy lifting and vigorous activities.

Clinical

Pain radiating into one or both limbs. Symptoms and signs are similar to those of an acute herniated disc (main differential).

Investigations

- *Radiology:* may show a small bone fragment (edge of ring apophysis) within the spinal canal. Rarely diagnosed on plain radiographs.
- *MRI or CT:* better at detecting bone fragments and are more likely to show the lesion.

Management

- *Non-operative:* usually unsuccessful.
- *Operative:* most patients require surgery to excise the disc and ring apophysis. Simple disc excision is inadequate.

Discitis

(See → Chapter 17, Adult orthopaedics: spine, pp. 558–563.)

Spondylolisthesis

(See → Chapter 17, Adult orthopaedics: spine, pp. 558–563.)

Deformity

Idiopathic scoliosis rarely causes pain. If a deformity is painful, consider syringomyelia, infection, osteoid osteoma, or neoplasm.

Scheuermann's disease

(See ➔ Chapter 7, Adult orthopaedics: spine, pp. 552–553.)

Traumatic back pain

Check for NAI. Fractures are usually painful, and post-traumatic kyphosis can cause severe back pain, particularly if there is progressive vertebral collapse.

Spinal neoplasm

Type of tumours

May be benign or malignant, and intra- or extraosseous. The commonest benign tumours involving the spine are osteoid osteoma, osteoblastoma, aneurysmal bone cyst, and eosinophilic granuloma. Malignant tumours include neuroblastoma, Ewing's sarcoma, and osteosarcoma. Children with acute lymphocytic leukaemia (ALL) sometimes present with back pain.

Clinical

Children with spinal tumours often present with back pain. Be suspicious of a tumour if the child is young (aged <10 years), the pain is constant (with or without night pain), or there is a neurological deficit.

Investigations

MRI is the investigation of choice, as some tumours causing back pain are extraosseous and unlikely to be detected with a bone scan.

Management

Depends on the type of tumour. The commonest tumours (osteoid osteoma and osteoblastoma) can be excised. An MDT approach (including a paediatric oncologist) should be adopted.

Further reading

Brown R, Hussain M, McHugh K, Novelli V, Jones D. Discitis in young children. *Journal of Bone and Joint Surgery (British Volume)*. 2001;**83**(1):106–11.

Garg S, Dormans JP. Tumors and tumor-like conditions of the spine in children. *Journal of the American Academy of Orthopaedic Surgeons*. 2005;**13**(6):372–81.

Ramirez N, Flynn JM, Hill BW, *et al*. Evaluation of a systematic approach to pediatric back pain: the utility of magnetic resonance imaging. *Journal of Pediatric Orthopaedics*. 2015;**35**(1):28–32.

Spinal infections in children

Spinal infections in children are uncommon.

Pyogenic infections

Pathology

Following colonization of the end plates by the causative organism, there is subsequent spread to the disc space, resulting in infection. Untreated, the infection spreads into the adjacent vertebral bodies, destroying bone and forming abscesses.

Clinical

Children may present at any age. Symptoms include fever, reluctance to walk, and back or abdominal pain. There are often reduced spinal movements, loss of lumbar lordosis, and local tenderness. There may be a positive SLR. Neurological deficits are uncommon.

Investigations

- *Laboratory:* FBC, ESR, and CRP. Results may be normal. Blood cultures may be positive.
- *Radiology:* plain radiographs—usually negative early in the disease but may be useful in excluding other pathology. Later, disc changes and bone destruction may be seen. MRI—imaging modality of choice, as can demonstrate bony and soft tissue changes.

Differential diagnosis

It includes pyogenic tuberculous infections and neoplasms, especially osteoblastoma.

Management

- *Non-operative:* early management is IV antibiotics covering *Staphylococcus aureus*; later, oral agents can be used. Bed rest and bracing are not indicated, unless there is vertebral collapse. IV antibiotics are most successful in patients with an identifiable organism (on blood cultures or biopsy).
- *Operative:* consider biopsy (may be image-guided) for identification of organism if blood culture does not yield results and empirical treatment is ineffective. Surgical debridement is indicated in patients with drainable collections or who respond poorly to antibiotic therapy.

Tuberculous osteomyelitis

Bone involvement, including that of vertebrae, is relatively common in children. The anterior spine is usually involved. The commonest site is the thoracolumbar junction.

Clinical

Back pain is the commonest presenting symptom. Children often have flu-like symptoms. Gait abnormalities occur due to psoas involvement or neurological deficits. Children with long-standing disease may present with an obvious spinal deformity. With involvement of the cervical spine, the child may have difficulty with swallowing or breathing due to pressure on adjacent structures by a paravertebral abscess. Children, unlike adults, are rarely paralysed by spinal TB.

Investigations
- *Radiographs:* may show extent of vertebral involvement. A deformity, usually kyphosis, may be seen and monitored with serial radiographs.
- *MRI:* to demarcate soft tissue involvement, associated collections, and impact of infection on neural elements (compression of cord or nerve roots).

Management
- *Non-operative:* primarily treated with long-term antituberculous chemotherapy (multiple agents).
- *Operative:* drainage, debridement, or stabilization (anterior, posterior, or both) may be required. Late deformity or development of neurological deficit may require reconstructive surgery.

Discitis in children

Benign, self-limiting infection or inflammation of the intervertebral disc or end plate. Considered part of the continuum of infective spondylitis.

Epidemiology
Discitis is uncommon in children. It usually affects children aged <10 years but is commoner in toddlers (1–3 years) than in older children. The lumbar spine is the commonest site.

Aetiology
Unclear. May represent a brisk host response to a low-grade pathogen that does not produce progressive vertebral osteomyelitis. Non-infective processes and trauma have been suggested.

Clinical
Non-specific features, including refusal to walk, back pain, inability to flex the lower back, and loss of lumbar lordosis. There are usually no systemic symptoms and children are typically afebrile. May present with hip or abdominal pain, a limp, or refusal to sit, stand, or walk. On examination, there is often tenderness over the spine and paravertebral muscle spasm, which results in loss of flexion and ↓ lumbar lordosis. It is often difficult to make a diagnosis in children aged under 3 years.

Differential diagnosis
Includes osteomyelitis, tuberculous spondylitis, and post-operative discitis.

Investigations
- *Laboratory:* may be unhelpful as WCC is often normal. ESR/CRP may be elevated. A significant proportion of blood cultures are sterile (50%), but when an organism is identified, it is usually *S. aureus*. Biopsy may be indicated for children who fail to respond to non-operative management, older children, adolescents in whom a non-staphylococcal infection is suspected, and those thought to have TB or tumour.
- *Radiographs:* normal early in disease. Later, disc space narrowing and irregularities of adjacent vertebral end plates are seen. In adults, vertebrae usually fuse, but in children, the disc space is usually preserved.
- *Bone scan:* demonstrates ↑ uptake of isotope in infected disc space— may be useful in early diagnosis of discitis (within 1 week of symptoms developing).

- *MRI:* more sensitive investigation than a bone scan in very early disease. May demonstrate a paravertebral inflammatory mass and epidural collections. Can prevent the need for biopsy by guiding management.

Management

Bed rest. If symptoms severe, an orthosis should be considered. Empirical oral or IV antibiotics are prescribed. If no organism is cultured, a broad-spectrum agent (e.g. cephalosporin) is commenced. Most children have a mobile, pain-free spine within 18–20 months of treatment being started.

Paediatric trauma

Growing bones

'Children should not simply be considered little adults.'

Mercer Rang

Unique properties of the immature skeleton include:
- Presence of growth plates (physis, epiphyseal plate)
- Great capacity to remodel, which is inversely proportional to age
- Different biomechanics from the adult musculoskeletal system.

Biomechanics

The immature skeleton has:
- More bone per unit area
- Enhanced vasculature
- Thicker periosteum
- Elastic properties.

The implications are:
- Different fracture patterns and propagation (e.g. greenstick, Torus/buckle)
- Greatly reduced healing times and much lower rates of non-union
- Intact periosteum which can aid in reduction and healing, but if torn and incarcerated in fracture, it will have the opposite effect and can inhibit healing
- Relatively more energy transfer to fracture the bone (thus greater local tissue damage than is seen in adults, e.g. rib fractures associated with lung contusion in a child, and visceral injury with pelvic fractures)
- Special fracture types (e.g. triplane ankle fracture reflects the course of physeal closure around adolescence, tibial spine avulsion the immature version of ACL rupture when the chondroepiphysis fails before the ligament).

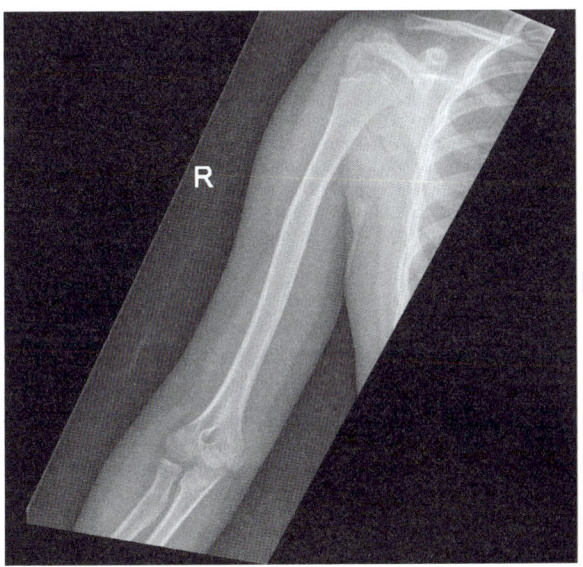

Physeal injuries

Due to accelerated growth, the physis can be an area of weakness where fracture can occur. Physeal fractures are the commonest cause of growth arrest, albeit rare but serious. The precise cell biology and healing responses of the physis are still not fully understood.

Salter and Harris in Toronto (Canada) established and popularized the principles of physeal fractures with their 1963 classification (Fig. 23.1), upon which current physeal fracture management is based:

- Fractures that do not disrupt the continuity of the germinal layer of the physis (types I and II) should not typically lead to growth arrest, although there is no guarantee of uneventful healing.
- Injuries that segment the growth plate and epiphysis (types III and IV) risk physeal arrest if not accurately reduced.
- Growth arrest after physeal injury is presumed to be due to bony bar forming across the physis of an unreduced fracture. Their work coincided with that of Langenskiold (1975), who identified the 'bony bridge'.

Harris lines are growth arrest lines described by Harris (radiodense lines parallel to the physis, moving away with time) that represent a previous self-limiting injury from which the growth plate has recovered (if straight), whereas a curved Harris line might indicate growth disturbance.

Growth arrest

If a discrete bony bar is identified on imaging (often CT or MRI) and can be resected, usually via the surgical creation of a metaphyseal window, then this may prove worthwhile if significant growth remains. Various materials, including fat and bone cement, are interposed to prevent reformation of the bony bar following resection.

Remember that longitudinal shortening alone is easier to correct (at skeletal maturity) than angular deformity. Thus, for a peripheral physeal bar causing eccentric growth arrest and angular deformity, if the child is nearing skeletal maturity, one can consider completing the epiphysiodesis if bar resection is not feasible, to avoid further eccentric growth. For paired bones (e.g. forearm, lower leg), it may be necessary to arrest growth of the other bone to prevent secondary joint deformity.

Non-traumatic physeal injury

The physis can be injured in other ways, including:

- Infection, especially meningococcal septicaemia
- Neurological disease
- Burns
- Malnutrition
- JIA
- Chemotherapy (side) effects
- Uraemia
- Endocrine disease
- Thalassaemia.

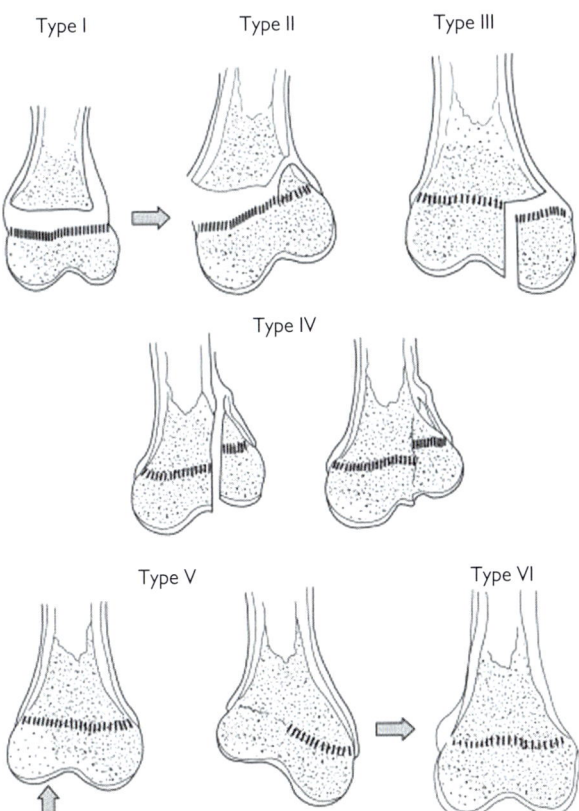

Fig. 23.1 Rang's modification of the Salter–Harris classification.

Reproduced from Bulstrode et al., *Oxford Textbook of Orthopaedics and Trauma*, with permission from Oxford University Press.

Salter–Harris classification of physeal injury
Mnemonic 'SALTER':
- Type I: through the physis (Slip)
- Type II: through the physis with metaphyseal fracture (Above physis)
- Type III: epiphyseal fracture (Lower than)
- Type IV: epiphyseal fracture extending across the physis to the metaphysis (Together/Through both sides)
- Type V: crush (comprEssion/cRush)
- Type VI: perichondral ring injury.

Further reading

Bush PG, Hall AC, Macnicol MF. New insights into function of the growth plate—review article. *Journal of Bone and Joint Surgery (British Volume)*. 2008;**90**:1541–7.

Salter TB, Harris WR. Injuries involving the epiphyseal plate. *Journal of Bone and Joint Surgery (American Volume)*. 1963;**45**:587–622.

Birth trauma

Injuries occurring during delivery are now less common due to improved obstetric care. Nonetheless, obstetric brachial plexus palsy/injury (OBPP/I) can be a cause of substantial subsequent morbidity with severe secondary shoulder dysplasia.

Factors associated with birth injuries

- Multiparous pregnancy.
- Breech presentation.
- Prolonged labour.
- Excessive birthweight >4kg (maternal diabetes).
- Shoulder dystocia.
- Osteogenesis imperfecta.

Clavicle fracture

Commonest injury, usually middle third. Causes pseudoparalysis of the upper limb, but beware 5% of cases are associated with brachial plexus injury. Treat expectantly and with reassurance. Heals within 1–2 weeks.

Brachial plexus injuries

Relatively uncommon (0.6–2.6 per 1000 live births) with improved obstetric care. Typically caused by distraction injury, primarily to the upper roots typically when the shoulders become stuck after the head has been delivered; this causes an upper plexus (C5/C6) injury. For patterns of injury, see Box 23.1. The majority recover spontaneously, but it can take up to 2 years for full recovery. Those without biceps function at 3 months have a poorer prognosis. Microsurgical plexus reconstruction in this group is controversial and rare, because of mixed results, and evidence advocates for early surgical intervention if required, with better outcomes observed with shorter grafts.

Internal rotation contracture of the affected shoulder is a sequela causing glenoid dysplasia and posterior dislocation. Options for the orthopaedic surgeon include:

- Early splintage in external rotation and abduction ± botulinum toxin injections to internal rotators of the shoulder
- Open or arthroscopic anterior release of the shoulder capsule, subscapularis, and rotator interval
- Transfer of tendons of latissimus dorsi and teres minor into rotator cuff external rotators
- Salvage derotational osteotomy of proximal humerus; brings the forearm away from the body but does not address the prominent humeral head dislocated posteriorly.

Humeral fracture

- Typically a transverse mid-shaft fracture pattern.
- Shortening or angulation will usually correct with remodelling.
- Treated by keeping the arm in a neutral position against the body under the neonate's clothing.
- Transphyseal separation at elbow and proximal humerus also possible and more significant due to injury to the physeal growth plate.

> **Box 23.1 Gilbert and Tassin classification of obstetric plexus palsy**
> - C5/6: full recovery in 90%
> - C5/6 + partial C7 injury: full recovery in 50–75%
> - C5/6/7 + partial C8/T1 injury: full recovery in 33%
> - C5/6/7/8/T1: full recovery not possible

Femoral fracture
- Mostly mid-shaft and transverse fracture patterns.
- Treat with Gallows traction, Pavlik harness, or strapping of the thigh to the chest (depending on age of the child).

Cervical injuries
- Cord injury may occur during breech delivery.
- May be a differential diagnosis for neuromuscular disorder in a 'floppy baby'.

Non-accidental injury

NAI is an injury that is purposefully inflicted upon a child. It is a form of physical child abuse, often affecting the skin and soft tissues. However, up to a third of NAIs may present as fractures.

Any clinician dealing with children must remain vigilant for signs of NAI to ensure prompt recognition, investigation, and protection of the child from further injury. Where doubt exists, admit the child for protection, pending further investigations via an MDT approach (with input particularly from the paediatric and children's safeguarding teams). Failure to recognize NAI carries a 20% risk of further injury and a 5% risk of permanent neurological damage or death.

Risk factors

Child
- First born.
- Unplanned pregnancy.
- Premature.
- Other significant chronic comorbidities (e.g. CP).

Parent
- Single-parent home.
- Recent social stressor.
- Unemployment.
- Substance and drug misuse.
- Personal history of abuse as a child.
- Lower socio-economic status.

Features in history
- Ninety per cent of cases in children aged <5 years.
- Delays in seeking treatment.
- Unwitnessed injury.
- Implausible or evolving story of injury mechanism.
- Pattern of injury inconsistent with mechanism described.
- Long bone fractures in a *non-ambulatory child*.
- Previous history of injuries.

Examination
- Be suspicious of the silent, watchful, abnormally still child, with poor interaction with their carer.
- Injuries of various ages.
- Bite marks, cigarette burns, scalds, fingertip bruises.
- Bruises on arm, leg, or face from gripping.
- Subconjunctival haemorrhage ('shaken baby').
- Posterior chest wall injuries.

Radiology
Either a skeletal survey (full-body radiographs in younger children, usually <2 years of age) or further focused radiographs are indicated if there is reasonable suspicion at this stage, looking for fractures at various stages of healing and injuries highly specific for NAI:

- Posterior rib fractures
- 'Corner' and 'bucket handle' metaphyseal fractures
- Complex or wide skull fracture
- Digital injury
- Lateral clavicle fracture
- Bilateral or multiple diaphyseal fractures.

Differential diagnosis

- Osteogenesis imperfecta.
- Juvenile osteoporosis.
- Caffey's disease—cortical hyperostosis resembling fracture with no history of injury.
- Haematological disorders—haemophilia, leukaemia.
- Congenital syphilis.

Management

Admit the child for protection from further injury, and refer to the paediatric team and alert the children's safeguarding team for further evaluation and referral to appropriate services. Be aware of any other vulnerable children or individuals in the household. Manage the individual injury as appropriate.

Further reading

Jayakumar P, Barry M, Ramachandran M. Orthopaedic aspects of paediatric non-accidental injury. *Journal of Bone and Joint Surgery (British volume)*. 2010;**92**(2):189–95.

Paediatric hand injuries

The hand is the commonest site of injury in children. It is central to function, and seemingly trivial injuries may have serious consequences.

Soft tissue injuries

- Crush injuries often are due to fingers trapped in doors or caught beneath heavy items.
- Fingertip or pulp amputations should be thoroughly irrigated, and the amputated part applied as a 'biological dressing' if clean enough.
- If amputation occurs proximal to the nail fold, refer to the hand surgeons for replantation or reconstruction, if indicated.
- Nail bed avulsion or lacerations should be repaired carefully under general anaesthesia to assess the germinal matrix; associated distal phalanx (tuft) fracture is an open injury and should be treated as such.

Tendon and nerve injuries

- Flexor tendon injuries should be repaired and protected (immobilized) post-operatively; stiffness is rarely a problem in children, so early active mobilization protocols are often not used.
- Extensor tendon injuries are rare, but a mallet finger (which is a Salter–Harris type III fracture of the distal phalanx extensor tendon insertion) should be splinted in hyperextension for 4–6 weeks.
- Nerve injuries should be referred for consideration of repair.

Fractures by anatomical location

- Metacarpal and phalangeal fractures are common after relatively minor trauma. Usually physeal injuries, but these often heal quickly and rarely cause growth disturbance.
- Distal phalanx fracture mallet finger as above; a variant in older adolescents is the *Seymour* fracture, a Salter–Harris type II injury of the distal phalanx (the physis is proximal, into which the extensor tendon inserts), commonly with disruption of dorsal skin. Needs washout and repair of the nail fold; always suspect open injury, especially if blood is seen.
- Proximal phalangeal fractures, usually Salter–Harris type II of base of proximal phalanx. In the little finger, abduction deformity may give the 'extra octave' sign. Reduce displaced fractures under nerve block with the MCPJ flexed (tightens collaterals to manipulate against), then buddy strap as for undisplaced.
- Boxers' fracture (fifth metacarpal), seen in adolescents; manage as for adults.
- Fracture of the thumb metacarpal is uncommon, may be: (1) metaphyseal and impacted (reduce closed and splint); (2) Salter–Harris type II with medial or lateral angulation (closed reduction and cast or percutaneous pinning as required); (3) type IV, which is the paediatric equivalent of a Bennett's intra-articular fracture–dislocation of the thumb base (requires anatomical reduction and stable fixation).

Paediatric wrist injuries

Distal radial fractures

The distal radius is a common site for injury, accounting for ~40% of all paediatric long bone fractures. It has significant remodelling potential due to proximity of the physis. Depending on energy transfer and fracture stability, up to 25° dorsal angulation in the sagittal plane and 1cm bayonet overlap can be accepted in children aged <10 years, and up to 15° in children aged >10 years (exact radiological parameters vary, with limited evidence to guide management). Coronal plane deformity (seen on AP films) remodels poorly. Skeletal maturity is presumed to occur at age 14 years in ♀ and at 16 years in ♂, so adult (anatomical) parameters should be attained in children within 2 years of skeletal maturity.

If the degree of deformity is beyond what is deemed acceptable, then closed reduction should be considered via manipulation, followed by cast immobilization. If the fracture is unstable, then surgical stabilization should be performed by using percutaneous k-wire(s), ORIF, or flexible intramedullary nails.

Torus (buckle) fractures are demonstrated by buckling of one cortex and preservation of the opposite cortex (i.e. failure in compression) (Fig. 23.2). These are usually inherently stable injuries and can be managed symptomatically in a splint for a short period (3 weeks).

Greenstick fractures occur due to failure on the tension side, with the compression-side periosteum remaining intact (i.e. an incomplete fracture) (Fig. 23.2). They therefore reduce easily but require careful 3-point moulding in cast to prevent redisplacement. Occasionally, further fixation is needed if the periosteum is torn during manipulation, resulting in instability.

Distal radius physeal injuries

- Most commonly Salter–Harris type II fractures.
- Reduce by traction and then gentle pressure in a distal and volar direction to minimize shear force across the physis (reduces risk of injury and growth arrest).

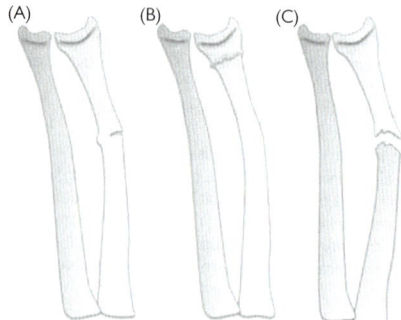

(A)   (B)   (C)

Fig. 23.2 (A) Greenstick fracture. (B) Buckle fracture. (C) Complete fracture.

- Avoid manipulation after 5–7 days (high risk of physeal injury). Most will remodel. If residual deformity or functionally deficient, can be addressed by later corrective osteotomy.
- Avoid remanipulation.
- Look critically for associated ulnar styloid fracture or ulnar physeal injury (high rate of ulnar physeal arrest).

Fractures and dislocations of the carpus

- Rare injuries in children.
- Commonest injured carpal bone is the scaphoid.
  - Scaphoid fractures are very rare before the age of 10 years.
  - Commonest site is the distal pole; this rarely results in osteonecrosis.
  - Diagnosis and treatment are as for adult scaphoid fractures.

Paediatric forearm injuries

The forearm comprises the radius and ulna bound together by the inter-osseous membrane. Although it is possible to break either of the bones in isolation, most commonly both bones break together. If only one bone appears broken, check carefully for dislocation or plastic deformation of the other.

Isolated fracture of the ulna

- Rare in children, results from a direct blow to the ulna.
- Usually managed non-operatively in cast (unlike adult nightstick fractures).

Fracture of both bones of forearm

- Can be plastic deformation, greenstick, or complete.
- Reduce by 3-point pressure centred on the apex of the deformity and cast likewise; commonly above-elbow plaster initially to control rotation.
- Residual ulna angulation influences forearm appearance; radial angulation reduces forearm rotation.
- Due to paediatric remodelling, often accept up to 15–20° angulation in children aged <10 years, and 10° in those aged over 9 years (aim for anatomical alignment of the forearm, including with open reduction and plate fixation, in older children, especially when within 2 years of skeletal maturity, as remodelling potential is very limited).
- Unstable fractures require fixation; intramedullary flexible nails are effective but may require limited open reduction to pass the fracture site.
- No definitive evidence for or against plate removal, but risk of nerve injury higher when removing plates. Flexible nails are generally removed but can be left *in situ*.
- Complications include refracture (higher risk with diaphyseal fracture and residual angulation, so avoid immediate return to impact sports and early removal of nails), compartment syndrome (recognize early and decompress), and nerve injury (usually neurapraxia).

Fracture–dislocations (Monteggia and Galeazzi)

(See ➲ Chapter 18, Adult forearm injuries, pp. 591–593.)

Elbow injuries in children

- Account for 7–10% of paediatric fractures.
- Clinical examination may be difficult due to a swollen elbow and an uncooperative child; try to establish whether tender medially, laterally, or both.
- Radiograph interpretation can be difficult in young children, as much of the elbow is cartilaginous. Look for displacement or absence of ossification centres; requires knowledge of sequence and rough timing of appearance.

Ossification centres

The mnemonic 'CRITOL' is helpful as an aide-memoire for the average age order in which the ossification centres appear (typically appear later in boys) (Fig. 23.3):

- Capitellum—1 year
- Radial head—3 years
- (Internal) medial epicondyle—5 years
- Trochlea—7 years
- Olecranon—9 years
- Lateral epicondyle—11 years.

Note the classic clinical picture of an elbow dislocation post-reduction, in which the humero-ulnar joint is less than congruent and the humeral trochlear ± olecranon centres are present, but the medial epicondylar centre is absent. In this scenario, the diagnosis is a medial epicondylar avulsion, with incarceration in the joint after reduction, which requires open reduction and fixation.

Supracondylar fracture

- Usually occurs following a fall onto the outstretched hand.
- Peak incidence is at age of 5–8 years. In younger children, transphyseal separation can occur (consider NAI in such cases), which is harder to identify radiographically.
- Vast majority are extension-type injuries (98%), which may have an intact posterior periosteal hinge against which to reduce. The remainder are either flexion or unstable injuries in both directions.
- Check for associated forearm fracture (up to 10%); high risk of compartment syndrome with double-level injury.
- Tenderness and swelling seen both medially and laterally.
- A 'pucker sign' suggests the proximal fragment has pierced the brachialis. This can be milked inferiorly at the time of reduction or may require an open procedure. Ecchymosis at the fracture is associated with the development of compartment syndrome.
- Neurovascular examination and documentation are imperative:
  - Risk of injury to brachial artery; check if radial pulse present, capillary refill time, and colour of hand (distinguish pink vs white).
  - Risk of nerve damage to median nerve (anterior interosseous branch—test for 'OK' sign, which requires thumb FPL flexion); ulnar nerve (vulnerable with medial placement of k-wires for fixation—test by crossing fingers); and radial nerve (especially in posteromedially displaced fractures—test by extending fingers).

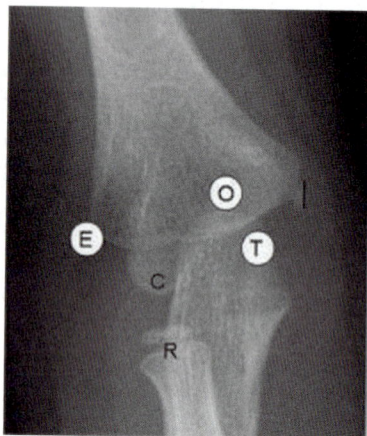

Fig. 23.3 'CRITOL'—radiograph showing the ossification centres around the elbow joint. The capitellum (C), radial head (R), and internal (medial) epicondyle (I) apophysis have ossified. The markers show the site of the trochlea (T), olecranon (O), and lateral (external) epicondyle (L), which are yet to ossify.

- A pale, pulseless hand warrants emergent surgical intervention with the availability of a vascular or plastic surgeon.
- A pink, pulseless hand can be treated by observation and surgical intervention on next suitable day-time list. The pulse usually returns upon reduction.
- Reduce by initial longitudinal traction, followed by aligning the fragments in the coronal plane, with correction of varus/valgus deformity and rotation, and then flexing up with gentle traction. Fracture occurs through thin bone surfaces like two thin edges; if rotation is not corrected, the blades will tilt (usually into cubitus varus, leading to 'gunstock' deformity).
- Another feared complication is compartment syndrome; this requires early diagnosis and emergent forearm fasciotomy.
- Check for colour of the hand and the radial pulse at the end of reduction; if lost and fails to return with elbow extension, consider exploration via an anterior approach with a vascular or plastic surgeon.
- The BOAST has a comprehensive guidance on management of supracondylar fractures.
- Supracondylar fractures are commonly classified using the Gartland classification (Box 23.2).

Box 23.2 Gartland classification of supracondylar fractures (extension-type)

- Type 1: undisplaced/minimally displaced—treat in above-elbow plaster or collar and cuff.
- Type 2: displaced with intact periosteal hinge—requires MUA ± k-wire. A line along the anterior humeral cortex should pass through the capitellum for satisfactory reduction on the lateral view.
- Type 3: complete displacement ('off-ended')—requires MUA + k-wire or ORIF. Two or three lateral wire configurations can help to avoid injury to/entrapment of the ulnar nerve.

MUA, manipulation under anaesthesia; ORIF, open reduction and internal fixation.

Lateral condylar mass fracture

- Lateral tenderness and swelling.
- Radiographs deceptive in younger child—cartilage fragment of the lateral condyle separates with a small sliver of metaphyseal bone. Internal oblique views can be diagnostic.
- Fracture is intra-articular, so only minimal displacement acceptable (unlike medial epicondylar fractures where greater displacement can be tolerated).
- Consider arthrography to assess whether the articular surface is intact. This can be performed intraoperatively to assess reduction if needed.
- Displaced fractures usually require open reduction with visualization of joint surface, anatomical reduction, and k-wire or screw fixation.

  Fig. 23.4 demonstrates a lateral condylar mass fracture.
- Non-union is a concern due to the intra-articular nature of the injury, especially in unstable patterns, so watch carefully during healing for displacement. Growth disturbance can occur, leading to cubitus valgus and a possible tardy ulnar nerve palsy.
- Various classifications exist, including the less useful Milch, or the more practical (and similar) Jakob (Box 23.3) or Weiss, systems.

Medial condylar fracture

- Rare pattern.
- Diagnosis and treatment similar to lateral condylar fractures.

Medial epicondylar fracture

- Third commonest fracture around the elbow in children.
- Peak age 11–12 years; commoner in boys than in girls.
- Fifty per cent have an associated elbow dislocation.
- Medial epicondyle traction apophysis for MCL (does not contribute to humeral growth).
- Generally managed non-operatively; intra-articular extension (medial condyle involvement), significant displacement (exact amount unclear; quoted displacement ranges from >2 to 15mm), associated elbow dislocation, and open fracture are relative indications for surgical fixation (mandatory if incarcerated in the joint post-reduction of a dislocated elbow).

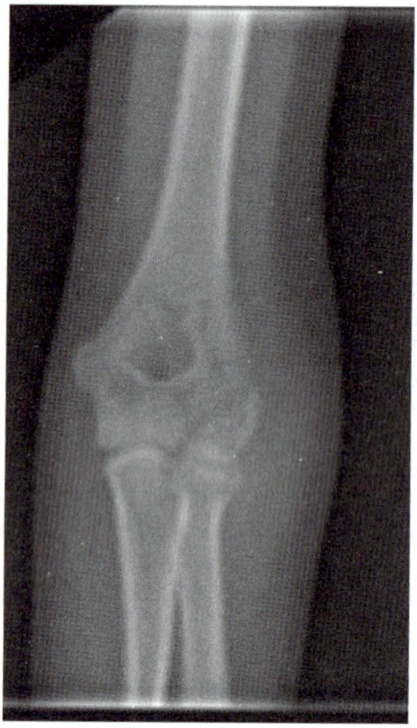

Fig. 23.4 A Jakob type 2 lateral mass fracture in the paediatric skeleton.

Box 23.3 Jakob's classification of lateral condylar mass fractures

- Type 1: <2mm displacement, indicating an intact cartilaginous hinge and an articular surface not significantly displaced—can be managed non-operatively
- Type 2: between 2 and 4mm displacement, articular surface displaced
- Type 3: >4mm displacement, displaced articular surface, and capitellum significantly displaced and rotated

Types 2/3 require operative intervention.

Radial head and neck fractures

- Most involve the neck of the radius.
- Pain on supination and pronation of the forearm.
- If <30° angulation, manage non-operatively.
- If >30° angulation, require MUA—various manoeuvres (e.g. 'Israeli' technique, direct k-wire ('joystick'), or intramedullary flexible nail ('Metaizeau' technique) to flip back the radial head into place.
- Avoid open reduction whenever possible; stiffness inevitable and risk of PIN injury. Sometimes required when radial head/neck buttonholes out through the capsule.

Olecranon fractures
- Rare in children. May be seen with osteogenesis imperfecta.
- Check for radial head dislocation (variant of Monteggia fracture).
- If displaced, may need ORIF.

Elbow dislocation
- Ninety per cent of posterior dislocations after a fall onto an outstretched hand.
- Most will reduce closed, with sedation. Then brief immobilization (1–2 weeks) and early motion.
- If there is an incarcerated bony fragment (usually medial epicondyle) or unstable fracture–dislocation, then ORIF is warranted.
- Complications include neurovascular injury, elbow stiffness, compartment syndrome, recurrent instability, and myositis ossificans.

Pulled elbow
- Injury results from traction to the arm, with the hand in pronation and the elbow extended; often when a child is lifted or swung by their arm.
- Radial head subluxes under the annular ligament.
- Radiographs unremarkable; diagnosis is clinical.
- Reduce closed by supinating the forearm, with the thumb over the radial head, followed by elbow flexion.

Further reading
British Orthopaedic Association. *BOA Standards for Trauma and Orthopaedics (BOASTs)*. Available from: ℘ www.boa.ac.uk/standards-guidance/boasts.html

Paediatric shoulder and arm injuries

Humeral shaft fractures

May occur as birth injuries or in older children secondary to trauma. Obstetric humeral and elbow fractures associated with pseudoparalysis that may mimic brachial plexus palsy. A spiral fracture of the humeral shaft should always alert the clinician to the possibility of NAI. Transverse fractures suggest a direct blow to the humerus.

The wide, multidirectional range of glenohumeral motion and circumferential muscle coverage of the humerus allow a good deal of angular and rotational deformity to be accepted without functional or cosmetic deficit. Consequently, most injuries can be managed non-operatively, usually in a sling or humeral brace.

Proximal humeral fractures

- Peak incidence of physeal injury in adolescents (sports injuries) and newborns (obstetric injury and NAI).
- Displacement usually anterolateral (muscle pull against intact posteromedial periosteum).
- Metaphyseal fractures common in 5- to 12-year age group.
- Eighty per cent of humeral growth from proximal physis, so remodelling potential is excellent.
- Almost always managed conservatively in a collar and cuff.
- In young children, up to 70° angulation may be acceptable due to huge remodelling potential; in adolescents, less deformity is acceptable and open reduction is occasionally indicated.
- Rare complications include humerus varus, axillary nerve injury, and osteonecrosis.

Clavicle fractures

- The clavicle is the first bone to ossify (intramembranous ossification) and the last to complete ossification.
- Mechanism of injury is a fall onto an outstretched hand or onto the shoulder.
- Eighty per cent occur in the shaft; 15% are in the lateral third.
- The lateral fragment is pulled down by the weight of the arm, whereas the medial fragment is pulled up by the SCM muscle.
- Neurovascular and respiratory examination is necessary to exclude injury to the brachial plexus or pneumothorax.
- Normally managed in a sling until pain-free (2–4 weeks).
- Open fractures (rare) require ORIF.
- Be wary of fractures with a medial spike that pierce the fascia and buttonholes through to become trapped. This can prevent union and may need surgical intervention.

Acromioclavicular joint injury

- Rare in children, as CC ligaments remain intact.
- Treatment as for adults.

Scapular fractures

- Rare in children.
- If present, usually indicate a significant injury—look for associated injury and consider NAI.
- Managed non-operatively, as surrounding musculature splints fragments with good vascular supply.

Anterior shoulder dislocation

- Rare in children, becoming commoner in adolescents with increasingly vigorous sports participation.
- Mechanism of injury is a fall with the arm in abduction, extension, and external rotation.
- Examination reveals squaring of the shoulder and an anteriorly palpable humeral head.
- Radiographs: axillary or scapular-Y view—confirm diagnosis.
- Neurovascular examination for axillary nerve injury (sensation over regimental patch and deltoid contraction post-reduction).
- Treatment is closed reduction under sedation, rest in broad arm sling, and then physiotherapy. Reduction should be as gentle as possible to prevent damage to the proximal humeral physis.
- Anterior dislocations in young athletes have a high risk of recurrence, increasing interest in early (or even acute) arthroscopic anterior repair of detached glenoid labrum and bone (Bankart repair).

Posterior dislocation

- Much less common than anterior. Associated with electrocution or epilepsy.
- Mechanism of injury is a fall with the shoulder adducted, flexed, and internally rotated or following an epileptic seizure.
- Examination reveals restricted external rotation.
- On AP X-ray, the humeral head may be the shape of a light bulb, with the head central on the shaft rather than offset medially (drumstick or lollipop sign).
- Posterior dislocation is easily missed; key to diagnosis are limited external rotation of the shoulder and careful review of the radiograph. Axillary view is diagnostic, and a modified axial view should always be possible.
- Reduce with traction applied to the shoulder in 90° abduction, followed by external rotation. Support with sling (usually broad arm), although an abduction brace may be useful in unstable cases.

Paediatric spinal injuries

Anatomy

In children:
- Vertebral column is mobile.
- Facet joints are shallow and oriented horizontally.
- Spinal ligaments and joint capsules can withstand significant stretching.
- Nuchal muscles are weak—↑ translation during flexion and extension.
- Large head-to-body ratio in children aged <8 years shifts the axis of rotation to the upper cervical spine (greatest movement is at C2/3, compared with C5/6 in adults).

Prevalence

Spinal injuries are rare in children: <1% of all fractures in children involve the spine. RTAs are the commonest mechanism of injury.

Clinical

Presenting symptoms are variable, but a spinal injury must be suspected when a child has:
- Loss of consciousness
- Pain related to the neck or back, guarding, rigidity, torticollis, numbness, weakness, or radicular symptoms
- Autonomic disturbances (bladder or bowel dysfunction)
- A neurological deficit (radicular or myelopathic) or unresolved pain within 1 or 2 weeks of an injury.

Injuries sustained include fractures, dislocations, and soft tissue injuries without significant bony or articular injury. The commonest injury to the spine is a fracture. Facet dislocations are uncommon in children, but when they occur, they are usually associated with neurological sequelae.

Partial SCIs are incomplete and may improve, but children with complete SCIs normally do not recover. Progressive neurological deficits can develop if instability is not recognized. Children with SCIs are at risk of developing scoliosis.

It is important clinically to establish which patients are at risk of having a significant spinal injury, and results of the NEXUS study are helpful.

NEXUS study

Low-risk patients must meet all five criteria:
- Absence of midline cervical tenderness
- No evidence of intoxication
- Normal level of alertness
- No focal neurological deficit, and
- No painful distracting injuries.

If a patient fulfils all five of the NEXUS criteria, plain radiographs are of marginal value. In this study, 1% of patients who did not meet the NEXUS criteria had a cervical spine injury. Therefore, serial assessment is important in managing children with cervical injuries.

Investigations

Differences in radiographs of children and adults

Synchondroses occur in all cervical vertebrae—there are three synchondroses at C2 that close between the ages of 3 and 7 years. That at the dens–arch is most prominent and is most frequently mistaken for a fracture. The distinguishing feature of the dens–arch synchondrosis from a fracture is that the synchondrosis is visible on an oblique, but not on a straight lateral, X-ray film. Subaxial vertebrae in young children have synchondroses between the posterior and anterior elements, and these can also be mistaken for fractures. Prominent vascular channels in the ossification centres have a similar appearance to fractures.

Pseudosubluxation: in the upper cervical spine of children, this is considered a normal finding. In 40% of children aged under 8 years, >3mm of anterior displacement is present at C2/3, and in 14% at C3/4.

Plain radiographs

AP, lateral, and odontoid views are often requested when a cervical injury is suspected. The value of an odontoid view in young children is of questionable value. Instability of the cervical spine is assessed by using flexion and extension views, but these should only be obtained if the child has no neurological deficit. If there is a neurological deficit, MRI is indicated.

CT

These are of limited value in children aged under 10 years, as most injuries in this age group are ligamentous. In children older than 10 years, 20% of cervical injuries are ligamentous and no fracture is identified. CT may be useful in planning surgery.

MRI

MRI can be used to 'clear' the cervical spine. If a child has neurological symptoms or signs and normal findings on plain radiographs and CT, MRI may show a ligamentous or disc injury that would otherwise be missed.

Evaluating cervical stability

In a normal imaging study, there should be <3.5mm displacement of one vertebral body relative to an adjacent vertebral body, and angular displacement between vertebral bodies should not exceed 11°. In children, flexion and extension views are not as reliable as in adults.

Spinal cord injury without radiographic abnormality (SCIWORA)

SCIWORA is found primarily in children. A child with this injury usually has signs of myelopathy, but with no evidence of a fracture or instability on plain radiographs or CT. Factors that predispose children to SCIWORA are a more tenuous spinal cord blood supply and greater elasticity in the vertebral column in relation to that of the spinal cord. Flexion or extension injuries are the commonest mechanism. MRI is best for evaluating patients with SCIWORA, as it will show ligamentous or disc injuries, spinal cord compression, spinal cord signal changes, and soft tissue or spinal cord haemorrhage.

Management

Most spinal injuries in children can be managed with immobilization of the injury (cervical collar, halo jacket, or thoracolumbar orthosis). With advances in surgical techniques and instrumentation, internal fixation surgery has become commoner. Surgical management is aimed at ensuring early stability of the vertebral column and protection of the spinal cord, facilitating early mobilization and return to normal activities. Indications for surgery include highly unstable injuries, significant deformities, progressive deformities, and compression of neural element (decompression and fixation).

Further reading

Cirak B, Ziegfeld S, Knight VM, Chang D, Avellino AM, Paidas CN. Spinal injuries in children. *Journal of Pediatric Surgery.* 2004;**39**(4):607–12.

Hoffman JR, Schriger DL, Mower W, Luo JS, Zucker M. Low-risk criteria for cervical-spine radiography in blunt trauma: a prospective study. *Annals of Emergency Medicine.* 1992;**21**(12):1454–60.

Paediatric pelvic injuries

Paediatric pelvic fractures are uncommon. In young children, the pelvis is predominantly cartilage; its higher elasticity implies higher-energy trauma if a fracture has occurred. Therefore, look first for other serious and potentially life-threatening injuries (head, chest, abdomen, and genitourinary). The majority of pelvic fractures will be managed non-operatively, with a good prognosis. In the acute setting, associated injuries are more important.

Other differences to adults are that children are more likely to injure intra-abdominal organs; single breaks in the pelvic ring can occur, and avulsion injuries (of vulnerable apophyseal cartilage plates) are common.

Fracture types

- *Avulsion:* of attached powerful muscle insertions, including the ischium (hamstring origin), ASIS (sartorius and ITB), anterior inferior iliac spine (AIIS) (rectus femoris), and iliac crest (hip abductors). Common in sporting adolescents. Treat with rest, crutches, and activity modification. Very displaced avulsions may require reduction and fixation.
- *Iliac wing or blade:* common pedestrian vs car injury. Adult problem of non-union not seen in children, fixation not required.
- *Pubis or ischium:* if pelvic ring not involved, then rest and activity modification only needed, but infers high-energy transfer, so the priority remains to look for, and manage, other serious injuries first.
- *Sacrum:* may be associated with anterior pelvic fractures. SIJ injuries are rare in isolation.
- *Pubic symphysis:* separation has differing normal limits according to age; stress views in lateral compression may be helpful.
- *Double breaks:*
  - *Straddle* (vertical pubic rami fractures): poorer prognosis due to associated injuries
  - *Malgaigne* (anterior and posterior pelvic ring injuries) may require fixation for severe displacement or external stabilization in older children with haemorrhage and haemodynamic instability
  - *Multiple crushing* injuries to pelvis (usually fatal).

Further imaging

- *CT:*
  - If doubt about diagnosis on plain radiograph
  - If operative intervention is planned.
- *MRI:*
  - Better delineation of soft tissue injuries
  - Absence of ionizing radiation exposure.

Complications

- Injury of triradiate cartilage leading to premature closure and risk of subsequent acetabular dysplasia.
- Heterotopic bone formation, especially where open reduction is required.
- Osteonecrosis if associated femoral head/neck fracture.
- Sciatic nerve palsy.
- Leg length discrepancy.

Signs of pelvic fracture

As described by Milch

- *Destot sign:* superficial haematoma beneath the inguinal ligament or in the scrotum.
- *Roux sign:* ↓ distance from the greater trochanter to the pubic spine on the affected side in lateral compression fractures.
- *Earle sign:* bony prominence or large haematoma and tenderness on rectal examination.

Associated injuries

- Skull, cervical, facial, and long bone fractures.
- Diaphragmatic rupture.
- Blunt chest trauma.
- Splenic/liver laceration.
- Damage to major blood vessels.
- Retroperitoneal bleeding.
- Rectal tears.
- Rupture or laceration of urethra/bladder.

Further reading

Hermans E, Cornelisse ST, Biert J, Tan EC, Edwards MJ. Paediatric pelvic fractures: how do they differ from adults? *Journal of Children's Orthopaedics*. 2017;**11**(1):49–56.

Shaath MK, Koury KL, Gibson PD, *et al*. Analysis of pelvic fracture pattern and overall orthopaedic injury burden in children sustaining pelvic fractures based on skeletal maturity. *Journal of Children's Orthopaedics*. 2017;**11**(3):195–200.

Hip fractures in children

Uncommon. Almost always associated with either high-energy trauma or a pathological lesion (e.g. fracture through bone cyst).

Tenuous blood supply predisposes to osteonecrosis (AVN), with rate determined by the type and degree of initial displacement. Physis of the hip contributes 3–4mm length growth per year.

The classification of Delbet is useful:
- Type I: fracture–separation of the epiphysis
- Type II: transcervical fracture of the femoral neck (commonest)
- Type III: basal (cervico-trochanteric) fracture
- Type IV: intertrochanteric fracture.

Type I has a strong association with hip dislocation; type II is the commonest pattern. Type IV has the best prognosis, with the lowest risk of AVN.

History

Ask about mechanism of injury, speed of impact if RTA, and other injuries. Antecedent hip symptoms if pathological fracture suspected.

Examination

Examine affected limb for deformity, posture, and pain on movement. Look for associated injuries, and assess neurovascular status of the limb.

Investigations

Plain radiographs will usually make the diagnosis; CT or MRI may be indicated for occult fracture.

Treatment

- Emergent if displaced or associated dislocation. May require prompt transfer to a specialist unit that manages major paediatric trauma.
- Closed or open reduction with internal fixation. The capital femoral physis may need to be crossed to achieve stable fixation (need to consider the age of the child).
- Children aged <4 years, undisplaced Delbet type I: can consider treatment with closed reduction and hip spica.

Complications

- AVN of femoral head: greatest in Delbet type I/II (20–50%) and in older children.
- Coxa vara: observe initially as many correct.
- Non-union: can treat this and coxa vara with subtrochanteric proximal valgus osteotomy.
- Physeal arrest, causing limb length discrepancy.

Femoral injuries in children

Shaft fractures

- These are not uncommon injuries. Beware NAI in children below walking age. In older children, these injuries are associated with higher-energy transfer, so remain vigilant for additional injuries.
- Management depends on age, fracture pattern, and patient factors, including socio-economic background.

Birth to age of 1 year

Immobilize in a Pavlik harness (hip spica may be used, but not required). Gallows traction (skin traction to overhead beam) can be used up to ~2 years, with a maximum weight of 12kg.

Up to age of 5 years

Reduction and hip spica application under general anaesthesia. Optimal position is hip flexed between 60° and 90° and 30° abduction, with moulding around the distal femoral condyle and buttock to maintain reduction. This can be performed acutely, with good effect and reduced inpatient stay. Another option is to apply skin traction and perform a delayed spica for up to 1 week to allow for early callus to form prior to spica application. Occasionally, this is preferred to allow better fracture control at the time of spica application.

Avoid excess traction and flexion of the knee beyond 90°. Ensure a smooth popliteal fossa to minimize the risk of compartment syndrome.

Acceptable results have been reported in this age group with flexible nailing, but this is usually unnecessary (may be indicated in certain situations such as polytrauma).

Age of 6–11 years (or up to 49kg)

Flexible intramedullary nails are the mainstay of treatment in fractures that are relatively stable. Unstable or very proximal and distal fractures may require open reduction or internal fixation with plate osteosynthesis. Always use two nails of symmetrical diameters to equalize the forces exerted within the intramedullary cavity.

Age of >11 years (or over 50kg)

Rigid intramedullary nailing is the preferred treatment method in older children, but there is a risk of femoral head AVN with the anterograde entry point (specialized adolescent nails should be used, avoiding the piriformis fossa entry point). Similar to younger children, very proximal or distal fractures or those with severe comminution may require ORIF methods instead.

Complications

- Leg length discrepancy; often overgrowth of fractured limb: poorly understood, may be ↑ vascularity at physis, but need to follow up for this. Between age 1 and 10 years, expect 9mm overgrowth (range 4–25mm); fracture shortening by this amount in closed treatment is therefore permitted.
- Angular deformity and rotational malunion: various guidelines propose differing acceptable limits. Can accept up to 30–40° varus/valgus or pro/recurvatum deformity, with lesser degrees of rotational deformity

up to age 2 years, with the expectation of remodelling. Less tolerance, particularly for rotation, with ↑ age. Age 2–10 years can allow up to 15° angulation, but avoid rotation.

Distal femoral physeal injuries

The distal femoral physis undulates, so traumatic separation associated with significant energy transfer ('cartwheel injury' is the historic name; may resemble knee dislocation on presentation). This is the body's largest and fastest growing physis, so even Salter–Harris type I/II injuries are not benign (angular deformity common after type II); the magnitude of displacement predicts the risk of growth disturbance.

Careful neurovascular examination is required. Oblique views may be helpful if minimally displaced.

Treat types I/II with closed reduction and pins (k-wires) or screws. Types III/IV require anatomical restoration of the articular surface and physis (may necessitate open reduction).

Observe for growth disturbance, including angular deformity or limb length discrepancy as a result of partial or complete physeal arrest.

Further reading

Poolman RW, Kocher MS, Bhandari M. Pediatric femoral fractures: a systematic review of 2422 cases. Journal of Orthopaedic Trauma. 2006;**20**(9):648–54.

Wright JG, Wang EE, Owen JL, et al. Treatments for paediatric femoral fractures: a randomised trial. The Lancet. 2005;**365**(9465):1153–8.

Knee injuries in children

Fracture of tibial intercondylar eminence

- In adolescents, rather than a cruciate ligament tear, the ACL avulses a bony fragment, commonest in the 8- to 13-year-old age group.
- Can follow a hyperextension injury, fall, or direct blow.
- Typically presents with pain and a large effusion, with inability to weight-bear.
- Radiographs will show a fragment in the centre of the knee. CT aids in assessment of displacement, and MRI can help to identify associated soft tissue injuries (e.g. meniscal tears). All three are recommended to fully assess the injury and manage appropriately.
- If undisplaced or the fragment reduces with knee extension, manage in a long leg cast in 10–15° flexion for 4–6 weeks.
- Not uncommonly, irreducible fragments may be flipped over a meniscal edge or an intermeniscal ligament; these need reduction and fixation with either a screw (without crossing the physis) or suture repair, often performed arthroscopically, although screw fixation can be performed via an arthrotomy if necessary. Avoid multiple drill passes through the physis (or altogether) if possible.

Tibial tubercle fractures

The tibial tubercle is part of the proximal tibial physis (traction apophysis). OS disease involves recurrent superficial microfractures of this region.

Injuries are common in adolescents. The usual mechanism is jumping or rapid quadriceps contraction with a flexed knee. Presentation is local pain, swelling, and difficulty with active knee extension.

Injury may be through the apophyseal secondary centre of ossification (type I), between this and the metaphysis (II), or intra-articular (III), according to Ogden classification. Fix displaced type I and II/III fractures after closed or open reduction with screws and washers.

There is a risk of genu recurvatum if anterior growth arrest follows.

Proximal tibial epiphyseal fractures

Uncommon injuries, but beware associated risk of popliteal artery damage (vessel closely apposed in the popliteal fossa and tethered by the anterior tibial branch passing anteriorly above the interosseous membrane). Moreover, anterior fractures can lead to anterior compartment syndrome. Salter–Harris type I/II injuries can usually be reduced closed and treated in cast; types III/IV require closed reduction and fixation with pins or screws, but open exploration is required if vascular compromise.

Patellar injuries

- Fractures are uncommon due to the high ratio of cartilage-to-bone in children.
- Beware *sleeve fractures*; radiographs show a small distal bony fragment only, which carries with it a large portion of the cartilaginous articular surface.
- Reduce and fix if >3mm separation of fragments; fixation or tension band wiring are options.

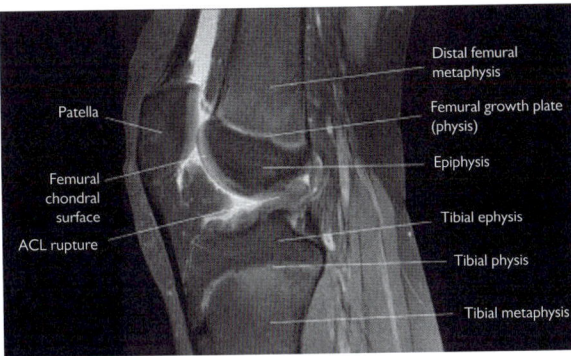

Fig. 23.5 Sagittal MRI of the paediatric knee with a complete anterior cruciate ligament rupture.

Patellar instability

Patellar instability can be:

- *True congenital:* usually dislocated at birth and often missed
- *Acute traumatic:* usually by direct trauma
- *Chronic laxity:* recurrent subluxations due to malalignment, typically in young ♀. Need to consider both passive and active stabilizers
- *Habitual:* usually painless and caused by proximal pathology such as tight lateral structures (ITB and vastus lateralis).

Patellar instability and dislocations can present with (tense) effusions and diffuse anterior pain. Plain long leg alignment view radiographs can help to identify the cause (e.g. abnormal Q angle, patella alta) and aid in identification of associated osteochondral fragment in the patellofemoral joint (skyline or Merchant view); if large and displaced, this will require reduction and fixation via arthrotomy. MRI may be indicated to demonstrate the true size of the fragment and examine the trochlear and patellar morphology (e.g. dysplasia); calculate the TT-TG distance and integrity of the MPFL to guide surgical intervention.

Knee soft tissue injuries

Meniscal injuries are uncommon in prepuberty, except in those with discoid meniscus.

Ligamentous injuries, such as true ACL ruptures, are ↑ in children/adolescents. Diagnosis is by clinical examination and imaging, usually with MRI (Fig. 23.5). Treatment is controversial, but surgical reconstruction takes into consideration the child's age and skeletal maturity, as per Tanner's classification, to minimize the impact to the physis and the risk of growth arrest. Various methods of reconstruction are available, depending on the amount of growth left, to avoid violating the physis.

Leg injuries in children

Tibial shaft fracture

- One of the commonest lower extremity injuries in children (15% of all paediatric fractures). Bimodal distribution, with lower-energy 'toddler's fractures' or higher-energy injuries in adolescents.
- Most closed tibial fractures can be treated by moulded plaster casting. The cast can be adjusted by removing wedges of plaster to adjust the alignment in subtle angulation.
- In children aged <10 years, up to 10° deformity in the coronal and sagittal planes may be tolerated. Up to 50% translation, but no malrotation, may also be acceptable.
- There is a tendency for more distal fractures to drift into recurvatum; this can be treated by casting with the ankle in equinus for 4 weeks— persistent stiffness is unusual in children, unless there is associated soft tissue injury.
- Surgical intervention in older children can facilitate earlier return to activities.

Indications for surgical intervention

- Soft tissue injury: open fracture, compartment syndrome.
- Polytrauma (including head injury).
- Floating knee.
- Failure to maintain adequate closed reduction.
- Unacceptable degree of angulation and/or displacement.

Operative treatment

- Rarely needed in toddler's fractures or undisplaced injuries.
- Closed manipulation and plaster cast application—this can be undertaken under general anaesthesia.
- Anterograde intramedullary flexible nailing, with an entry point posterior to the apophysis to prevent injury and resultant recurvatum from the medial and lateral sides. Flexible nails exert 3-point fixation within the medullary canal and splint the fracture.
- External fixator—severe or open soft tissue injury are the main indications. Application is quick, although monolateral constructs may be unstable, with issues including pin site infection, delayed union, and psychological impacts. Stress shielding and risk of refracture after frame removal.
- Plating—take care to ensure good soft tissue coverage.
- k-wires—can be used in distal tibial fractures in younger children. Can be removed after 3–4 weeks once callus has started to form.

Proximal tibial metaphyseal fracture

- Commonly occurs in children aged 2–8 years, typically with a low-energy valgus force.
- Treatment is usually long leg cast with a varus mould, with the aim of slight overcorrection of the valgus deformity.
- Rarely requires open reduction. This is usually only indicated if soft tissue interposition, preventing closed reduction.
- Cast wedging can be used to correct any early deformity.

- Cozen's phenomenon is described as a late valgus deformity (of unknown aetiology), most pronounced at 12–18 months post-injury, occurring in as many as 50–90% of cases. Generally, this resolves at 3 years, so the patient and parents must be appropriately counselled. In those with ongoing deformity and functional issues, corrective osteotomy or medial proximal tibial epiphysiodesis may be required.

Further reading

Baldwin KD, Babatunde OM, Russell Huffman G, Hosalkar HS. Open fractures of the tibia in the pediatric population: a systematic review. *Journal of Children's Orthopaedics*. 2009;**3**(3):199–208.

Sankar WN, Jones KJ, David Horn B, Wells L. Titanium elastic nails for pediatric tibial shaft fractures. *Journal of Children's Orthopaedics*. 2007;**1**(5):281–6.

Ankle injuries in children

The Salter–Harris classification is the most widely used descriptive system for ankle injuries in children. The Dias–Tachdjian classification is the Lauge–Hansen classification modified for the paediatric population (Fig. 23.6). It is based on the mechanism of injury and can help to identify the direction of applied force.

Special consideration needs to be made for the juvenile Tillaux and triplane fracture variants of adolescence; anatomical reduction of the physis is generally less important at the age at which these fractures occur, but the joint surface must be reduced anatomically. CT can help to diagnose these fracture variants and guide surgical fixation.

Implanted subchondral metalwork should be removed after fracture healing to prevent ↑ local stress on the overlying cartilage, which may predispose to OA.

Distal tibial fractures

- The distal tibial physis accounts for 35–40% of overall distal tibial longitudinal growth (at ~3mm/year).
- *Salter–Harris types I and II:* closed reduction and casting if displaced. Allow weight-bearing after 3–4 weeks. Occasionally need reduction and pinning if unstable.
- *Salter–Harris types III and IV:* truly undisplaced fractures can be treated as above, but require weekly follow-up with radiographs to check for displacement. Displaced fractures require closed reduction and cannulated screw fixation. Occasionally may require open reduction due to incarcerated periosteum or soft tissues.
- Eccentric physeal injuries should be followed for partial growth arrest causing angular deformity.

Juvenile Tillaux and triplane injuries

The distal tibial physis closes around a central 'bump', beginning in an anteromedial direction. The posterior and lateral portions of the physis are the last to fuse. As adolescents approach skeletal maturity, physeal injuries occur around this partially fused physis. An anterolateral fragment (of Tillaux) and sometimes a posterior (coronal) spike can be created. The

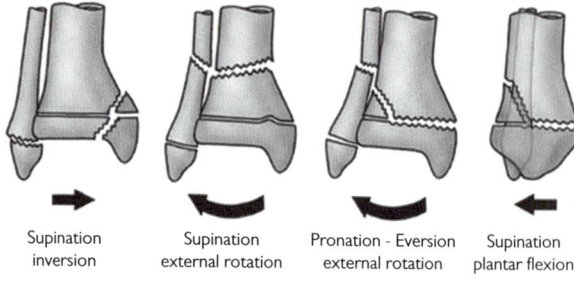

| Supination inversion | Supination external rotation | Pronation - Eversion external rotation | Supination plantar flexion |

Fig. 23.6 Dias–Tachdjian ankle fracture classification.

combination of the two is called triplane because the fracture plane is sagittal in the epiphysis, axial in the physis, and coronal in the metaphysis (i.e. a Salter–Harris type IV injury overall, appearing as a Salter–Harris type III on the AP radiograph and a Salter–Harris type II on the lateral view). There are many variants of the triplane fracture pattern, and CT is indicated to assess the fracture configuration and assist in the operative reduction and fixation of these fracture fragments, ensuring articular congruence.

Distal fibular fractures

The usual injury is a Salter–Harris type I fracture; this is a diagnosis of suspicion, unless there is a small metaphyseal fragment indicating a type II injury. Treatment is usually in a walking cast/boot until symptoms subside. If displacement is present, then MUA ± k-wire fixation through the physis is an acceptable form of treatment.

Foot injuries in children

Significant fractures of the foot are uncommon in the paediatric population. In older children (e.g. adolescents), diagnosis and management generally mirror those of the adult population.

Fractures of the talus

This is a rare injury in children and is usually related to high-energy trauma. Undisplaced injuries usually only require a non-weight-bearing cast until union (usually 6–8 weeks). Displaced neck fractures should be treated surgically, with closed reduction if possible, followed by stabilization with percutaneous screws. AVN (osteonecrosis) is the commonest complication, usually occurring within 6 months. Fractures of the talar body and head are very rare.

Fractures of the os calcis

Rare injury. Usually occur after a fall from height (axial load). Undisplaced and extra-articular fractures are usually treated in a cast. Occasionally, open reduction/internal fixation or percutaneous pin fixation is required if there is significant displacement.

Tarso-metatarsal injuries

Excessive foot swelling, ecchymosis, and inability to weight-bear are clues to the diagnosis of an injured Lisfranc (tarso-metatarsal) joint. Order AP, lateral, and oblique (the medial border of the fourth metatarsal should line up with that of the cuboid) *weight-bearing* plain radiographs. May need CT to diagnose if doubt remains or for surgical planning. There may be an associated fracture of the cuboid. For displaced injuries, it is critical to reduce the second metatarsal base into its recessed position relative to those on either side (usually held there by the Lisfranc ligament, running from its base to the medial cuneiform), and fixation may be necessary to maintain the coronal arch of the foot. There is negligible movement at the rigid medial TMTJs (vs the more flexible lateral side), but arch restoration is critical for foot shape.

Metatarsal fractures

Relatively common injuries. Most are treated with a walking cast, as even moderate displacement remodels well. Fifth metatarsal base fractures can be difficult to diagnose because of the apophysis and sesamoids present at this level. Fixation is indicated in significant displacement and considered in athletes for speed to return to sports.

Phalangeal fractures

Treated by neighbour strapping. Likewise, dislocations of MTPJs and IPJs are neightbour-strapped after closed reduction to restore gross deformity and angulation.

Puncture wounds

Puncture wounds should always be well irrigated to prevent infection. If there is surrounding cellulitis, treat with antibiotics. *Pseudomonas* ('trainer sole' contaminant) should be covered. Consider surgical exploration for 'dirty' mechanisms/contamination or for puncture wounds that do not settle after 2–3 days of antibiotic treatment.

Lawnmower injuries

Typically occur when a child is playing too close to a lawnmower on a wet, sloping surface. Usually severe soft tissue and bone destruction, or even traumatic amputation, with highly contaminated wounds. Require cephalosporin and aminoglycoside antibiotic cover ± penicillin for agricultural dirt. Multiple debridement (vacuum dressings useful in between) and plastic coverage are usually required. May need to counsel the parents and child for amputation. These injuries are best treated in conjunction with plastic surgeons.

Further Reading

Numerous scoring, classification, and assessment systems exist. References to a few commonly used examples are provided below:

- American Spinal Injury Association (ASIA) Impairment Scale: Standardised documentation of neurological injury status. ℘ https://asia-spinalinjury.org/wp-content/uploads/2019/04/ASIA-ISCOS-IntlWorksheet_2019.pdf
- Ganga Hospital Open Injury Score (GHOISS): Prognosticatication of limb salvage and outcome measures in open tibia fractures. ℘ https://gangascore.com.
Rajasekaran S, Naresh Babu J, Dheenadhayalan J, Shetty AP, Sundararajan SR, Kumar M, Rajasabapathy S. A score for predicting salvage and outcome in Gustilo type-IIIA and type-IIIB open tibial fractures. J Bone Joint Surg Br. 2006 Oct;88(10):1351–60. doi: 10.1302/0301-620X.88B10.17631. PMID: 17012427.
- Mangled extremity severity score (MESS): Applied to mangled extremities to determine which may require amputation. Johansen K, Daines M, Howey T, Helfet D, Hansen ST Jr. Objective criteria accurately predict amputation following lower extremity trauma. J Trauma. 1990 May;30(5):568–72; discussion 572-3. doi: 10.1097/00005373-199005000-00007. PMID: 2342140.
- Laboratory Risk Indicator for Necrotizing Fasciitis (LRINEC): Clinical tool for differentiating necrotizing fasciitis from non-necrotizing infections. Wong CH, Khin LW, Heng KS, Tan KC, Low CO. The LRINEC (Laboratory Risk Indicator for Necrotizing Fasciitis) score: a tool for distinguishing necrotizing fasciitis from other soft tissue infections. Crit Care Med. 2004 Jul;32(7):1535–41. doi: 10.1097/01.ccm.0000129486.35458.7d. PMID: 15241098.
- Spinal Instability Neoplastic Scale (SINS) Score: Evaluates the degree of spinal instability in patients with spinal tumours. Fisher CG, DiPaola CP, Ryken TC, Bilsky MH, Shaffrey CI, Berven SH, Harrop JS, Fehlings MG, Boriani S, Chou D, Schmidt MH, Polly DW, Biagini R, Burch S, Dekutoski MB, Ganju A, Gerszten PC, Gokaslan ZL, Groff MW, Liebsch NJ, Mendel E, Okuno SH, Patel S, Rhines LD, Rose PS, Sciubba DM, Sundaresan N, Tomita K, Varga PP, Vialle LR, Vrionis FD, Yamada Y, Fourney DR. A novel classification system for spinal instability in neoplastic disease: an evidence-based approach and expert consensus from the Spine Oncology Study Group. Spine (Phila Pa 1976). 2010 Oct 15;35(22):E1221–9. doi: 10.1097/BRS.0b013e3181e16ae2. PMID: 20562730.
- Thoracolumbar Injury Classification and Severity Scale (TLICS): Assesses the integrity of the posterior ligamentous complex, injury morphology, and neurological status of the patient. Vaccaro AR, Lehman RA Jr, Hurlbert RJ, Anderson PA, Harris M, Hedlund R, Harrop J, Dvorak M, Wood K, Fehlings MG, Fisher C, Zeiller SC, Anderson DG, Bono CM, Stock GH, Brown AK, Kuklo T, Oner FC. A new classification of thoracolumbar injuries: the importance of injury morphology, the integrity of the posterior ligamentous complex, and neurologic status. Spine (Phila Pa 1976). 2005 Oct 15;30(20):2325–33. doi: 10.1097/01.brs.0000182986.43345.cb. PMID: 16227897.
- Neurologic, oncologic, mechanical, and systemic (NOMS): Decision-making framework to determine the optimal treatment for patients with spine metastases. Laufer I, Rubin DG, Lis E, Cox BW, Stubblefield MD, Yamada Y, Bilsky MH. The NOMS framework: approach to the treatment of spinal metastatic tumors. Oncologist. 2013 Jun;18(6):744–51. doi: 10.1634/theoncologist.2012-0293. Epub 2013 May 24. PMID: 23709750; PMCID: PMC4063402.

Index

For the benefit of digital users, indexed terms that span two pages (e.g., 52–53) may, on occasion, appear on only one of those pages.

Tables, figures, and boxes are indicated by an italic t, f, and b following the page number.

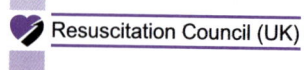

Resuscitation Council (UK)

Adult Advanced Life Support Algorithm

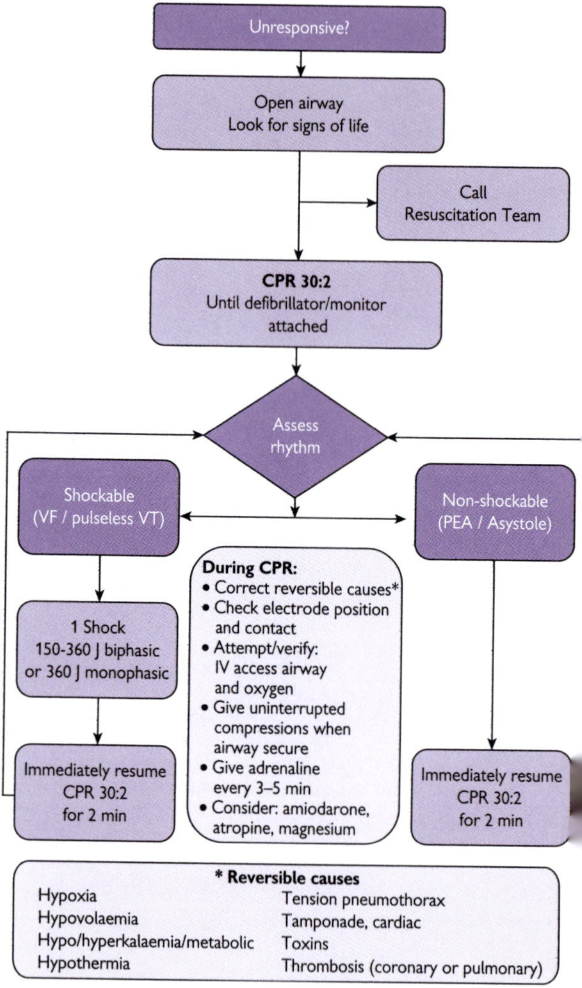
Unresponsive?
Open airway
Look for signs of life
Call
Resuscitation Team
CPR 30:2
Until defibrillator/monitor
attached
Assess
rhythm
Shockable
(VF / pulseless VT)
Non-shockable
(PEA / Asystole)
1 Shock
150-360 J biphasic
or 360 J monophasic
During CPR:
• Correct reversible causes*
• Check electrode position
and contact
• Attempt/verify:
IV access airway
and oxygen
• Give uninterrupted
compressions when
airway secure
• Give adrenaline
every 3–5 min
• Consider: amiodarone,
atropine, magnesium
Immediately resume
CPR 30:2
for 2 min
Immediately resume
CPR 30:2
for 2 min
* Reversible causes
Hypoxia
Hypovolaemia
Hypo/hyperkalaemia/metabolic
Hypothermia
Tension pneumothorax
Tamponade, cardiac
Toxins
Thrombosis (coronary or pulmonary)

UK Adult Basic Life Support Algorithm 2005. Reproduced with permission from the Resuscitation Council UK (2005). *Resuscitation Guidelines*. London: Resuscitation Council available from ⚲ www.resus.org.uk. CPR, cardiopulmonary resuscitation; IV, intravenous; PEA, pulseless electrical activity; VF, ventricular fibrillation; VT, ventricular tachycardia.